Revision *and* Complex Shoulder Arthroplasty

Revision *and* Complex Shoulder Arthroplasty

EDITORS

Robert H. Cofield, MD
Professor of Orthopaedic Surgery
Orthopaedic Department
Mayo Clinic
Rochester, Minnesota

John W. Sperling, MD, MBA
Professor of Orthopaedic Surgery
Orthopaedic Department
Mayo Clinic
Rochester, Minnesota

Michael A. King
Illustrations and Design
Mayo Clinic
Rochester, Minnesota

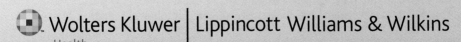

Wolters Kluwer | Lippincott Williams & Wilkins
Health

Philadelphia • Baltimore • New York • London
Buenos Aires • Hong Kong • Sydney • Tokyo

Acquisition Editor: Robert Hurley
Managing Editor: Dave Murphy
Marketing Director: Sharon Zinner
Project Manager: John Larkin
Design Manager: Teresa Mallon
Production Services: Maryland Composition

Printed in China

Library of Congress Cataloging-in-Publication Data

Cofield, Robert H. (Robert Hahn), 1943–
Revision and complex shoulder arthroplasty / Robert H. Cofield, John W. Sperling.
    p. ; cm.
Includes bibliographical references.
ISBN 978-0-7817-7747-6
1. Shoulder joint—Surgery. 2. Artificial shoulder joints. 3. Arthroplasty. I. Sperling,
John W. II. Title.
[DNLM: 1. Arthroplasty—adverse effects. 2. Shoulder—surgery. 3. Arthroplasty—methods.
4. Prosthesis Failure. 5. Reoperation—methods. 6. Treatment Failure. WE 810 C675r 2009]
  RD557.5.C62 2009
  617.5′72059—dc22

                                                                    2008026615

Care has been taken to confirm the accuracy of the information presented and to describe generally accepted practices. However, the authors, editors, and publisher are not responsible for errors or omissions or for any consequences from application of the information in this book and make no warranty, expressed or implied, with respect to the currency, completeness, or accuracy of the contents of the publication. Application of the information in a particular situation remains the professional responsibility of the practitioner.

The authors, editors, and publisher have exerted every effort to ensure that drug selection and dosage set forth in this text are in accordance with current recommendations and practice at the time of publication. However, in view of ongoing research, changes in government regulations, and the constant flow of information relating to drug therapy and drug reactions, the reader is urged to check the package insert for each drug for any change in indications and dosage and for added warnings and precautions. This is particularly important when the recommended agent is a new or infrequently employed drug.

Some drugs and medical devices presented in the publication have Food and Drug Administration (FDA) clearance for limited use in restricted research settings. It is the responsibility of the health care provider to ascertain the FDA status of each drug or device planned for use in their clinical practice.

To purchase additional copies of this book, call our customer service department at (800) 638-3030 or fax orders to (301) 223-2320. International customers should call (301) 223-2300.

Visit Lippincott Williams & Wilkins on the Internet: at LWW.com. Lippincott Williams & Wilkins customer service representatives are available from 8:30 am to 6 pm, EST.

10 9 8 7 6 5 4 3 2 1

Dedication and Acknowledgments

We would like to dedicate this book to all the authors who have contributed their time, knowledge, skills and insights into developing this text. We deeply appreciate these works on subjects the authors embrace with enthusiasm but of necessity, consume precious time that could be directed to other work or personal activities.

Michael King, the illustrator of most of the drawings in this text, is to be especially acknowledged for not only his technical skills but for his in-depth understanding of the shoulder. These clear illustrations make understanding the material, the written word, so much easier to appreciate and are in addition delightful to the eye.

There are many people who have offered important essential contributions to the development of the editors' interests and focus in this area of orthopedic surgery. At our institution Doctor Patrick Kelly lead us in applying the scientific method to orthopedic surgery. Doctor Mark Coventry had the insight to formulate a joint registry approach to understanding the benefits or limitations of prosthetic arthroplasty. Doctor Edward Henderson clearly defined the need for developing special expertise in our practice in the area of shoulder surgery, and stimulated us to do so. Doctor Ron Linscheid was an earlier advocate of refining the care for people with complex shoulder problems. So many people from outside the institution have served as our mentors at a distance. Notably, Doctor Charles Neer practicing in New York City exhibited for us the extreme dedication to the patient and such a thorough understanding of orthopedic principles applied to shoulder surgery. Without his guidance these editors and many involved in this field would not be able to offer the patient care that we can consistently and effectively do today.

We have been so fortunate in our work to have the collaboration of so many orthopedic surgery colleagues, residents, and fellows who share in our patient care activities and stimulate us to further read, study, and write about problems and solutions in shoulder arthroplasty.

Our families of course are the core to whom we are so grateful, our fathers and mothers who ceaselessly supported us in our education, who gave us unendingly sound advice and served as fine examples for life, our dear wives who sacrifice so much while we carry on with professional lives, and our magnificent children who continually reward us with their love and accomplishments. It is a special treat for us to acknowledge them.

Thank you so very, very much.

Robert H. Cofield, MD
John W. Sperling, MD

Contents

PART I: The Problems in Failed Shoulder Arthroplasty

PART II: Techniques in Revision Shoulder Arthroplasty

PART III: Specific Types of Reconstruction

Contributors

Samuel A. Antuña, MD, PhD, FEBOT
Department of Orthopedic Surgery
La Paz University Hospital
Madrid, Spain

Elie F. Berbari, MD
Division of Infectious Diseases
Department of Internal Medicine
Mayo Clinic College of Medicine
Rochester, MN

Louis U. Bigliani, MD
Chairman of Orthopedic Surgery
Columbia University Medical Center
New York, NY

Pascal Boileau, MD
Department of Orthopaedic Surgery
Hôpital de l'Archet
Nice, France

John G. Bowsher, PhD
Assistant Professor of Orthopaedic Research
Department of Orthopaedic Surgery
Loma Linda University, School of Medicine
Loma Linda, CA

Emilie V. Cheung, MD
Assistant Professor
Department of Orthopaedic Surgery
Stanford University
Stanford, CA

Akin Cil, MD
Assistant Professor of Orthopaedics
Department of Orthopaedic Surgery
University of Missouri Kansas City
Truman Medical Center
Kansas City, MO

Robert H. Cofield, MD
Professor of Orthopaedic Surgery
Orthopaedic Department
Mayo Clinic
Rochester, MN

David M. Dines, MD
Assistant Attending Orthopaedic Surgeon
Hospital for Special Surgery
New York, NY

Jonathan T. Finnoff
Senior Associate Consultant of Physical Medicine and Rehabilitation
Mayo Clinic
Rochester, MN

Evan L. Flatow, MD
Lasker Professor and Chairman
Leni and Peter May Department of Orthopaedic Surgery
Mount Sinai School of Medicine
New York, NY

Mark A. Frankle, MD
Florida Orthopaedic Institute
Temple Terrace, FL

Tyler J. Fox, MD
Orthopedic Department
Mayo Clinic
Rochester, MN

Matthew H. Griffith, MD
Hospital for Special Surgery
New York, NY

Konrad I. Gruson, MD
Shoulder Fellow
Leni and Peter May Department of Orthopaedic Surgery
Mount Sinai School of Medicine
New York, NY

Steven J. Hattrup, MD
Assistant Professor of Orthopedics
Mayo Clinic Arizona
Phoenix, AZ

Pierre J. Hoffmeyer MD
Professor of Orthopaedic Surgery
Head Division of Orthopaedics
Chairman Department of Surgery
University Hospital of Geneva
Geneva, Switzerland

Jason L. Hurd, MD
Clinical Instructor
Section of Orthopaedic Surgery
Sanford School of Medicine
University of South Dakota
Sioux Falls, SD

Eiji Itoi, MD
Professor and Chairman
Department of Orthopaedic Surgery
Tohoku University School of Medicine
Sendai, Japan

Christopher M. Jobe, MD
Professor of Orthopaedic Surgery
School of Medicine
Loma Linda University
Loma Linda, CA

Matthew Kippe, MD
Post Doctoral Clinical Fellow
New York Presbyterian
Columbia University
New York, NY

Todd J. Kowalski, MD
Section of Infectious Diseases
Department of Internal Medicine
Gundersen Lutheran Medical Center
La Crosse, WI

William N. Levine, MD
Professor of Clinical Orthopedic Surgery
Center for Shoulder, Elbow, and Sports Medicine
Columbia University Medical Center
New York, NY

Joachim F. Loehr, MD
ENDO-Klinik Hamburg GmbH
Hamburg, Germany

Joseph R. Lynch, MD
Acting Instructor and Senior Fellow
Department of Orthopaedics and Sports Medicine
University of Washington Medical Center
Seattle, WA

Pierre Mansat, MD, PhD
Service d'Orthopédie-Traumatologie
Centre Hospitalier Universitaire Toulouse / PURPAN
Toulouse, France

Michel Mansat, MD
Centre Hospitalier Universitaire Toulouse / PURPAN
Toulouse, France

Frederick A. Matsen III, MD
Professor and Chairman
Department of Orthopaedics and Sports Medicine
University of Washington Medical Center
Seattle, WA

Benjamin W. Milne, MD
Orthopaedic Department
Royal North Shore Hospital
Saint Leonards, NSW
Australia

Daniel Molé, MD
Clinique de Traumatologie et d'Orthopedie
Nancy, France

Mark E. Morrey, MD
Orthopaedic Department
Mayo Clinic
Rochester, MN

Lionel Neyton, MD
Centre Orthopédique Santy
Lyon, France

Duong Nguyen, MD
Post Doctoral Clinical Fellow
New York Presbyterian
Columbia University
New York, NY

Shawn W. O'Driscoll, PhD, MD
Professor of Orthopedics
Department of Orthopedics
Mayo Clinic
Rochester, MN

Douglas R. Osmon MD, MPH
Division of Infectious Diseases
Department of Internal Medicine
Mayo Clinic College of Medicine
Rochester, MN

Steve A. Petersen, MD
Co-Director, Division of Shoulder Surgery
Department of Orthopaedic Surgery
Johns Hopkins Medicine
Lutherville, MD

Wesley P. Phipatanakul, MD
Assistant Clinical Professor
Department of Orthopaedic Surgery
Loma Linda University School of Medicine
Loma Linda, CA

Herbert Resch, MD
Chairman
Traumatology and Sport Injuries
University Hospital of Salzburg
Salzburg, Austria

Joaquin Sanchez-Sotelo, MD, PhD
Associate Professor of Orthopaedics
Department of Orthopaedic Surgery
Mayo Clinic Rochester
Rochester, MN

Hirotaka Sano, MD
Assistant Professor
Department of Orthopaedic Surgery
Tohoku University School of Medicine
Sendai, Japan

Francois Sirveaux, MD, PhD
Clinique de Traumatologie et d'Orthopedie
Nancy, France

David H. Sonnabend, MD
Orthopaedic Department
Royal North Shore Hospital
Saint Leonards, NSW
Australia

John W. Sperling, MD, MBA
Professor of Orthopaedic Surgery
Orthopaedic Department
Mayo Clinic
Rochester, MN

Jay Smith, MD, FACSM
Associate Professor of Physical Medicine and Rehabilitation
Mayo Clinic College of Medicine
Rochester, MN

Scott P. Steinmann, MD
Associate Professor of Orthopedics
Department of Orthopedic Surgery
Mayo Clinic
Rochester, MN

Mark Tauber, MD
Department of Traumatology and Sports Injuries
Paracelsus Medical University
Salzburg, Austria

Christian J. H. Veillette, MD
Division of Orthopaedic Surgery
Toronto Western Hospital
Toronto, ON

Gilles Walch, MD
Centre Orthopédique Santy
Lyon, France

Brent B. Wiesel, MD
Attending Surgeon, Chief Shoulder Service
Department of Orthopaedic Surgery
Georgetown University Hospital
Washington, DC

Gerald R. Williams Jr., MD
The Rothman Institute
Thomas Jefferson University Hospital
Philadelphia, PA

Thomas W. Wright, MD
Professor of Orthopaedic Surgery
Department of Orthopaedics and Rehabilitation
University of Florida
Gainesville, FL

Joseph Zuckerman, MD
Walter A.L. Thompson Professor and
Chairman of Orthopaedic Surgery
Department of Orthopedic Surgery
NYU Hospital for Joint Diseases
New York, NY

Preface and Purpose

Surgeons at our institution developed a serious, focused, and continued interest in total shoulder arthroplasty since its inception in the 1970s. As a part of that activity, a Joint Registry was developed to allow consistent patient contact and ongoing evaluation. A team approach has emerged over the years with a section of six individuals interested in and focusing on shoulder and elbow surgery. This included development of fellowship opportunities that have now extended over 20 years. The clinical practice has been expansive in this area, and scientific publications now approach 100 in number with many more presentations at scientific meetings.

This wealth of experience has allowed the development of understanding of details that go into assessment of the problems in shoulder arthroplasty, have created techniques for the surgical treatment of complex and revision shoulder arthroplasty, and have refined specific issues for the various specialized types of shoulder reconstruction requiring prosthetic arthroplasty. This information is, of course, essential for complex and revision surgery but is also very much needed to address the nuances of primary arthroplasty itself.

We have been fortunate with our practice and education programs to develop a cadre of professional associates at our institution, nationally, and internationally who have participated in this work and who are contributing to this text. Certainly, the foundation of this information emulates from the Mayo Clinic experience but is expanded by knowledge that has accrued to others throughout the world. We feel this will offer a valuable further step in carrying information past the fundamentals in managing shoulder arthritis and complex trauma into the more difficult areas of shoulder arthroplasty and the reconstructive requirements for revision surgery—a topic which has typically been ignored or addressed in a single chapter in current publications on this subject.

The Problems in Failed Shoulder Arthroplasty

Joseph R. Lynch
Frederick A. Matsen III

CHAPTER

1

Unsatisfactory Outcomes of Primary Shoulder Arthroplasty

INTRODUCTION

Arthroplasty, as a treatment alternative for painful and disabling conditions of the shoulder, has evolved considerably with time. Yet, from the beginning, the practice of shoulder arthroplasty has been challenged by the occurrence of unsatisfactory outcomes. In fact, the first "total shoulder" procedure performed in 1983 by Péan, a French surgeon, had to be removed because of infection and mechanical failure. Neer pioneered modern shoulder arthroplasty beginning in 1953 with the use of prostheses for the management of complex proximal humerus fractures. Shoulder arthroplasty is now most commonly used as a treatment alternative for the management of both degenerative and inflammatory conditions of the shoulder.[1,2] As indications for its use evolve and the number of procedures performed annually increase, it is imperative that we document the effectiveness and carefully track the outcomes of this procedure as a treatment alternative for common conditions of the shoulder.[3–5] Additionally, it is equally important that we learn from the instances in which shoulder arthroplasty has failed to yield the result anticipated by the patient.[6]

Few individuals were as forward-thinking as Ernest Codman, who promoted the idea of the "end result system" in the early 1900s—an idea that gave rise to what we know today as outcomes research. It was his pursuit to follow clinical outcomes and use the data collected from both his successes and failures to improve the care he provided to future patients. In fact, he stated, "Every hospital should follow every patient it treats long enough to determine whether the treatment has been successful, and then to inquire 'if not, why not' with a view to preventing similar failures in the future."[8]

Despite the introduction of this concept in the early 1900s, and the recent emphasis on evidence-based medicine, our methodological tracking of the long-term outcomes of shoulder arthroplasty has been limited. Outcomes for shoulder arthroplasty are very much determined by the nature and severity of the pathology being treated, as well as by the surgeon's experience.[7,9,10] Moreover, it is a technically challenging procedure with perhaps a greater potential for technical errors and complications than other commonly performed arthroplasties.[4,5,11]

Short-term results have suggested that this procedure is highly effective in restoring joint function and alleviating pain.[11–17] Very few studies, however, have systematically evaluated the long-term results of shoulder arthroplasty.[11,13,18–20] And even fewer have concerned themselves with the causes and prevention of shoulder arthroplasty failure.[3,6,7,21]

In 1997, Torchia et al[20] evaluated the long-term results of 89 shoulders (mean follow-up 12.2 years) for the diagnoses of osteoarthritis, rheumatoid arthritis, and secondary arthritis, demonstrating survivorship of 93% and 87% based on the need for prosthetic revision at 10 and 15 years, respectively. In 1998, Sperling et al[22] estimated the survival of shoulder arthroplasty based on 114 patients and demonstrated 84% and 73% survival for total shoulder arthroplasty and hemiarthroplasty at 15 years, respectively. More recent long-term data were published by Deshmukh et al[13] in 2005, reviewing their experience with 72 shoulder arthroplasties with a minimum 10-year follow-up performed for the diagnoses of rheumatoid arthritis, osteoarthritis, and juvenile rheumatoid arthritis, demonstrating survivorship with revision as the end point of 93%, 88%, and 85% at 10, 15, and 20 years, respectively.

These studies, considered in concert, suggest that shoulder arthroplasty has proved to be a reliable treatment alternative for common degenerative, inflammatory, and traumatic conditions of the shoulder, with results that last well into the second decade. They also indicate, however, that one in ten patients has an unsatisfactory outcome, even in the hands of expert surgeons. Additionally, it has been suggested that the published literature tends to overestimate the success of this procedure.[4–7] It is possible that patients with unsatisfactory outcomes are lost to follow-up and thus underrepresented in most published series.[23] It is therefore evident not only that unsatisfactory outcomes exist, but that they may occur more often than previously suspected. Furthermore, all of the current outcome data concerning shoulder arthroplasty are published by high-volume subspecialty surgeons, even though it is recognized that most of these procedures are done by surgeons who perform fewer than three shoulder arthroplasties per year.[10,24] It has also been demonstrated that the results from these low-volume surgeons are poorer than those of their high-volume counterparts.[10,24] Thus the outcomes of the majority of total shoulder arthroplasties never appear in the literature and are essentially unknown. The result of this fact is that the published literature may not be a valid reflection of the overall experience of patients and surgeons with shoulder arthroplasty.

As advocated by Codman in the early 1990s, there is much, if not more, to learn from the study of failures than from the reports of successes. By learning from the cases in which shoulder arthroplasty failed to yield a satisfactory outcome, we will be better positioned to avoid unsatisfactory outcomes in the future.

DEFINITION OF AN UNSATISFACTORY OUTCOME

An unsatisfactory outcome following shoulder arthroplasty can be defined from the perspective of the surgeon, the patient, or both. The vast majority of outcomes research concerning the topic of shoulder arthroplasty defines success or failure based on the interpretation of the treating surgeon.[11–13,15–20,25] Commonly, this body of literature describes outcomes as excellent, satisfactory, or unsatisfactory based on objective criteria measured in the clinician's office. These criteria often include variables such as strength, range of motion, and radiographic criteria (component alignment and fixation integrity). In addition to the criteria previously mentioned, many authors consider the presence or absence of perioperative complications in the determination of a successful or unsuccessful result.[3–5,26] Clearly, as in cases of persistent pain or stiffness after a shoulder arthroplasty, it is possible to have an unsatisfactory result without a complication. However, complications such as persistent infection, neurological injury, deltoid dysfunction, and recurrent instability would be considered failures by many treating surgeons, despite the fact that most of the conventional outcomes tools used to evaluate shoulder arthroplasty do not specifically consider these variables within their scoring systems.[27]

Long-term outcomes are sometimes characterized on the basis of implant survival.[3–5,26] The need for revision surgery characterizes a shoulder arthroplasty as a success or a failure, irrespective of subjective complaints such as pain and stiffness and objective findings such as strength and range of motion. Very few long-term outcome studies determine survivorship based on anything other than the need for revision surgery, despite evidence that suggests that nearly a quarter of all failed arthroplasties do not proceed to revision surgery, perhaps because the patient is unwilling to undertake the risks of another procedure.[6,7]

Outcomes assessment after shoulder arthroplasty, as defined by the surgeon, has focused on objective, condition-specific measures that often fail to account adequately for patient satisfaction.[27] Moreover, subjective assessment of patient satisfaction may be disparate from results obtained by objective measures. Sperling et al[18] found that half of patients with a total shoulder arthroplasty and nearly half of patients with a hemiarthroplasty graded their result as unsatisfactory or unsuccessful, despite survivorship estimates, as determined by traditional criteria, suggesting 84% and 73% survival, respectively, at 15 years. Similarly, Skutek et al,[28] reviewing a series of patients with proximal humerus fractures, found that although the mean Hospital for Special Surgery Score was 69 points for those treated with a Neer II prosthesis, 85% of patients rated their results as good or excellent using a visual analog scale designed to assess patient satisfaction. Although many of the

common rating systems include both subjective domains (symptoms, activities of daily living, pain) and objective domains (range of motion, strength, stability, radiographic parameters), the relative contributions of each of these domains vary by the scoring system used. Moreover, patient satisfaction is often a minor component of the assessment and has relatively little impact on overall scoring.[27] Finally, it is evident that points for pain, range of motion, function, and satisfaction cannot be meaningfully combined into a single numerical score any more than one can meaningfully combine pounds, miles per hour, lumens, and amperes.

In an investigation by Hasan et al[7] reviewing 139 consecutive failed shoulder arthroplasties, a failure was defined as an arthroplasty that did not meet the expectations of the patient. They found that many of these patients who were unsatisfied with their original shoulder arthroplasty did not meet many of the previously accepted criteria for failure. Moreover, the prevalence of revision surgery—a traditional benchmark for success or failure used by most long-term outcome studies—underestimated the prevalence of failure by 23%.[7] A more recent observational study performed by Franta et al[6] focusing on a larger cohort of failed shoulder arthroplasties emphasized the importance of patient self-assessment in determining failure. In this series the authors reviewed 282 consecutive patients who were referred for the reason of dissatisfaction with the results of a previous shoulder arthroplasty. The most common characteristics associated with a failed shoulder arthroplasty were the presence of pain and stiffness. Two hundred forty-one shoulders (85%) presented with pain as a principal complaint, and 141 (50%) complained of stiffness—numbers that rivaled the prevalence of glenoid failure for both total shoulder arthroplasty (65%) and hemiarthroplasty (63%)—a characteristic that is traditionally thought of as the most common reason for long-term failure. These findings demonstrate the importance of documenting the clinical effectiveness of arthroplasty in terms of the improvement in patient-assessed comfort and function.

As the importance of patient self-assessment is recognized in the evaluation of the success or failure of a particular treatment, it is essential that the approach to outcome assessment be modified accordingly. The necessity for improving study design, defining the important constituents of outcome measurement, and increasing validity of orthopaedic clinical research has been emphasized by several authors.[6,27,29–31] It has been suggested that the current emphasis of orthopaedic clinical studies should be directed toward outcomes research that documents the effect of treatment on the health of those treated and the subsequent quality of their lives.[30] As we develop a better understanding of what determines an unsatisfactory outcome as defined by the patient as well as by the surgeon, we will begin to improve our ability to address these challenging problems.

CHARACTERISTICS ASSOCIATED WITH UNSATISFACTORY ARTHROPLASTIES

In an effort to better understand and prevent unsatisfactory outcomes, it is important to document the factors that are commonly associated with them and that may play a role in their causation. These factors can be considered in three broad categories: (a) patient characteristics, (b) disease characteristics, and (c) surgical characteristics. It is apparent from much of the current literature focusing on failed shoulder arthroplasty that causes of unsatisfactory outcomes are both complex and multifactorial.[3–7,9] In what is considered the largest review of failed shoulder arthroplasties to date, the average patient had four or five potential causative factors of failure,[6] suggesting that assigning an unsatisfactory result to one cause is often not possible. For instance, as used as an example by Franta et al,[6] excessive humeral retroversion may be associated with failure, but it is not necessarily the cause of an unsatisfactory outcome in patients with this finding; instead it may be a marker of surgeon inexperience that is reflected in patient selection or postoperative management. Similarly, a malaligned humeral component or the presence of lucent lines surrounding the glenoid component may not necessarily preclude an excellent functional result. From the perspective of the patient, unsatisfactory outcomes tend to manifest as poor shoulder function and subjective complaints such as pain, stiffness, and weakness. From the perspective of the surgeon, however, failure may manifest as objective findings such as diminished range of motion, poor component position, poor component fixation, and the presence of surgical complications. Many of these attributes will coexist in the unsatisfactory shoulder arthroplasty, and none is necessarily exclusive of another. Nevertheless, identification of variables that are associated with poor or unfavorable outcomes can be helpful because this will aid clinical decision making for prospective patients who present with similar characteristics.

PATIENT CHARACTERISTICS

SUBJECTIVE COMPLAINTS

Patients with unsatisfactory shoulder arthroplasties usually complain of pain and stiffness. Pain is recognized as the most common subjective sign of a failed shoulder arthroplasty and is the most common reason for patients with shoulder problems to seek evaluation by a physician.[6,7] In one of the largest series of failed shoulder arthroplasties, pain was the most common presenting complaint and was present 85% of the time.[6] However, in relatively few patients (6%) was pain the *only* presenting symptom. Stiffness was the second most common complaint. Additional presenting complaints included weakness, instability, and crepitus. Very few individuals complained of complications such as fracture (1%) or infection (5%). Additionally, more than half of patients presented with more than one chief complaint.

Chen et al[27] investigated the determinants of patient satisfaction following shoulder arthroplasty and found a correlation between patient satisfaction and pain at the time of evaluation. These authors demonstrated that patient satisfaction was significantly decreased for patients who complained of pain at rest, pain with activities, and pain requiring narcotic or anti-inflammatory medication following a shoulder arthroplasty, emphasizing the importance of pain with respect to unsatisfactory outcomes, despite concerns regarding its subjective characteristics.

SHOULDER FUNCTION

Poor shoulder function is a prominent finding in failed shoulder arthroplasties. In addition, function appears to be related to patient gender, diagnosis, type of arthroplasty, and general

health status.[6,7] The worst shoulder function among a population of failed shoulder arthroplasties was found in women and in shoulders that received a hemiarthroplasty. Similarly, diagnoses such as nonunion, cuff tear arthropathy, rheumatoid arthritis, and fracture were all associated with a worse functional outcome among failed shoulder arthroplasties. Of interest, although patients who have undergone prior revision arthroplasty surgery tended to demonstrate worse functional results at the time of failure, no functional difference was demonstrated between those who had received prior nonarthroplasty surgery before their index shoulder arthroplasty and those who did not receive such surgery.[6,7]

In a review by Hasan et al,[7] 82% (107 of 131) with failed shoulder arthroplasties indicated that they could not sleep comfortably and 23% indicated that they could not perform any of the 12 essential shoulder functions tested by the Simple Shoulder Test (SST). Fifty-seven percent of patients answered "No" to all questions assessing shoulder mobility, and 71% answered "No" to all questions assessing shoulder strength. In this cohort of patients the mean number of shoulder functions performable on the SST was 2.5 of 12. These findings of severe limitation in shoulder function are supported by a more recent analysis of 282 failed shoulder arthroplasties in which the authors demonstrated similar deficits among a population of failed shoulder arthroplasties; the mean SST score was 2.6 of 12 for the entire cohort.[6] This is in stark contrast to the observation that on average patients after shoulder arthroplasty for the diagnosis of osteoarthritis can perform nine of these functions.[14] Chen et al[27] demonstrated significant associations between functional capacities and patient satisfaction. Those patients who indicated functional difficulty with work, recreation, fitness programs, and sporting activities—in addition to those functions assessed by the SST—demonstrated significantly worse overall satisfaction as assessed by an ordinal scale.

Shoulder function among failed shoulder arthroplasty appears to be influenced by overall patient health.[6,7] Patients who are healthy typically demonstrate greater self-assessed function, as measured by the SST, compared to those with poor health. Similarly, patients' self-perceived general health appears to be worse in cases of failure of prosthetic shoulder arthroplasty. In a cohort of failed shoulder arthroplasties, the scores for all eight domains assessed by the Short Form-36 (SF-36) were significantly lower than those of age- and sex-matched controls.[7] The normalized scores were lowest for the physical role function and pain domains.

DISEASE CHARACTERISTICS

The most common diagnoses for which shoulder arthroplasty is performed include osteoarthritis, inflammatory arthritis, capsulorrhaphy arthropathy, rotator cuff tear arthropathy, secondary degenerative joint disease, and fracture. Each of these glenohumeral joint diseases implicates specific factors that may have a substantial impact on the perceived outcome of shoulder arthroplasty. The influence of disease on outcome following shoulder arthroplasty has been studied by Parsons et al.[32] In this study the authors reviewed self-assessed deficits in comfort, function, and health status before and after total shoulder arthroplasty for four different diagnoses (osteoarthritis, secondary arthritis, rheumatoid arthritis, and capsulorrhaphy arthropathy). These authors demonstrated significant differences among diagnoses for preoperative and postoperative functional deficits. Patients with osteoarthritis and capsulorrhaphy arthropathy were most improved in the category of motion, whereas those with secondary arthritis and rheumatoid arthritis were most improved in the category of comfort. There was also a statistically significant difference in five of the eight domains of the preoperative SF-36 among diagnoses. Understanding the effectiveness and shortfalls of arthroplasty in restoring functional deficits is important in counseling patients about the anticipated benefits of surgery. In addition, recognizing the impact of diagnosis on the quality of the outcomes may encourage surgeons to establish focused surgical strategies that might address the specific challenges associated with each condition.

OSTEOARTHRITIS

Although introduced first as a salvage procedure for the management of tuberculosis arthritis, shoulder arthroplasty is now most commonly used as the treatment for many of the different arthritic and degenerative conditions about the shoulder. Currently one of the most common indications for shoulder arthroplasty is osteoarthritis.[11,13,14,20,22,33–35] In many short- and long-term series the treatment of osteoarthritis with shoulder arthroplasty has demonstrated superior results compared to the use of shoulder arthroplasty in the management of other forms of arthritis, such as secondary arthritis, inflammatory arthritis, and rotator cuff tear arthropathy.[14,18,20,34,36] Torchia et al[20] studied the long-term results of shoulder arthroplasty for the diagnoses of osteoarthritis, rheumatoid arthritis, and secondary arthritis and found a greater percentage of excellent or satisfactory results among those patients treated with osteoarthritis (71%) compared to those with rheumatoid arthritis (67%) and secondary arthritis (56%) at a mean of 12.2 years. Hettrich et al[34] reviewed the outcomes of hemiarthroplasty and found that patients with the diagnosis of rheumatoid arthritis, capsulorrhaphy arthropathy, and cuff tear arthropathy demonstrated the least functional improvement, whereas those with osteonecrosis (p = 0.0004) and primary (p = 0.02) and secondary degenerative joint disease (p = 0.03) had the greatest improvement.

Osteoarthritis of the shoulder typically manifests with the triad of anterior capsular contracture, posterior glenoid wear, and posterior humeral subluxation.[8] Each of these characteristics presents its own challenges in the management of this disease that can potentially affect patient satisfaction and outcome. Anterior capsular contracture, if severe enough, can predispose the shoulder to limited external rotation, subscapularis weakness, stiffness, and potential failure secondary to excessive tension on the subscapularis repair. Similarly, posterior glenoid wear presents a challenge for both humeral hemiarthroplasty and total shoulder arthroplasty. A posteriorly worn, or biconcave, glenoid predispose the patient to posterior instability resulting from increased retroversion of the glenoid surface. In the setting of humeral hemiarthroplasty a posteriorly worn or biconcave glenoid provides an irregular and painful surface for articulation with the prosthetic humerus; however, in the setting of total shoulder arthroplasty a posteriorly worn and excessively retroverted glenoid surface may compromise the proper seating of a glenoid component because of challenges with proper glenoid preparation and the need for excessive reaming. Levine et al[37] demonstrated an association with glenoid configuration and

patient outcomes. Outcomes correlated significantly with the degree of posterior glenoid wear. Patients with concentric, type I glenoid achieved 86% satisfactory results, whereas patients with nonconcentric, type II glenoid had only 63% satisfactory results. Other authors have also found an association between posterior glenoid wear and poorer functional outcome following humeral hemiarthroplasty.[34,37–40]

Other characteristics that predict unsatisfactory outcomes following shoulder arthroplasty for the diagnosis of osteoarthritis include prior surgery and large rotator cuff tears. Sperling et al[18,22] provided what may be the longest follow-up study on shoulder arthroplasty. In their series of 114 shoulder arthroplasties followed for a period of 20 years, they noted that age younger than 50 years and a history of prior shoulder surgery (as well as a preoperative diagnosis of secondary arthritis) were significantly associated with an unsatisfactory outcome and increased risk for revision surgery. Hettrich el al[34] also found that a history of prior surgery was associated with poorer functional outcome for a population of hemiarthroplasties. In addition, shoulders with an intact rotator cuff showed significantly (p < 0.05) greater improvement in the ability to lift weight above shoulder level after hemiarthroplasty. Patient age and gender did not significantly affect outcome.

Others have clearly documented the influence of rotator cuff tears in the setting of primary shoulder arthroplasty by demonstrating strong associations with unsatisfactory outcomes.[11,41–44] Most studies report the prevalence of rotator cuff tears at the time of shoulder arthroplasty to range between 12% and 46%.[41,42,44] Hasan et al[7] noted that 21% of unsatisfactory shoulder arthroplasties were associated with rotator cuff tears. In a multicenter investigation of 555 shoulder arthroplasties performed for primary osteoarthritis, Edwards et al observed that small, minimally retracted tears of the rotator cuff noted at the time of surgery did not affect objective or subjective outcome. However, larger degenerative tears and those associated with fatty degeneration were associated with poorer objective outcome and decreased patient satisfaction.[42]

INFLAMMATORY ARTHRITIS

The management of inflammatory arthritis with shoulder arthroplasty presents unique challenges for the patient and the surgeon. Large clinical series suggest that the outcomes of shoulder arthroplasty for the management of inflammatory arthritis demonstrate less functional improvement compared to other diagnoses, such as degenerative arthritis.[20,34,45–48] Inflammatory arthritis may involve not only the glenohumeral joint but also surrounding articulations such as the acromioclavicular joint, sternoclavicular joint, elbow, wrist, and hand—all of which may limit perceived functional improvement from a well-performed shoulder arthroplasty.[8]

A characteristic manifestation of inflammatory arthritis involving the glenohumeral joint is medial glenoid erosion. In a natural history study performed by Lehtinen et al,[49] the authors demonstrated that erosive involvement of the glenohumeral joint occurred in 48% of patients. In addition, inflammatory arthritis is known for its association with osteopenia and bilateral involvment.[8] Moreover, the soft tissues, including the rotator cuff, may be swollen, contracted, weakened, or torn. In two series of patients with rheumatoid arthritis treated with total shoulder arthroplasty, full-thickness rotator cuff tears were identified in 42% and 52% of shoulders.[50,51] In the latter study, repair of the torn tendon was possible in fewer than half of the treated patients and the quality of the rotator cuff repair correlated significantly with postoperative outcome.[51]

Other variables to consider in patients with inflammatory arthritis include the current forms of pharmacotherapy. Many of these patients are receiving disease-modifying agents and immunosuppressants, such as tumor necrosis factor-alpha antagonists, prednisone, and methotrexate, which may increase the prevalence of postoperative infection.[52] The prevalence of infection in total joint arthroplasty is approximately 2.6 times greater in patients with rheumatoid arthritis than in patients with osteoarthritis.[53] In addition, the typical drug regimen, which includes disease-modifying agents and immunosuppressants, has the potential to adversely affect wound healing.[52] Finally, the involvement of other joints and the trend to limit antirheumatic medications around the time of surgery may tend to exacerbate patients' underlying condition, ultimately affecting their ability to fully participate in an active rehabilitation program.[52] These variables considered in concert may negatively affect the outcome of shoulder arthroplasty.[45,46–48]

CAPSULORRHAPHY ARTHROPATHY

Joint destruction is a well-recognized complication of surgery for the treatment of shoulder instability. Capsulorrhaphy arthropathy is the term used to describe the subset of patients who develop secondary degenerative joint disease related to a prior surgery for recurrent dislocations.[8,54] Glenohumeral arthritis developing subsequent to prior instability surgery presents several potential challenges related to the relative age of the patient, soft-tissue contracture, scarring, altered anatomy from prior surgery, and potential bone loss—typically involving the posterior glenoid resulting from chronic posterior humeral subluxation. Lusardi et al[55] retrospectively reported on a series of patients who had been managed for severe loss of external rotation of the glenohumeral joint after previous anterior capsulorrhaphy for recurrent instability. All patients noted severe restriction of motion, and 85% reported significant pain. In addition, 35% of the shoulders had been dislocated or subluxated posteriorly and 80% developed glenohumeral arthritis. Sperling et al[54] presented the long-term results of shoulder arthroplasty in patients who had undergone a prior surgery for glenohumeral instability. These authors reviewed 31 patients, two thirds of whom underwent total shoulder arthroplasty and a third underwent humeral hemiarthroplasty. Shoulder arthroplasty was associated with significant pain relief and improvement in external rotation at a mean follow-up of 7 years. However, according to a modified Neer system an unsatisfactory outcome was observed in more than half of the patients (62% unsatisfactory results for total shoulder arthroplasty and 40% for humeral hemiarthroplasty). Survival of the implant was estimated as 86% at 5 years and 61% at 10 years, an estimate that is considerably worse than that reported by most long-term outcome studies for shoulder arthroplasty performed for other diagnoses.[13,18,22,20] Bigliani et al,[56] as well as Green and Norris,[57] reported on the results of shoulder arthroplasty in the treatment of capsulorrhaphy arthropathy. In each of these series the mean patient age was in the mid-40s and severe internal rotation contracture, posterior glenoid deficiency, and altered anatomy from previous surgery were complicating

factors in achieving a stable and functional prosthetic reconstruction. The series by Bigliani's group[56] reported a 23% rate of unsatisfactory outcomes at a follow-up of 3 years, whereas Sperling et al[54] noted unsatisfactory results in 62% of patients at a mean of 7 years after surgery.

ROTATOR CUFF TEAR ARTHROPATHY

The characteristics of rotator cuff tear arthropathy were described by Neer et al[58] in 1983. These authors described the pathological changes in 26 patients with this disease and noted the presence of the following characteristics: massive rotator cuff tearing, glenohumeral instability, loss of articular cartilage of the glenohumeral joint, humeral head collapse, and related bone loss. These attributes present a significant challenge for the surgeon because these shoulders typically lack normal bone stock and do not offer reconstructable rotator cuff tissue. In addition, as suggested by Matsen et al[8] in the setting of rotator cuff tear arthropathy, the shoulder is deprived of several major stabilizing structures such as (a) the normal cuff muscle force vector compressing the humeral head into the glenoid; (b) the superior lip of the glenoid concavity, which is typically worn away by chronic superior subluxation; and (c) the cuff tendon interposed between the humeral head and the coracoacromial arch. If the coracoacromial arch has been sacrificed by prior acromioplasty, the risk of instability is much greater.

All of these factors lend to a situation in which the shoulder can become superiorly unstable, presenting a unique challenge for traditional unconstrained shoulder arthroplasty. This was made evident by the case series reported by Franklin et al[43] in 1988. In this review the authors evaluated a series of total shoulder arthroplasties that exhibited accelerated glenoid failure with the purpose of identifying factors associated with glenoid loosening. The average time from arthroplasty was 30 months (range, 14 to 44 months). A strong association was observed between incompletely reconstructable rotator cuff tears present at the time of surgery, the amount of superior migration of the humeral component, and the degree of glenoid loosening.

Results of hemiarthroplasty in these situations demonstrated only modest improvement. Sanchez-Sotelo et al[59] reviewed 33 shoulders treated with hemiarthroplasty for cuff tear arthropathy, with an average follow-up of 5 years. Anterosuperior instability occurred in more than 20% of patients in their series and was associated with a history of subacromial decompression.[59] Successful results based on Neer's limited-goals criteria were achieved in only two thirds of their patient population. The authors concluded that hemiarthroplasty, although a reconstructive option for these patients, may be complicated by instability and progressive bone loss.

SECONDARY ARTHRITIS

Shoulders with secondary degenerative joint disease often present specific challenges that may predispose a patient to an unsatisfactory outcome. Often a shoulder that has received significant trauma has complex pathology that requires difficult surgical management.[60,61] Challenges in managing patients with secondary degenerative joint disease are related to the presence of deformity, muscle contractures, scarring, malunion, nonunion, bone loss, and humeral shortening. Although there are no recent studies reporting on the results of shoulder arthroplasty for an isolated series of patients with secondary arthritis, many authors have demonstrated that a preoperative diagnosis of secondary osteoarthritis can negatively affect shoulder function after arthroplasty.[18,22,34,62,63] Factors associated with this diagnosis clearly have a substantial impact on the results of prosthetic reconstruction. In a review by Parsons et al[32] characterizing the effect of diagnosis on outcomes following shoulder arthroplasty, only 26% of patients with secondary degenerative joint disease had improved across all functional categories.

ARTHROPLASTY FOR FRACTURE

Treatment of proximal humeral fractures with prosthetic replacement has been recognized as a challenge and is associated with limited outcomes compared to those in other common diagnoses such as primary osteoarthritis.[64] These cases are often associated with altered anatomy, compromised soft tissues (torn rotator cuff), neurological injury, and predisposition to instability—characteristics that may predict an unsatisfactory outcome in most series. In addition, a challenge that is unique to the arthroplasty for fracture is tuberosity management. Demirhan et al[65] retrospectively reviewed prognostic factors associated with functional outcomes of prosthetic replacement for acute proximal humerus fractures and found that preoperative delay, problems of tuberosity fixation, and position of the tuberosities were the strongest parameters influencing clinical outcome. Of their patients, 50% had problems with the tuberosities, all of which negatively affected clinical outcome. Additionally, shoulders with high positioning of the prosthesis had poorer functional outcomes.

Reliable replication of normal proximal humeral anatomy is an important goal of shoulder arthroplasty for acute proximal humeral fractures. Malrotation of the prosthesis or rotational malposition of the tuberosities can result in decreased motion.[66,67] Instability following prosthetic replacement for proximal humerus fractures has also been reported as a common complication affecting outcome.[68–70] In addition, infection and neurological injury are thought to occur more readily in the setting of trauma than during elective surgery.[69,71] Meticulous soft tissue technique, secure placement of the prosthesis with proper version and height, firm tuberosity reconstruction, careful rotator cuff repair, and proper rehabilitation are all important factors that affect patient outcome following shoulder arthroplasty for proximal humeral fractures.

SURGICAL CHARACTERISTICS

VARIABLES ASSOCIATED WITH PLACEMENT OF THE PROSTHESIS

Technical factors such as component malpositioning, glenohumeral malalignment, and glenoid failure are among the most common characteristics associated with failed shoulder arthroplasties.[6,7] Malpositioning of the humeral and glenoid prostheses refers to the position of these implants in relation to the humerus and glenoid, respectively.[6] Glenohumeral malalignment refers to the relationship between the center of the humeral head and the center of the glenoid, commonly descried as glenohumeral register.[8] Glenoid failure manifests in multiple ways. For humeral hemiarthroplasty, glenoid failure occurs most commonly by progressive glenoid arthrosis or glenoid erosion. In the setting of total shoulder arthroplasty, glenoid failure most commonly involves loosening, fracture, displacement, or wear of the polyethylene glenoid component.

Malposition and Malalignment

Neer was one of the first to recognize component position and alignment as a potential cause of failure in shoulder arthroplasties.[72,73] More recent data from a large series of failed shoulder arthroplasties demonstrated that humeral component malposition and glenohumeral malalignment were the most common technical problems seen among this population of failed arthroplasties (65% and 67%, respectively).[6] Within this series of 282 patients, those with the diagnosis of secondary degenerative joint disease demonstrated the highest percentage of humeral component malposition and glenohumeral malalignment. Superior placement of the humeral component in relation to the greater tuberosity was the most common problem with component positioning.

Recent studies have stressed the need for anatomic reconstruction of the proximal humerus.[74] Figgie et al[75] correlated the functional outcome with position of the glenoid and humeral components. They noted that when the humeral head was positioned slightly above the greater tuberosity, and the glenoid and humeral offsets were restored, there was an improved range of motion, a reduced incidence of glenoid lucent lines, and decreased glenoid component failure compared with the findings in those in whom the correct alignment had not been completely restored.[75] Hsu et al[76] also concluded that the humeral head offset and the position of the tuberosities were of particular importance in restoring the abductor lever arm and therefore the range of elevation and abduction of the shoulder. In addition, many studies have demonstrated an association with superior humeral migration after total shoulder arthroplasty and glenoid loosening, as well as between glenohumeral malalignment and erosion of the glenoid.[3,4,5,11,38,43,77]

Glenoid Failure

The orthopaedic literature would suggest that the long-term problems with shoulder arthroplasty often relate to problems with the glenoid.[3,4,5,8,9] For humeral arthroplasty this manifests as medial glenoid erosion and progressive glenohumeral arthritis requiring revision. For total shoulder arthroplasty this manifests as loosening, wear, fracture, and displacement. All of these characteristics have been associated with poor outcomes following shoulder arthroplasty.

The prevalence of glenoid erosion following humeral hemiarthroplasty has been estimated to be as high as 100%.[78] In addition, glenoid erosion has been associated with unsatisfactory results and the need for conversion to total shoulder arthroplasty in many studies.[6,10,26,37,78] Among a population of failed hemiarthroplasties, the greatest prevalence of glenoid erosion was found among those patients treated for degenerative conditions of the glenohumeral joint (64%), whereas glenoid erosion was less prevalent among those individuals treated for proximal humeral fractures (46%) and proximal humeral nonunions (29%).[6] Erosion affected the superior portion of the glenoid most commonly. In addition, the presence of erosion was significantly related to humeral component malposition and glenohumeral malalignment, findings that have been supported by others.[6,38]

Failure of the prosthetic glenoid in total shoulder arthroplasty is thought to be the most common prosthesis-related variable associated with the need for revision surgery.[3–5,79,80] In addition, failure of the glenoid component has been associated with both increased pain and decreased patient satisfaction in long-term studies.[79] Within a population of 136 unsatisfactory total shoulder arthroplasties, 63% had a loose glenoid component. Surgical technique, instability, rotator cuff tears, and heavy use have all been implicated in glenoid loosening. Lazarus et al[81] suggest that proper seating and cementing of the glenoid component is technically difficult. Although most surgeons have intuitively suspected the significance of these lucent lines to be signs of impending loosening, the absence of long-term results in excess of 10 years failed to confirm the suspicion until recently, when Torchia et al[20] reported a 5- to 17-year follow-up study and demonstrated the progression of these lucent lines to symptomatic loosening. Of the patients in their series, 84% demonstrated radiolucencies at a mean of 12 years. In addition, data from this series demonstrated a strong association between glenoid component loosening and subjective pain.

SURGICAL COMPLICATIONS

Complications associated with total shoulder arthroplasties can be multiple and include glenohumeral instability, periprosthetic fracture, muscle dysfunction (rotator cuff and deltoid), neural injury, and infection. The prevalence of complications reported in the literature is highly variable, ranging between 0 and 62%.[3–5,8] In an analysis of 18 reports on total shoulder arthroplasty with a minimum of 2-years follow-up, Matsen et al[8] observed a mean complication rate of 16%. These authors identified the following factors in order of decreasing frequency: component loosening, instability, rotator cuff tear, periprosthetic fracture, infection, implant failure, and deltoid dysfunction. Wirth and Rockwood[4] reported a similar prevalence of surgical complications (14%) following a review of 1,459 arthroplasties from 23 series. In this report the prevalence of complications following hemiarthroplasty and total shoulder arthroplasty was 16% and 10%, respectively.

Instability

Instability is the most commonly reported complication following unconstrained shoulder arthroplasty.[3–5,8,82] Its prevalence has been reported to be as high as 35% among primary arthroplasties, and it is thought to represent nearly 40% of all complications.[3,8] Anterior instability is typically associated with subscapularis and capsular failure, whereas posterior failure has been attributed to excessive retroversion of the humeral or glenoid components.[8,82,83] Inferior instability commonly results from failure to restore humeral length, such as in the setting of arthroplasty for fracture or tumor, and superior instability is typically encountered in the setting of cuff-tear arthropathy and deficiency of the coracoacromial arch. Moeckel et al[83] reported one of the first series of patients with instability following primary shoulder arthroplasty. These authors observed that treatment of instability following shoulder arthroplasty is associated with loss of motion compared to motion before the episode of instability, and that proper balancing of the soft

tissues and positioning of the components are essential to a satisfactory outcome.

Periprosthetic Fractures

Periprosthetic fractures, though infrequent, present difficult technical challenges. These fractures may involve the humerus or glenoid and represent approximately 20% of all complications associated with shoulder arthroplasty.[8] The vast majority of periprosthetic fractures involve the humerus (86%); a lesser number of fractures are seen involving the glenoid (12%). Additionally, the majority of fractures occur in the perioperative period (62%) as opposed to the postoperative period (48%). Perioperative humerus fractures are most commonly related to errors in surgical technique such as overzealous reaming, aggressive impaction, and excessive manipulation.[3–5,8] Fractures of the glenoid may also occur and predispose the arthroplasty to failure by means of instability or poor glenoid fixation. Bone grafting in glenoid defects has been performed; however, it is technically challenging and associated with a higher prevalence of complications and poorer outcomes compared to uncomplicated primary shoulder arthroplasties.[84]

Rotator Cuff Tears

Injury to the rotator cuff can be related to technical aspects of the operation or can occur postoperatively. During the operation the posterior rotator cuff tendon is vulnerable when the humeral head is being excised. Excising too large a segment of the head or excising the head in too much retroversion can place the posterior cuff at significant risk.[85] If damage during this portion of the procedure is recognized, salvaging the injured tendon is necessary. Repairable full-thickness tears of the rotator cuff isolated to the supraspinatus tendon in two series did not affect outcome.[3,86] Although these tears were not traumatically induced at the time of surgery secondary to poor surgical technique, this does support the idea that small reparable cuff defects may not present a large challenge for patients if managed properly. Hettrich et al[34] found greater improvement with respect to self-assessed function and level of comfort in patients who did not have full-thickness rotator cuff tears who were treated with hemiartroplasty. Similarly, Edwards et al[42] in reviewing 555 shoulders in 514 patients demonstrated that small, reparable, supraspinatus tears were not found to influence the postoperative outcome with respect to the total Constant score, active mobility, subjective satisfaction, radiographic result, or rate of complications; however, shoulders with moderate fatty degeneration and those with severe degeneration of the infraspinatus were associated with poorer results than those with no degeneration with respect to the total Constant score ($p < 0.0005$), active external rotation ($p < 0.0005$), active forward flexion ($p = 0.001$), and subjective satisfaction ($p = 0.031$).

Tearing of the rotator cuff following shoulder arthroplasty in the postoperative period is said to occur in 2% of treated patients.[3,8] Symptoms are usually minimal and reflect the natural history of rotator cuff disease in the general population.[8] Nonoperative, as well as operative, treatment has been used successfully in these situations. In stark contrast, however, postoperative ruptures of the subscapularis represent significant challenges for the patient that may lead to pain, weakness, instability, and an unsatisfactory outcome. Ruptures of the subscapularis are said to represent half (53%) of the tears following shoulder arthroplasty.[3] Characteristics that have been associated with this complication include prior operations, aggressive physical therapy (particularly external rotation), and tendon lengthening techniques.[87-89] In a series of 119 patients treated with shoulder arthroplasty, Miller et al[89] found the prevalence of subscapularis ruptures to be 6%, and all required operative repair. More importantly, arthroplasties that were complicated by postoperative subscapularis failure demonstrated lower American Shoulder and Elbow Surgeons (ASES) and patient satisfaction scores.

Neural Injuries

Neural injury is a significant, but rare, complication associated with shoulder arthroplasty. Injuries commonly manifest as neurapraxias of either the axillary nerve or brachial plexus. The vast majority of these injuries (77%) resolve with expectant management.[3] Very rarely does actual transection of a nerve occur.[3-5,8] Nevertheless, neural injury can be associated with unsatisfactory outcomes following shoulder arthroplasty. Despite a well-performed arthroplasty, patients with neural injuries may experience a delay in appropriate rehabilitation and may be concerned about the extent of the paralysis and the uncertainty associated with a lengthy of recovery. Stiffness and chronic neural pain may result from these injuries. Because this complication is relatively rare, there are no good clinical studies analyzing the influence of neural injury on outcome data following shoulder arthroplasty. Nevertheless, the challenges associated with rehabilitation following neural injury and the potential psychological stressors that may accompany this complication may easily affect overall patient satisfaction.

Infection

One of the more devastating complications associated with unsatisfactory outcome following shoulder arthroplasty is the development of prosthetic infection.[3,8] Prevalence of infection following shoulder arthroplasty based on the current published series is estimated to be less than 1%.[3] Infection has been associated with inflammatory arthritis, diabetes mellitus, advanced age, remote sites of infection, malnutrition, and immunosupression.[3,90] Coste et al[91] retrospectively reviewed 49 patients with prosthetic infections associated with shoulder arthroplasty. These authors noted strong associations with pain, limited motion, and radiological loosening in the majority (88%) of patients. In addition, the antibiotics chosen and the length of treatment for these patients was considered to be suboptimal in 50% of the patients in their series, emphasizing the challenges associated with identifying and implementing the appropriate treatment regimen in many of these complex situations. Unexplained pain after shoulder arthroplasty should always cause concern about the possibility of infection. Low-virulence organisms, such as *Propionibacterium acnes* and *Staphylococcus epidermidis* are relatively common offenders in this context.[6]

Deltoid Muscle Dysfunction

Deltoid function is critical to the outcome of shoulder arthroplasty. Catastrophic loss of shoulder function is the end result of deltoid dysfunction secondary to axillary nerve injury or deltoid muscle detachment.[3,8] Clinical investigation of this complication has demonstrated significant disability and persistent pain.[8] Deltoid integrity is essential for proper function of both unconstrained and constrained shoulder arthroplasties. Reconstruction attempts for a denervated or detached deltoid are not commonly successful. Without proper function, shoulder arthrodesis is a consideration as a salvage attempt to improve comfort, stability, and function.

SUMMARY

Unsatisfactory outcomes following primary shoulder arthroplasty are unfortunately common, affecting approximately one in ten patients having this procedure. The potential contributing factors include the patient, the disease, technical factors, and the experience of the surgeon performing the procedure. The patient's subjective view of the success of the procedure may be different from the views of the surgeon or from an objective evaluation of shoulder function and radiographs.

As shoulder surgeons, it is our challenge to focus not on the instances in which shoulder arthroplasty yields a result pleasing to patient and surgeon but on those instances in which our procedure fails to deliver its potential improvement in the quality of life of our patients. As Codman admonished, ask "Why not?" if the result is not satisfactory. Only by holding our collective feet to the fire of the end result will we learn how to better prevent future unsatisfactory results. Hopefully we will learn the lessons needed for questions such as (a) When is a patient not a good candidate for shoulder arthroplasty? (b) When is a glenoid component not a good idea for the particular patient? (c) When does the postoperative plan need to be altered to reduce the risk of failure? (d) When is a reverse total shoulder arthroplasty a better choice than an anatomic arthroplasty? (e) When is a particular surgeon not the best person to do the arthroplasty? (f) How can we best inform our patients about the risk for an unsatisfactory result?

REFERENCES

1. Lugli T. Artificial shoulder joint by Péan (1893): the facts of an exceptional intervention and the prosthetic method. *Clin Orthop Relat Res* 1978;133:215–218.
2. Neer CS, Brown TH Jr, McLaughlin HL. Fracture of the neck of the humerus with dislocation of the head fragment. *Am J Surg* 1953;85:252–258.
3. Bohsali KI, Wirth MA, Rockwood CA Jr. Complications of total shoulder arthroplasty. *J Bone Joint Surg Am* 2006;88:2279–2292.
4. Wirth MA, Rockwood CA Jr. Complications of shoulder arthroplasty. *Clin Orthop Relat Res* 1994;307:47–69.
5. Wirth MA, Rockwood CA Jr. Complications of total shoulder-replacement arthroplasty. *J Bone Joint Surg Am* 1996;78:603–616.
6. Franta AK, Lenters TR, Mounce D, et al. The complex characteristics of 282 unsatisfactory shoulder arthroplasties. *J Shoulder Elbow Surg* 2007;16:555–562.
7. Hasan SS, Leith JM, Campbell B, et al. Characteristics of unsatisfactory shoulder arthroplasties. *J Shoulder Elbow Surg* 2002;11:431–441.
8. Matsen FA 3rd, Rockwood CA Jr, Wirth MA, et al. *Glenohumeral Arthritis and Its Management.* Vol 2. 3rd ed. Philadelphia, Pa: Saunders; 2004:879–1007.
9. Chin PY, Sperling JW, Cofield RH, et al. Complications of total shoulder arthroplasty: are they fewer or different? *J Shoulder Elbow Surg* 2006;15:19–22.
10. Hasan SS, Leith JM, Smith KL, et al. The distribution of shoulder replacement among surgeons and hospitals is significantly different than that of hip or knee replacement. *J Shoulder Elbow Surg* 2003;12:164–169.
11. Barrett WP, Franklin JL, Jackins SE, et al. Total shoulder arthroplasty. *J Bone Joint Surg Am* 1987;69:865–872.
12. Cofield RH. Total shoulder arthroplasty with the Neer prosthesis. *J Bone Joint Surg Am* 1984;66:899–906.
13. Deshmukh AV, Koris M, Zurakowski D, et al. Total shoulder arthroplasty: long-term survivorship, functional outcome, and quality of life. *J Shoulder Elbow Surg* 2005;14:471–479.
14. Fehringer EV, Kopjar B, Boorman RS, et al. Characterizing the functional improvement after total shoulder arthroplasty for osteoarthritis. *J Bone Joint Surg Am* 2002;84:1349–1353.
15. Frich LH, Moller BN, Sneppen O. Shoulder arthroplasty with the Neer Mark-II prosthesis. *Arch Orthop Trauma Surg* 1988;107:110–113.

16. Kelly IG, Foster RS, Fisher WD. Neer total shoulder replacement in rheumatoid arthritis. *J Bone Joint Surg Br* 1987;69:723–726.
17. Weiss AP, Adams MA, Moore JR, et al. Unconstrained shoulder arthroplasty: a 5-year average follow-up study. *Clin Orthop Relat Res* 1990;257:86–90.
18. Sperling JW, Cofield RH, Rowland CM. Neer hemiarthroplasty and Neer total shoulder arthroplasty in patients 50 years old or less: long-term results. *J Bone Joint Surg Am* 1998;80:464–473.
19. Stewart MP, Kelly IG. Total shoulder replacement in rheumatoid disease: 7- to 13-year follow-up of 37 joints. *J Bone Joint Surg Br* 1997;79:68–72.
20. Torchia ME, Cofield RH, Settergren CR. Total shoulder arthroplasty with the Neer prosthesis: long-term results. *J Shoulder Elbow Surg* 1997;6:495–505.
21. Cofield RH, Edgerton BC. Total shoulder arthroplasty: complications and revision surgery. *Instr Course Lect* 1990;39:449–462.
22. Sperling JW, Cofield RH, Rowland CM. Minimum 15-year follow-up of Neer hemiarthroplasty and total shoulder arthroplasty in patients aged 50 years or younger. *J Shoulder Elbow Surg* 2004;13:604–613.
23. Norquist BM, Goldberg BA, Matsen FA III. Challenges in evaluating patients lost to follow-up in clinical studies of rotator cuff tears. *J Bone Joint Surg Am* 2000;82:838–842.
24. Jain N, Pietrobon R, Hocker S, et al. The relationship between surgeon and hospital volume and outcomes for shoulder arthroplasty. *J Bone Joint Surg Am* 2004;86:496–505.
25. Brenner BC, Ferlic DC, Clayton ML, et al. Survivorship of unconstrained total shoulder arthroplasty. *J Bone Joint Surg Am* 1989;71:1289–1296.
26. Sperling JW, Cofield RH. Revision total shoulder arthroplasty for the treatment of glenoid arthrosis. *J Bone Joint Surg Am* 1998;80:860–867.
27. Chen AL, Bain EB, Horan MP, et al. Determinants of patient satisfaction with outcome after shoulder arthroplasty. *J Shoulder Elbow Surg* 2007;16:25–30.
28. Skutek M, Fremerey RW, Bosch U. Level of physical activity in elderly patients after hemiarthroplasty for three- and four-part fractures of the proximal humerus. *Arch Orthop Trauma Surg* 1998;117:252–255.
29. Cutler SJ, Ederer F. Maximum utilization of the life table method in analyzing survival. *J Chronic Dis* 1958;8:699–712.
30. Gartland JJ. Orthopaedic clinical research: deficiencies in experimental design and determinations of outcome. *J Bone Joint Surg Am* 1988;70:1357–1364.
31. Rudicel S, Esdaile J. The randomized clinical trial in orthopaedics: obligation or option? *J Bone Joint Surg Am* 1985;67:1284–1293.
32. Parsons IMT, Campbell B, Titelman RM, et al. Characterizing the effect of diagnosis on presenting deficits and outcomes after total shoulder arthroplasty. *J Shoulder Elbow Surg* 2005;14:575–584.
33. Adams JE, Sperling JW, Hoskin TL, et al. Shoulder arthroplasty in Olmsted County, Minnesota, 1976–2000: a population-based study. *J Shoulder Elbow Surg* 2006;15:50–55.
34. Hettrich CM, Weldon E 3rd, Boorman RS, et al. Preoperative factors associated with improvements in shoulder function after humeral hemiarthroplasty. *J Bone Joint Surg Am* 2004;86:1446–1451.
35. Matsen FA III, Antoniou J, Rozencwaig R, et al. Correlates with comfort and function after total shoulder arthroplasty for degenerative joint disease. *J Shoulder Elbow Surg* 2000;9:465–469.
36. Lynch JR, Franta AK, Montgomery WH Jr, et al. Self-assessed outcome at 2 to 4 years after shoulder hemiarthroplasty with concentric glenoid reaming. *J Bone Joint Surg Am* 2007;89:1284–1292.
37. Levine WN, Djurasovic M, Glasson JM, et al. Hemiarthroplasty for glenohumeral osteoarthritis: results correlated to degree of glenoid wear. *J Shoulder Elbow Surg* 1997;6:449–454.
38. Carroll RM, Izquierdo R, Vazquez M, et al. Conversion of painful hemiarthroplasty to total shoulder arthroplasty: long-term results. *J Shoulder Elbow Surg* 2004;13:599–603.
39. Edwards TB, Boulahia A, Kempf JF, et al. Shoulder arthroplasty in patients with osteoarthritis and dysplastic glenoid morphology. *J Shoulder Elbow Surg* 2004;13:1–4.
40. Walch G, Boulahia A, Boileau P, et al. Primary glenohumeral osteoarthritis: clinical and radiographic classification. The Aequalis Group. *Acta Orthop Belg* 1998;64(suppl 2):46–52.
41. Arntz CT, Jackins S, Matsen FA 3rd. Prosthetic replacement of the shoulder for the treatment of defects in the rotator cuff and the surface of the glenohumeral joint. *J Bone Joint Surg Am* 1993;75:485–491.
42. Edwards TB, Boulahia A, Kempf JF, et al. The influence of rotator cuff disease on the results of shoulder arthroplasty for primary osteoarthritis: results of a multicenter study. *J Bone Joint Surg Am* 2002;84:2240–2248.
43. Franklin JL, Barrett WP, Jackins SE, et al. Glenoid loosening in total shoulder arthroplasty: association with rotator cuff deficiency. *J Arthroplasty* 1988;3:39–46.
44. Zeman CA, Arcand MA, Cantrell JS, et al. The rotator cuff-deficient arthritic shoulder: diagnosis and surgical management. *J Am Acad Orthop Surg* 1998;6:337–348.
45. Boyd AD Jr, Aliabadi P, Thornhill TS. Postoperative proximal migration in total shoulder arthroplasty: incidence and significance. *J Arthroplasty* 1991;6:31–37.
46. Matsen FA 3rd, Smith KL, DeBartolo SE, et al. A comparison of patients with late-stage rheumatoid arthritis and osteoarthritis of the shoulder using self-assessed shoulder function and health status. *Arthritis Care Res* 1997;10:43–47.
47. Sneppen O, Fruensgaard S, Johannsen HV, et al. Total shoulder replacement in rheumatoid arthritis: proximal migration and loosening. *J Shoulder Elbow Surg* 1996;5:47–52.
48. Sojbjerg JO, Frich LH, Johannsen HV, et al. Late results of total shoulder replacement in patients with rheumatoid arthritis. *Clin Orthop Relat Res* 1999;366:39–45.
49. Lehtinen JT, Kaarela K, Belt EA, et al. Incidence of glenohumeral joint involvement in seropositive rheumatoid arthritis: a 15-year endpoint study. *J Rheumatol* 2000;27:347–350.
50. Cofield RH. Unconstrained total shoulder prostheses. *Clin Orthop Relat Res* 1983;97–108.
51. Rozing PM, Brand R. Rotator cuff repair during shoulder arthroplasty in rheumatoid arthritis. *J Arthroplasty* 1998;13:311–319.
52. Howe CR, Gardner GC, Kadel NJ. Perioperative medication management for the patient with rheumatoid arthritis. *J Am Acad Orthop Surg* 2006;14:544–551.
53. Luessenhop CP, Higgins LD, Brause BD, et al. Multiple prosthetic infections after total joint arthroplasty: risk-factor analysis. *J Arthroplasty* 1996;11:862–868.
54. Sperling JW, Antuna SA, Sanchez-Sotelo J, et al. Shoulder arthroplasty for arthritis after instability surgery. *J Bone Joint Surg Am* 2002;84:1775–1781.
55. Lusardi DA, Wirth MA, Wurtz D, et al. Loss of external rotation following anterior capsulorrhaphy of the shoulder. *J Bone Joint Surg Am* 1993;75:1185–1192.
56. Bigliani LU, Weinstein DM, Glasgow MT, et al. Glenohumeral arthroplasty for arthritis after instability surgery. *J Shoulder Elbow Surg* 1995;4:87–94.
57. Green A, Norris TR. Shoulder arthroplasty for advanced glenohumeral arthritis after anterior instability repair. *J Shoulder Elbow Surg* 2001;10:539–545.
58. Neer CS 2nd, Craig EV, Fukuda H. Cuff-tear arthropathy. *J Bone Joint Surg Am* 1983;65:1232–1244.
59. Sanchez-Sotelo J, Cofield RH, Rowland CM. Shoulder hemiarthroplasty for glenohumeral arthritis associated with severe rotator cuff deficiency. *J Bone Joint Surg Am* 2001;83:1814–1822.
60. Mehlhorn AT, Schmal H, Sudkamp NP. Clinical evaluation of a new custom offset shoulder prosthesis for treatment of complex fractures of the proximal humerus. *Acta Orthop Belg* 2006;72:387–394.
61. Wiater JM, Flatow EL. Posttraumatic arthritis. *Orthop Clin North Am* 2000;31:63–76.
62. Levy O, Copeland SA. Cementless surface replacement arthroplasty of the shoulder: 5- to 10-year results with the Copeland mark-2 prosthesis. *J Bone Joint Surg Br* 2001;83:213–221.
63. Norris BL, Lachiewicz PF. Modern cement technique and the survivorship of total shoulder arthroplasty. *Clin Orthop Relat Res* 1996;328:76–85.
64. Compito CA, Self EB, Bigliani LU. Arthroplasty and acute shoulder trauma: reasons for success and failure. *Clin Orthop Relat Res* 1994:27–36.
65. Demirhan M, Kilicoglu O, Attinel L, Eralp L, Akalin Y. Prognostic factors in prosthetic replacement for acute proximal humerus fractures. *J Orthop Trauma*. 2003;17:181–188.
66. Frankle MA, Greenwald DP, Markee BA, et al. Biomechanical effects of malposition of tuberosity fragments on the humeral prosthetic reconstruction for four-part proximal humerus fractures. *J Shoulder Elbow Surg* 2001;10:321–326.
67. Hempfing A, Leunig M, Ballmer FT, et al. Surgical landmarks to determine humeral head retrotorsion for hemiarthroplasty in fractures. *J Shoulder Elbow Surg* 2001;10:460–463.
68. Boileau P, Caligaris-Cordero B, Payeur F, et al. Prognostic factors during rehabilitation after shoulder prostheses for fracture [in French]. *Rev Chir Orthop Reparatrice Appar Mot* 1999;85:106–116.
69. Muldoon MP, Cofield RH. Complications of humeral head replacement for proximal humeral fractures. *Instr Course Lect* 1997;46:15–24.
70. Rietveld AB, Daanen HA, Rozing PM, et al. The lever arm in glenohumeral abduction after hemiarthroplasty. *J Bone Joint Surg Br* 1988;70:561–565.
71. Cofield RH. Comminuted fractures of the proximal humerus. *Clin Orthop Relat Res* 1988;49–57.
72. Neer CS 2nd, Kirby RM. Revision of humeral head and total shoulder arthroplasties. *Clin Orthop Relat Res* 1982;170:189–195.
73. Neer CS 2nd, Watson KC, Stanton FJ. Recent experience in total shoulder replacement. *J Bone Joint Surg Am* 1982;64:319–337.
74. Pearl ML. Proximal humeral anatomy in shoulder arthroplasty: implications for prosthetic design and surgical technique. *J Shoulder Elbow Surg* 2005;14:99S–104S.
75. Figgie HE III, Inglis AE, Goldberg VM, et al. An analysis of factors affecting the long-term results of total shoulder arthroplasty in inflammatory arthritis. *J Arthroplasty* 1988;3:123–130.
76. Hsu HC, Luo ZP, Stone JJ, et al. Correlation between rotator cuff tear and glenohumeral degeneration. *Acta Orthop Scand* 2003;74:89–94.
77. Collins D, Tencer A, Sidles J, et al. Edge displacement and deformation of glenoid components in response to eccentric loading: the effect of preparation of the glenoid bone. *J Bone Joint Surg Am* 1992;74:501–507.
78. Parsons IMT, Millett PJ, Warner JJ. Glenoid wear after shoulder hemiarthroplasty: quantitative radiographic analysis. *Clin Orthop Relat Res* 2004;120–125.
79. Boileau P, Krishnan SG, Tinsi L, et al. Tuberosity malposition and migration: reasons for poor outcomes after hemiarthroplasty for displaced fractures of the proximal humerus. *J Shoulder Elbow Surg* 2002;11:401–412.
80. Rodosky MW, Bigliani LU. Indications for glenoid resurfacing in shoulder arthroplasty. *J Shoulder Elbow Surg* 1996;5:231–248.
81. Lazarus MD, Jensen KL, Southworth C, et al. The radiographic evaluation of keeled and pegged glenoid component insertion. *J Bone Joint Surg Am* 2002;84:1174–1182.
82. Sanchez-Sotelo J, Sperling JW, Rowland CM, et al. Instability after shoulder arthroplasty: results of surgical treatment. *J Bone Joint Surg Am* 2003;85:622–631.
83. Moeckel BH, Altchek DW, Warren RF, et al. Instability of the shoulder after arthroplasty. *J Bone Joint Surg Am* 1993;75:492–497.
84. Hill JM, Norris TR. Long-term results of total shoulder arthroplasty following bone-grafting of the glenoid. *J Bone Joint Surg Am* 2001;83:877–883.
85. Pearl ML, Volk AG. Retroversion of the proximal humerus in relationship to prosthetic replacement arthroplasty. *J Shoulder Elbow Surg* 1995;4:286–289.
86. Iannotti JP, Norris TR. Influence of preoperative factors on outcome of shoulder arthroplasty for glenohumeral osteoarthritis. *J Bone Joint Surg Am* 2003;85:251–258.
87. Bonutti PM, Hawkins RJ. Fracture of the humeral shaft associated with total replacement arthroplasty of the shoulder: a case report. *J Bone Joint Surg Am* 1992;74:617–618.
88. Brems JJ. Complications of shoulder arthroplasty: infections, instability, and loosening. *Instr Course Lect* 2002;51:29–39.
89. Miller BS, Joseph TA, Noonan TJ, et al. Rupture of the subscapularis tendon after shoulder arthroplasty: diagnosis, treatment, and outcome. *J Shoulder Elbow Surg* 2005;14:492–496.
90. Sperling JW, Kozak TK, Hanssen AD, et al. Infection after shoulder arthroplasty. *Clin Orthop Relat Res* 2001;382:206–216.
91. Coste JS, Reig S, Trojani C, et al. The management of infection in arthroplasty of the shoulder. *J Bone Joint Surg Br* 2004;86:65–69.

Robert H. Cofield

John W. Sperling

Tyler J. Fox

Akin Cil

Christian J. H. Veillette

CHAPTER

2

Mayo Clinic Registry Experience with Shoulder Arthroplasty

INTRODUCTION

Joint replacement registries can be quite powerful, offering many benefits but also having certain limitations.[1-7] There are several practical considerations, including the considerable effort, time, and expense required to maintain a registry; the necessity of maintaining a data set that is somewhat limited in scope; incomplete participation by those potentially involved; lack of complete follow-up information; and fear of distorted analysis of the information collected. The benefits, though, are also many. One can analyze patient demographics in many ways, leading to a better understanding of the epidemiology of diseases and their treatment; large numbers of patients can be entered; patients can be followed for a long time; exclusion criteria in ordinary studies are largely eliminated; trends can be identified and followed; and developing problems may be recognized earlier. The prospective follow-up of patients after surgery can form the basis of detailed retrospective analyses, and recommendations can be given relative to various arthroplasty designs both from a quality and patient care standpoint and for improvement in the finances of healthcare delivery.[1]

A common analytic method for joint registries is survivorship analysis. Various end points for failure have been recommended and used, the most common being revision or removal of the prosthetic implant. The Kaplan-Meier survivorship curve seemingly represents, if not the best, the standard estimate used for the probability of survivorship.[8] This is usually presented with confidence intervals defining the variability of the estimate. More than 15 years ago, Brenner et al[9] reported on the survivorship of unconstrained total shoulder arthroplasty for several diagnoses and two prosthetic types.[9] They used several end points, including the time when the surgeon decided that revision arthroplasty was necessary because of loosening of the components and the patient found the pain was the same or worse than it had been before operation. With these criteria, survivorship of unconstrained total shoulder arthroplasty was 75% at 11 years. More recently, in 2005 Deshmukh et al[10] reported on the survivorship of 220 consecutive total shoulder arthroplasties performed between 1974 and 1988. Six types of

implants were used, but 90% were Neer II implants. These were performed in patients with a variety of diagnoses, but 74% had rheumatoid arthritis. The survival rate at 1 year was 99%, at 5 years 98%, at 10 years 93%, at 15 years 88%, and at 20 years 85%. The end point represented freedom from revision surgery. There were 15 revisions for component loosening, 8 for periprosthetic fractures, 4 for glenohumeral dislocation, and 3 for deep joint infection.

Outside the United States, Norway has established a joint registry for all artificial joints, but to our knowledge has not reported specifically on shoulder implants.[11] In Scotland a registry of shoulder arthroplasty has been developed; it was started in 1996.[12] The goals were to accurately define the epidemiology of arthroplasty, provide timely information to the orthopedic community on outcomes, and identify risk factors for a poor outcome. The registry has been moderately effective but at best has collected only 53% of all the arthroplasties performed in Scotland. They have recognized, of course, that the value of the registry is dependent on the completeness of the data in addition to its accuracy, again demonstrating that although there are many benefits of a registry, there are deficiencies too. A new shoulder arthroplasty registry began in Australia in 2006. They have identified that shoulder arthroplasty use has risen and the reverse type of implant has become quite commonly used. They plan to focus on prosthesis outcome, with revision as the primary end point. Thus far, reporting is rather incomplete; activities are underway to increase this level of participation and establish clear-cut goals for analysis.[13]

The Swedish Shoulder Arthroplasty Register is probably the most complete national registry. It began in 1999 and has been able to categorize the types of diseases being treated, the types of implants being used, and, of course, revision rates. In this registry the revision rate for hemiarthroplasty between 1999 and 2006 was 5.7% and for total arthroplasty was 4.1%. The reasons for revisions in hemiarthroplasty were glenoid erosion and pain in most cases. In the total shoulder arthroplasties the reasons were varied. Most notably, the most common reason for revision was instability and the second was infection. Glenoid and humeral component loosening was less frequent. They noted that modern implants have a revision rate of approximately 2% to 3%. The older implant revision rates are higher, as are the revision rates for the reverse and bipolar prostheses. Of those entered in the Registry between 1999 and 2001, approximately half of 616 patients completed a self-evaluation score. The score for total arthroplasty was higher than for hemiarthroplasty. The best score was in osteoarthritis and the worst score in nonunion. Men had a higher median score. Yet again, one can identify quite useful information emerging from a registry such as this, even in the early days of development.[14–16]

MAYO CLINIC JOINT REGISTRY

The Total Joint Registry at the Mayo Clinic was established in 1969.[1] Space and personnel were allocated for this purpose. Standardized forms for recording data were developed for collecting preoperative, operative, and postoperative information. There is a systematic mechanism that triggers follow-up evaluation at regular intervals. If patients cannot return for personal assessment of their situation, including examination and radiographs, a standardized letter including a questionnaire has been developed and a standard telephone questionnaire formulated. The information obtained on these mailed or telephone-acquired questionnaires has been compared with the information obtained during on-site interview and found to be essentially equivalent for the hip, knee, and shoulder.[17,18] Every effort is made to contact patients who would be lost to follow-up. This includes obtaining information and radiographs for patients if they received care, particularly reoperations, at facilities other than the Mayo Clinic. Ongoing analysis has indicated that clinical follow-up at each time interval approaches 95%.[1]

This database has allowed investigators to perform multiple retrospective analyses of this prospectively collected data, such as the identification of early hospital care issues,[19] mortality,[20] the identification of all complications,[21] the study of specific complications,[22,23] the assessment of outcomes for the defined population group,[24] or for a specific diagnosis.[25]

The long-term nature of this data collection methodology has provided the opportunity to create long-term survivorship analysis with a specific type of prosthesis,[26] with a defined diagnosis,[27] or, for example, with a defined age-group.[28,29] It also makes possible population-based studies for outcome or survivorship analysis.[30]

The information collected includes patient identifying information, age, sex, height, weight, and side of involvement. Recorded are a history of previous operations, the surgery date, operative diagnosis, operative time, surgeon, catalog number of the implants, use of bone cement, and use of bone grafting. The complications and their dates are identified. The patients are routinely assessed at 2, 5, 10, 15, 20, and 25 years. Information is recorded relative to patient interview, examination, and images. Reoperation dates and type are recorded, and date of death is defined should that occur. Given the wealth of this material, we have felt obligated to report survivorship analysis of shoulder arthroplasty components performed over past decades. This report analyzes the glenoid and humeral components separately, with several subanalyses. This methodology not only will allow the understanding of the outcome for the various kinds of components used, but also will lead to a better understanding of the effect of patient and diagnostic characteristics on survivorship.

SURVIVORSHIP ANALYSIS OF THE GLENOID COMPONENT

The Mayo Clinic Joint Registry database was searched, identifying all patients who had a primary total shoulder arthroplasty between January 1, 1984 and December 31, 2004.[31] There were 1,542 total shoulder arthroplasties in 1,337 patients. Of these, 121 shoulders were revised for mechanical failure or loosening of the glenoid component. Survival curves are displayed for the six types of glenoid components (Figs. 2.1 to 2.6). Survival rates for each of the six types of glenoid components used are reported in the figure legends, along with 95% confidence intervals. In addition to the 121 shoulders with glenoid revisions or removals, there were 51 shoulders undergoing a reoperation

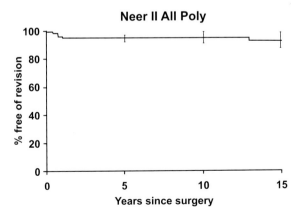

Figure 2.1. Survival free of glenoid component revision or removal for the 99 Neer II polyethylene glenoid components. The 5-, 10-, and 15-year survivals with confidence intervals are 5-year 96% CI (92–100), 10-year 96% (92–100), and 15-year 94% (89–100).

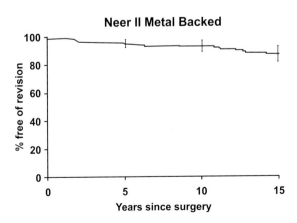

Figure 2.2. Survival free of glenoid component revision or removal for the 254 Neer II metal-backed glenoid components. The 5-, 10-, and 15-year survivals with confidence intervals are 5-year 96% CI (94–99), 10-year 94% (91–97), and 15-year 89% (85–94).

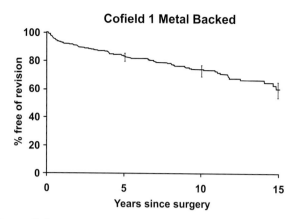

Figure 2.3. Survival free of glenoid component revision or removal for the 316 Cofield 1 metal backed glenoid components. The 5-, 10-, and 15-year survivals with confidence intervals are 5-year 86% CI (82–90), 10-year 79% (74–84), and 15-year 67% (59–76).

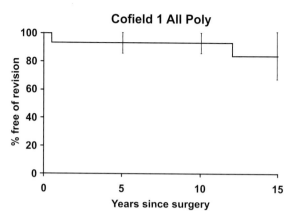

Figure 2.4. Survival free of glenoid component revision or removal for the 18 Cofield 1 all-polyethylene glenoid components. The 5-, 10-, and 15-year survivals with confidence intervals are 5-year 94% CI (84–100), 10-year 94% (84–100), and 15-year 87% (71–100).

for other reasons with retention of the glenoid component. These 51 shoulders are not reflected in the component failure analysis reported here.

In comparing the survival rate among the six types of components used, the metal-backed uncemented glenoid design (Cofield 1 metal-backed) suffered higher revision rates than the cemented glenoid components ($p < 0.001$). The more recently used all-polyethylene, cemented pegged, glenoid component (Cofield 2 all-polyethylene pegged) had an improved survival rate compared with the older Neer II all-polyethylene, cemented glenoid at the 5-year analysis point ($p = 0.03$).

When assessing gender, age, and diagnosis, survivorship was lower among men ($p < 0.001$). Patients younger than age 65 were at a higher, although not significant, risk of revision ($p = 0.17$). In a multiple variable model, operative diagnosis affected survival. Relative to osteoarthritis, posttraumatic arthritis and osteonecrosis were associated with a greater risks for revision ($p = 0.02$, $p = 0.06$).

The reasons for glenoid revision or removal are displayed in Table 2.1. Infection occurred in 19 of these shoulders, requiring glenoid revision or removal (1.2%). It was typically a late or chronic infection. Component loosening requiring revision surgery occurred in 51 shoulders (3.3%). To this point in time, loosening occurred in 24 of 316 metal-backed tissue ingrowth shoulders (7.6%), in 12 of 254 metal-backed Neer II cemented shoulders (4.7%), and in only 15 of 972 all-polyethylene cemented components of various types (1.5%). Revision of the glenoid component related to instability was almost exclusively limited to the metal-backed tissue ingrowth type of component. Polyethylene wear requiring revision surgery was limited to metal-backed glenoid components, with the uncemented metal-backed component dominating in that area. Several pieces of information have emerged from this large, long-term analysis of glenoid components and their survival. Clearly, the design of metal-backed tissue ingrowth glenoid component (Cofield 1 metal-backed) did not fare as well as the other types of glenoid

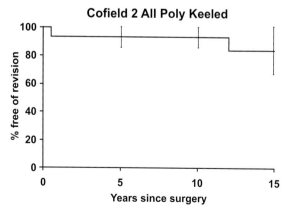

Figure 2.5. Survival free of glenoid component revision or removal for the 497 Cofield 2 all-polyethylene keeled glenoid components. The 5-, 10-, and 12-year survivals with confidence intervals are 5-year 99% CI (98–100), 10-year 94% (91–98), and 12-year 89% (79–100).

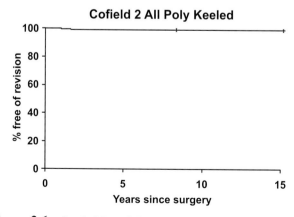

Figure 2.6. Survival free of glenoid component revision or removal for the 358 Cofield 2 all-polyethylene pegged glenoid components. The 5-year survival with confidence intervals is 99% CI (98–100).

TABLE 2.1	Reasons for Glenoid Component Revision and Removal					
Component	No.	Acute Infection (<3 Months)	Late or Chronic Infection	Loosening	Instability	Wear (Metal/Poly)	Total
Neer II all-polyethylene	99	0	0	5	2	0	7
Neer II metal-backed	254	0	6	12	0	3	21
Cofield 1 metal-backed	316	1	6	24	20	23	74
Cofield 1 all-polyethylene	18	0	0	2	0	0	2
Cofield 2 all-polyethylene keeled	497	1	4	7	3	0	15
Cofield 2 all-polyethylene pegged	358	0	1	1	0	0	2
Total		2	17	51	25	26	121

components used with cement fixation. Considering all groups, the patient factors of age, sex, and diagnostic category do play a role in implant survival. Glenoid revision surgery for infection at just above 1% does not seem strikingly different from results with other major elective orthopedic procedures. Revision of the glenoid component or its removal for loosening is very uncommon for all-polyethylene cemented glenoid components. A cemented metal-backed glenoid component has no advantage in this regard, and metal-backed tissue ingrowth components did not fare so well relative to component loosening. Similarly, revision or removal of the glenoid component for polyethylene wear occurred only in metal-backed components. Glenoid revision surgery for instability was almost never necessary except in the presence of the metal-backed tissue ingrowth component.

SURVIVORSHIP ANALYSIS OF THE HUMERAL COMPONENT

The Mayo Clinic Joint Registry database was searched to identify hemiarthroplasties or total shoulder arthroplasties that were done between January 1, 1984 and December 31, 2004.[32] Among the 1,584 primary shoulder replacements in 1,423 patients,

472 were hemiarthroplasties and 1,112 were total shoulder arthroplasties. Of these shoulders, 108 had humeral component revision and 17 had humeral component removal. Survivorship by stem type is displayed in Figures 2.7 to 2.9. Statistical comparisons of survival rates indicated that better survival was achieved with Neer II and Cofield 2 components. Survival with hemiarthroplasty proved to be better than with total shoulder arthroplasty ($p = 0.005$). Survival is also improved with cement fixation of the component ($p = 0.007$). The reasons for revision or removal of the three types of humeral stems is tabulated in Table 2.2. Survival was worse in those younger than 65 years ($p = 0.03$), in men ($p = 0.001$), and in those having surgery for posttraumatic arthritis ($p = 0.005$).

SUMMARY, CONCLUSIONS, AND RECOMMENDATIONS

Strikingly, only 1.5% of cemented all-polyethylene glenoid components have required revision or removal to date. Also, quite dramatically, the metal-backed ingrowth components did not fair nearly as well as their cemented counterparts. The cemented Neer II all-polyethylene glenoid components fared quite well, as

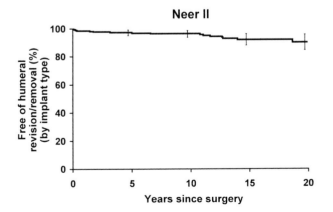

Figure 2.7. Survival free of humeral component revision or removal for the 244 Neer II humeral components. The 5-, 10-, 15-, and 20-year survivals with confidence intervals are 5-year 97% CI (95–100), 10-year 97% (94–99), 15-year 92% (88–96), and 20-year 90% (85–96).

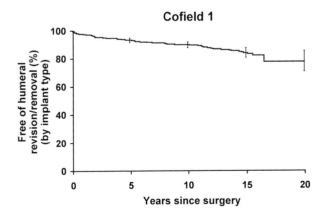

Figure 2.8. Survival free of humeral component revision or removal for the 869 Cofield 1 humeral components. The 5-, 10-, 15-, and 20-year survivals with confidence intervals are 5-year 93% CI (92–95), 10-year 90% (88–92), 15-year 84% (81–88), and 20-year 78% (71–86).

	Type	
Reoperation Diagnosis	Hemiarthroplasty	TSA
Glenoid Issues		
Arthritis	8	0
Arthritis + humeral loosening	2	0
Arthritis + rotator cuff tear	3	0
Loosening	0	14
Loosening + humeral component fracture	0	1
Loosening + humeral loosening	0	19
Loosening + instability	0	1
Malposition + instability	0	1
Polyethylene dislocation	0	3
Polyethylene dislocation + humeral loosening	0	1
Polyethylene dislocation + instability	0	2
Polyethylene wear	0	4
Humerus issues		
Loosening	1	3
Loosening + glenoid polyethylene wear	0	7
Loosening + instability	0	2
Malposition + glenoid polyethylene wear	0	1
Infection	4	10
Instability	2	28
Instability + glenoid polyethylene wear	0	4
Periprosthetic fracture	1	2
Periprosthetic fracture + glenoid polyethylene wear	0	1
Total	21	104

TABLE 2.2   Reasons for Humeral Component Revision and Removal

is easily recognized. The cemented Cofield II pegged components have a somewhat statistically better survival at 5 years, but the difference is not dramatic.

Survival of the humeral component is highly dependent on the condition of the glenoid or the glenoid component. Over half of the revisions or removals of humeral components occurred in relation to a glenoid or glenoid component problem. Survival was better for hemiarthroplasties than it was for humeral components associated with total shoulder arthroplasty. Survival was better if the humeral component was cemented. Survival was better for Neer II and Cofield 2 components than for Cofield 1 components, with in-growth tissue limited to the undersurface of the humeral head.

For both humeral and glenoid components there was a protective factor with a lower rate of component revision or removal for older age, female gender, and diagnoses other than those related to trauma.

Overall, the results of total shoulder arthroplasty related to survivorship are very reasonable. These data identify additional design features, diagnostic implications, and patient factors that will allow a surgeon to assess the predictability of proposed shoulder arthroplasty surgery.

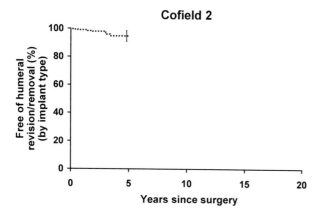

Figure 2.9. Survival free of humeral component revision or removal for the 471 Cofield 2 humeral components. The 5-year survival with confidence intervals are 5-year 95% CI (91–99).

REFERENCES

1. Berry DJ, Kessler M, Morrey BF. Maintaining a hip registry for 25 years: Mayo Clinic experience. *Clin Orthop* 1997;344:61–68.
2. Gioe TJ, Killeen KK, Mehle S, et al. Implementation and application of a community total joint registry: a 12-year history. *J Bone Joint Surg Am* 2006;88:1399–1404.
3. Kärrholm J, Garellick G, Lindahl H, et al. Improved analyses in the Swedish Hip Arthroplasty Register. Presented at the Scientific Exhibition of the Annual Meeting of the American Academy of Orthopaedic Surgeons, February 14–18, 2007, San Diego, CA. Swedish Hip Arthroplasty Register, Göteborg, Sweden: Swedish Orthopaedic Association, 2007:2–7.
4. Kolling C, Simmen BR, Labek G, et al. Key factors for a successful National Arthroplasty Register. *J Bone Joint Surg Br* 2007;89:1567–1573.
5. Kop AM, Swarts E. Selection of primary hip and knee arthroplasties for public hospitals in Western Australia: a clinical evidence approach. *ANZ J Surg* 2006;76:1068–1074.
6. Philipson MR, Westwood MJ, Geoghegan JM, et al. Shortcomings of the National Joint Registry: a survey of consultants' review. *Ann R Coll Surg Eng* 2005;87:109–112; discussion 112.
7. Robertsson O. Knee arthroplasty registers. *J Bone Joint Surg Br* 2007;89:1–4.
8. Dorey F, Amstutz HC. Survivorship analysis in the evaluation of joint replacement. *J Arthroplasty* 1986;1:63–69.

9. Brenner BC, Ferlic DC, Clayton ML, et al. Survivorship of unconstrained total shoulder arthroplasty. *J Bone Joint Surg* 1989;71:1289–1296.

10. Deshmukh AV, Koris M, Jurakowski D, et al. Total shoulder arthroplasty: long-term survivorship, functional outcome, and quality of life. *J Shoulder Elbow Surg* 2005;14:471–479.

11. Haveli LI. The Norwegian Joint Registry. *Bull Hosp Joint Dis* 1999;58:139–147.

12. Sharma S, Dreghorn CR. Registry of shoulder arthroplasty: the Scottish experience. *Ann R Coll Surg Engl* 2006;88:122–126.

13. Page R. A National Australian Shoulder Joint Registry: where we are up to and where we are going. *Proceedings of the 10th International Congress of Shoulder and Elbow Surg*, São Paulo, Brazil, September 16–19, 2007:202, poster 251.

14. Rahme H, Jacobsen MB, Salomonsson B. The Swedish Elbow Arthroplasty Register and The Swedish Shoulder Arthroplasty Register: two new Swedish arthroplasty registers. *Act Orthop Scand* 2001;72:107–112.

15. Salomonsson B, Lillkrona U, Nordqvist A, et al. The Swedish Shoulder Arthroplasty Register: an analysis of 255 reoperations on arthroplasties reported to the registry. *Proceedings of the 10th International Congress of Shoulder and Elbow Surg*, São Paulo, Brazil, September 16–19, 2007:87, poster 113.

16. Salomonsson B, Lillkrona U, Nordqvist A, et al. The Swedish Shoulder Arthroplasty Register: 5-year follow-up by Woos-score in 616 primary shoulder arthroplasties. *Proceedings of the 10th International Congress of Shoulder and Elbow Surg*, Brazil, September 16–19, 2007: 224, poster 344.

17. McGrory BJ, Morrey BF, Rand JA, et al. Correlation of patient questionnaire responses and physician history in grading clinical outcome following hip and knee arthroplasty: a prospective study of 201 joint arthroplasties. *J Arthroplasty* 1996;11:47–57.

18. Smith AM, Barnes SA, Sperling JW, et al. Patient and physician-assessed shoulder function after arthroplasty. *J Bone Joint Surg Am* 2006;88:508–513.

19. Sperling JW, Duncan SFM, Cofield RH, et al. Incidence and risk factors for blood transfusion in shoulder arthroplasty. *J Shoulder Elbow Surg* 2005;14:599–601.

20. White CB, Sperling JW, Cofield RH, et al. Ninety-day mortality after shoulder arthroplasty. *J Arthroplasty* 2003;18:886–888.

21. Chin PYK, Sperling JW, Cofield RH, et al. Complications of total shoulder arthroplasty: are they fewer or different? *J Shoulder Elbow Surg* 2006;15:19–22.

22. Hattrup SJ, Cofield RH, Cha SS. Rotator cuff repair after shoulder replacement. *J Shoulder Elbow Surg* 2006;15:78–83.

23. Sanchez-Sotelo J, Sperling JW, Rowland CM, et al. Instability after shoulder arthroplasty: results of surgical treatment. *J Bone Joint Surg Am* 2003;85:622–631.

24. Adams JE, Sperling JW, Schleck CD, et al. Outcomes of shoulder arthroplasty in Olmsted County, Minnesota. *Clin Orthop* 2006;455:176–182.

25. Koch LD, Cofield RH, Ahlskog JE. Total shoulder arthroplasty in patients with Parkinson disease. *J Shoulder Elbow Surg* 1997;6:24–28.

26. Torchia ME, Cofield RH, Settergren CR. Total shoulder arthroplasty with the Neer prosthesis: long-term results. *J Shoulder Elbow Surg* 1997;6:495–505.

27. Rispoli DM, Sperling JW, Athwal GS, et al. Humeral head replacement for the treatment of osteoarthritis. *J Bone Joint Surg Am* 2006;88:2637–2644.

28. Sperling JW, Cofield RH, Rowland CM. Neer hemiarthroplasty and Neer total shoulder arthroplasty in patients 50 years old or less. *J Bone Joint Surg Am* 1998;80:464–473.

29. Sperling JW, Cofield RH, Rowland CM. Minimum 15-year follow-up of Neer hemiarthroplasty and total shoulder arthroplasty in patients aged 50 years or younger. *J Shoulder Elbow Surg* 2004;13:605–613.

30. Adams JE, Sperling JW, Hoskin TL, et al. Shoulder arthroplasty in Olmsted County, Minnesota, 1976–2000: a population-based study. *J Shoulder Elbow Surg* 2006;15:50–55.

31. Fox TJ, Cil A, Sperling JW, et al. Survivorship analysis of the glenoid component in total shoulder arthroplasty. Submitted for consideration of publication, 2007.

32. Cil A, Veillette CJH, Fox TJ, et al. Humeral component revisions and removals in shoulder replacement surgery: a registry-based analysis. Submitted for consideration of publication, 2007.

Francois Sirveaux
Daniel Molé

Failures of the Reverse Prosthesis: Identifying the Problems

INTRODUCTION

The concept of the reverse prosthesis was conceived in the 1970s and rapidly abandoned because of a high complication rate. It was revived by Paul Grammont 15 years ago, with a new concept of lowering and medializing the prosthetic center of rotation to minimize the complications attributed to previous designs. Since that time, this prosthesis has demonstrated encouraging results, which has allowed an expansion of its use from primary surgery to more complex revision cases. However, the enthusiasm initially prevalent has been moderated by the occurrence of specific problems related to the constrained design of this prosthesis, which remains used primarily for elderly patients and in salvage situations. This chapter identifies the issues that can be encountered with the reverse prosthesis and develops specific solutions to these problems.

Determining the global complication rate of the reverse prosthesis depends on the method used to calculate the complications, as well as how one defines a "complication." Including patients who have had a reoperation and a revision of a prosthesis, Wall et al[1] reported a 19% complication rate. In this study, the authors reported 24.1% of humeral fractures in revision cases, although these events were not considered to be complications of the reverse prosthesis itself because they were related to the revision surgery. Werner et al[2] reported a 50% complication rate in a series of 58 cases of painful pseudo-paralytic shoulders resulting from irreparable massive rotator cuff tears. In this series, the authors included a postoperative hematoma as a complication, because it had been treated by aspiration or open revision, although the hematoma was not thought to affect the ultimate outcome. Others, such as Bohsali et al,[3] consider the glenoid notching to be a complication, although it is regarded by many authors to be a radiographic anomaly. Moreover, those patients who have sustained multiple, simultaneous, or successive complications present an additional difficulty because the complication rate can vary according to the manner in which authors account for these cases. Indeed, in his series of 60 cases, Frankle[4] reported 13 complications (21.6% complication rate) occurring in 10 patients (17% complication rate). In the SOFCOT symposium[5] on 484 reverse prostheses for osteoarthritis with a rotator cuff tear and minimum 2-year follow-up, the global complication rate was of 21%. Among patients with complications, 70% had only one complication and 30% had between two and five complications.

Considering the differences in methods and definitions of the complications in the literature, it is difficult to compare the overall complication rate. Whatever the type of complication, prevention, diagnosis, and appropriate treatment are of the utmost importance because the occurrence of at least one complication may significantly affect the final functional result.[6]

PROBLEMS RELATED TO IMPLANT DESIGN

CONCEPTUAL ERRORS

The Grammont prosthesis was the first new generation of reverse arthroplasty designs. However, Grammont was not the first to use a reverse implant to attempt to solve the issue of arthritis with a rotator cuff tear. Neer-Averill's[7] prosthesis and those of Reeves,[8] Kolbel,[9] KESSEL,[10] Fenlin,[11] and Gerard,[12] developed in the 1970s, were also based on a reverse design. However, they were all abandoned because of mobility or loosening problems. All of these prostheses had a glenoid sphere with a lateral center of rotation in relation to the scapula, with avulsion forces at the start of the elevation, endangering fixation of the implant. The originality of Grammont's concept is based on the existence of a center of rotation that is medial and lower, generating compression forces around the interface between the glenoid baseplate and the bone, from initial elevation.

IMPACT DEFECT AND GLENOID DISSOCIATION

Until 1995, the Grammont prosthesis used a screw system to assemble the sphere on the baseplate. This system was exposed to a risk for unscrewing of the sphere, which was reported in seven cases in the series reported by Sirveaux et al.[13] This anomaly, linked to the implant, imposes regular monitoring of patients with this kind of prosthesis.[14] In some cases, the unscrewing will remain stable, without consequences on the clinical result. However, it can also evolve and lead to the dislocation of the implant[15] (Fig. 3.1). The unscrewing of the old sphere

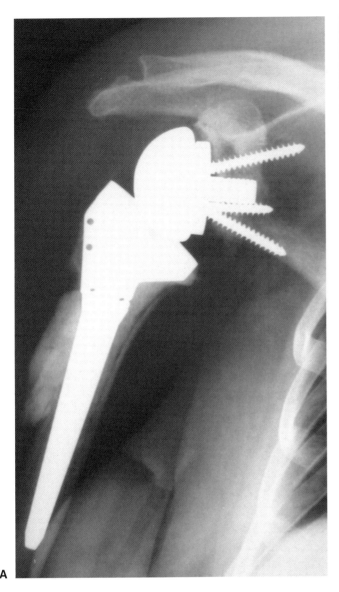

A

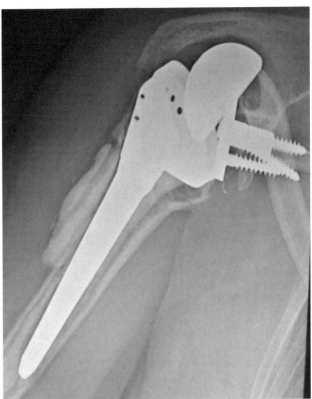

B

Figure 3.1. Example of impact defect on a Morse taper prosthesis with full unscrewing and bipolar dissociation of the prosthesis.

designs can also bring about a fracture of the central peg, which will thus make it necessary to change the entire glenoid implant (Fig. 3.2).

The assembling system by Morse taper does not allow for the definite disappearance of the sphere/baseplate assembling issue. Improper seating of the sphere on the baseplate has been reported in five cases by Wall et al.[1] None of the prosthesis required revision, and no effect was shown on the clinical results.

Middernacht and al[16] recently analyzed the radiographs of 499 reverse prostheses with an average follow-up of 2.8 years. In 16 cases (3.2%), they noticed a seating defect of the sphere on the baseplate. The dissociation is diagnosed when a visible gap between the baseplate and the sphere is found on the anteroposterior or axillary view. In three cases, the dissociation led to a fracture of the central screw that required revision. Spontaneous reassembling of the sphere was noticed in three cases. In this series, dissociation was not associated with a lower functional score. Considering this potential complication, one must perform adequate reaming of the glenoid surface and pay

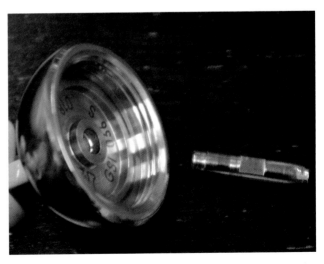

Figure 3.2. Fracture of the central screw of the sphere secondary to sphere unscrewing in the original model of the Grammont prosthesis.

particular attention to avoid soft tissue and bone interposition during fitting of the Morse taper. It is recommended to obtain postoperative radiographs to detect assembling defects as early as possible and to plan close monitoring in case of an anomaly. If the dissociation evolves, another surgery should be strongly considered. Considering the risk of dissociation between the sphere and the baseplate, Frankle et al[4] modified their reverse prosthesis by adding a 3.5-mm retaining screw and augmenting the Morse taper.

POLYETHYLENE DISSOCIATION

The reverse design of the Grammont prosthesis induces serious and asymmetrical stress on the polyethylene, imposing the necessity to ensure a secure fixation in the epiphysis. De Wilde and Walch[17] reported a case of dissociation of the polyethylene, which led to abnormal metal-metal contact and loosening of the humeral component. Werner et al[2] reported one case of polyethylene dissociation treated by polyethylene replacement and complicated by secondary infection. In cases of polyethylene dissociation, another surgery is likely necessary and should be performed as soon as possible, to avoid the rapid degradation of the humeral and glenoid components.

Levy et al[18] reported four cases of polyethylene dissociation or fracture in reverse arthroplasty for revision after failed

hemiarthroplasty. They considered that this complication was related to the lack of proximal humeral bone support in revision surgery.

HUMERAL DISSOCIATION

Cases of dissociation between the epiphyseal component and the prosthetic stem have been reported in various studies.[3,17,19,20] This type of complication can occur when there is a proximal bone defect in cases of revision or reverse prosthesis for tumors. De Wilde and Walch[17] hypothesized that the epiphysis can be blocked against the anterior wall of the glenoid, in maximal internal rotation, and that the torque exerted by the flexed forearm can lead to unscrewing. This is a rare complication (3 of 399 cases in the Nice multicenter series[20]), which can lead to dislocation (Fig. 3.3). In cases of revision, it is possible to adapt the retroversion of the epiphysis by adding a metal washer of appropriate thickness to connect the stem, so as to avoid diaphyseal revision.[17]

For the same reasons, the unscrewing can also occur between the metaphyseal metal extension and the epiphysis.[17] In that case, it is possible to reposition the extension device without necessarily having to change the humeral component. This complication can be avoided by ensuring, as much as possible, that the assembling of the prosthetic pieces are secure.

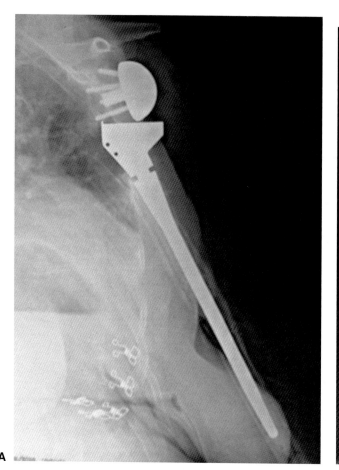
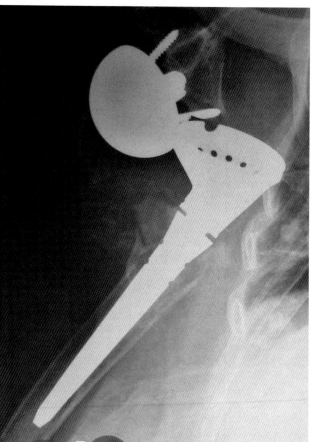

A   B

Figure 3.3.   Two cases of humeral dissociation with (**A**) or without (**B**) dislocation.

PROBLEMS RELATED TO THE GLENOID AND SCAPULA

GLENOID INSUFFICIENCY

The preoperative assessment of the bone stock around the glenoid is imperative, whether concerning a reverse prosthesis for a first intervention or a revision prosthesis. For cuff tear arthropathy, the glenoid erosion is assessed according to Favard's classification,[13] which includes four types of glenoid erosion in the frontal plane (Fig. 3.4).

Type E3 is defined by a large erosion of the top of the glenoid that can reach the bottom of the coracoid process. In that case, the bone defect is such that it may compromise the primary fixation of the glenoid baseplate, exposing it to a risk of early dislocation. This risk is even more important considering that there is often asymmetrical erosion associated in the sagittal plane. On the preoperative computed tomography (CT) image it is imperative to assess the glenoid bone stock. Asymmetrical erosion of the glenoid increases the risk that the baseplate may be positioned with a superior tilt, especially if a superior approach has been used—the wrong initial position of the glenoid implant being in fact the main cause of early loosening.[6] If the baseplate is settled in this position, the risk for notching in the scapula pillar and of dislocation of the shoulder increases. In that case, it is preferable to use a bone transplant around the glenoid and to lateralize the joint using, if necessary, a baseplate with a long peg.[21] The insufficiency of the bone stock in cases of reverse prosthesis is indeed a major issue; it is necessary to warn the patient of the possibility of a bone graft in one or two steps.[21,22]

GLENOID FRACTURE

The risk of glenoid fracture while placing a reverse prosthesis is approximately 2%. It is associated with scapula osteoporosis and subchondral bone sclerosis, which makes the bone more fragile during the drilling phase.[23] Most of these fractures are partial and do not compromise the final result. Molé et al[23] reported a 2% rate of intraoperative fractures, of which only 0.5% were complete fractures. The situation sometimes impedes the possibility to consider placing a glenoid implant, and a hemiarthroplasty may be a good salvage solution.

ASEPTIC GLENOID LOOSENING

The rate of aseptic glenoid loosening as reported in the literature is quite low if one takes into account the constrained nature of the prosthesis. In the SOFCOT multicenter study[5] of 527 cases of reverse prosthesis for cuff tear arthropathy, with an average follow-up of 52 months, glenoid loosening was observed in 22 cases, 4.1% of the series. In four cases, the loosening was linked to an infection, which corresponds to a 3.4% aseptic loosening rate. The statistical study showed that the loosening concerned younger subjects, mostly women, and that it was more frequent among patients who underwent a superolateral approach compared to those who had a deltopectoral approach. Loosening was an early complication that occurred, in more than half of the cases, during the first 2 years postoperatively. Glenoid loosening was linked to a technical error in the initial positioning of the implant (11 cases)—it was set too high, there was a superior or anterior tilt, or there was a deficient fixation of the baseplate with too short of a central peg. It was also linked to an error in the initial indication (three cases)—severe Parkinson disease for a patient in a wheelchair, balance troubles and frequent falls for the second patient, and a history of radiation treatment in the third patient. According to Frankle et al,[4] superior tilt is responsible for early mechanical failure. They recommend that the baseplate be inserted at a 10- to 15-degree inferior tilt to minimize the shear forces across the bone-baseplate interface. Moreover, they moved to a more medialized sphere design for patients with poor bone quality.

Delloye[15] reported two cases of aseptic loosening of the sphere-baseplate block, with a 6-year follow-up. The authors noticed medial erosion of the polyethylene, with contact between the baseplate's inferior screw and the medial part of the metaphysis. According to Delloye et al,[15] this mechanical conflict is responsible for the notching that weakens the fixation of the baseplate and leads to loosening of the glenoid component. Until now, no clinical series has established a link between the occurrence of notching and glenoid loosening.

In cases of revision for glenoid loosening, it is often difficult to reimplant a reverse prosthesis in one stage. The prosthesis can be converted in hemiarthroplasty definitively or while waiting for the healing of a glenoid graft before reimplantation of a baseplate.[22]

SCAPULA NOTCHING

The notching of the scapula pillar is a frequent radiographic finding after a Grammont reverse prosthesis has been placed. It is linked to the medial center of rotation, which brings the proximal humerus and the scapula pillar closer. Notching has not been observed after a reverse design prosthesis with a lateralized rotation center has been placed.[4,24] The rate of notching observed in the published series varies between 20% and 70%.[5,25–29] The size of the scapula notch is currently analyzed on anteroposterior radiography according to the classification we reported previously[13] (Fig. 3.5). A bone defect limited to the pillar corresponds to grade 1; it is considered to be grade 2 when the defect is in contact with the lower screw, grade 3 when it is over the lower screw, and grade 4 when it extends under the baseplate. The rate of scapula notching at revision is influenced by the etiology. The highest prevalence has been reported in cuff tear arthropathy and the lowest in traumatic cases.[29]

Levigne et al[29] demonstrated that accurate evaluation of notching is not easy. They recommended the use of fluoroscopy

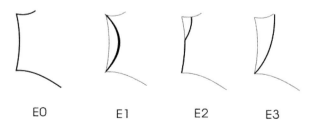

EO   E1   E2   E3

Figure 3.4. Favard's classification of glenoid erosion in the frontal plane.

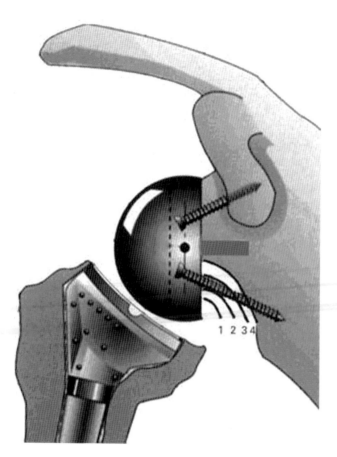

Figure 3.5. Scapular notch classification.

to adapt the radiographic view to the individual variation. By including 461 cases of osteoarthritis with massive cuff tear, reviewed at an average follow-up of 51 months, the multicenter study demonstrated a 68% rate of scapula notching. Some preoperative factors were correlated with the notch at revision: active patients, Hamada stage IV and V arthropathies, preoperative fatty infiltration of the subscapularis, and preoperative superior erosion of the glenoid. The approach and the size of the sphere did not influence the occurrence of the notch, whereas the rate of notching was lowered by using a lateralized polyethylene insert rather than a standard insert. The frequency of the notch and its size increased according to the follow-up. Generally, the notch appeared within the first year postoperatively and the prevalence of a notch gradually increased with time. In this series, the notch did not significantly influence the functional results, except for the strength and range of motion in anterior elevation. The significant correlation between the rate of radiolucent lines around the humeral stem and the occurrence of the notch supports the hypothesis of an osteolysis related to polyethylene debris, as had been assumed by Nyffeler et al.[30] In this large series, there was no evidence of a direct link between the failure of glenoid fixation and scapula notching, as suspected by Delloye et al[31] and Vanhove and Beugnies.[32] According to Delloye et al,[31] notching is an evolving process that is directly related to a mechanical impingement between the humerus and the scapula pillar. They consider that the notch is responsible for glenoid implant loosening. Different and new configurations of the glenoid implant may be available

on the market in the future to avoid the notch, but, at the present time, there are no clinical data to support the efficiency of such new designs in relation to the risk for scapula notching. Scapula notching is a major concern for long-term survival of the prosthesis. For the moment, the only way to decrease the risk for notching is to place the glenoid component 2 to 4 mm more distally, as demonstrated by Nyffeler and al[33] in their experimental study.

The high rate of scapula notching is a significant factor limiting the indication of the reverse prosthesis for elderly patients and as a salvage procedure for younger patients.

ACROMIAL FRACTURES

Placing a reverse prosthesis induces a lowering and an increased lateral offset of the humerus, which leads to a tensioning of the deltoid. Frequently, the acromion is weakened preoperatively, because of osteoporosis linked to age, extensive immobilization (in fracture sequelae), corticosteroid use (in rheumatoid polyarthritis[34]), or repeated contact with the humeral head in cuff tear arthropathy (CTA). Mottier et al[35] analyzed preoperative lesions of the acromion before a reverse prosthesis could be implanted. Among 457 cases of reverse shoulder arthroplasties, they found 5% of preoperative os acromiale (meso-acromion type). The preoperative os acromiale did not compromise the result of the operation, whatever approach was used. Fracture or fragmentation of the acromion was reported in 3.7% of cases. In most cases, the acromial fragment tilted after implantation of the reverse prosthesis but it did not interfere with the final functional results. In the SOFCOT series,[5] the rate of postoperative acromial tilting was higher after a deltopectoral approach (6%) than after a superior approach (1.5%), without a difference in the clinical results. Osteosynthesis or resection of the fragment is not recommended. On the contrary, the postoperative fracture of the scapula spine jeopardizes definitively the clinical results (Fig. 3.6). This complication was previously reported by Werner et al[2] and Frankle et al.[4] It should be suspected when the rehabilitation progresses slowly and with pain or when it deteriorates suddenly within the first year. Considering the risk of secondary displacement, nonunion, and poor final results, these authors recommended early surgical fixation of the postoperative spine fracture.

PROBLEMS RELATED TO THE HUMERUS

FRACTURE

The risk of humeral fracture is high in revision surgery. Of 28 humerus fractures reported in the multicenter study, 26 were noted in cases of revision.[6] In 16 cases, the fracture required an osteosynthesis with cerclage during the intervention. In 22 cases the humerus healed without consequence on the clinical and radiological result. Three cases evolved toward loosening of the humeral implant, and in three cases a radiolucent line (>2 mm wide) was noted at revision. In revision cases, it is better to perform a humeral osteotomy immediately to access the cement rather than to induce an unexpected fracture. In this series, 12 cases of late humeral fracture were noticed. Eight of these cases healed after conservative treatment. In four cases the prosthesis was revised by using a longer stem.

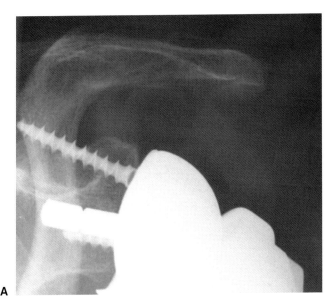
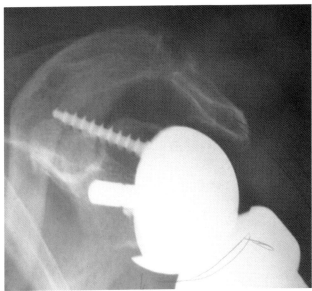

Figure 3.6.   Example of a secondary scapula spine fracture that compromises the deltoid lever arm.

LOOSENING

In the absence of infection, subsidence of the uncemented humeral stem is rare.[2,5,20] We have reported five cases of gross aseptic loosening (1%) that led to subsidence of the stem.[5] In nonseptic cases, we defined seven radiographic zones around the stem and measured the width of the radiolucent lines on the anteroposterior view (Fig. 3.7). The humeral component was considered to be "subsided" when the stem migrated (1%), as "at risk" for loosening when a radiolucent line more than 2 mm wide was noticed in more than two zones (18.5%), or to be "stable." The follow-up differed significantly depending on the group: 49 months for the "stable" stem, 60 months for the "at-risk" stem, and 84 months for the "subsided" stem. Werner et al[2] stopped implanting the uncemented stem because of subsidence in one case, but in the multicenter series we found an 11% occurrence of "subsided or at-risk" stems when using an uncemented humeral component, compared with 27% when using the cemented stem. The rate of scapular notching on the glenoid side was lower in the "stable" group compared with the "subsided or at-risk" groups (63% versus 90%).

The parallel between the anomalies around the humerus and in the glenoid area can be explained by the existence of polyethylene deposits, which are responsible for resorption granuloma, as has been reported on explanted prosthesis.[31] Delloye et al[31] noticed proximal osteolysis in five patients operated with the first generation of Grammont prosthesis. They assumed that the proximal cortical defect could compromise the fixation of the humeral implant. Chuinard et al[20] considered that the reverse design transfers the prosthetic constraints from the glenoid to the humerus and that the fixation of the humeral implant remained a real concern for survivability.

TUBEROSITY

In the multicenter study,[5] we noticed 26% of greater tuberosity disappearance on the radiograph at revision. The absence of the tuberosities affects slightly but significantly the Constant score (58 points versus 63 points in average, $p = 0.01$). The active external rotation was 4 degrees compared to 13 degrees ($p < 0.05$) with a hornblower sign in 43% of the cases, compared to 25% when the tuberosities had healed. After a deltopectoral approach, 37% of the tuberosities disappeared compared to 17% after a superior approach for a cohort of 246 paired patients with equivalent follow-up ($p = 0.01$). Considering these findings, we concluded that the surgeon should preserve the greater tuberosity as much as possible when implanting a reverse prosthesis.

In fracture cases the recovery of active external rotation is best when the tuberosities are fixed around the prosthesis.[26,36] To improve tuberosity healing, we recommend that the tuberosity be secured to the proximal humerus as in hemiarthroplasty for fractures, as well as the use of a cemented stem with an uncemented metaphysis (Fig. 3.8).

INFECTION

The overall infection rate after reverse arthroplasty reported in the literature is between 3% and 5%.[2,5,6] This rate is higher than the rate currently reported in unconstrained shoulder arthroplasty. The infection rate is higher in cases of reverse for revision surgery (7%) and rheumatoid arthritis (11%) than in primary cases, and the most common pathogen is *Propionibacterium acnes*.[37] The risk for infection could be related to the general poor health status of the patient—diabetes, alcoholism, obesity, age, corticosteroid use, and so forth. The hematoma that fills the dead space around the reverse prosthesis paves the way for infection. Moreover, the risk for infection is increased when the prosthesis has to be revised for postoperative complications.

In the case of acute infection (within 2 months of surgery), the infection is isolated and can be treated conservatively by debridement and antibiotics. Debridement and antibiotics are also recommended in acute hematogenous infection.[38]

In the SOFCOT series,[5] among 20 cases of chronic infection of the reverse prosthesis, 6 were treated conservatively (one

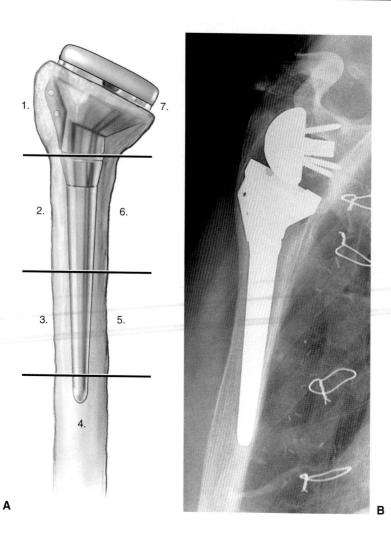

A

B

Figure 3.7. **(A)** Definition of the humeral zone on anteroposterior view. **(B)** Example of subsided uncemented humeral stem.

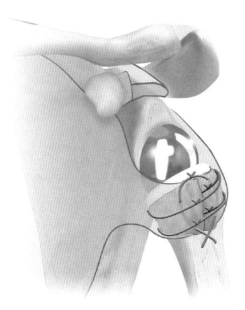

Figure 3.8. Technique of tuberosities fixation in reverse for fracture.

success) and a two-stage procedure was performed in 14 cases by using a temporary cemented spacer. It was possible to reimplant a prosthesis in 12 cases. Definitive resection arthroplasty is a salvage procedure that can successfully eradicate infection in elderly patients.

In revision cases, shoulders with multiple steroid injections, and cases with a large preoperative effusion, it is recommended to obtain culture specimens and maintain the cultures for several weeks to allow growth of the slow-growing organisms. Some authors advocate the use antibiotic-laden cement in all cases.[4,39]

DISLOCATION

Postoperative instability of the reverse prosthesis is the most frequent complication reported in large series that takes all of the etiologies into account.[1,28,40] The overall rate of instability was 4.8% in the French multicenter study.[5] A higher risk for instability has been reported with the reverse in revision surgery (10.7%), in proximal humerus tumors (10%), and for the sequelae of fractures (9.2%). Whatever the etiology, the risk for postoperative instability is higher when the patient already has a surgical history concerning the affected shoulder, before reverse replacement. Preoperative fatty infiltration of the subscapularis muscle on the CT scan has been identified as a risk factor for postoperative instability. In the literature, most patients experiencing reverse instability had been operated on using the deltopectoral approach[5,40] and a 36-mm-diameter sphere. For Nove-Josserand et al[40] the risk for dislocation associated with the deltopectoral approach can be explain by the larger anterior and inferior release. So far, there are no data to demonstrate that subscapularis repair can obviate the risk for dislocation.

It is important to differentiate early (within the first 3 months) from late dislocation. In the SOFCOT study,[5] closed reduction failed in 50% of the early cases, but no recurrence was found in cases of dislocation that had occurred after 1 year. Early dislocation can be due to loss of deltoid tension or to medial abutment against the scapula neck. Loss of deltoid tension is induced by humeral shortening, especially in revision or tumor cases. The length of the humerus can then be improved by adding a humeral metal spacer or increasing the height of the polyethylene insert. The dislocation is rarely due to rotational malposition of the humeral stem, but excessive humeral anteversion has been reported as a factor of dislocation and may prompt a revision of the stem.[26] The medial abutment of the prosthesis against the scapula pillar and the triceps tendon modifies the relationship between the sphere and the humeral cup, which can create lateral instability in maximal adduction. During the procedure, it is important to test the stability of the trial component before placing the final implant. Inferior capsular release prevents soft tissue impingement. Moreover, the medial impingement can be avoided by lateralizing the prosthesis. This can be obtained by grafting the glenoid in the case of revision or glenoid bone loss or by increasing the sphere's diameter. Some reverse design prostheses include a lateral offset into the design of the sphere, to avoid abnormal medial contact[4] and improve mobility. Other glenoid implants extend inferiorly to avoid medial bony contact and the risk for lateral instability. At the end of the procedure, if there is any doubt about the stability, it is better to immobilize the shoulder and delay shoulder rehabilitation program to allow healing of the periprosthetic soft tissue.

Late dislocation occurs less frequently than early dislocation and may be successfully treated by closed reduction and immobilization. According to Nyffeler et al,[33] late instability of the reverse prosthesis can be linked to medial polyethylene.

Whatever the delay of the instability onset, dislocation is a rare but dramatic complication. Overall results of the SOFCOT study[5] showed that 54% of the unstable prosthesis had to undergo a second operation. Of these unstable prostheses, 40% remained unstable after revision and 40% of revision procedures were complicated by infection.

SOFT TISSUE

HEMATOMA

The high risk for postoperative hematoma has been reported by Werner et al.[2] They considered the hematoma to be a genuine complication, even if they did not report any consequence on the final functional results. The rate of postoperative hematoma was 20% in this series, and 40% of the hematomas were treated by open revision. The risk for postoperative hematoma is much more important than in standard shoulder replacement because of the dead space around the prosthesis. Careful hemostasis and suction drainage are recommended for prevention. Early postoperative hematoma prevents soft tissue healing around the prosthesis and improves the risk for instability and infection.

OSSIFICATIONS

Postoperative subacromial ossification was reported in 13% of cases following reverse replacement.[5] This rate is lower than the rate of heterotopic ossification reported by Boehm et al,[41] who found 36.4% heterotopic ossification in primary unconstrained arthroplasty for cuff tear arthropathy. The occurrence of subacromial ossification is higher when the shoulder had prior surgical treatment. In the SOFCOT series,[5] we found a significant loss of function in the case of subacromial ossification (Constant score: 54 versus 64 points). The occurrence of postoperative ossification was not influenced by surgical approach. This type of ossification must be distinguished from the migration of a fragmented acromion, which does not influence the clinical results. It may be prevented by washing the subacromial space before deltoid closure, to remove all the bone particles. The rate of periprosthetic ossifications seems higher after reverse prosthesis for fracture.[25]

Further heterotopic ossifications are currently found at the lower margin of the glenoid.[28,38] This type of ossification was noticed in 36% of the cases by Renaud et al[38] and 45% of the cases by Hatzidakis et al.[28] In these studies, cases with large glenoid ossification tended to have greater restriction in range of motion. This has to be distinguished from a bony spur at the inferior margin of the scapula, which was noted in 63% of cases and has always been associated with a scapular notch.

DELTOID

The reverse prosthesis relies on the deltoid muscle to restore power elevation of the arm, and some surgeons do not use the superior approach because of concerns about violating the deltoid. Nevertheless, among a large series of 95 cases operated with a superior approach, we did not observe any complications related to the deltoid[6] using this approach.

Bufquin et al[25] reported one case of deltoid failure following a reverse arthroplasty for acute fracture, operated on through a superior approach. This was revised after 17 months by suturing the deltoid flap to the acromial process, with no further complications. Seebauer et al[42] described the onset of postoperative dehiscence of the deltoid resulting from early increase of range of motion and early exercises against resistance. They recommended immediate revision for reattachment of the muscle.

The analysis of the results of the reverse prosthesis for proximal humerus tumors showed that the range of motion in elevation was not affected by the partial resection of the anterior deltoid, corresponding to the approach for biopsy.[43] Moreover, a history of prior anterior deltoid detachment for cuff surgery is not a contraindication for reverse replacement, as long as the middle and posterior deltoid remain functional (Fig. 3.9). In that case, a preoperative electromyelographic assessment is useful. In our experience, the reverse prosthesis can be used after failure of a deltoid flap, but the results tend to be lower in terms of mobility.[13] Four of the five patients who had undergone a deltoid flap procedure to reverse prosthesis replacement were subjectively satisfied at revision, and their Constant score was, on average, 58 points.[5]

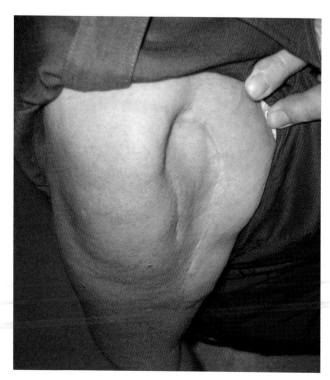

Figure 3.9. Example of anterior deltoid atrophy in patient operated through superior approach for cuff repair and later through deltopectoral approach for reverse replacement.

NEUROLOGICAL COMPLICATION

The risk for neurological complication after a reverse shoulder replacement is equivalent to the risk reported after an unconstrained prosthesis has been placed. In most cases, it resolves spontaneously. In the SOFCOT series,[5] neurological complications were observed in 1.1% of cases after reverse replacement. They could be attributed to the stretching of the brachial plexus during surgical exposure. Moreover, the caudal displacement of the humerus related to the migration of the center of rotation can reveal preoperative latent nerve compression syndrome.[42] One case has been reported of temporary radial nerve palsy related to cement extravasation during a revision surgery to convert a failed hemiarthroplasty into a reverse.[44] The upper or posterior screw of the baseplate can damage the suprascapular nerve while drilling the posterior cortex.[33] Bufquin et al[25] reported a higher rate of nerve complication after reverse for fracture (12%) with five cases (three median, one axillary, and one ulnar). In the case of early postoperative dysesthesia or paralysis, it is logical to immobilize the shoulder in 30-degree flexion-abduction and internal rotation to relax the neural structures.

LOSS OF ROTATION

INTERNAL ROTATION

The improvement in internal rotation is very low with the reverse prosthesis.[13] The patient must be informed of the risk for difficulties with perineal care, particularly in case of bilateral reverse arthroplasty. In the study of Wall et al,[1] patients with repair of the subscapularis had greater improvement in the amount of internal rotation (from L5 to L4) than did those without repair (from the sacrum to L5). For De Wilde et al,[45] the limitation can be explained by excessive retroversion on the humeral implant, which can impinge with the glenoid in internal rotation. They recommended implanting the humeral stem in neural rotation to enable perineal care. Theoretically, the use of a larger sphere could improve the mobility in internal rotation.

EXTERNAL ROTATION

The absence of active external rotation recovery can be found in most reverse prosthesis series[1,2,5,6,13,46–48] It is mostly linked to the preoperative state of the minor teres. In the SOFCOT multicenter series,[5] the average active external rotation, elbow to the side, was 4 degrees when the minor teres was atrophied or absent, compared to 15 degrees, on average, when it was present or hypertrophic. In the abduction position, active external rotation was, respectively, 34 and 52 degrees, on average. The preoperative state of the minor teres is assessed preoperatively by examining for the hornblower sign and by CT scan. In that same series, detailed analysis of active external rotation showed that 27% of patients had lost some external rotation compared with their preoperative state, and 13% had a negative or no external rotation. This is why Boileau and Trojani[49] and Gerber et al[47] suggested adding a latissimus dorsi to the reverse prosthesis when there is a preoperative deficiency of the external rotators.

According to some authors, the loss of external rotation is due to humeral retroversion. Placing the humeral prosthesis in 0 degree retroversion could, in theory, improve external rotation.[38] In fracture cases, the loss of active external rotation can be due to failure of greater tuberosity healing after fixation. Of the 36 shoulders studied by Bufquin[25] in which the tuberosities had been fixed, 19 (53%) suffered secondary displacement, leading to malunion for five of them (13.8%) and nonunion for the other 14 (38.8%).

Analyzing a retrieved prosthesis, Nyffeler et al[30] hypothesized that the loss of active external rotation could be attributed to suprascapular nerve damage secondary to the perforation of the posterior cortex by the drill or the posterior screw. When the infraspinatus is intact, the nerve should be protected during surgery to preserve active external rotation. According to Frankle and al,[4] the use of a larger sphere could improve the arc of motion in rotation.

If the disappearance of external rotation muscles can explain active rotation deficiency, it is likely that the respective positioning of the humeral implant and of the glenoid implant can have repercussions on the passive arc of motion.

PROBLEMS RELATED TO THE PATIENT

The reverse prosthesis is frequently used in elderly patients, who often present with many associated medical pathologic conditions. A thorough preoperative assessment of the associated pathologic states is essential to assess the risk for complications among this particularly fragile population. The thromboembolic risk for a shoulder arthroplasty is approximately 0.5% and is thought to increase with age.[50] It is also in this age-group that postoperative psychological troubles are noted, including disori-

TABLE 3.1		Influence of Prior Procedures on Postoperative Complication Rates				
Procedure	Infection (%)	Instability (%)	Humeral Complications (%)	Glenoid Complications (%)	At Least One Complication (%)	Reoperation (%)
No prior surgery (293 cases)	2.7	3.8	2.4	2.7	12.6	5.6
Revision arthroplasty (94 cases)	6.4	10.6	10.6	1	27.7	21.3
Prior nonprosthetic surgery (70 cases)	0	1.4	4.3	1.4	8.6	5.7

From Walch G, Wall B, Mottier F. Complications and revision of the reverse prosthesis: a multicenter study of 457 cases. In: Walch G, Boileau P, Molé D, et al, eds. *Reverse Shoulder Arthroplasty: Clinical Results, Complications, Revision*. Montpellier, France: Sauramps Médical; 2006:335–342.

entation and agitation, exposing the patients to the risk for dislocation and periprosthetic fracture. These specific risks must be investigated before the intervention (Table 3.1).

In a multicenter study, the complication rate was 25% in hemiarthroplasty revisions, and 37% in total shoulder prosthesis revision, with reoperation rates, respectively, of 16.9% and 29%.[6] Nevertheless, subjective results and satisfaction rates were not influenced by complications or reoperations when the prosthesis had been retained.[2]

In the SOFCOT multicenter study,[5] 20 patients presented with a poor functional result defined by a Constant score of 40 points or less. This concerned 13 massive cuff tears and 7 rotator cuff arthropathy patients. Fifteen of these patients were disappointed or displeased. Nine of them presented with a history of previous surgery (45%), and 12 (60%) presented with a postoperative complication. The age of these patients at intervention was 66 ± 9.6 years compared to 72 ± 7.2 years for the rest of the series ($p = 0.0001$). Thus they were younger patients, which confirms, if ever necessary, that the reverse shoulder prosthesis must be reserved for elderly patients—above 70 years of age, in theory. The Constant score and active anterior elevation did not improve. Moreover, they lost some external and internal rotation.

Analyzing the results of the reverse prosthesis for specific indications as presented at the Nice Shoulder Course, June 1–3, 2006, Nice, France, allowed us to isolate erroneous indications for a reverse prosthesis. Among these erroneous indications are rheumatoid polyarthritis, a painful yet still mobile shoulder, a painful shoulder after failure of rotator cuff surgery, and a nonunion of the surgical neck. The prosthesis must be considered a salvage solution in young and active subjects who have undergone multiple operations and after all other solutions have failed, with the patient warned of the high failure risk.

CONCLUSION

The availability of the reverse prosthesis was a significant evolution in the treatment of arthropathies with rotator cuff tears and in revision prosthetic surgery. Nevertheless, and even in the most experienced hands, the complication rate is high and must be well known to the surgeon.[51] The operative technique and the choice of implants must be adapted to each case. Postoperative monitoring must be close and extended, so that postoperative complications can be detected as quickly as possible in order to take appropriate measures.

ACKNOWLEDGMENT

The authors would like to acknowledge John Sperling, who assisted in the preparation of this chapter.

REFERENCES

1. Wall B, Nove-Josserand L, O'Connor DP, et al. Reverse total shoulder arthroplasty: a review of results according to etiology. *J Bone Joint Surg Am* 2007;89:1476–1485.
2. Werner CM, Steinmann PA, Gilbart M, et al. Treatment of painful pseudoparesis due to irreparable rotator cuff dysfunction with the Delta III reverse-ball-and-socket total shoulder prosthesis. *J Bone Joint Surg Am* 2005;87:1476–1486.
3. Bohsali KI, Wirth MA, Rockwood CA Jr. Complications of total shoulder arthroplasty. *J Bone Joint Surg Am* 2006;88:2279–2292.
4. Frankle M, Siegal S, Pupello D, et al. The reverse shoulder prosthesis for glenohumeral arthritis associated with severe rotator cuff deficiency: a minimum 2-year follow-up study of 60 patients. *J Bone Joint Surg Am* 2005;87:1697–1705.
5. Molé D, Favard L. Excentered scapulohumeral osteoarthritis. *Rev Chir Orthop* 2007;93 (Suppl 6):37–94.
6. Walch G, Wall B, Mottier F. Complications and revision of the reverse prosthesis: a multicenter study of 457 cases. In: Walch G, Boileau P, Mole D, et al, eds. *Reverse Shoulder Arthroplasty: Clinical Results, Complications, Revision*. Montpellier, France: Sauramps Médical; 2006:335–342.
7. Neer C. Glenohumeral arthroplasty. In: Neer C, ed. *Shoulder Reconstruction*. Philadelphia, Pa: WB Saunders; 1990:143–269.
8. Reeves B, Jobbins B, Flowers M. Biomechanical problems in the development of a total shoulder endoprosthesis. *J Bone Joint Surg Br* 1972;54:193.
9. Kolbel R, Friedebold G. Moglichkeiten der alloarthroplastik an der schulter. *Arch Orthop Unfallchir* 1973;76:31–39.
10. Broström L, Wallenstein R, Olsson E, et al. The KESSEL prosthesis in total shoulder arthroplasty. *Clin Orthop* 1992;277:155–160.
11. Fenlin J. Total glenohumeral joint replacement. *Orthop Clin North Am* 1975;6:565–583.
12. Gerard Y, Leblanc J, Rousseau B. Une prothèse totale d'épaule. *Chirurgie* 1973;99:655–663.
13. Sirveaux F, Favard L, Oudet D, et al. Grammont inverted total shoulder arthroplasty in the treatment of glenohumeral osteoarthritis with massive rupture of the cuff: results of a multicentre study of 80 shoulders. *J Bone Joint Surg Br* 2004;86:388–395.
14. Boileau P, Watkinson DJ, Hatzidakis AM, et al. Grammont reverse prosthesis: design, rationale, and biomechanics. *J Shoulder Elbow Surg* 2005;14:147S–161S.
15. Delloye C, Joris D, Colette A, et al. Mechanical complications of total shoulder inverted prosthesis [in French]. *Rev Chir Orthop Reparatrice Appar Mot* 2002;88:410–414.
16. Middernacht B, De Wilde L, Molé D, et al. Glenosphere disengagement: a potentially serious default in reverse shoulder surgery. *Clin Orthop Relat Res* 2008;466:892–898.
17. De Wilde L, Walch G. Humeral prosthetic failure of reversed total shoulder arthroplasty: a report of three cases. *J Shoulder Elbow Surg* 2006;15:260–264.
18. Levy JC, Virani N, Pupello D, Frankle M. Use of the reverse shoulder prosthesis for the treatment of failed hemiarthroplasty in patients with glenohumeral arthritis and rotator cuff deficiency. *J Bone Joint Surg Br* 2007;89(2):189–95.
19. Kaplan E, Meier P. Nonparametric estimation for incomplete observations. *J Am Stat Assoc* 1958;53:457–481.
20. Chuinard C, Trojani C, Brassard N, et al. Humeral problems in reverse total shoulder arthroplasty. In: Walch G, Boileau P, Molé D, et al, eds. *Reverse Shoulder Arthroplasty: Clinical Results, Complications, Revision*. Montpellier, France: Sauramps Médical; 2006: 275–288.
21. Neyton L, Boileau P, Nove-Josserand L, et al. Glenoid bone grafting with a reverse design prosthesis. *J Shoulder Elbow Surg* 2007;16:S71–S78.
22. Norris TR, Kelly J, Humphrey C. Management of glenoid bone defects in revision shoulder arthroplasty: a new application of the reverse total shoulder prosthesis. *Tech Shoulder Elbow Surg* 2007;8:37–46.
23. Molé D, Navez G, Garaud P. Reverse shoulder prosthesis, problems related to the glenoid. In: Walch G, Boileau P, Molé D, et al, eds. *Reverse Shoulder Arthroplasty: Clinical Results, Complications, Revision*. Montpellier, France: Sauramps Médical; 2006:289–301.

24. Levy J, Frankle M, Mighell M, et al. The use of the reverse shoulder prosthesis for the treatment of failed hemiarthroplasty for proximal humeral fracture. *J Bone Joint Surg Am* 2007;89:292–300.

25. Bufquin T, Hersan A, Hubert L, et al. Reverse shoulder arthroplasty for the treatment of three- and four-part fractures of the proximal humerus in the elderly: a prospective review of 43 cases with short term follow-up. *J Bone Joint Surg Br* 2007;89:516–520.

26. Cazeneuve JF, Cristofari DJ. Grammont reversed prosthesis for acute complex fracture of the proximal humerus in an elderly population with 5 to 12 years follow-up [in French]. *Rev Chir Orthop Reparatrice Appar Mot* 2006;92:543–548.

27. Valenti P, Boutens D, Nerot C. Delta 3 reversed prosthesis for arthritis with massive rotator cuff tear: long-term results. In: Walch G, Boileau P, Molé D, eds. *2000 Shoulder Prosthesis: Two to Ten Years Follow-up.* Montpellier, France: Sauramps Médical; 2001:253–259.

28. Hatzidakis AM, Norris TR, Boileau P. Reverse shoulder arthroplasty: indications, techniques, and results. *Tech Shoulder Elbow Surg* 2005;6:135–149.

29. Levigne C, Boileau P, Favard L, et al. Scapular notching in reverse shoulder arthroplasty. In: Walch G, Boileau P, Molé D, et al, eds. *Reverse Shoulder Arthroplasty: Clinical Results, Complications, Revision.* Montpellier, France: Sauramps Médical; 2006:353–372.

30. Nyffeler RW, Werner CM, Simmen BR, et al. Analysis of a retrieved delta III total shoulder prosthesis. *J Bone Joint Surg Br* 2004;86:1187–1191.

31. Delloye C, Joris D, Colette A, et al. Complications mécaniques de la prothèse totale inversée de l'épaule. *Rev Chir Orthop* 2002;88:410–414.

32. Vanhove B, Beugnies A. Grammont's reverse shoulder prosthesis for rotator cuff arthropathy: a retrospective study of 32 cases. *Acta Orthop Belg* 2004;70:219–225.

33. Nyffeler RW, Werner CM, Gerber C. Biomechanical relevance of glenoid component positioning in the reverse Delta III total shoulder prosthesis. *J Shoulder Elbow Surg* 2005;14:524–528.

34. Rittmeister M, Kerschbaumer F. Grammont reverse total shoulder arthroplasty in patients with rheumatoid arthritis and nonreconstructible rotator cuff lesions. *J Shoulder Elbow Surg* 2001;10:17–22.

35. Mottier F, Wall B, Liotard JP, et al. Pathologic acromion in reverse shoulder arthroplasties. In: Walch G, Boileau P, Molé D, et al, eds. *Reverse Shoulder Arthroplasty: Clinical Results, Complications, Revision.* Montpellier, France: Sauramps Médical; 2006:261–274.

36. Sirveaux F, Navez G, Favard L, et al. Reverse prosthesis for acute proximal humerus fracture, the multicentric study. In: Walch G, Boileau P, Molé D, et al, eds. *Reverse Shoulder Arthroplasty: Clinical Results, Complications. Revision.* Montpellier, France: Sauramps Médical; 2006:73–80.

37. Jacquot N, Chuinard C, Boileau P. Results of deep infection after a reverse shoulder arthroplasty. In: Walch G, Boileau P, Molé D, et al, eds. *Reverse Shoulder Arthroplasty: Clinical Results, Complications. Revision.* Montpellier, France: Sauramps Médical; 2006:303–313.

38. Renaud P, Wahab H, Bontoux L, et al. Prothèse totale inversée de l'épaule et insuffisance de la coiffe des rotateurs: évaluation et approche de paramètres anatomiques prédictifs d'une bonne fonctionnalité—à propos de 21 cas. *Ann Réadapat Med Phys* 2001; 44:273–280.

39. Matsen FA 3rd, Boileau P, Walch G, et al. The reverse total shoulder arthroplasty. *J Bone Joint Surg Am* 2007;89:660–667.

40. Nove-Josserand L, Walch G, Wall B. Instability of the reverse prosthesis. In: Walch G, Boileau P, Molé D, eds. *Reverse Shoulder Arthroplasty: Clinical Results, Complications, Revision.* Montpellier, France: Sauramps Médical;2006:247–260.

41. Boehm TD, Wallace WA, Neumann L. Heterotopic ossification after primary shoulder arthroplasty. *J Shoulder Elbow Surg* 2005;14:6–10.

42. Seebauer L. Reverse prosthesis through a superior approach for cuff tear arthropathy. *Tech Shoulder Elbow Surg* 2006;7:13–26.

43. Sirveaux F, Favard L, Boileau P, et al. Reverse prosthesis for tumors of the proximal humerus. In: Walch G, Boileau P, Molé D, et al, eds. *Reverse Shoulder Arthroplasty: Clinical Results, Complications, Revision.* Montpellier, France: Sauramps Médical; 2006:185–197.

44. Levy JC, Virani N, Pupello D, et al. Use of the reverse shoulder prosthesis for the treatment of failed hemiarthroplasty in patients with glenohumeral arthritis and rotator cuff deficiency. *J Bone Joint Surg Br* 2007;89:189–195.

45. De Wilde LF, Plasschaert FS, Audenaert EA, et al. Functional recovery after a reverse prosthesis for reconstruction of the proximal humerus in tumor surgery. *Clin Orthop Relat Res* 2005;430:156–162.

46. Seebauer L, Walter W, Keyl W. Reverse total shoulder arthroplasty for the treatment of defect arthropathy. *Oper Orthop Traumatol* 2005;17:1–24.

47. Gerber C, Pennington SD, Lingenfelter EJ, et al. Reverse Delta-III total shoulder replacement combined with latissimus dorsi transfer: a preliminary report. *J Bone Joint Surg Am* 2007;89:940–947.

48. Favard L, Lautman S, Sirveaux F, et al. Hemiarthroplasty versus reverse arthroplasty in the treatment of osteoarthritis with massive rotator cuff tear. In: Walch G, Boileau P, Molé D, eds. *2000 Shoulder Prosthesis: Two to Ten Year Follow-up.* Montpellier, France: Sauramps Médical; 2001:261–268.

49. Boileau P, Trojani C. Latissimus dorsi and teres major transfer with reverse total shoulder arthroplasty for a combined loss of elevation and external rotation. *Tech Shoulder Elbow Surg* 2007;8:13–22.

50. Lyman S, Sherman S, Carter TI, et al. Prevalence and risk factors for symptomatic thromboembolic events after shoulder arthroplasty. *Clin Orthop Relat Res* 2006;448:152–156.

51. Rockwood CA Jr. The reverse total shoulder prosthesis: the new kid on the block. *J Bone Joint Surg Am* 2007;89:233–235.

Pierre J. Hoffmeyer

Clinical Assessment of Failed Shoulder Arthroplasty

INTRODUCTION

Contemporary shoulder replacement is reliable and long lasting.[1-15] Shoulder arthroplasty ensures pain relief, improves range of motion, and enhances function, with results similar to those in total hip replacement. Survivorship analysis of unconstrained total shoulder replacements projected survival rates of 96% at 2 years, 92% at 5 years, and 88% at 10 years.[16,17] However, a proportion of shoulder replacements will fail and will pose important difficulties for patients and surgeons alike because of increasing absolute numbers of shoulder arthroplasties and heightened functional demands from younger and more active patients. The type and frequency of complications that plague shoulder arthroplasty procedures are continuously evolving. Chin et al[18] compared two series of shoulder arthroplasties performed over a span of 25 years. The first is a published series of 419 unconstrained total shoulder arthroplasties performed between 1975 and 1989.[19] In this early series, 130 shoulders (31% of the 419 reported) presented with a major complication and 95 of the arthroplasties required reoperation. The most frequent complication was found, in this early series, to be joint subluxation, followed in order of frequency by rotator cuff tearing, glenoid loosening, glenohumeral dislocation, humeral stem loosening, and infection. In 2006 the same authors published a series of 431 total shoulder arthroplasties performed between 1990 and 2000.[18] In total in this later series, 53 surgical complications occurred in 53 patients (12%). Of these complications, 32 (7.4%) were major, with 17 shoulders requiring reoperation. For this series the complications included, in order of frequency, rotator cuff tearing, postoperative glenohumeral instability, and periprosthetic humeral fracture. It is noteworthy that glenoid and humeral component loosening requiring reoperation occurred in only one shoulder in the later series.[18] The lesson of this study is that the learning curve for shoulder arthroplasty has progressed over the years and is flattening, with certain specific types of complications still in need of a solution. It must be remembered, however, that these published data concern high-volume institutions and that for lower volume surgeons and institutions the learning curve has yet to flatten.[20] Also, as with all types of arthroplasties, length of follow-up entails an increasing incidence of failure

and studies with short follow-ups have, understandably, fewer complications than longer follow-up studies.[21-23]

FAILURE MODES OF SHOULDER ARTHROPLASTIES

Because shoulder arthroplasty surgery is a complex and delicate undertaking, meticulous attention must be paid to the particulars of each situation in which a foreseeable failure of the arthroplasty is a serious risk to be avoided. In addition, successful revision of a failed arthroplasty entails the necessary identification of the problems encountered because these may involve all of the structures constitutive of the shoulder arthroplasty, including the surrounding capsulotendinous soft tissue, the osseous structures, and the prosthetic components.[24-26] The most commonly reported failure modes for total shoulder arthroplasty are joint subluxation, followed in order of frequency by rotator cuff tearing, glenoid loosening, dislocation, humeral loosening, and infection.[14,17,18,23,24,27-31] Knowledge of these typical and frequent failure modes should guide the investigation in cases of suspected shoulder arthroplasty failure.

The notion of the failure as pertaining to shoulder arthroplasty is also in need of precise definition and criteria for determining when failure actually occurs and which investigations will be the most fruitful for diagnosis. From the patient's viewpoint the salient features recognized as identifying clinical failure are onset of pain, loss of motion, and failing strength.[32] These features are analyzed in the major shoulder scoring systems: the Guidelines of Neer and Cofield,[10,16] ASES score,[33] Constant score,[34] Simple Shoulder test,[35] UCLA score,[36] and visual analog scores. However, these clinically oriented scoring systems do not incorporate imaging and laboratory criteria such as the presence of component loosening, progressive thinning of the rotator cuff with subacromial space loss, glenohumeral subluxation, and elevated C-reactive protein levels. All of these signs may signify impending failure, but they play little or no role in the clinical scores. It is therefore important to include regular radiographic examination in the follow-up of patients, even in those without subjective complaints, to avoid major and catastrophic failures with irreparable losses of bone stock and musculotendinous soft tissues because of tardy diagnosis.

Different types of prosthetic designs have different failure modes. Earlier designs included constrained prostheses with a specific failure pattern; these prostheses have been discarded for the more reliable nonconstrained prosthesis.

For *constrained prostheses* the listed causes for failure are glenohumeral instability and mechanical loosening, along with material failures such as implant breakage, polyethylene wear, deformation, ectopic ossification, nerve injury, joint ankylosis, and component loosening.[23,37,38] Because of these shortcomings entailing prohibitive failure rates, the constrained prostheses have progressively fallen out of favor in recent years.[37,39]

For *unconstrained prostheses*, Bohsali et al,[40] Lynch et al,[41] and Wirth and Rockwood[23] listed the following complications in order of decreasing frequency: loosening; glenohumeral instability; rotator cuff tear; periprosthetic fracture; infection; and failure of the implant, including disassociation of modular prostheses and weakness or dysfunction of the deltoid. According to Neer,[12,42] there are at least four special problems that must be considered in the face of a failed arthroplasty and in which revisions may need to be optimally addressed: (a) humeral head or glenoid bone deficiency, (b) a defective rotator cuff, (c) a deficient deltoid, and (d) chronic instability.

HISTORY

THE PREOPERATIVE SITUATION

To minimize the advent of complications and ultimate failure of the arthroplasty, the individual patient must be thoroughly evaluated before undertaking the implantation of a shoulder arthroplasty.

General Medical Condition

The surgeon must first delve into the medical history, presenting history, and complaints to determine whether risk factors exist that will negatively influence the outcome of the intervention.

Before the operation the surgeon must address, in priority, the expectations of the patient. A low-demand patient whose only aims are pain relief and peaceful sleep will not be expected to have the same outcome in terms of functional ability as a very active patient waiting only for his painful shoulder to be relieved by the arthroplasty to resume his professional, recreational, and sports activities.[42–44] In all patients the level and type of professional activities must be assessed. The examining surgeon will also want to know precisely the type of performance expected from the patient in his or her profession. For example, it is not enough to know that the patient is engaged in secretarial work; the amount of carrying and lifting at or above shoulder level must be defined and quantified. Sports and recreational activities must also be described with precision as to intensity and duration. Although this is especially true for activities engaging the upper extremities, such as tennis, golfing, swimming, or other types of activities, such as jogging, cycling, and horseback riding, although seemingly less demanding of the upper extremities, also exert stress on the shoulders.[43,45]

Comorbidities such as hypertension, diabetes, and obesity play an important role in the outcome of shoulder arthroplasties, and the appropriate preoperative measures must be taken before the intervention if these risks are to be minimized.[46] Inflammatory diseases,[29,47,48] osseous necrosis (alcohol, sickle cell, etc.), cardiac pathology (coronary artery bypass graft, artificial valves, pacemakers), or heavy smoking may also compromise mid- or long-term results and outcomes.[49,50] Hemophilic arthropathy is also a condition in which expert and specialized advice must be obtained before contemplating replacement surgery.[51,52] A precise preoperative assessment of any existing neurological conditions, whether peripheral (plexus) or central (stroke), should be performed. The surgeon should be wary of patients prone to peripheral neuropathies with predisposing diseases such as diabetes, alcoholism, hereditary neuropathy with liability to pressure palsies, or Bell's palsy, to cite the most common.[46,53] Careful interrogation must identify any underlying pathology, and the patient should be specifically, and at length, informed of the risk for developing a postoperative complication such as a total or partial plexular lesion. Severe preoperative neurological conditions impairing motor or sensory functions, such as syringomyelia or multiple sclerosis, need special attention; surgical techniques and implants may have to be adapted to the particular situation of the individual patient.[54]

Patients with previous irradiation to the shoulder region or axillary lymph node dissection after mastectomy for breast cancer must also be warned of the possibility of soft tissue and skin healing difficulties. If postradiation bone necrosis is visible on radiography, caution should be exercised and the patient warned of possible early loosening and increased risk for sepsis in this situation.[55]

Wheelchair-bound patients are a special cohort, with specific overuse shoulder pathology leading to the need for arthroplasty.[56] These patients must be monitored carefully, especially in the immediate postoperative course. Forceful soliciting of the shoulder arthroplasty for chair to bed or chair to car transfers should be avoided until complete soft tissue healing if early failure is to be avoided.[57]

Specific Shoulder Condition

Concerning more specifically the affected shoulder, careful preoperative physical examination appraisal along with standard radiological evaluation will yield valuable information as to the future performance of the planned arthroplasty. The clinical examination with its accompanying clinical tests will help in determining the status of the potential shoulder presenting for surgery and will be of invaluable help in identifying potential problems needing to be specifically dealt with by the surgeon. Specific imaging studies will be essential in understanding the morphology of the osseous skeleton, as well as the surrounding soft tissues, and will be critical for orienting the choice of the surgical technique and choosing the appropriate implant.[15] The success or failure of the arthroplasty will therefore largely depend on a meticulous appraisal of the preoperative situation.

Iannotti and Norris[58] reported on a multicentric series of 128 shoulder arthroplasties for osteoarthritis evaluated at a minimum of 24 months and for a mean of 46 months postoperatively. These authors concluded that severe loss of preoperative passive external rotation had a significantly negative effect on outcome of shoulder arthroplasty. For Franta et al[32] pain and loss of function are the two main patient complaints that motivate investigation for failed arthroplasty. A detailed history of invasive procedures about the involved glenohumeral joint, including frequency of intra-articular steroid injections and repetition of invasive imaging procedures (arthrography, computed tomography [CT] arthrography, magnetic resonance imaging [MRI] arthrography, and arthroscopic procedures) must be obtained. It may reasonably be surmised that these invasive procedures are liable to augment the risk of inoculation of organisms, more specifically, fastidious and slow-growing organisms, such as *Propionibacterium acnes*, into the shoulder joint. Chronic skin conditions such as eczema, severe acne, hypersensitivity to metals, and psoriasis may also augment the postoperative risk of infection and early loosening, and specialized dermatological consultation should be obtained before surgery.[59,60]

Deficient glenoid bone stock, such as is commonly encountered in the posterior wear of osteoarthritis, the erosive wear of rheumatoid arthritis, the bone loss and fragility resulting from profound osteoporosis or posttraumatic alteration, or the deformation characteristic of congenital dysplasia, must be rigorously analyzed and classified.[61–67] These deficiencies of the glenoid can lead to technical difficulties, including early loosening and humeral component subluxation or dislocation, that will compromise the outcome of the arthroplasty. If untoward results are to be avoided, rigorous and meticulous preoperative examination and planning using all available and relevant imaging techniques will allow a precise characterization of the morphological anomalies, thereby avoiding surprises in the operating room and disappointments to surgeon and patient alike.[15,63,68,69] Some situations, such as shoulder arthroplasty for fixed anterior dislocation after shoulder instability or in the postinfectious setting, have a poorer prognosis, with many postoperative complications, so the surgeon must be alert to these instances.[70–73]

Rotator cuff status must be accurately assessed; reparable tears do not compromise outcome, but irreparable or massive tears will certainly play a role and the surgical technique must be adapted to the situation and the type of implant.[32,74] In some situations, a total shoulder arthroplasty will give predictably good results; in others, different implants, such as hemiarthroplasties or reverse arthroplasties, will be best indicated.[12,75]

The factors described indicating a predictably poorer outcome of shoulder arthroplasty need to be preoperatively considered and the patient adequately informed of the risks if disappointments are to be avoided.

THE POSTOPERATIVE SITUATION

Once the failure has declared itself, it will be again up to the surgeon to determine, through history, current status, and appropriate adjunctive testing and imaging, the exact nature of the problem.[76,77] All of the necessary steps must be undertaken so that the patient will benefit from the best possible preoperative preparation before undertaking surgical revision of the arthroplasty, because this procedure is fraught with danger and risk, especially for the unprepared.

History of Present Complaints

A careful history must elicit the circumstances of onset of the symptoms related to the shoulder arthroplasty and to its mode

of failure so as to rapidly identify the category or the type of failure with which the surgeon is confronted. The complaints may be varied, such as pain, instability, loss of motion, or deformity. A detailed description of the complaints must be obtained and special attention given to time of onset and manner of onset, whether abrupt, acute, or insidious. Accurate descriptions of associated signs, such as malaise, paresthesias, fever, night sweats, chills, swelling, or redness, must also be elicited. It is well documented that risk for infection increases in patients with comorbidities such as diabetes mellitus, psoriatic arthritis, rheumatoid arthritis, and sickle cell anemia; organ transplant recipients; patients undergoing renal dialysis or steroid therapy; and immunosuppressed patients.[14,28,35,40] Furthermore, the history will guide to the identification of the specific problems at hand. According to Dines et al,[24] failure of shoulder arthroplasty leading to reoperation may be categorized into two broad categories—osseous or implant-related problems and soft tissue deficiencies. The category with osseous or implant-related problems may be subdivided as follows: glenoid component loosening, glenoid arthrosis after hemiarthroplasty, humeral stem loosening, and periprosthetic fractures. In the soft tissue deficiencies category the following are found: rotator cuff tearing, failed tuberosity reconstruction, cuff tear arthropathy, instability, and infection.[78]

Pain

Pain is a nonspecific but highly sensitive indicator of failure of shoulder arthroplasty.[1,32] The onset of pain can be immediate and persistent right after the implantation of the prosthesis or may appear after a pain-free interval. Pain in the shoulder when accompanied by fever is an ominous sign, and an acute infectious process must be immediately suspected.

IMMEDIATE AND PERSISTENT PAIN. Obviously, a careful clinical examination will reveal an immediate postoperative complication, such as an enlarging hematoma caused by an unrecognized laceration of a vascular structure, acute immediate dislocation resulting from early failure of the subscapularis suture, implant malposition, or a neurological injury, such as an elongation of the brachial plexus. Acute infection is also a cause for pain and will be accompanied by the usual inflammatory signs. Persisting postoperative pain beginning immediately after the operation can also stem from an unrecognized fracture, usually of the proximal humerus involving the tuberosities or the shaft. Component disassociation should also be evaluated and the appropriate radiographs ordered.[79,80] In a situation of immediate onset and persisting pain in the postoperative period, a careful physical examination accompanied by simple appropriate diagnostic measures such as routine laboratory blood work, standard plain radiographs, technetium-99 bone scan, and perhaps electromyographic examination will be adequate in the great majority of cases to elucidate the causes of concern.

In the event the clinical examination and the standard diagnostic measures described remain inconclusive and if the characteristics of the pain are similar to those in the preoperative state, the initial working diagnosis must be questioned. Rarely, in this situation, even with pre-existing radiological arthrosis, pain at the shoulder may be referred from elsewhere, and its origin must be elucidated by further examination, testing, and imaging. Commonly encountered causes may stem from painful acromioclavicular or sternoclavicular joints, a herniated cervical disc, or even a thoracic or abdominal condition masquerading as pain of shoulder origin.[81]

A very infrequent cause for persistent pain after the implantation of a shoulder arthroplasty may be related to an allergic phenomenon resulting from intolerance to the cement or to the metallic components.[60] All implanted materials may give rise to an allergy, and definitive diagnosis in this situation will require the aid of an astute allergologist. Treatment, however, may be rather complex, ranging from local medication to chelating agents to implant removal, depending on the severity of symptoms.

PAIN-FREE INTERVAL. Failed shoulder arthroplasty most commonly is associated with pain appearing after a symptom-free interval.[32] The mode of onset of pain can be an important clue to the underlying disorder, which may be infectious, inflammatory, mechanical, or neurological.[82] An acute onset is usually associated with an infectious process with a rapidly growing organism (*Staphylococcus, Streptococcus,* or gram-negative microorganisms). A slowly evolving painful condition usually of low intensity, not associated with motion, and exacerbated at night is a sign of an inflammatory condition possibly caused by a slow-growing organism such as *Propionibacterium.*[30,83] Pain associated with a visible deformity of the shoulder can be the sign of a dislocation that may be superior, anterior, or posterior. A painful subacromial mass can also testify to the presence of a distended and inflamed subacromial bursa secondary to cuff rupture or sepsis. Progressive pain associated with a loss of active range of motion and strength should make one suspect rotator cuff tearing. Glenoid component loosening is also associated with pain.[19] Wirth and Rockwood[23] report that humeral component loosening is rare and not specifically associated with pain. Pain can also reflect osteolysis resulting from particle release.[84]

PHYSICAL EXAMINATION

AGE

Very young patients are not good candidates for a total shoulder arthroplasty. Most reported series show that in patients younger than 30 years, the rate of success is low and accompanied by a high revision rate. In this younger population, suspicion of failure must be heightened if symptoms such as pain or instability occur.[18,61,67] Shoulder arthroplasty for dislocation arthropathy is reported to have a higher rate of aseptic failure resulting from glenoid and humeral loosening occurring in more active patients in a younger age bracket.[67]

BODY HABITUS

The habitus of the patient is generally indicative of the level of the patient's physical activity. Although the literature is silent on the subject, it may be surmised that thin, highly active, muscular patients are more likely to be prone to aseptic loosening of the components. These patients also tend to erode the rotator cuff and damage the tendons through overuse. The overweight patient is more prone to infection of arthroplasties and complications of regional anaesthesia.[85,86] Although these

considerations are of a very general nature, they may be helpful in guiding the first steps of an investigation into a painful shoulder arthroplasty.

Integument

Meticulous observation of the patient is the obligatory first step in establishing the diagnosis of failed shoulder arthroplasty. Obviously an erythematous and tender area adjacent to the surgical scar, a draining surgical scar, a draining sinus, or an abscess in the vicinity of the surgical approach all point to an infectious process. Inspection of the skin may reveal the thickened or atrophic scarring characteristic of previous treatment by irradiation for cancer of the breast, for example, a well-known cause of bone necrosis leading to early loosening or tendon ruptures. Multiple scarring is indicative of multiple surgical procedures, which tends to augment the risk for a postoperative infection. Chronic dermatological conditions also put the patient at risk for developing infectious complications. There is, for example, a positive correlation between prosthetic joint infections and the existence of psoriatic lesions.[59]

Shoulder Contour

An inflammatory condition of any etiology, such as infection, rheumatoid arthritis, or rotator cuff tearing, will cause synovial thickening or bursal effusion. This will alter the contour of the shoulder with an arthroplasty. A deformed shoulder contour may also be associated with instability and dislocation of the shoulder arthroplasty. The observed deformity is caused by the displaced and protruding humeral head. Instability and dislocation are the leading causes of failure of glenohumeral arthroplasty, and the reported prevalence of postoperative unstable or dislocated shoulder arthroplasties reaches 29% in some series.[23] In the event of a suspected dislocation, careful inspection of the shoulder contour, usually harboring anomalous, disgraceful, and salient bulges and hollows, will immediately orient the examiner to the type and direction of the underlying dislocation.

When the protruding bulge of the humeral head is anterior or anteroinferior with a posterior hollow, this usually indicates an anterior dislocation associated most probably with a rupture of the subscapularis or detachment of the infraspinatus, which may be caused by overgenerous section of the humeral neck at the time of surgery. Sometimes the humeral head is reducible with external maneuvers, but the reduction is usually short-lived, the head tending to return to the dislocated position.

When the bulging head lies anterosuperiorly, this signifies that the prosthetic head has passed through a large cuff breach, eroding through the coracoacromial arch and destroying, in passing, the barrier represented by the coracohumeral ligament.[87] These anterosuperior protrusions are as a rule passively reducible by simply applying traction to the arm. The patient can actively accentuate the phenomenon on contracting the deltoid, which aggravates the superior displacement (Fig. 4.1).

When the bulging head is posterior, with a matching anterior hollow and an easily palpable and salient coracoid, the dislocation is posterior.

Dislocation is a frequent complication, and when soft tissue problems or neurological injury are excluded, implant malposition with excessive glenoid or humeral head version are most commonly incriminated.[74] Incorrect sizing of the humeral

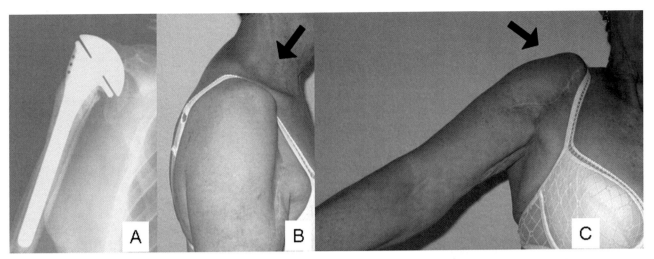

Figure 4.1. Failed hemiarthroplasty for a four-part fracture dislocation (**A**). As a result of tuberosity malunion and massive cuff destruction, the bulging prosthetic head (arrow) protrudes anterosuperiorly, signifying that the prosthetic head has passed anterior to coracoacromial arch altering the contour of the shoulder (**B**) and accompanied by a major limitation of the range of motion (**C**).

head, either too small or too large, is also a cause for instability and dislocation.[88]

Muscle Atrophy

Inspection with palpation of the shoulder will reveal the existence of atrophy of scapulohumeral muscular groups. Global atrophy including deltoid, trapezius, pectoralis, and cuff musculature is indicative of long-standing disuse and stiffness associated with painful loosening or low-grade infection. Anterior deltoid muscle atrophy may be the result of a surgical section of the distal axillary nerve after a deltopectoral approach or a transdeltoid approach. Atrophy of the supraspinatus and the infraspinatus fossae is a sign of long-standing tendinous rupture.[89] Atrophy of the pectoralis muscle with loss of the normal contour of the axillary fold is a consequence of a pectoralis muscle detachment, possibly resulting from overzealous release procedures.

CLINICAL TESTING

SENSORY TESTING

Sensory testing of the shoulder yields important information and is an integral part of the physical examination. The axillary nerve's sensory distribution dermatome is subacromial and lies over the middle deltoid area in an area extending 20 to 30 cm², depending on the individual's size and habitus. The musculocutaneous nerve dermatome lies on the medial forearm. Testing of the plexus must be carefully performed, and the individual rami, cords, and nerve trunks must be meticulously evaluated. Reasons for nerve injury can be poor surgical positioning or injurious intraoperative maneuvers. Forceful extension or excessive posterior humeral translation for glenoid exposure are notorious for overstretching fragile nerve structures. Anesthetic procedures, such as scalene blocks, may at times be incriminated in the cause of these types of neurological complications.[90]

MUSCLE STRENGTH TESTING

The integrity of the rotator cuff and its musculature plays a major role in the results of a shoulder arthroplasty, and good rotator cuff function is usually associated with a successful arthroplasty.[29] Most muscles around the shoulder may be readily observed, and atrophy will be the principal witness testifying to loss of strength when evaluating a patient with a suspected arthroplasty failure.[91] However, muscles such as the supraspinatus, infraspinatus, and teres minor are not so easily individually tested in the face of a painful shoulder and interpretation is often moot. One muscle that remains hidden from the examiner's view is the subscapularis muscle. Evaluating the strength of the subscapularis is especially important when faced with an anterior subluxation or dislocation, both situations implicating the integrity of the subscapularis muscle-tendon unit. Specific clinical tests have been developed that allow the examiner to evaluate the function of the subscapularis. The belly-press test, the lift-off test, the bear-hug test, and comparative internal rotation strengths have all been validated and are helpful in determining the subscapularis muscle-tendon unit's integrity[91–93] (Fig. 4.2).

RANGE OF MOTION

Most patients in published series have an improvement over their preoperative range of motion after a shoulder arthroplasty for long-standing degenerative disease such as osteoarthritis. Range of motion improvement depends on implant positioning and soft tissue integrity.[94,95] The improvement after arthroplasty is approximately 30 degrees from the preoperative range of motion.[16,17,96,97] This general statement does not hold true, however, for posttraumatic shoulder arthroplasty, in which most patients tend to loose some amount of range of motion postoperatively.[98,99] Range of motion will also tend to be diminished in most, if not in all, cases of failed shoulder arthroplasty. If the loss of range of motion or joint stiffness is of sudden onset, with the development of a stiff and painful shoulder over a short period, acute sepsis must be suspected. In aseptic failure, passive range

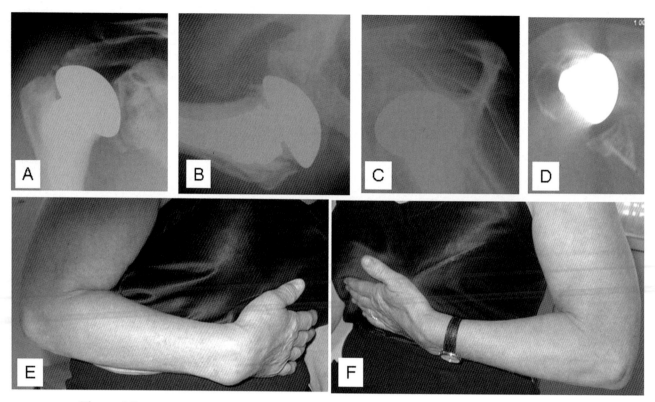

Figure 4.2. Anterior subluxation due to subscapularis failure and insufficient humeral head retroversion. **(A)** Anteroposterior view. **(B)** Axillary view. **(C)** Neer view. **(D)** Computed tomography image. **(E)** Positive belly press test. The patient is asked to forcefully press her hand on her abdomen: Notice flexed wrist and inability to bring elbow forward. **(F)** Belly-press test. Comparative normal side; wrist is extended and elbow brought forward.

of motion will be preserved in the face of a diminishing active range unless an acute mechanical cause such as dislocation or a component disassembly is present. In those cases the shoulder will be stiff and painful both passively and actively. Common causes for progressive loss of range of motion include thinning and tearing of the rotator cuff or loosening of the glenoid or humeral components.[91]

ADJUNCTIVE TESTING

Laboratory Tests (Blood, Periprosthetic Aspirate, Tissue Biopsy)

Laboratory tests are not diagnostic in the case of mechanical failure such as dislocation, periprosthetic fracture, or component disassociation. In the face of a painful arthroplasty, laboratory tests are essential to establish a definitive diagnosis and notably to rule out or to ascertain an infectious complication or a hypersensitivity reaction.

INFECTION. The most common mode of failure that may be successfully diagnosed with laboratory blood-based testing is an infectious process. Infection is relatively infrequent in primary total shoulder arthroplasty, and reported incidence oscillates between 0% and 3.9% according to the published reports for nonconstrained prostheses and up to 15% for constrained arthroplasties. Suspicion must be high in the case of a revised shoulder arthroplasty in which the incidence is an order of magnitude greater. Long-standing oral steroid use, a history of

malignancy, and diabetes mellitus tend to be associated with higher rates of infection. Rheumatoid arthritis has also been found to be an important factor increasing the incidence of postoperative infections.[83] All of the organisms usually associated with postoperative infections, such as *Staphylococcus aureus* or coagulase-negative *Staphylococcus*, may be involved. More specifically, in the shoulder, *P. acnes* is found more often than expected, in up to 60% of cases, as the infecting organism in shoulder arthroplasties compared to the other major joint arthroplasties.[100] No satisfactory explanation for this fact has yet emerged, yet it may be surmised that the skin of the axilla, being a reservoir harboring this anaerobic grampositive bacterium, may be the source for this infecting organism.[100] Another hypothesis may be the fact that many patients who have undergone total shoulder arthroplasty have had preoperative invasive procedures such as steroid injections or arthrograms associated with CT or MRI. These diagnostic or therapeutic maneuvers may have caused silent inoculations into the shoulder joint of dormant *Propionibacterium* organisms. The surgical intervention may then induce a *locus minoris resistentiae*, or an environment favorable for bacterial proliferation, in a zone of local tissue injury such as is present at the operative site. This is compounded by the presence of inert foreign material suitable for biofilm production.[30]

In the investigation of a suspected infectious process associated with a painful arthroplasty there are many laboratory tests and investigations, such as biomarkers, joint aspiration, or implant sonication, available for the detection and identification of the offending micro-organism.[76]

Biomarkers for Bacterial Infection. Erythrocyte sedimentation rate (ESR) and white blood cell count are helpful in the diagnosis and follow-up of clinically overt infections and are the primary investigations associated with a suspected infection.[82] These tests, however, are not specific enough for determining the presence of low-grade infectious conditions such as those commonly encountered in painful shoulder arthroplasties.[30,100]

Although disputed by some,[100] in the context low-grade infection it is deemed that the most effective screening biomarker is a measure of the serum C-reactive protein (CRP) level.[28] As a rule the CRP level returns to normal values 3 weeks after prosthetic implantation.[28] An elevated CRP level after that period augments the likelihood of bacterial infection in the face of a painful arthroplasty. However, an elevated CRP level is not specific and inflammatory conditions of any origin may cause elevation of the CRP, so the results must be considered with other information such as clinical examination and imaging studies.[28]

ESR and CRP taken individually are nonspecific tests but when used in combination and when within the normal range will tend to rule out the presence of infection.[101,102] Newer biomarkers such as procalcitonin, tumor necrosis factor–alpha, and interleukins are also found to be promising in providing indirect evidence of periprosthetic bacterial infections, but this needs further evaluation.[77]

Joint Aspiration. Joint aspiration of the periprosthetic fluid in case of suspected acute or chronic infection is both sensitive and specific and accurately ascertains the existence of an infection in the presence of an arthroplasty.[27,76,101,102] In aspirated synovial fluid the pathogen can be detected in 45% to 100% of cases. In a recent study, a synovial fluid leukocyte count of more than 1,700 per cubic millimeter or a finding of more than 65% neutrophils had sensitivities for infection of 94% and 97%, respectively, and specificities of 88% and 98%, respectively, in patients without underlying inflammatory joint diseases.[103] *Propionibacterium* is a fastidious organism, and cultures may take many days before becoming positive. Cultures of a superficial wound or sinus tract are often positive because of microbial colonization from the surrounding skin and should therefore be avoided.

Periprosthetic Tissue Biopsy. In some cases the joint aspiration procedure may be augmented by a synovial biopsy obtained through an arthroscopic technique or intraoperatively with an open biopsy during the revision procedure. The definition of acute inflammation in periprosthetic tissue varies in studies from 1 to 10 or more neutrophils per high-power field at a magnification of 400. Gram staining of synovial fluid and periprosthetic tissue has a high specificity, that is, more than 97%, but a low sensitivity of less than 26%.[104] Histopathological examination has a sensitivity of more than 80% and a specificity of more than 90%.[103,105,106]

Polymerase Chain Reaction. Polymerase chain reaction (PCR) is a technique of amplification of nucleic acids found in the periprosthetic tissues to identifying remnants of bacterial DNA in the face of fastidious organisms or inadequate and blind preoperative antibiotic administration, to identify micro-organisms that are difficult to grow. Unfortunately, the accuracy of this procedure has not been shown sufficient to be clinically useful.[103,107]

Sonication. In the case of an exchange arthroplasty in which infection is strongly suspected, but with biomarkers such as ESR and CRP remaining noncontributive, and in the absence of positive bacteriological cultures even after repeated preoperative cultures of joint aspirates, whole-implant sonication techniques are recommended. After surgical removal, the whole implant is subjected to ultrasonic treatment to dislodge any existing bacteria, encased in their protective polymeric matrix biofilm and clinging to the metallic implants.[30] This will make the organisms amenable to culture and identification, which in turn will let a specifically targeted antimicrobial treatment be introduced. Using this technique, Trampuz et al[108] studied 79 prosthetic joint infections with a sensitivity of sonicate fluid cultures of 78.5% and a specificity of 98.8%. For patients previously treated with antimicrobial therapy the sensitivity fell to 45.0% and the specificity to 75.0%. These results are significant, and sonication is a promising technique for establishing positive bacteriological diagnosis in cases of infection with recalcitrant organisms.[108]

Metal or Cement Allergy or Hypersensitivity

In some cases of unexplained ongoing pain related to an arthroplasty, some authors have incriminated allergic or hypersensitivity reactions to metals (nickel, chrome, cobalt, titanium) and in some cases to bone cement, including acrylates and additives, such as benzoyl peroxide, N,N-dimethyl-p-toluidine, hydroquinone, or antibiotics, particularly gentamicin.[60,109] It may be of help to proceed with thorough investigations using sophisticated immunoallergological testing techniques. In the case of positive results, adequate measures must be proposed to the patient; these may involve antihistamine medication providing symptomatic relief or steroidal agents in more severe cases; in some rare cases, resorting to chelating agents to remove the offending systemically distributed metallic molecules may be needed. In very severe cases, implant removal and exchange for components not containing the hypersensitivity-inducing agents may be the only solution.

Particulate Matter–Induced Osteolysis

Aseptic osteolysis not associated with visible wear may be induced by periprosthetic particulate matter of metallic or polyethylene origin initiating macrophage activation through complex biological mechanisms.[109–111] Examination of periprosthetic fluid or tissue obtained by aspiration or synovial biopsy may shed light on the diagnosis if particulate matter is present. This situation must be considered after all other causes for chronic pain, stiffness, or loosening have been ruled out. Newer agents such as biphosphonates to arrest macrophage activity are in the testing phase.

ELECTROMYOGRAPHIC EXAMINATION

Electromyography (EMG) examination is a helpful adjunctive testing modality used to assess peripheral neurological symptoms associated with a painful shoulder arthroplasty. The incidence of neurological injury after shoulder arthroplasty has been reported to be between 1% and 4.3%.[112–114] The position of the arm during the operation plays a role in the occurrence of these injuries. To prepare the proximal humerus for prosthesis insertion when using the long deltopectoral approach, the shoulder is placed in extreme external rotation and extension. With this same approach, preparation for the insertion of the glenoid component also puts the plexus at risk because the metaphysis must be translated behind the posterior glenoid rim and simultaneously the arm is internally rotated and abducted. This combined maneuver will cause plexular stretching. Multiply operated shoulders with scarring and stiffened tissues also place the patient at risk for neurological stretching injuries. Nagda et al[114] have shown alteration in EMG readings in up to 57% of patients during intraoperative monitoring. This study demonstrates that plexular stretching is common during an arthroplasty procedure and that although the majority of the alterations are infraclinical, patients are at serious risk for injury. In some instances of unexplained pain after shoulder arthroplasty, this may be the explanation. In Lynch's series of 417 shoulder arthroplasties in 368 patients,[113] a subset of 17 (4.3%) patients were found to present neurological injury postoperatively. Although the authors state that statistically no correlations were found for age and body mass index (BMI), the average age of the patients with neurological lesions was somewhat younger (54 years versus 62 years) and the average calculated BMI was slightly less (24 versus 26) in the patient group with neurological lesions than in the group without neurological lesions. Nagda et al[114] found a positive correlation with the use of a long deltopectoral incision not detaching the deltoid and the preoperative use of methotrexate. Plexular or truncular compression signs may also theoretically arise from mechanical causes in the case of chronic dislocation or component disassociation. Soft tissue inflammation may also cause compression or irritation of the neurological structures about the shoulder because of thickened synovial membranes or bursal enlargement.[114]

IMAGING STUDIES

STANDARD RADIOGRAPHY

Plain, standard radiography is indisputably the most useful tool available for diagnosing and documenting the causes of a failed arthroplasty.[115] Standard radiographic examinations are useful not only for diagnosing gross events, such as dislocation, component disassociation, or breakage, but also more subtle changes, including signs of early loosening or rotator cuff damage, can also be well appreciated on plain radiographs, which must always include two planes.[31,79,80,116,117] A true anteroposterior-plane film must be taken of the shoulder, along with an axillary view; this is especially important if the glenoid component is to be correctly visualized and the bone-implant interface well analyzed.[118] In cases of contemplated revision surgery, films showing the entire humerus and scapula must be obtained. However, before attempting to commit to a diagnosis based on plain radiographs, the examiner must be aware of the particulars of the arthroplasty in place, and, in case of doubt, perusal of the operative report, when obtainable, is of invaluable help.

Hemiarthroplasty

Hemiarthroplasty and bipolar hemiarthroplasty prostheses have no glenoid component, but attention must be directed toward

the native glenoid in some cases. Loss of joint space is indicative of cartilage thinning and usually accompanied by subchondral sclerosis.[119,120] This a worrisome sign signifying loss of the cartilage surface because of lysis resulting from infection or ongoing mechanical wear leading to arthrosis.[121] Progressively symptomatic glenoid arthrosis has been commonly reported after hemiarthroplasty.[24] In a short-term retrospective study, Sperling and Cofield[120] report on 18 shoulders treated with glenoid replacement because of painful glenoid arthrosis following prosthetic replacement of the humeral head. Although the patients' satisfaction with pain relief after the revision was excellent, seven patients were not satisfied with the result of the surgery because of a decreased range of motion and/or the need for a subsequent operation[120] (Fig. 4.3).

Glenoid Component Appearance

In the total shoulder arthroplasty, complications related to the glenoid component in the form of loosening, fragmentation, dislodging, and wear are the most commonly reported causes of poor outcome of shoulder arthroplasty, and up to 44% of glenoids show signs of loosening.[27,84,122–127] Familiarity with radiographic appearance of the glenoid component is necessary if these complications are to be detected and identified with standard radiographic examination. The glenoid component may be metal-backed or not, its back may be flat or convex, and

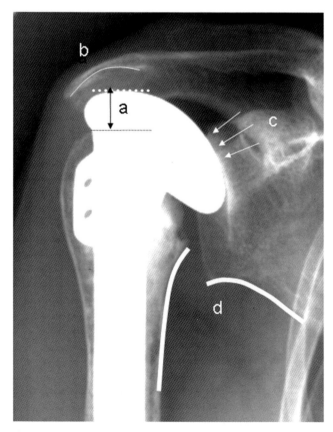

Figure 4.3. Hemiarthroplasty for fracture 2 years postoperatively. Proud head in relation to the tuberosity (*a*), thinned and concave acromion indicative of massive cuff tear (*b*), loss of glenoid cartilage and arthrosis (*c*), and humeral ascension interrupting the scapulo-humeral line (*d*).

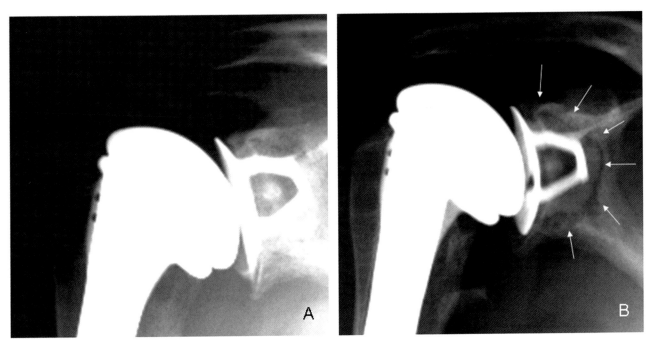

Figure 4.4. **(A)** Metal-backed cemented glenoid (Neer). **(B)** Asymptomatic radiolucent line indicating loosening after 5 years.

its surface may be anatomic or oval.[128] In the case of an all-polyethylene component it may be pegged or keeled. These components are usually cemented in place, so radiolucent lines around the mantle of cement must be carefully analyzed and described.[68,129–132] (Fig. 4.4).

When metal-backed glenoid implants with pegs and screws are used, the implant bone interface must be scrutinized to detect anomalies at that level.[3,133] Some glenoid components will have been augmented with an autologous bone graft screwed into place because of a bony deficiency, and only an astute observer cognizant of the procedures used will pick up loosening, necrosis, or other anomalies associated with this construct combining a polyethylene liner, a metal-backed component with screws, an autologous bone graft, and a cement mantle.[63,134] In 1982, Neer et al[9] reported a 30% prevalence of radiolucent lines around the glenoid component in a series of 194 shoulders. More than 90% of the radiolucent lines were observed on the initial postoperative radiographs and were attributed to poor cementing technique. More optimistically, in a recent report, Neer[10] reviewed the results for 46 shoulders that had been evaluated radiographically and had been followed for more than 10 years after a total shoulder arthroplasty, all without evidence of clinical loosening. In 1984, Cofield reported the results of 73 Neer total shoulder arthroplasties at 2 to 6 years of follow-up.[16] Although the clinical results were excellent and compared favorably with those of other studies, 52 shoulders had radiolucent lines at the bone-cement interface and 8 had radiographic evidence of loosening of the component, as defined by a shift in the position of the component or a circumferential radiolucent line at the bone-cement interface that was at least 1.5 mm wide.[135]

Antuna et al[62] retrospectively reviewed the results of glenoid revision in 48 patients, 30 of whom had a new glenoid component implanted and 18 of whom underwent resection and bone-grafting. Overall, the shoulders had significant improvements ($p < 0.05$) in pain relief, active elevation, and external rotation, but patients who had undergone resection were less satisfied than those who had a new glenoid component implanted ($p = 0.01$). Twelve patients (eight treated with reimplantation and four treated with glenoid resection) required a subsequent revision.[62] Although no radiolucent lines were observed around the glenoid component on the radiographs made immediately postoperatively, the lines developed within 3 years after the operation in 25 shoulders. Broström et al[136] reported that the development of radiolucent lines around the glenoid was associated with a slight decrease in function and a mild increase in pain.

The debate of keel versus pegs is still not settled, and early loosening is ascribed to either implant type, according to authors.[131,137] It is recommended, on the basis of cadaveric studies, to insert the cement under pressure into the holes with a syringe rather than just with finger-packing and to place some cement on the back of the glenoid to avoid immediate radiolucent lines. For many authors, surgical technique certainly plays a major role for the prevention of early loosening.[10,131,137] (Fig. 4.5).

Thinning of the polyethylene liner of the glenoid component is well appreciated on a two-plane radiograph series, with a progressive disappearance of the space between the glenoid and the metallic plate if a metal-backed component is used or if an all-polyethylene component is used between the bony scapular face and the humeral head component.

Relative Position of Implants

When examining radiographs of a conventional shoulder arthroplasty, the relationships between the skeletal structures and the components of the arthroplasty must be recognized; as

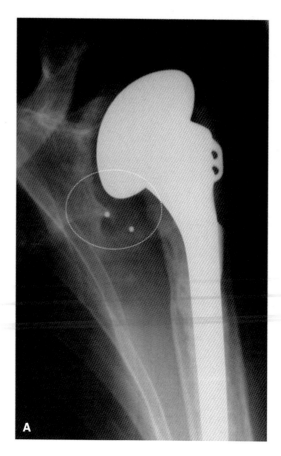

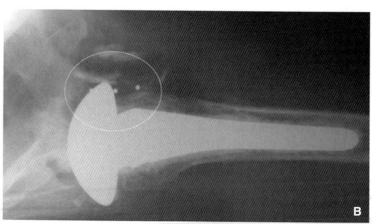

Figure 4.5.   Dislodged pegged glenoid in anteroposterior (**A**) and axillary views (**B**). The dotted ovals highlight the embedded markers in the glenoid polyethylene, testifying to the anomalous position of the glenoid component.

a rule when these relationships are not respected, a dysfunctional joint is at hand.[138] In the "normal" glenohumeral joint, the distance between the apex of the humeral head and the top of the greater tuberosity averages 7 mm, and the offset between the tip of the greater tuberosity and the glenoid face averages 55 mm.[78,139–142] The normal distance between the apex of prosthetic head and the acromion or acromiohumeral space should measure approximately 7 mm or more depending on the prosthetic model and the head shape. This space of 7 mm (or more) represents approximately the thickness of the supraspinatus tendon.[139,142–144] Acromiohumeral space thinning, leading to head contact with the undersurface of the acromion, is a sure sign of cuff alteration or rupture, as demonstrated by anteroposterior radiographs in internal, neural, and external rotation.[143]

Prosthetic Head

Many types of humeral components exist—monobloc stems with head and stem in one piece or modular components with heads of different sizes adapted onto stems of varying diameters. In some models, the Morse taper socket is on the modular head, usually eccentrically positioned, allowing adjustment of the head rotated to the appropriate position onto the shank on the baseplate of the stem. The Morse taper is then cold-welded with the head in the desired position in the usual fashion with a short mallet blow. In other prostheses, the Morse taper is reversed, with the shank set in the back of the cephalic component and the socket machined into the baseplate of the humeral component. Head size, head shape (ovoid, spherical, conch shaped), radius of curvature, and diameter also vary among manufacturers, as well as head-stem angulation (variable in some implants and fixed in others) and stem length and diameter. The examiner must be aware of these characteristics of the individual prosthesis for correct interpretation of the radiographic images.[2,145,146]

The size of the head must be evaluated, and close approximation to the anatomic situation is desirable.[144,147] However, no objective rules exist as to how to evaluate the ideal prosthetic head size intraoperatively in a given situation. The examiner, however, on reviewing the appropriate imaging studies, will rapidly come to a conclusion as to the adequacy of the head size, taking into account the overall morphology and incorporating parameters such as ideal head diameter and height ratio between tuberosity and harmonious scapulohumeral line.[141,146–148] "Overstuffing" is defined by the use of a head too large for its osteoligamentous environment or an excessive "high" proximal positioning of the head.[138,144] This will produce stiffness and cuff destruction. On the contrary, "understuffing" signifies that the head is too small or too "low," and this will also cause pain and cuff damage from excessive translation and wear.[88,138]

Stem Appearance

Prosthetic stems may be cemented or noncemented, and the cement may or may not be radiotransparent. When a noncemented stem is used, its surface may be fully or partially covered with osteoinductive and osteoconductive textures.[149,150] Some stems are coated with variable thicknesses of hydroxyapatite layers for the purpose of obtaining fixation by secondary bony ingrowth.[151] Periprosthetic radiopaque hydroxyapatite debris seen on plain films may signify stem loosening or loss of fixation. Examination of the stem-cement-bone interface is more thorough if the humerus is divided into distinct sectors and each sector assessed independently, similar to the examination of Gruen zones.[150–152]

Loosening of the humeral component, with radiolucencies, subsidence, cement mantle breakage, and cortical osteolysis, is much less common than glenoid loosening, and despite high rates of radiographic changes around the stem, loosening is rarely a cause for revision surgery.[150,153,154] Torchia et al[155] reported a high rate of subsidence of press-fit humeral prostheses; however, they noted no association between stem loosening and pain in their study. This is confirmed by Wirth et al,[23] for whom humeral component loosening is rare and not specifically associated with pain.

Resurfacing prostheses are stemless, and the metaphyseal bone needs careful analysis for signs of failure, including lucencies, sclerosis, or bone loss in the symptomatic patient.[48,156]

Instability

Postarthroplasty instability remains a very difficult problem. Along with loosening of the glenoid component, instability is the reason for the majority of total shoulder replacement revisions.[26,157,158] Moeckel et al[157] reported ten cases of shoulder instability in a total of 236 controlled shoulder arthroplasties.

The direction of the dislocation, whether superior, anterior, or posterior, may be without doubt ascertained on plain radiographs. Component orientation may also be evaluated with standard anteroposterior and axillary radiographs. Malpositioning, such as excessive or insufficient retroversion of the humeral component or excessive tilting of the glenoid component, is also accurately diagnosed on plain films, and CT scanning is invaluable for the exact determination of the torsion defects.[94,159–161]

Infection

In the case of infection the radiological signs include new subperiosteal bone growth and transcortical sinus tracts that are specific for infection; however, migration or shifting of implants and periprosthetic osteolysis can also occur without infection. Foci of osteolysis, areas of sclerosis, and generalized bone resorption can also occur but are not specific signs of an infectious process.[162]

Heterotopic Ossification

Periarticular ossification is a relatively common complication after shoulder arthroplasty according to one study and is easily diagnosed with plain radiography.[163,164]

Periprosthetic Fracture

After a traumatic event in a patient with a shoulder arthroplasty, a fracture of the scapula or of the tuberosity may be diagnosed using plain radiography (Fig. 4.6).

The reported rate of humeral fracture after shoulder arthroplasty is approximately 1.6% and 2.4%.[98,165–169] Treatment outcomes can often be attributed to the location and configuration of the fracture. Kumar et al[166] retrospectively reviewed the treatment results of 16 periprosthetic humeral fractures. Ten of the fractures were managed operatively, and all healed. On the other hand, Kim et al[170] report good results using functional bracing in this situation.

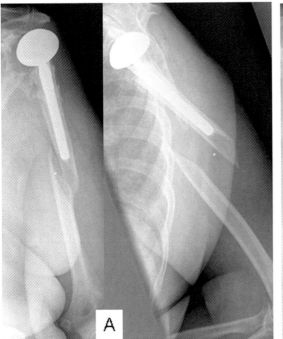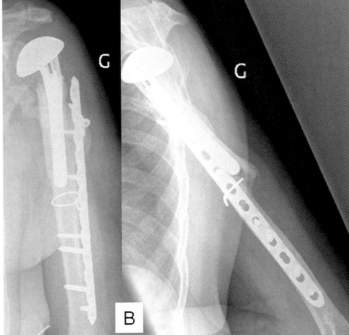

Figure 4.6. **(A)** Periprosthetic fracture at the distal tip of the stem. **(B)** Plate fixation and union obtained after 3 months in spite of migration of a proximal screw resulting from poor bone quality.

Radiology of Reverse Arthroplasty

The reverse arthroplasty developed by Grammont poses special problems for the interpretation of radiographs.[75,171–182] The radiological appearance is different from that of previous shoulder arthroplasties. A certain familiarity with this implant is necessary if one is to accurately diagnose the signs of failure and complications associated with this particular implant, which are reported as to be as high as 50% by some authors.[182] The reverse shoulder arthroplasty uses a new concept based on the medialization and lowering of the center of rotation of the glenohumeral joint, thereby enhancing the moment arm of the deltoid muscle. To achieve this goal, a hemispheric component is screwed onto the glenoid face and a cup is mounted on a stem implanted into the humeral diaphysis. The glenoid implant consists of a series of components, the metaglene, or baseplate fixed generally with a central peg and augmented with two sagittal and two transverse screws. The two sagittal screws either have a fixed angle or may be oriented to enter into the pillars of the scapula. A hemispheric component, the glenosphere, is then screwed onto the baseplate.[183] The glenosphere articulates with a polyethylene cup clipped into a metaphyseal component, itself screwed onto a humeral stem.[178] The radiograph shows a relatively impressive distance separating the acromion from the top of the glenosphere of up to 2 cm or more. The glenoid and humeral components may appear incongruent when the arm is at rest in adduction; however, the center of the glenosphere must be aligned with the center of the cup and stem in both the anteroposterior and lateral views. Coaptation of both components will occur when the shoulder is actively abducted. Anomalies around the stem such as radiolucencies and subsidence indicative of loosening are easily appreciated on plain radiographs. The same is true for

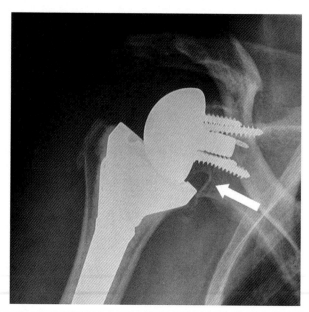

Figure 4.7.   Glenoid notching in a reverse prosthesis (arrow). In this case there are aggravating factors: upward tilting and superior placement of glenosphere and metaglene components.

disassociation or dislocation of the prosthetic components: The glenosphere can unscrew itself from the metaglene, and the metaphyseal component can also unscrew itself from the stem. Inferior scapular notching, commonly seen in the evolution of the reverse prosthesis is also well analyzed on plain anteroposterior radiographs (Fig. 4.7). Dislocation is usually anterosuperior, the humerus being attracted upward by the deltoid muscle (Fig. 4.8). Exact positioning of the glenoid components and

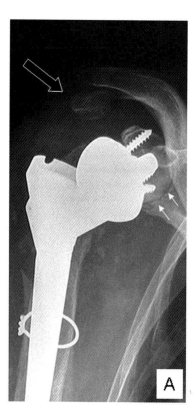

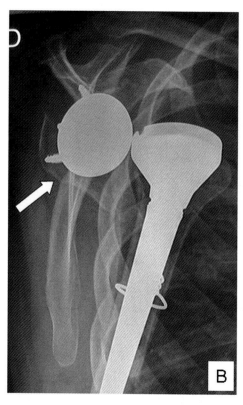

Figure 4.8.   Dislocated reverse total shoulder arthroplasty. **(A)** Fracture of the acromion (black arrow), loose metaglene with concomitant lucent line on the scapula (small arrows). **(B)** Detachment of a proximal metaphysis fragment (white arrow).

screws is more difficult to determine, however, and more sophisticated transverse imaging modalities such as CT may be necessary to assess the true position of these implants. The anterior, superior, and posterior screws can be bicortical in the scapula, but the inferior screw should be entirely within the inferior scapular pillar. Ideally, the glenosphere should be placed flush to the native glenoid, as low as possible and inclined slightly inferiorly; this should diminish the incidence of inferior scapular notching.[75,171,178,179,180,184]

COMPUTED TOMOGRAPHY

Many conditions involving soft tissue alterations and some bony anomalies are difficult to diagnose using plain radiography. CT with fast multichannel detectors enhanced by advances in postprocessing software and sophisticated workstations with multislicing and three-dimensional capacity have considerably improved imaging possibilities.[159,185] Prostheses will alter and degrade the images obtained because of beam hardening or projection data noise resulting from their metallic nature and the particular geometry of the implants. Tubular stems will interfere less with the image than complex spherical shapes such as the humeral head or the glenoid, especially if metal-backed implants are used. Titanium is more amenable to imaging than stainless steel or cobalt chrome alloys.[186] Even though artefacts cannot be completely avoided, many periprosthetic osseous anomalies can be detected, such as osteolysis or stress fractures. Yiang et al[187] determined that CT was more sensitive for detecting osteolysis at the bone-cement interface than plain fluoroscopy-guided radiographs in a series of 47 cemented

pegged glenoid components. CT can also aid in determining torsion of the humeral component with precision, and glenohumeral subluxation may be precisely appreciated[188] (Fig. 4.9).

Soft tissue anomalies such as periprosthetic fluid collections or rotator cuff intratendinous or full-thickness tearing are also well appreciated. Furthermore, CT allows evaluation and quantification of fatty muscle degeneration of the muscles of the rotator cuff.[89]

MAGNETIC RESONANCE IMAGING

MRI is a powerful diagnostic tool that unfortunately has drawbacks for the examination of metallic arthroplasties.[189] Metal composition and implant architecture play an important role in the generation of artefacts. Titanium tends to generate little distortion, whereas stainless steel and metallic alloys with ferromagnetic properties induce major artefactual changes. Implant morphology plays a role; as with CT, tubular implants such as stems are also better visualized than more complex shapes such as cephalic components or metal-backed glenoids.[186] High-strength 3-tesla magnetic fields tend to produce more artefacts in the presence of metallic implants than lower strength fields (0.5 or 1.0 tesla), and these are therefore preferred in this indication. The radiologist performing the examination must be thoroughly cognizant about and informed on the implant characteristics if adequate techniques and sequences are to be used to obtain optimal images. MRI can pick up periprosthetic fatigue fractures, but, more important in shoulder arthroplasty, it is able to show tendon anomalies and tearing, muscle atrophy, heterotopic ossification, and periprosthetic fluid collections.[190]

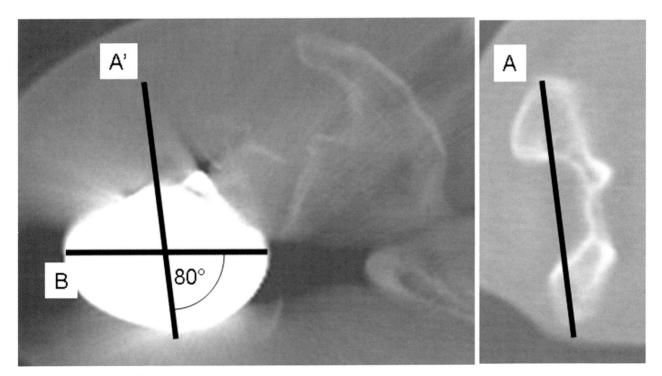

Figure 4.9. Computed tomography examination with cuts at proximal and distal humerus depicting posterior dislocation of prosthetic head, excessive retroversion of the humeral head measured at 80 degrees, and greater and lesser tuberosity malposition. **(A)** A′, Transepicondylar axis. **(B)** Transverse prosthetic head axis.

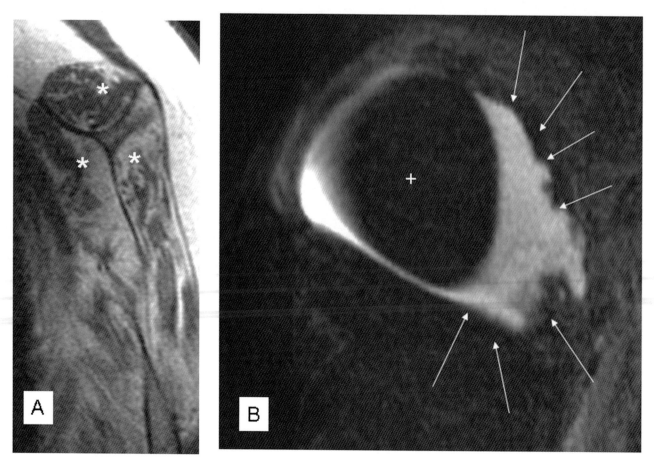

Figure 4.10. Magnetic resonance imaging imaging (1.5 tesla field) of dislocated reverse total shoulder arthroplasty (see Fig. 4.8). **(A)** Dystrophic scapular musculature (*). **(B)** Liquid-filled bursa (*arrows*) surrounding the dislocated humeral component (+).

(Fig. 4.10). Sperling et al[191] report a series of 21 MRI studies for painful shoulder arthroplasties that subsequently underwent surgical exploration and revision. In this study, MRI identified correctly 10 of the 11 full-thickness rotator cuff tears found at surgery, of which 8 were subscapularis tears. MRI also correctly identified 8 of the 10 shoulders with an absence of rotator cuff tearing.[191]

ULTRASONOGRAPHY

CT and MRI are not always diagnostic in the presence of metallic or ferromagnetic devices because of the major image distortions discussed previously. Ultrasound is an adjunctive imaging modality useful when a metallic implant is in place. Ultrasound can depict periprosthetic soft tissue conditions such as rotator cuff tendinopathy or tearing, bursal edema or thickening, fluid collections, hematomas, or abscesses, and it can also help to guide joint aspiration and needle biopsy procedures. The subscapularis is particularly well analyzed with ultrasonography because it is a relatively superficial structure, well amenable to this imaging modality. An advantage of ultrasonography over all other imaging techniques is the ability to provide dynamic images that can, for example, show tendon interactions with the implanted components. A serious drawback is that ultrasonog-

raphy is very operator dependent and requires a skilled sonographist versed in implant imaging, to reproducibly establish the essential information needed for the assessment of a painful or failed arthroplasty.[186]

NUCLEAR MEDICINE IMAGING STUDIES

Radionuclide imaging techniques and procedures have progressed and diversified, with many types of scanning procedures available.

Technetium-99m–Labeled Phosphonate

The uptake of technetium-99m–labeled phosphonate, a bone-seeking radiopharmaceutical, depends on tissue perfusion and vascular permeability. This imaging modality differentiates areas of high or low metabolic activity. Cameras may either cone down on a particular area or give a general image of the whole skeleton with low radiation exposure to the patient. Although the image obtained is not detailed, the high activity areas are accurately delineated. ^{99m}Tc-labeled phosphonate scans are triphasic, with a rapid vascular or perfusion phase, followed some minutes later by a blood pooling phase and some hours later by a bone metabolism phase. Bone scans are very sensitive in detecting osteoblastic activity resulting from loosening or infection in the periprosthetic bone; it may be stated that if there is no activity at all, the prosthesis is neither loose nor infected. However, bone scans are not specific and activity can persist normally for months and up to years after prosthetic implantation. Also, bone scans cannot differentiate between septic and aseptic processes, such as mechanical loosening, reflex dystrophy, or bacterial infection around the implant; however, bone scans have a high negative predictive value; that is, if the bone scan is negative, the probability for infection is low.[81,192,193]

Indium-111

Indium-111–labeled leukocytes or immunoglobulins migrating to sites of infection are very sensitive. Studies have not shown any advantage over ^{99m}Tc scans in the case of an infected arthroplasty, however, so they lose their value in terms of clarifying the diagnostic dilemma of suspected low-grade infection in a painful arthroplasty. Scher et al[194] conclude, after a study involving 143 patients, that ^{111}In scans have a limited indication and that a negative scan might be, at most, helpful only in suggesting the absence of infection. Some authors contend that ^{99m}Tc-HMPAO–labeled leukocytes have been used with success in detecting infectious processes.[195]

Technetium-99m–Labeled Monoclonal Anti–NCA-90 Antibody Fab' Fragments

Because ^{111}In scans are fastidious and time consuming, they have been replaced in some regions by ^{99m}Tc–labeled monoclonal anti–NCA-90 antibody Fab' fragments scans. This imaging modality is reported to have a high accuracy, up to 81% for detecting periprosthetic infections.[196]

Gallium-67

Gallium-67 is an isotope that binds to transferrin or other iron-transporting molecules in the serum and accumulates in the tissue because of the increased vascularity associated with inflammation. Itasaka et al[192] report a series of 48 hip arthroplasties that were revised for infection. ^{67}Ga scans in this study had a sensitivity of 67%, a specificity of 100%, and an accuracy of 96%. Other authors, Kraemer et al,[197] found a sensitivity of 38% and a specificity of 100% in detection of an infected arthroplasty and concluded that ^{67}Ga scanning had no added value over other diagnostic modalities.

Single-Photon Emission Computed Tomography

Single-photon emission computed tomography (SPECT) is a modality fast becoming a tool in the diagnosis of periprosthetic infections. Studies have shown that when coupled with CT for better spatial localization the accuracy is enhanced. Clinical experience is still lacking over large series for this technique to become a routine investigational tool, however.[198,199]

^{18}F-Fluoro-Deoxyglucose Positron Emission Tomography

A promising new technique is ^{18}F-fluoro-deoxyglucose positron emission tomography. This imaging modality depicts the metabolic activity of glucose, which tends to accumulate in areas of inflammation at the molecular level in the tissues. Although it may be possible in the future to differentiate the origin of the osteolysis, whether infectious or wear debris response, this is not yet confirmed. Studies show a high sensitivity, and if the scan remains negative, the likelihood of infection is nonexistent; however, if positive, it is not specific enough to consistently differentiate between periprosthetic infection and aseptic loosening.[200,201] Love et al[202] concluded that ^{18}F-fluoro-deoxyglucose positron emission tomography when compared to ^{111}In-labeled leukocytes scan is less accurate in detecting infection. These techniques are still in process of evaluation; they hold great promise but should be used and interpreted with care.[202,203]

ARTHROSCOPY

Arthroscopy can be, in experienced hands, an adjunctive technique useful to evaluate or even to treat the painful shoulder arthroplasty. Hersch and Dines[204] described 13 arthroscopic procedures for pain after shoulder arthroplasty. All of these patients had soft tissue pathology involving various degrees of rotator cuff tearing, retracted capsulitis, or biceps tendon involvement. Closed or mini-open cuff repairs, biceps tenodesis, and adhesive scarring takedown using arthroscopically aided techniques were successful and brought about significant relief to the patients. The authors warn, however, that if complications are to be minimized, careful attention must be paid to surgical technique, including using blunt trocars, traction to decoapt the joint, and administration of prophylactic antibiotics. In some rare cases, arthroscopic surgery may act directly on the implants. O'Driscoll et al[205] reports an arthroscopic removal of a loose and damaged glenoid component.

SUMMARY

The failed shoulder arthroplasty is an infrequent condition with multiple origins and causes. As a first approach, prevention of failure is an important step, and care must be taken to identify preoperatively the factors known to lead to a poor result in the future, such as young age, unrealistic patient expectations, neuromuscular deficits, and major loss of bone stock. When the patient presents with pain and a functional deficit in the course of a shoulder arthroplasty, a detailed history and a careful physical examination will most often yield the cause of the failure. Standard radiographic examination will be the most useful tool to further the diagnosis. CT and MRI can also be of use to delineate the morphological situation. Infection is the most dreaded complication because it entails the undertaking of major procedures for the patient. In cases of early infection without bone destruction or reaction it poses a particularly difficult diagnostic challenge, and this is where adjunctive techniques such as direct joint aspiration and nuclear-based imaging scans are the most useful. The newer imaging techniques sensitive to metabolic activity as opposed to simple depiction of morphology hold great promise for the future but need further clinical evaluation. A proposed algorithm outlining the main steps of investigation is presented in Figure 4.11.

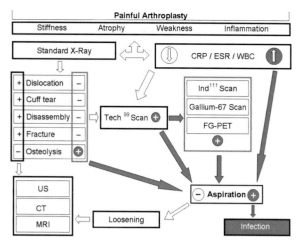

Figure 4.11. Algorithm to determine an investigational pathway into the painful arthroplasty. Clinical assessment, standard radiography, technetium bone scanning, and joint aspiration will generally be diagnostic. If these investigations do not answer the question, then more sophisticated examinations may be necessary to elucidate rarer causes of failure such as allergic conditions or neurological problems. If all is negative, then it may not be the shoulder and further more general causes must be identified.

REFERENCES

1. Chen AL, Bah EB, Horan MP, et al. Determinants of satisfaction with outcome after shoulder arthroplasty. *J Shoulder Elbow* 2007;16:25–30.
2. Churchill RS, Kopjar B, Fehringer EV, et al. Humeral component modularity may not be an important factor in the outcome of shoulder arthroplasty for glenohumeral osteoarthritis. *Am J Orthop* 2005;34:173–176.
3. Hill JM, Norris TR. Long-term results of total shoulder arthroplasty following bone-grafting of the glenoid. *J Bone Joint Surg Am* 2001;83:877–883.
4. Levy O, Copeland S. Cementless surface replacement arthroplasty (Copeland CSRA) for osteoarthritis of the shoulder. *J Shoulder Elbow Surg* 2004;13:266–271.
5. Mackay DC, Hudson B, Williams JR. Which primary shoulder and elbow replacement? A review of the results of prostheses available in the UK. *Ann R Coll Surg Engl* 2001;83: 258–265.
6. Mansat P, Mansat M, Bellumore Y, et al. Mid-term results of shoulder arthroplasty for primary osteoarthritis [in French]. *Rev Chir Orthop Reparatrice Appar Mot* 2002;88:544–552.
7. Mileti J, Sperling JW, Cofield RH, et al. Monoblock and modular total shoulder arthroplasty for osteoarthritis. *J Bone Joint Surg Br* 2005;87:496–500.
8. Neer CS II. Articular replacement for the humeral head. *J Bone Joint Surg Am* 1955;37: 215–228
9. Neer CS, Watson KC, Stanton FJ. Recent experience in total shoulder replacement. *J Bone Joint Surg Am* 1982;64:319–337.
10. Neer CS. Glenohumeral arthroplasty. In: Neer, CS, ed. *Shoulder Reconstruction*. Philadelphia: WB Saunders; 1990:181–185.
11. Neer CS. Indications for replacement of the proximal humeral articulation. *Am J Surg* 1955;89:901–907.
12. Neer CS. Shoulder reconstruction. In: Neer CS, ed. *Shoulder Reconstruction*. Philadelphia, WB Saunders, 1990.
13. Norris TR, Iannotti JP. Functional outcome after shoulder arthroplasty for primary osteoarthritis: a multicenter study. *J Shoulder Elbow Surg* 2002;11:130–135.
14. Sperling JW, Cofield RH, Rowland CM. Minimum 15-year follow-up of Neer hemiarthroplasty and total shoulder arthroplasty in patients aged 50 years or younger. *J Shoulder Elbow Surg* 2004;13:604–613.
15. Walch G, Boulahia A, Boileau P, et al. Primary glenohumeral osteoarthritis: clinical and radiographic classification. The Aequalis Group. *Acta Orthop Belgica* 1998;64(suppl 2):46–52.
16. Cofield RH. Total shoulder arthroplasty with the Neer prosthesis. *J Bone Joint Surg Am* 1984;66:899–906.
17. Deshmukh AV, Koris M, Zurakowski D, et al. Total shoulder arthroplasty: long-term survivorship, functional outcome, and quality of life. *J Shoulder Elbow Surg* 2005;14:471–479.
18. Chin PY, Sperling JW, Cofield RH, et al. Complications of total shoulder arthroplasty: are they fewer or different? *J Shoulder Elbow Surg* 2006;15:19–22.
19. Cofield RH, Chang W, Sperling JW. Complications of shoulder arthroplasty. In: Iannotti JP, Williams GR, editors. *Disorders of the Shoulder: Diagnosis and Management*. Philadelphia: Lippincott Williams & Wilkins; 1999:571–193.
20. Jain NB, Pietrobon R, Hocker S, et al. The relationship between surgeon and hospital volume and outcomes for shoulder arthroplasty. *J Bone Joint Surg Am* 2004;86:496–505.
21. Brems JJ. Complications of shoulder arthroplasty: infections, instability, and loosening. *Instr Course Lect* 2002;51:29–39.
22. Hasan SS, Leith JM, Campbell B, et al. Characteristics of unsatisfactory shoulder arthroplasties. *J Shoulder Elbow Surg* 2002;11:431–441.
23. Wirth MA, Rockwood CA. Complications of total shoulder-replacement arthroplasty. *J Bone Joint Surg Am* 1996;78:603–616.
24. Dines JS, Fealy S, Strauss EJ, et al. Outcomes analysis of revision total shoulder replacement. *J Bone Joint Surg Am* 2006;88:1494–500.
25. Kelly JD Jr, Norris TR. Decision making in glenohumeral arthroplasty. *J Arthroplasty* 2003;18:75–82.
26. Petersen SA, Hawkins RJ. Revision of failed total shoulder arthroplasty. *Orthop Clin North Am* 1998;29:519–533.
27. Ali F, Wilkinson JM, Cooper JR, et al. Accuracy of joint aspiration for the preoperative diagnosis of infection in total hip arthroplasty. *J Arthroplasty* 2006;21:221–226.
28. Schmalzried T. The infected hip: telltale signs and treatment options. *J Arthroplasty* 2006;21(suppl 1):97–100.
29. Trail IA, Nuttall D. The results of shoulder arthroplasty in patients with rheumatoid arthritis. *J Bone Joint Surg Br* 2002;84:1121–1125.
30. Zimmerli W, Trampuz A, Ochsner PE. Prosthetic-joint infections. *N Engl J Med* 2004;14: 1645–1654.
31. Zuckerman JD, Shapiro JA, Moghtaderi S, et al. Fatigue failure of a shoulder hemiarthroplasty stem: a case report. *J Shoulder Elbow Surg* 2003;12:635–636.
32. Franta AK, Lenters TR, Mounce D, et al. The complex characteristics of 282 unsatisfactory shoulder arthroplasties. *J Shoulder Elbow Surg* 2007;16:555–562.
33. Sallay PI, Reed L. The measurement of normative American Shoulder and Elbow Surgeons scores. *J Shoulder Elbow Surg* 2003;12:622–627.
34. Constant CR, Murley AGH. A clinical method of functional assessment of the shoulder. *Clin Orthop Rel Res* 1987;214:160–164.
35. Lippitt SB, Harryman DT, Matsen FA. A practical tool for evaluating function: the simple shoulder test. In: Matsen FA III, Fu FH, Hawkins RJ, eds. *The Shoulder: A Balance of Mobility and Stability*. Rosemont, Ill: American Academy of Orthopaedic Surgeons; 1993: 501–518.
36. Ellman H, Kay SP. Arthroscopic subacromial decompression for chronic impingement: 2- to 5-year results. *J Bone Joint Surg Br* 1991;73:395–398.
37. Post M. Constrained arthroplasty of the shoulder. *Orthop Clin North Am* 1987;18:455–462.
38. Wretenberg PF, Wallensten R. The Kessel total shoulder arthroplasty: a 13- to 16-year retrospective follow-up. *Clin Orthop Relat Res* 1999;365:100–103.
39. Kessel L, Bayley I. Prosthetic replacement of shoulder joint: preliminary communication. *J R Soc Med* 1979;72:748–752.
40. Bohsali KI, Wirth MA, Rockwood CA. Complications of total shoulder arthroplasty. *J Bone Joint Surg Am* 2006;88:2279–2292.
41. Lynch JR, Franta AK, Montgomery WH Jr, et al. Self-assessed outcome at 2 to 4 years after shoulder hemiarthroplasty with concentric glenoid reaming. *J Bone Joint Surg Am* 2007;89:1284–1292.
42. Neer CS. Neer hemiarthroplasty and Neer total shoulder arthroplasty in patients 50 years old or less: long-term results. *J Bone Joint Surg Am* 1998;80:464–473.
43. Clifford PE, Mallon WJ. Sports after total joint replacement. *Clin Sports Med* 2005;24: 175–186.
44. Healy WL, Iorio R, Lemos MJ. Athletic activity after joint replacement. *Am J Sports Med* 2001;29:377–388.
45. Jensen KL, Rockwood CA. Shoulder arthroplasty in recreational golfers. *J Shoulder Elbow Surg* 1998;7:362–367.
46. Jain NB, Guller U, Pietrobon R, et al. Comorbidities increase complication rates in patients having arthroplasty. *Clin Orthop Relat Res* 2005;435:232–238.
47. Thomas S, Price AJ, Sankey RA, et al. Shoulder hemiarthroplasty in patients with juvenile idiopathic arthritis. *J Bone Joint Surg Br* 2005;87:672–676.
48. Thomas SR, Wilson AJ, Chambler A, et al. Outcome of Copeland surface replacement shoulder arthroplasty. *J Shoulder Elbow Surg* 2005;14:485–491.
49. Collins DN, Harryman DT, Wirth MA. Shoulder arthroplasty for the treatment of inflammatory arthritis. *J Bone Joint Surg Am* 2004;86:2489–2496.
50. Lau MW, Blinder MA, Williams K, et al. Shoulder arthroplasty in sickle cell patients with humeral head avascular necrosis. *J Shoulder Elbow Surg* 2007;16:129–134.
51. Heyworth BE, Su EP, Figgie MP, et al. Orthopedic management of hemophilia. *Am J Orthop* 2005;34:479–486.
52. Luck JV, Silva M, Rodriguez-Merchan EC, et al. Hemophilic arthropathy. *J Am Acad Orthop Surg* 2004;12:234–245.
53. Simonetti S. Lesion of the anterior branch of axillary nerve in a patient with hereditary neuropathy with liability to pressure palsies. *Eur J Neurol* 2000;7:577–579.
54. Crowther MA, Bell SN. Neuropathic shoulder in syringomyelia treated with resurfacing arthroplasty of humeral head and soft-tissue lining of glenoid: a case report. *J Shoulder Elbow Surg* 2007;16:e38–40.
55. Andrews LR, Cofield RH, O'Driscoll SW. Shoulder arthroplasty in patients with prior mastectomy for breast cancer. *J Shoulder Elbow Surg* 2000;9:386–388.
56. Ambrosio F, Boninger ML, Souza AL, et al. Biomechanics and strength of manual wheelchair users. *J Spinal Cord Med* 2005;28:407–414.
57. Garreau De Loubresse C, Norton MR, et al. Replacement arthroplasty in the weight-bearing shoulder of paraplegic patients. *J Shoulder Elbow Surg* 2004;13:369–372.
58. Iannotti JP, Norris TR. Influence of preoperative factors on outcome of shoulder arthroplasty for glenohumeral osteoarthritis. *J Bone Joint Surg Am* 2003;85:251–258.
59. Stern SH, Insall JN, Windsor RE, et al. Total knee arthroplasty in patients with psoriasis. *Clin Orthop Relat Res* 1989;248:108–110; discussion 111.
60. Thomas P, Schuh A, Summer B, et al. Allergy toward bone cement. *Orthopäde* 2006;35:956, 958–960.
61. Antuna S, Sperling JW, Cofield RH. Reimplantation of a glenoid component after component removal and allograft bone grafting: a report of three cases. *J Shoulder Elbow Surg* 2002;11:637–641.

62. Antuna SA, Sperling JW, Cofield RH, et al. Glenoid revision surgery after total shoulder arthroplasty. *J Shoulder Elbow Surg* 2001;10:217–224.

63. Cofield RH. Bone grafting for glenoid bone deficiencies in shoulder arthritis: a review. *J Shoulder Elbow Surg* 2007;16:S273–281.

64. Cofield RH. Revision procedures in shoulder arthroplasty. In: Morrey BF, editor. *Reconstructive Surgery of the Joints.* 2nd ed. New York: Churchill Livingstone; 1996:789.

65. Gagey O, Pourjamasb B, Court C. Revision arthroplasty of the shoulder for painful glenoid loosening: a series of 14 cases with acromial prostheses reviewed at 4-year follow up [in French]. *Rev Chir Orthop Reparatrice Appar Mot* 2001;87:221–228.

66. Hopkins AR, Hansen UN, Amis AA, et al. The effects of glenoid component alignment variations on cement mantle stresses in total shoulder arthroplasty. *J Shoulder Elbow Surg* 2004;13:668–675.

67. Sperling JW, Antuna SA, Sanchez-Sotelo J, et al. Shoulder arthroplasty for arthritis after instability surgery. *J Bone Joint Surg Am* 2002;84:1775–1781.

68. Baumgarten KM, Lashgari CJ, Yamaguchi K. Glenoid resurfacing in shoulder arthroplasty: indications and contraindications. *Instr Course Lect* 2004;53:3–11.

69. Sperling JW, Cofield RH, Steinmann SP. Shoulder arthroplasty for osteoarthritis secondary to glenoid dysplasia. *J Bone Joint Surg Am* 2002;8:541–546.

70. Matsoukis J, Tabib W, Guiffault P, et al. Primary unconstrained shoulder arthroplasty in patients with a fixed anterior glenohumeral dislocation. *J Bone Joint Surg Am* 2006;88:547–552.

71. Matsoukis J, Tabib W, Guiffault P, et al. Shoulder arthroplasty for osteoarthritis after prior surgery for anterior instability: a report of 27 cases [in French]. Rev *Chir Orthop Reparatrice Appar Mot* 2003;89:580–592.

72. Matsoukis J, Tabib W, Mandelbaum A, et al. Shoulder arthroplasty for nonoperated anterior shoulder instability with secondary osteoarthritis [in French]. *Rev Chir Orthop Reparatrice Appar Mot* 2003;89:7–18.

73. Mileti J, Sperling JW, Cofield RH. Shoulder arthroplasty for the treatment of postinfectious glenohumeral arthritis. *J Bone Joint Surg Am* 2003;85:609–614.

74. Iannotti JP, Spencer EE, Winter U, et al. Prosthetic positioning in total shoulder arthroplasty. *J Shoulder Elbow Surg* 2005;14(1 suppl S):111S–121S.

75. Grammont P, Trouilloud P, Laffay J, et al. Etude et réalisation d'une nouvelle prothèse d'épaule. *Rhumatologie* 1987;39:407–418.

76. Bernard L, Lübbeke A, Stern R, et al. Value of preoperative investigations in diagnosing prosthetic joint infection: retrospective cohort study and literature review. *Scand J Infect Dis* 2004;36:410–416.

77. Bhatia BD, Basu S. Newer diagnostic tests for bacterial diseases. *Indian J Pediatr* 2007;74: 673–677.

78. Boileau P, Krishnan SG, Tinsi L, et al. Tuberosity malposition and migration: reasons for poor outcomes after hemiarthroplasty for displaced fractures of the proximal humerus. *J Shoulder Elbow Surg* 2002;11:401–412.

79. Cooper RA, Brems JJ. Recurrent disassembly of a modular humeral prosthesis: a case report. *J Arthroplasty* 1991;6:375–377.

80. Levy O, Copeland SA. Rotational dissociation of glenoid components in total shoulder prosthesis: an indication that sagittal torque forces may be important in glenoid component. *J Shoulder Elbow Surg* 1999;8:279–280.

81. Castro WHM, Jerosh J, Grossman TW. *Examination and Diagnosis of Musculoskeletal Disorders: Clinical Examination, Imaging Modalities.* Stuttgart: Georg Thieme Verlag; 2001:1–74.

82. Ince A, Seemann K, Frommelt L, et al. One-stage exchange shoulder arthroplasty for periprosthetic infection. *J Bone Joint Surg Br* 2005;87:814–818.

83. Sperling JW, Kozak T, Hanssen AD, et al. Infection after shoulder arthroplasty. *Clin Orthop Rel Res* 2001;382:206–216.

84. Buckingham BP, Parsons IM, Campbell B, et al. Patient functional self-assessment in late glenoid component failure at 3 to 11 years after total shoulder arthroplasty. *Shoulder Elbow Surg* 2005;14:368–374.

85. Lübbeke A, Stern R, Garavaglia G, et al. Differences in outcomes of obese women and men undergoing primary total hip arthroplasty. *Arthritis Rheum* 2007;15;57:327–334.

86. Schwemmer U, Papenfuss T, Greim C, et al. Ultrasound-guided interscalene brachial plexus anaesthesia: differences in success between patients of normal and excessive weight. *Ultraschall Med* 2006;27:245–250.

87. Hockman DE, Lucas GL, Roth CA. Role of the coracoacromial ligament as restraint after shoulder hemiarthroplasty. *Clin Orthop Relat Res* 2004;419:80–82.

88. Harryman DT, Sidles JA, Harris SL, et al. The effect of articular conformity and the size of the humeral head component on laxity and motion after glenohumeral arthroplasty: a study in cadavers. *J Bone Joint Surg Am* 1995;77:555–563.

89. Goutallier D, Postel JM, Bernageau J, et al. Fatty muscle degeneration in cuff ruptures: pre- and postoperative evaluation by CT scan. *Clin Orthop Relat Res* 1994;304:78–83.

90. Bishop JY, Sprague M, Gelber J, et al. Interscalene regional anesthesia for shoulder surgery. *J Bone Joint Surg Am* 2005;87:974–979.

91. Becker R, Pap G, Machner A, et al. Strength and motion after hemiarthroplasty in displaced four-fragment fracture of the proximal humerus: 27 patients followed for 1 to 6 years. *Acta Orthop Scand* 2002;73:44–49.

92. Gerber C, Hersche O, Farron A. Isolated rupture of the subscapularis tendon: results of operative repair. *J Bone Joint Surg Am* 1996;78:1015–1023.

93. Barth JR, Burkhart SS, De Beer JF. The bear-hug test: a new and sensitive test for diagnosing a subscapularis tear. *Arthroscopy* 2006;22:1076–1084.

94. Oosterom R, Herder JL, van der Helm FC, et al. Translational stiffness of the replaced shoulder joint. *J Biomech* 2003;36:1897–1907.

95. Orfaly RM, Rockwood CA Jr, et al. A prospective functional outcome study of shoulder arthroplasty for osteoarthritis with an intact rotator cuff. *J Shoulder Elbow Surg* 2003;12: 214–221.

96. Bryant D, Litchfield R, Sandow M, et al. A comparison of pain, strength, range of motion, and functional outcomes after hemiarthroplasty and total shoulder arthroplasty in patients with osteoarthritis of the shoulder: a systematic review and meta-analysis. *J Bone Joint Surg Am* 2005;87:1947–1956.

97. Haines JF, Trail IA, Nuttall D, et al. The results of arthroplasty in osteoarthritis of the shoulder. *J Bone Joint Surg Br* 2006;88:496–501.

98. Plausinis D, Greaves C, Regan WD, et al. Ipsilateral shoulder and elbow replacements: on the risk of periprosthetic fracture. *Clin Biomech (Bristol, Avon)* 2005;20:1055–1063.

99. Prakash U, McGurty DW, Dent JA. Hemiarthroplasty for severe fractures of the proximal humerus. *J Shoulder Elbow Surg* 2002;11:428–430.

100. Topolski MS, Chin PY, Sperling JW, et al. Revision shoulder arthroplasty with positive intraoperative cultures: the value of preoperative studies and intraoperative histology. *J Shoulder Elbow Surg* 2006;15:402–406.

101. Jerosch J, Schneppenheim M. Management of infected shoulder replacement. *Arch Orthop Trauma Surg* 2003;123:209–214.

102. Spangehl MJ, Masri BA, O'Connell JX, et al. Prospective analysis of preoperative and intraoperative investigations for the diagnosis of infection at the sites of 202 revision total hip arthroplasties. *J Bone Joint Surg Am* 1999;81:672–683.

103. Trampuz A, Hanssen AD, Osmon DR, et al. Synovial fluid leukocyte count and differential for the diagnosis of prosthetic knee infection. *Am J Med* 2004;117:556–562.

104. Trampuz A, Steckelberg JM, Osmon DR, et al Advances in the laboratory diagnosis of prosthetic joint infection. *Rev Med Microbiol* 2003;14:1–14.

105. Banit DM, Kaufer H, Hartford JM. Intraoperative frozen section analysis in revision total joint arthroplasty. *Clin Orthop Relat Res* 2002;401:230–238.

106. Pandey R, Drakoulakis E, Athanasou NA. An assessment of the histological criteria used to diagnose infection in hip revision arthroplasty tissues. *J Clin Pathol* 1999;52:118–123.

107. Panousis K, Grigoris P, Butcher I, et al. Poor predictive value of broad-range PCR for the detection of arthroplasty infection in 92 cases. *Acta Orthop* 2005;76:341–346.

108. Trampuz A, Piper KE, Jacobson MJ, et al. Sonification of removed hip and knee prostheses for diagnosis of infection. *N Engl J Med* 2007;357:654–663.

109. Looney RJ, Schwarz EM, Boyd A, et al. Periprosthetic osteolysis: an immunologist's update. *Curr Opin Rheumatol* 2006;18:80–87.

110. Mabrey JD, Afsar-Keshmiri A, Engh GA, et al. Standardized analysis of UHMWPE wear particles from failed total joint arthroplasties. *J Biomed Mater Res* 2002;63:475–483.

111. Purdue PE, Koulouvaris P, Potter HG, et al. The cellular and molecular biology of periprosthetic osteolysis. *Clin Orthop Relat Res* 2007;454:251–261.

112. Boardman ND, Cofield RH. Neurologic complications of shoulder surgery. *Clin Orthop Relat Res* 1999;368:44–53.

113. Lynch NM, Cofield RH, Silbert PL, et al. Neurologic complications after total shoulder arthroplasty. *J Shoulder Elbow Surg* 1996;5:53–61.

114. Nagda SH, Rogers KJ, Sestokas AK, et al. Neer Award 2005: peripheral nerve function during shoulder arthroplasty using intraoperative nerve monitoring. *J Shoulder Elbow Surg* 2007;16(3 suppl):S2–S8.

115. Green A, Norris TR. Imaging techniques for glenohumeral arthritis and glenohumeral arthroplasty. *Clin Orthop Relat Res* 1994;307:7–17.

116. Manicom O, Mseddi M, Karoubi M, et al. Radiographic diagnosis of dislocated inverted shoulder prosthesis: two cases of unrecognized dislocation [in French]. *Rev Chir Orthop Reparatrice Appar Mot* 2006;92:266–268.

117. Sisto DJ, France MP, Blazina ME, et al. Disassembly of a modular humeral prosthesis: a case report. *J Arthroplasty* 1993;8:653–655.

118. Havig MT, Kumar A, Carpenter W, et al. An in vitro assessment of radiolucent lines about the glenoid: a radiographic study. *J Bone Joint Surg Am* 1997;79:428–432.

119. Duranthon LD, Augereau B, Thomazeau H, et al. Bipolar arthroplasty in rotator cuff arthropathy: 13 cases [in French]. *Rev Chir Orthop Reparatrice Appar Mot* 2002;88:28–34.

120. Sperling JW, Cofield RH. Revision total shoulder arthroplasty for the treatment of glenoid arthrosis. *J Bone Joint Surg Am* 1998;80:860–867.

121. Radnay CS, Setter KJ, Chambers L, et al. Total shoulder replacement compared with humeral head replacement for the treatment of primary glenohumeral osteoarthritis: a systematic review. *J Shoulder Elbow Surg* 2007;16:396–402.

122. Churchill RS, Boorman RS, Fehringer EV, et al. Glenoid cementing may generate sufficient heat to endanger the surrounding bone. *Clin Orthop Relat Res* 2004;419:76–79.

123. Farron A, Terrier A, Buchler P. Risks of loosening of a prosthetic glenoid implanted in retroversion. *J Shoulder Elbow Surg* 2006;15:521–526.

124. Lazarus MD, Jensen KL, Southworth C, et al. The radiographic evaluation of keeled and pegged glenoid component insertion. *J Bone Joint Surg Am* 2002;84:1174–1182.

125. Phipatanakul WP, Norris TR. Treatment of glenoid loosening and bone loss due to osteolysis with glenoid bone grafting. *J Shoulder Elbow Surg* 2006;15:84–87.

126. Rahme H, Mattsson P, Larsson S. Stability of cemented all-polyethylene keeled glenoid components: radiostereometric study with a 2-year follow-up. *J Bone Joint Surg Br* 2004;86: 856–860.

127. Scarlat MM, Matsen FA. Observations on retrieved polyethylene glenoid components. *J Arthroplasty* 2001;16:795–801.

128. Williams GR, Abboud JA. Total shoulder arthroplasty: glenoid component design. *J Shoulder Elbow Surg* 2005;14(1 suppl S):122S–128S.

129. Boileau P, Avidor C, Krishnan SG, et al. Cemented polyethylene versus uncemented metal-backed glenoid components in total shoulder arthroplasty: a prospective, double-blind, randomized study. *J Shoulder Elbow Surg* 2002;11:351–359.

130. Martin SD, Zurakowski D, Thornhill TS. Uncemented glenoid component in total shoulder arthroplasty: survivorship and outcomes. *J Bone Joint Surg Am* 2005;87: 1284–1292.

131. Nyffeler RW, Meyer D, Sheikh R, et al. The effect of cementing technique on structural fixation of pegged glenoid components in total shoulder arthroplasty. *J Shoulder Elbow Surg* 2006;15:106–111.

132. Roche C, Angibaud L, Flurin PH, et al. Glenoid loosening in response to dynamic multi-axis eccentric loading: a comparison between keeled and pegged designs with an equivalent radial mismatch. *Bull Hosp Jt Dis* 2006;63:88–92.

133. Sperling JW, Cofield RH, O'Driscoll SW, et al. Radiographic assessment of ingrowth total shoulder arthroplasty. *J Shoulder Elbow Surg* 2000;9:507–513.

134. Neyton L, Walch G, Nove-Josserand L, et al. Glenoid corticocancellous bone grafting after glenoid component removal in the treatment of glenoid loosening. *J Shoulder Elbow Surg* 2006;15:173–179.
135. Torchia ME, Cofield RH. Long-term results of Neer total shoulder arthroplasty. *Orthop Trans* 1994;18:977.
136. Broström LÅ, Kronberg M, Wallensten R. Should the glenoid be replaced in shoulder arthroplasty with an unconstrained Dana or St. Georg prosthesis? *Ann Chir Gynaecol* 1992;81:54–57.
137. Gartsman GM, Elkousy HA, Warnock KM, et al. Radiographic comparison of pegged and keeled glenoid components. *J Shoulder Elbow Surg* 2005;14:252–257.
138. Nyffeler RW, Sheikh R, Jacob HA, et al. Influence of humeral prosthesis height on biomechanics of glenohumeral abduction: an in vitro study. *J Bone Joint Surg Am* 2004;86:575–580.
139. Lervick GN, Carroll RM, Levine WN. Complications after hemiarthroplasty for fractures of the proximal humerus. *Instr Course Lect* 2003;52:3–12.
140. Plausinis D, Kwon YW, Zuckerman JD. Complications of humeral head replacement for proximal humeral fractures. *Instr Course Lect* 2005;54:371–380.
141. Takase K, Yamamoto K, Imakiire A, et al. The radiographic study in the relationship of the glenohumeral joint. *J Orthop Res* 2004;22:298–305.
142. Weiner DS, Macnab I. Superior migration of the humeral head: a radiological aid in the diagnosis of tears of the rotator cuff. *J Bone Joint Surg Br* 1970;52:524–527.
143. Saupe N, Pfirrmann CW, Schmid MR, et al. Association between rotator cuff abnormalities and reduced acromiohumeral distance. *AJR Am J Roentgenol* 2006;187:376–382.
144. Thomas SR, Sforza G, Levy O, et al. Geometrical analysis of Copeland surface replacement shoulder arthroplasty in relation to normal anatomy. *J Shoulder Elbow Surg* 2005;14:186–192.
145. Pearl ML, Kurutz S. Geometric analysis of commonly used prosthetic systems for proximal humeral replacement. *J Bone Joint Surg Am* 1999;81:660–671.
146. Pearl ML. Proximal humeral anatomy in shoulder arthroplasty: implications for prosthetic design and surgical technique. *J Shoulder Elbow Surg* 2005;14(1 suppl S):99S–104S.
147. Hertel R, Knothe U, Ballmer FT. Geometry of the proximal humerus and implications for prosthetic design. *J Shoulder Elbow Surg* 2002;11:331–338.
148. Harding WG. The scapulohumeral line revisited. *Am J Orthop* 1999;28:313–315.
149. Matsen FA, Iannotti JP, Rockwood CA Jr. Humeral fixation by press-fitting of a tapered metaphyseal stem: a prospective radiographic study. *J Bone Joint Surg Am* 2003;85:304–308.
150. Sanchez-Sotelo J, O'Driscoll SW, Torchia ME, et al. Radiographic assessment of cemented humeral components in shoulder arthroplasty. *J Shoulder Elbow Surg* 2001;10:526–531.
151. Sanchez-Sotelo J, Wright TW, O'Driscoll SW, et al. Radiographic assessment of uncemented humeral components in total shoulder arthroplasty. *J Arthroplasty* 2001;16:180–187.
152. Mileti J, Boardman ND, Sperling JW, et al. Radiographic analysis of polyethylene glenoid components using modern cementing techniques. *J Shoulder Elbow Surg* 2004;13:492–498.
153. Amstutz HC, Thomas BJ, Kabo JM, et al. The Dana total shoulder arthroplasty. *J Bone Joint Surg Am* 1988;70:1174–182.
154. Klimkiewicz JJ, Iannotti JP, Rubash HE, et al. Aseptic loosening of the humeral component in total shoulder arthroplasty. *J Shoulder Elbow Surg* 1998;7:422–426.
155. Torchia ME, Cofield RH, Settergen CR. Total shoulder arthroplasty with the Neer prosthesis: long-term results. *J Shoulder Elbow Surg* 1997;6:495–505.
156. Fink B, Singer J, Lamla U, et al. Surface replacement of the humeral head in rheumatoid arthritis. *Arch Orthop Trauma Surg* 2004;124:366–373.
157. Moeckel BH, Altchek DW, Warren RF, et al. Instability of the shoulder after arthroplasty. *J Bone Joint Surg Am* 1993;75:492–497.
158. Sanchez-Sotelo J, Sperling JW, Rowland CM, et al. Instability after shoulder arthroplasty: results of surgical treatment. *J Bone Joint Surg Am* 2003;85:622–631.
159. Nyffeler RW, Jost B, Pfirrmann CW, et al. Measurement of glenoid version: conventional radiographs versus computed tomography scans. *J Shoulder Elbow Surg* 2003;12:493–496.
160. Nyffeler RW, Sheikh R, Atkinson TS, et al. Effects of glenoid component version on humeral head displacement and joint reaction forces: an experimental study. *J Shoulder Elbow Surg* 2006;15:625–629.
161. Spencer EE, Valdevit A, Kambic H, et al. The effect of humeral component anteversion on shoulder stability with glenoid component retroversion. *J Bone Joint Surg Am* 2005;87: 808–814.
162. Coste JS, Reig S, Trojani C, et al. The management of infection in arthroplasty of the shoulder. *J Bone Joint Surg Br* 2004;86:65–69.
163. An HS, Ebraheim N, Kim K, et al. Heterotopic ossification and pseudoarthrosis in the shoulder following encephalitis: a case report and review of the literature. *Clin Orthop Relat Res* 1987;219:291–298.
164. Kjaersgaard-Andersen P, Frich LH, Sõjbjerg JO, et al. Heterotopic bone formation following total shoulder arthroplasty. *J Arthroplasty* 1989;4:99–104.
165. Boyd AD, Thornhill TS, Barnes CL. Fractures adjacent to humeral prostheses. *J Bone Joint Surg Am* 1992;74:1498–504.
166. Kumar S, Sperling JW, Haidukewych GH, et al. Periprosthetic humeral fractures after shoulder arthroplasty. *J Bone Joint Surg Am* 2004;86:680–689.
167. McDonough EB, Crosby LA. Periprosthetic fractures of the humerus. *Am J Orthop* 2005;34:586–591.
168. Williams GR Jr, Iannotti JP. Management of periprosthetic fractures: the shoulder. *J Arthroplasty* 2002;17(4 suppl 1):14–16.
169. Worland RL, Kim DY, Arredondo J. Periprosthetic humeral fractures: management and classification. *J Shoulder Elbow Surg* 1999;8:590–594.
170. Kim DH, Clavert P, Warner JJ. Displaced periprosthetic humeral fracture treated with functional bracing: a report of two cases. *J Shoulder Elbow Surg* 2005;14:221–223.
171. Boileau P, Watkinson D, Hatzidakis AM, et al. Neer Award 2005: the Grammont reverse shoulder prosthesis—results in cuff tear arthritis, fracture sequelae, and revision arthroplasty. *J Shoulder Elbow Surg* 2006;15:527–540.
172. Boileau P, Watkinson DJ, Hatzidakis AM, et al. Grammont reverse prosthesis: design, rationale, and biomechanics. *J Shoulder Elbow Surg* 2005;14(1 suppl S):147S–161S.
173. De Wilde L, Mombert M, Van Petegem P, et al. Revision of shoulder replacement with a reversed shoulder prosthesis (Delta III): report of five cases. *Acta Orthop Belg* 2001;67: 348–353.
174. De Wilde L, Walch G. Humeral prosthetic failure of reversed total shoulder arthroplasty: a report of three cases. *J Shoulder Elbow Surg* 2006;15:260–264.
175. Delloye C, Joris D, Colette A, et al. Mechanical complications of total shoulder inverted prosthesis [in French]. *Rev Chir Orthop Reparatrice Appar Mot* 2002;88:410–414.
176. Frankle M, Siegal S, Pupello D, et al. The reverse shoulder prosthesis for glenohumeral arthritis associated with severe rotator cuff deficiency: a minimum 2-year follow-up study of 60 patients. *J Bone Joint Surg Am* 2005;87:1697–1705.
177. Guery J, Favard L, Sirveaux F, et al. Reverse total shoulder arthroplasty: survivorship analysis of 80 replacements followed for 5 to 10 years. *J Bone Joint Surg Am* 2006;88: 1742–1747.
178. McFarland EG, Sanguanjit P, Tasaki A, et al. The reverse shoulder prosthesis: a review of imaging features and complications. *Skeletal Radiol* 2006;35:488–496.
179. Simovitch RW, Zumstein MA, Lohri E, et al. Reverse total shoulder replacement predictors of scapular notching in patients managed with the Delta III. *J Bone Joint Surg Am* 2007;89: 588–600.
180. Sirveaux F, Favard L, Oudet D, et al. Grammont inverted total shoulder arthroplasty in the treatment of glenohumeral osteoarthritis with massive rupture of the cuff: results of a multicentre study of 80 shoulders. *J Bone Joint Surg Br* 2004;86:388–395.
181. Wall B, Nové-Josserand L, O'Connor DP, et al. Reverse total shoulder arthroplasty: a review of results according to etiology. *J Bone Joint Surg Am* 2007;89:1476–1485.
182. Werner CM, Steinmann PA, Gilbart M, et al. Treatment of painful pseudoparesis due to irreparable rotator cuff dysfunction with the Delta III reverse-ball-and-socket total shoulder prosthesis. *J Bone Joint Surg Am* 2005;87:1476–1486.
183. Karelse A, Kegels L, De Wilde L. The pillars of the scapula. *Clin Anat* 2007;20:392–399.
184. Nyffeler RW, Werner CM, Simmen BR, et al. Analysis of a retrieved Delta III total shoulder prosthesis. *J Bone Joint Surg Br* 2004;86:1187–1191.
185. Pressel T, Lengsfeld M, Leppek R, et al. Bone remodelling in humeral arthroplasty: follow-up using CT imaging and finite element modeling—an in vivo case study. *Arch Orthop Trauma Surg* 2000;120:333–335.
186. Sofka CM, Adler RS. Original report: sonographic evaluation of shoulder arthroplasty. *AJR Am J Roentgenol* 2003;180:1117–1120.
187. Yiang EH, Werner CM, Nyffeler RW, et al. Radiographic and computed tomography analysis of cemented pegged polyethylene glenoid components in total shoulder replacement. *J Bone Joint Surg Am* 2005;87:1928–1936.
188. Buckwalter KA, Parr JA, Choplin RH, et al. Multichannel CT imaging of orthopedic hardware and implants. *Semin Musculoskelet Radiol* 2006;10:86–97.
189. Naraghi AM, White LM. Magnetic resonance imaging of joint replacements. *Semin Musculoskelet Radiol* 2006;10:98–106.
190. Potter HG, Foo LF. Magnetic resonance imaging of joint arthroplasty. *Orthop Clin North Am* 2006;37:361–73,vi–vii.
191. Sperling JW, Potter HG, Craig EV, et al. Magnetic resonance imaging of painful shoulder arthroplasty. *J Shoulder Elbow Surg* 2002;11:315–321.
192. Itasaka T, Kawai A, Sato T, et al. Diagnosis of infection after total hip arthroplasty. *J Orthop Sci* 2001;6:320–326.
193. Iyengar KP, Vinjamuri S. Role of ^{99m}Tc Sulesomab in the diagnosis of prosthetic joint infections. *Nucl Med Commun* 2005;26:489–496.
194. Scher DM, Pak K, Lonner JH, et al. The predictive value of indium-111 leukocyte scans in the diagnosis of infected total hip, knee, or resection arthroplasties. *J Arthroplasty* 2000;15: 295–300.
195. Wolf G, Aigner RM, Schwarz T, et al. Localization and diagnosis of septic endoprosthesis infection by using ^{99m}Tc-HMPAO labelled leucocytes. *Nucl Med Commun* 2003;24:23–28.
196. Ivancevic V, Perka C, Hasart O, et al. Imaging of low-grade bone infection with a technetium-99m labelled monoclonal anti-NCA-90 Fab' fragment in patients with previous joint surgery [erratum appears in *Eur J Nucl Med Mol Imaging* 2002;29:835]. *Eur J Nucl Med Mol Imaging* 2002;29:547.
197. Kraemer WJ, Saplys R, Waddell JP, et al. Bone scan, gallium scan, and hip aspiration in the diagnosis of infected total hip arthroplasty. *J Arthroplasty* 1993;8:611–616.
198. Kaisidis A, Megas P, Apostolopoulos D, et al. Diagnosis of septic loosening of hip prosthesis with LeukoScan: SPECT scan with ^{99m}Tc-labeled monoclonal antibodies. *Orthopäde* 2005;34:462.
199. Ingui CJ, Shah NP, Oates ME. Infection scintigraphy: added value of single-photon emission computed tomography/computed-tomography fusion compared with traditional analysis. *J Comput Assist Tomogr* 2007;31:375–380.
200. Delank KS, Schmidt M, Michael JW, et al. The implications of 18F-FDG PET for the diagnosis of endoprosthetic loosening and infection in hip and knee arthroplasty: results from a prospective, blinded study. *BMC Musculoskelet Disord* 2006;3:20.
201. Mumme T, Reinartz P, Alfer J, et al. Diagnostic values of positron emission tomography versus triple-phase bone scan in hip arthroplasty loosening. *Arch Orthop Trauma Surg* 2005;125:322–329.
202. Love C, Marwin SE, Tomas MB, et al. Diagnosing infection in the failed joint replacement: a comparison of coincidence detection 18F-FDG and 111In-labeled leukocyte/99mTc-sulfur colloid marrow imaging. *J Nucl Med* 2004;45:1864–1871.
203. Reinartz P, Mumme T, Hermanns B, et al. Radionuclide imaging of the painful hip arthroplasty: positron-emission tomography versus triple-phase bone scanning. *J Bone Joint Surg Br* 2005;87:465–470.
204. Hersch JC, Dines DM. Arthroscopy for failed shoulder arthroplasty. *Arthroscopy* 2000;16: 606–612.
205. O'Driscoll SW, Petrie RS, Torchia ME. Arthroscopic removal of the glenoid component for failed total shoulder arthroplasty: a report of five cases. *J Bone Joint Surg Am* 2005;87: 858–863.

Todd J. Kowalski
Elie F. Berbari
Douglas R. Osmon

Medical Evaluation and Treatment for Infection in Shoulder Arthroplasty

INTRODUCTION

Shoulder arthroplasty infection presents diagnostic and therapeutic challenges. Complex factors must be considered when approaching a patient suspected or proven to have shoulder arthroplasty infection. Such patients are best approached in a multidisciplinary fashion, often benefiting from the input and care of orthopedic, infectious disease, and internal medicine physicians, physical and occupational therapists, and, in select circumstances, other subspecialists. The medical evaluation and treatment for shoulder arthroplasty infection involves (a) diagnostic evaluations, (b) assessing local and systemic host factors, (c) antimicrobial and surgical therapy, (d) outcome monitoring, and (e) prevention. Surgical management strategies and options are directly influenced by medical factors (e.g., host factors may limit surgical options). Conversely, the surgical treatment strategy chosen largely dictates the antimicrobial therapeutics applied in any specific situation. Hence, cooperative management is essential to optimizing outcomes.

ESTABLISH THE DIAGNOSIS

Ideally, the diagnosis of shoulder arthroplasty infection and the microbiological etiology of the infection can be confirmed before any surgical intervention. This facilitates optimal surgical and perioperative antimicrobial planning during and immediately after the procedure. Several diagnostic modalities assist in establishing the diagnosis. First one relies on the history and physical examination of the patient. Key aspects of the history include assessment of functional status of the patient; joint prosthesis history, including type of prior prostheses; date of prior joint prosthesis placement; perioperative wound healing problems and other perioperative complications; and the use of antimicrobial-impregnated material to fixate the prosthesis, because this may have an impact on subsequent antimicrobial resistance patterns and yield of intraoperative cultures.[1,2] In addition the results of previous joint aspiration cultures, imaging studies, and the type and duration of any previously administered systemic antimicrobial therapy should be identified.[3,4] Lastly, the patient should be asked about any possible sources of hematogenous seeding of the prosthesis, such as any recent infections (e.g., pneumonia) and risk factors for unusual pathogens (such as the use of immunosuppressant medications or exposure to organisms such as *Mycobacterium tuberculosis*).

Symptom duration and nature (e.g., nocturnal, with activity, etc.), assessment of systemic symptoms (e.g., fevers, chills, night sweats) and the presence of any concomitant or recent localizing infection are also crucial. Pain (95%), stiffness (38%), and fever (22%) are clinical symptoms in patients with shoulder arthroplasty infection but nonspecific.[5] In one series, notable physical examination findings included a draining sinus (47%), shoulder erythema (38%), and effusion (34%).[5] Except for pain, all of the signs and symptoms of shoulder arthroplasty infection occur in fewer than 50% of patients, particularly in patients diagnosed with intraoperative cultures after revision shoulder arthroplasty.[4] This highlights the need to have a high index of suspicion for infection in shoulder arthroplasty patients who present with only persistent discomfort, particularly when there is not an obvious mechanical reason for the discomfort.

Laboratory values are frequently used but are often of limited value in establishing the diagnosis. Erythrocyte sedimentation rates (ESR) and leukocyte counts lack diagnostic sensitivity and specificity. In one series they were elevated in 14 of 24 (58%) and 2 of 29 patients (7%), respectively.[5] Therefore one should not be dissuaded from the diagnosis of shoulder arthroplasty infection in a suggestive clinical setting because of normal laboratory values. C-reactive protein (CRP) may be more sensitive for prosthetic joint infection than ESR,[6] though it too suffers from nonspecificity. To maximize diagnostic sensitivity, we typically obtain both ESR and CRP values when assessing patients for prosthetic joint infection because there is occasionally discordance between tests.

A variety of imaging studies have been used in diagnosing shoulder arthroplasty infection. Plain radiographs should always be obtained and may show evidence of loosening, dislocation, or associated osteomyelitis[7] but suffer from poor sensitivity and specificity. Aseptic loosening cannot easily be distinguished from septic loosening. Radionuclide studies may be helpful. Technetium-99 bone scan is a highly sensitive but nonspecific test for prosthetic joint infection in patients with total knee arthroplasties.[8] Limited information on accuracy in infected shoulder arthroplasty exists. In two series of shoulder arthroplasty infection combined, 12 of 22 scans were positive, 6 of 22 equivocal, and 4 of 22 normal among patients with proven infection.[5,9] The specificity of the scans for prosthetic joint infection is increased by leukocyte labeling methodology (i.e., indium-labeled white blood cell scan).[8] If the diagnosis remains in doubt despite clinical, laboratory, and radiographic assessment, indium-labeled white blood cell scans may provide useful information.

A synovial fluid total leukocyte count greater than 1.7 × 10^9/L and neutrophil percent greater than 65% have been shown recently to be very sensitive and specific in identifying chronic total knee arthroplasty infection.[10,11] Of interest, to achieve this excellent sensitivity and specificity a much lower cutoff for the presence of infection is used compared to that in native joint septic arthritis. Recent data from the Mayo Clinic, however, suggest that the same is not true for the sensitivity of these tests in diagnosing total shoulder arthroplasty infection because synovial fluid leukocyte counts and differentials were not predictive of infection.[12]

Establishing a pathogen is crucial in confirming the diagnosis of shoulder arthroplasty infection. Knowledge of the microbiology of the infection before surgical intervention aids in choosing an appropriate antimicrobial agent with which to impregnate cement spacers or other local antimicrobial delivery devices (if applicable) and allows appropriate postoperative antimicrobials to be initiated. Preoperative pathogen identification may also affect decision making when choosing a surgical strategy. Therefore preoperative joint aspiration to identify a pathogen is warranted when shoulder arthroplasty infection is suspected. In hip and knee prosthetic joint infection, a positive culture from a preoperative joint aspiration is only moderately sensitive (55% to 86%) but quite specific (94% to 96%).[8] Considering five studies in shoulder arthroplasty infection, 33 of 50 (66%) preoperative joint aspirations were positive.[5,13–16] Unfortunately, this number is significantly less (1 of 11, 9%) in patients diagnosed with shoulder arthroplasty infection after revision surgery with intraoperative cultures.[4] Obtaining adequate samples, culturing for both aerobic and anaerobic organisms, and, in select circumstances, fungi, mycobacterium, and other atypical organisms may maximize aspirate culture yields. We recommend cultures for fungi and mycobacterial species if prior aspirates or surgical specimens have been unrevealing but infection is suspected or if epidemiological factors place patients at higher risk for atypical infectious organisms (e.g., patient with advanced immunosuppression, patients with history of latent tuberculosis, etc.). Of importance, patients should be off of antimicrobials, ideally for at least 14 days before joint aspiration if clinically feasible. to maximize culture yield.[17]

Patients undergoing surgery for possible shoulder arthroplasty infection should have intraoperative samples obtained for culture. Although the optimal number of tissue specimens to obtain for aerobic and anaerobic culture is unknown, at least three and up to six have been recommended to diagnose total hip arthroplasty and total knee arthroplasty infection.[1] Obtaining this number of specimens potentially prevents sampling error and can prove useful in interpreting the pathological importance of a single positive culture of a common skin commensal. This is of particular importance in shoulder arthroplasty infection, because the most common pathogens (coagulase-negative staphylococci and *Propionibacterium* species) are common skin commensals and laboratory contaminants.[4,5] To optimize yield, anaerobic cultures should be obtained and observed for at least 7 days. Fungal and mycobacterial cultures should be performed in select circumstances, including in immunocompromised patients, patients with multiple prior shoulder surgeries, and if initial cultures are negative.

A recent report suggests culture yield may be enhanced by sonicating and then culturing removed prostheses, particularly if patients had received recent antimicrobial therapy.[17] Other newer microbiological approaches such as immunofluorescence microscopy, 16S rRNA amplification, and species-specific polymerase chain reaction have shown promise to increase diagnostic yield even greater, but remain largely investigational at this time.[18]

Histopathology can provide useful information regarding the presence or absence of infection in culture-negative cases[19,20] and may suggest the presence of an atypical organism if granulomatous inflammation is discovered or specific tissue stains for mycobateria and fungi are performed and are positive. Demonstrating five neutrophils per high-power field from pathological specimens has been shown to be sensitive (82% to 84%) and specific (93% to 96%) in hip and knee prosthetic joint infection.[19–21] Limited data on the usefulness of histopathology in large unselected series of total shoulder arthroplasties undergoing revision are available. Shoulder arthroplasty infection diagnosed with intraoperative culture, however, rarely (7 of 73, 9%) is diagnosed using intraoperative frozen section results.[4]

DEFINING THE HOST

It is essential to define the general medical status of the host, including fitness to undergo one or more surgical interventions. The presence and severity of cardiovascular disease, pulmonary disease, malignancy, and other comorbid conditions affect patients' ability to safely and successfully tolerate one or more surgical interventions. Therefore a thorough medical evaluation to assess the presence and severity of significant comorbid cardiovascular, pulmonary, and other pertinent disease processes that influence the overall health and functional status of the host should be performed. The baseline general functional status of the patient affects the goals of revision shoulder surgery. The presence of comorbid diseases or severely compromised functional status may dictate a different set of goals when approaching the treatment of shoulder arthroplasty infection. Subspecialist input from cardiology, internal medicine, pulmonary, and other areas may be appropriate to accurately gauge perioperative risk in select patients. After assessing these broad medical factors and determining the appropriateness of surgery in a given host, a thorough evaluation of host factors that increase the risk for recurrent infection or treatment failure is warranted.

Host risk factors for prosthetic joint infection include immunosuppression,[22] diabetes mellitus,[16] inflammatory skin conditions (e.g., psoriasis),[23] malignancy,[24] distant foci of infection,[16] malnutrition,[16] prior revisions and infections,[24] and high National Nosocomial Infections Surveillance (NNIS) scores.[24,25] The presence of one or more of these risk factors modifies the probability of successful outcomes. The underlying original indication for which the patient received the shoulder arthroplasty is also of importance. Rheumatoid arthritis, prior native joint septic arthritis, and prior arthroplasty have been implicated as risk factors for treatment failure in hip and knee prosthetic joint infection.[24]

Immunosuppression, which may include regular use of corticosteroids or other immune-modulating medications, human immune deficiency virus (HIV) infection or recent chemotherapy, may have an impact on successful outcomes of prosthetic joint infection management. In some instances, reducing doses of immunosuppressive medications or treating the underlying condition can temporarily mitigate immunosuppression (e.g., diabetes mellitus, HIV infection). These interventions to boost the host's immune status should be attempted before elective surgery. Similarly, nutrition should be assessed and optimized in at-risk patients. Chronic skin conditions such as psoriasis may increase the risk of subsequent infection and should be aggressively optimized before elective revision surgery if possible. Occasionally, shoulder arthroplasty infection is related to systemic infection (e.g., infective endocarditis) or is accompanied by concomitant distant sites of infection. Therefore one should investigate for foci of infection distant to the shoulder arthroplasty by careful history and examination followed by focused diagnostic studies as indicated. Eradication of distant foci of infection should be completed before reimplanting a new shoulder prosthesis.

When assessing the host, one must consider the suspected duration of infection when considering treatment options. Longer duration of symptoms before diagnosis has been shown to be an independent risk factor for treatment failure in patients with hip and knee prosthetic joint infection treated with debridement and prosthesis retention.[26] Experience with hip and knee prosthesis infections suggests acute symptomatology of 10 to 14 days or less may be treated with prosthesis retention, although outcomes are still variable and dependent on host and microbiological factors. However, most cases of shoulder arthroplasty infection present late (>1 year after implantation) and rarely with acute symptomatology.[5] The presence of a sinus tract, also a marker of chronic infection, is an independent risk factor for treatment failure.[26] A final important factor in defining the host is assessing the patient's medication allergies and current medications. If patients are reported to be allergic to an antimicrobial agent, careful history to determine the nature of the reaction and review of supporting documentation helps clarify whether the allergy is "true" or not. Referral to an allergist can be helpful in defining these allergies.[27] Finally, some drug interactions need to be considered when choosing which antimicrobial agent to use because occasionally current medications need to be discontinued or an alternative antimicrobial drug chosen on these grounds.

After the host has been thoroughly assessed, the surgical risks considered, and modifiable risk factors addressed, surgical and attendant medical treatment plans can be established.

MEDICAL THERAPY OF SHOULDER ARTHROPLASTY INFECTION

Choosing and optimizing medical therapy for shoulder arthroplasty infection is dependent on the surgical treatment strategy to be employed. Resection arthroplasty and prosthesis reimplantation either at the time of resection (one-stage or direct exchange) or delayed (two-stage exchange), debridement and prosthesis retention, and resection arthroplasty represent surgical options for treatment. In addition to the overall fitness of the patient for surgical intervention and technical considerations (i.e., condition of bone stock, soft tissue envelope, etc.) that may influence surgical options, the etiological pathogen and antimicrobial susceptibilities, timing of infection onset after implantation, and duration of symptoms before diagnosis all have an impact on surgical and medical management strategies.

The microbiology of shoulder arthroplasty is similar to that of lower extremity prosthetic joint infection, with a notable exception. *Staphylococcus aureus* and coagulase-negative staphylococci cause the majority of infections in most reported series.[3,5,13,28,29] However, in contrast to lower extremity prosthetic joint infection, *Propionibacterium acnes,* an anaerobic gram-positive bacillus, is a relatively common cause of late shoulder arthroplasty infection, accounting for as much as 16% to 18% of infections.[5,12] Prosthetic joint infections caused by *Staphylococcus aureus* and aerobic gram-negative bacilli have been associated with increased risk of treatment failure.[26] Fungal prosthetic joint infection is rare, usually resulting from *Candida* species, and often requires resection arthroplasty with delayed reimplantation to achieve optimal results.[30] Therefore infections caused by *S. aureus,* gram-negative rods, or fungi warrant careful consideration before retaining the implant.

Shoulder arthroplasty infections usually present late with chronic symptoms. This limits the number of patients suitable for debridement and implant retention relative to lower extremity prosthetic joint infection. In lower extremity prosthetic joint infection, early-onset infections after implantation (<4 weeks) and acute hematogenous infections with short symptom duration (<10–14 days) are commonly treated with debridement and prosthesis retention, with variable results (18% to 83% infection free).[8] A similar approach has been recommended in shoulder arthroplasty infection.[28] However, there is scant published experience with outcomes of debridement and retention of shoulder arthroplasty.[5,13,28] Lower extremity *S. aureus* prosthetic joint infection treated with debridement and prosthesis retention commonly results in high rates of failure,[26] but outcomes may be better in patients with streptococcal prosthetic joint infection.[31] Published experience with resection arthroplasty with immediate implant replacement (one-stage or direct exchange) for shoulder arthroplasty infection is also limited. One-stage implant replacement is most commonly used in Europe for lower extremity prosthetic joint infection, and results have been encouraging, with failure rates of 0 to 25%.[8] Of 17 patients with shoulder arthroplasty infection treated with this strategy, 4 subsequently underwent resection arthroplasty for either reinfection (1), periprosthetic fracture (1), acromial pseudoarthrosis (1), or recurrent dislocation.[5,13,14] None of the remaining 13 patients were thought to have residual infection at last follow-up examination. Direct exchange is therefore an attractive strategy for patients whose general medical health or functional goals discourage multiple surgeries. Further experience, ideally in clinical trials, is necessary before advocating widespread use.

As in lower extremity prosthetic joint infection in the United States,[8] two-stage shoulder replacement arthroplasty has emerged as the preferred surgical modality to achieve optimal functional status in hosts with permissible general health and amenable bone stock and soft tissues.[3,5,9] Successful eradication of infection for lower extremity prosthetic joint infection is reported to be 87% for this strategy.[8] In shoulder arthroplasty infection, limited data suggest infection-free outcomes equivalent to those in resection arthroplasty but improved functional outcomes with two-stage reimplantation.[3,5,9] It is widely accepted to use antimicrobial-impregnated cement spacers in patients requiring a two-stage surgical strategy.[15,32] If the microbiology is known preoperatively, it is crucial to choose an antimicrobial agent with activity against the pathogen. If the antimicrobial agent is not tailored to the infecting organism, the cement may serve as a foreign body that hinders clearance of infection instead of an antimicrobial delivery device that assists in eradication. One should choose an antimicrobial agent to which the patient does not have an allergy and monitor for systemic toxicity, although adverse events occur rarely.[33]

Resection arthroplasty is typically used as a salvage procedure in patients with uncontrollable infections, the inability to tolerate multiple procedures, if bone stock and soft tissues are not conducive to two-stage reimplantation, or for persistent infection.[34,35] Infection is typically cured with this strategy, and pain is usually much improved also, but functional outcomes may be undesirable.[5,9,35] Figures 5.1 and 5.2 summarize the general approach to decision making in the medical assessment and treatment strategies involved in shoulder arthroplasty infection.

Organism-appropriate antimicrobial therapy is essential regardless of the surgical treatment strategy. Analogous to treatment in lower extremity prosthetic joint infection, prolonged intravenous therapy for at least 4 to 6 weeks is recommended. In some series, systemic antimicrobial therapy was reported to be less than 2 weeks,[14] and others treated for over 3 months[3] or until normalization of CRP.[35] Antimicrobial agents should be chosen based on the pathogen's susceptibility, host allergies, and ease of outpatient administration. Patient selection criteria and guidelines for monitoring prolonged outpatient parenteral antimicrobials are published.[36] Key components include regular physician and home health care nurse visits and at least weekly drug monitoring to evaluate for medication toxicity and response.[36] Infectious disease physicians experienced in outpatient parenteral antimicrobial therapy may provide useful assistance in choosing the most appropriate antimicrobial and monitoring for adverse events. Selected pathogen-specific antimicrobial recommendations are shown in Table 5.1.

Oral antimicrobial therapy has been used primarily as adjunctive therapy following prolonged parenteral treatment courses. The use of prolonged oral antimicrobial combinations that include rifampin and a quinolone have been shown to be effective in one small series of device-associated staphylococcal infections,[37] but data on the use of rifampin in shoulder arthroplasty infection are lacking. In cases of debridement and retention or single-stage exchange, rifampin is often used to enhance eradication of organisms in retained prosthetic biofilms.[37,38] Long term and in select circumstances, indefinite oral suppressive antimicrobial therapy is often used when implants are retained. In some instances the host may be too frail or refuse to undergo surgery, and in those instances suppressive antimicrobial therapy may provide symptomatic relief and prevent overt clinical signs and symptoms of infection in the absence of cure. Table 5.2 summarizes important information related to oral antimicrobials used for suppression.

In addition to systemic antimicrobial therapy, antimicrobials are commonly administered locally as a clinician-directed,

non–Food and Drug Administration (FDA)–approved application in antimicrobial-impregnated bone cement spacers or used for prosthesis fixation at the time of reimplantation. High local tissue concentrations of an antimicrobial agent can be achieved with this approach, delivered via antimicrobial-impregnated cement, polymethylmethacrylate (PMMA), or other spacer materials. In two-stage exchanges, spacers serve the additional role of maintaining soft tissue tension to facilitate reimplantation.[15,33] Experience in lower extremity prosthetic joint infection suggests benefit of local antimicrobial agent delivery in one- and two-stage exchanges.[8] Vancomycin and aminoglycosides are the most commonly used agents.[8] The FDA has approved a variety of aminoglycoside-impregnated antimicrobial bone cements for use at the time of the second-stage reimplantation for total joint replacement infection. A high rate of aminoglycoside resistance among staphylococcal prosthetic joint infection isolates has been reported.[39] It is unknown whether the high local tissue concentrations of aminoglycosides achieved with antibiotic-impregnated bone cement allows for effective prophylaxis and treatment of these aminoglycoside-resistant isolates.

In summary, local antimicrobial delivery is widely used as part of one- and two-stage exchange strategies in shoulder arthroplasty infection,[14,15,28,29] but further research as to its optimal use and potential limitations and toxicities is still needed.

OUTCOME ASSESSMENT AND PREVENTION

Assessing the outcome of the infection involves clinical, functional, laboratory, and, sometimes, pathology assessments. All patients should be assessed for resolution of systemic evidence of infection, as well as for functional abilities during follow-up. In patients who undergo a two-stage exchange strategy, intraoperative inspection, frozen pathology specimens, and the collection of at least three intraoperative aerobic and aerobic cultures at the time of reimplantation arthroplasty can provide useful information regarding the success of infection eradication that may influence either the decision to reimplant or subsequent antimicrobial therapy. ESR and CRP laboratory tests should also be obtained preoperatively and before reimplantation, although data on the utility of these tests to predict infection eradication are limited. CRP levels tend to drop sooner than ESR levels and tend to be more sensitive and specific for prosthetic joint infection.[6]

Systemic antimicrobial prophylaxis should be used at the time of reimplantation. Data recommending its use are extrapolated from data from total hip arthroplasty and total knee arthroplasty infection prevention.[40] Cefazolin is the agent recommended most commonly because of its activity against the common organisms causing infection and favorable toxicity profile. Optimal dosing, timing, and duration of systemic prophylaxis recently have been discussed elsewhere, and the interested reader is referred to these sources for an up-to-date discussion of this topic.[40,41]

The routine use of antibiotic-impregnated cement to prevent infection (other than in the setting of reimplantation arthroplasty following resection arthroplasty for prosthetic joint infection) is controversial. Use of antibiotic cement for this indication currently remains a clinician-directed, non-FDA

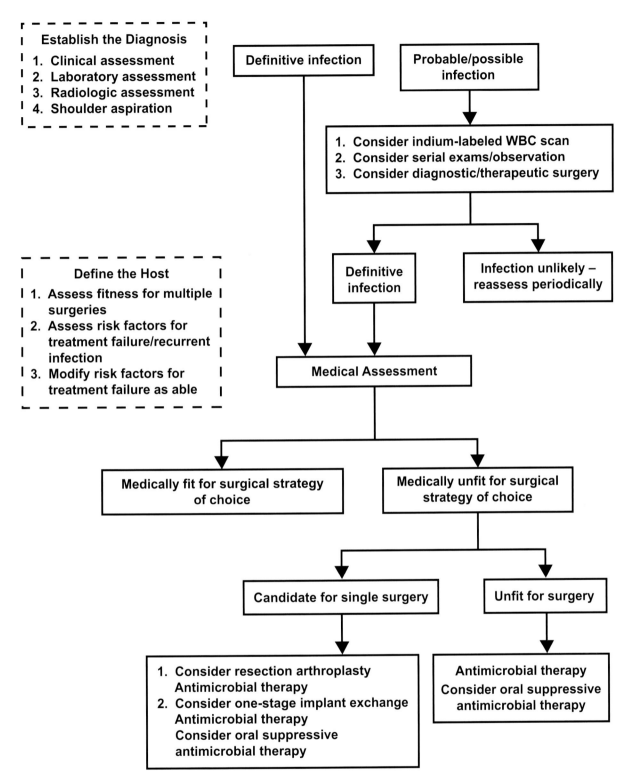

Figure 5.1.   Diagnosis and medical assessment in total shoulder arthroplasty infection.

approved, application. The advantages and disadvantages of using antibiotic-impregnated cement in this setting have recently been discussed. We agree with Jiranek et al[42] that low-dose antibiotic-loaded bone cement in primary or uninfected revision joint arthroplasty cannot be routinely recommended at this time because of issues regarding resistance and cost.

The use of antimicrobial prophylaxis to prevent hematogenous infection following high-risk procedures (e.g., dental extractions) to prevent reinfection of a shoulder arthroplasty is controversial. Current recommendations suggest patients with a high risk for prosthetic joint infection undergoing dental procedures with a high incidence of bacteremia (e.g., extractions,

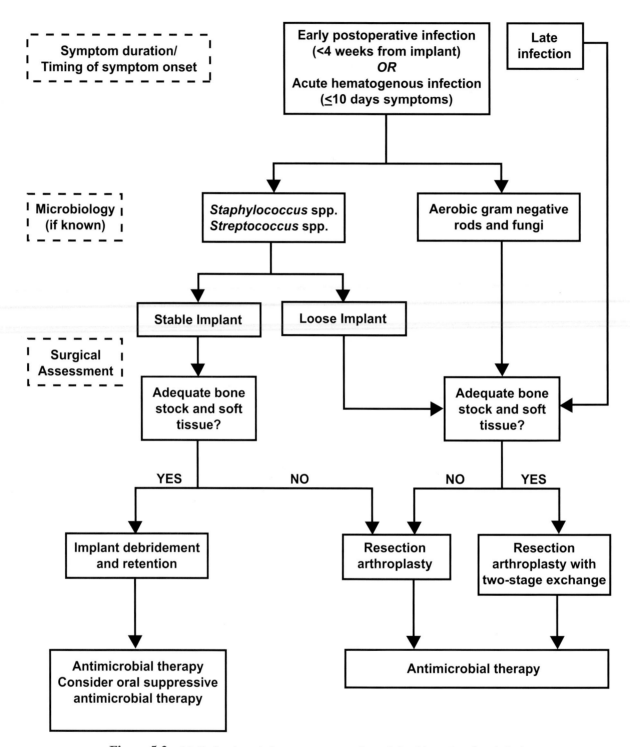

Figure 5.2.   Medical and surgical treatment strategy in total shoulder arthroplasty infection.

periodontal surgery, placement of dental implants, teeth cleaning with expected bleeding) should be considered to receive antimicrobial prophylaxis.[40,43] Amoxicillin or a first-generation cephalosporin, or clindamycin in patients allergic to penicillin, 1 hour before the procedure is recommended. Professional societies have also issued recommendations for patients undergoing endoscopy and urological procedures. Routine antimicrobial prophylaxis was not recommended.[44,45] Specific high-risk patients undergoing high-risk urological procedures may benefit from antimicrobial therapy.[40,44] Ampicillin and gentamicin, or ciprofloxacin, or levofloxacin in patients allergic to penicillin, were recommended. Guidelines for the prevention of infective endocarditis using antimicrobial prophylaxis, however, have recently undergone dramatic changes, and far fewer patients are

TABLE 5.1	Suggested Antimicrobial Treatment of Common Pathogens Causing Prosthetic Joint Infections	
Microorganism	First Choice[a]	Alternative[a]
Staphylococcus spp., oxacillin-susceptible	Nafcillin sodium 1.5–2 g IV q4h or cefazolin 1–2 g IV q8h	Vancomycin 15 mg/kg IV q12h or levofloxacin 500–750 mg PO or IV q24h + rifampin 300–450 mg PO q12h[b]
Staphylococcus spp., oxacillin-resistant	Vancomycin 15 mg/kg IV q12h	Linezolid 600 mg PO or IV q12h or daptomycin 6 mg/kg IV q24h or levofloxacin 500–750 mg PO or IV q24h + rifampin 300–450 mg PO q12h[b]
Enterococcus spp., penicillin-susceptible[c]	Aqueous crystalline penicillin G 24–30 million units IV q24h continuously or in six divided doses or ampicillin sodium, 12 g IV q24h continuously or in six divided doses	Vancomycin 15 mg/kg IV q12h
Enterococcus spp., penicillin-resistant[c]	Vancomycin, 15 mg/kg IV q12h	Linezolid 600 mg PO or IV q12h
Pseudomonas aeruginosa[d]	Cefepime 1–2 g IV q12h or meropenem 1 g IV q8h or imipenem 500 mg IV q6–8h	Ciprofloxacin 750 mg PO or 400 mg IV q12h or ceftazidime, 2 g IV q8h
Enterobacter spp.	Meropenem 1 g IV q8h or imipenem 500 mg IV q6–8h or ertapenem 1 g IV q24h	Cefepime 1–2 g IV q12h or ciprofloxacin 750 mg PO or 400 mg IV q12h
β-Hemolytic streptococci	Aqueous crystalline penicillin G, 20–24 million units IV q24h by continuous infusion or in six divided doses or ceftriaxone 1–2 g IV q24h	Vancomycin 15 mg/kg IV q12h
Propionibacterium acnes and Corynebacterium spp.	Aqueous crystalline penicillin G 20–24 million units IV q24h by continuous infusion or in six divided doses or ceftriaxone 1–2 g IV q24h or vancomycin 15 mg/kg IV q12h	Clindamycin 600–900 mg IV q8h

[a]Dose adjustment necessary for renal impairment assumes in vitro susceptibility and as known antibiotic allergies or intolerances.
[b]Levofloxacin-rifampin combination therapy for patients managed by debridement with retention. See reference regarding prolong duration of therapy.
[c]Addition of aminoglycoside for bactericidal synergy is optional. Considerations in choice of an agent are similar to those noted for treatment of enterococcal endocarditis.*
[d]Addition of an aminoglycoside is option.
*Baddour LM, Wilson WR, Bayer AS, et al. Infective endocarditis: diagnosis, antimicrobial therapy, and management of complications: a statement for healthcare professionals from the Committee on Rheumatic Fever, Endocarditis, and Kawasaki Disease, Council on Cardiovascular Disease in the Young, and the Councils on Clinical Cardiology, Stroke, and Cardiovascular Surgery and Anesthesia, American Heart Association. Endorsed by the Infectious Diseases Society of America. Circulation 2005;111:e394–e434.
Modified from Sia IG, Berbari EF, Karchmer AW. Prosthetic joint infections. Infect Dis Clin North Am 2005;19:885–914, with permission.

TABLE 5.2	Selected Side Effects and Considerations Regarding Antimicrobials of Potential Use for Chronic Suppressive Therapy
Antimicrobial	Long-Term Side Effects and Cautions
Minocycline	Photosensitivity, discoloration of skin; permanent discoloration of teeth when used in early childhood; drug-induced lupus erythematosus; dizziness, light-headedness, vertigo; rarely, pseudotumor cerebri; should not be taken with antacids or iron-containing preparations; caution with concurrent anticoagulant therapy; may decrease contraceptive efficacy
Trimethoprim-sulfamethoxazole	Myelosuppression; elevated creatinine; nephrotoxicity, crystalluria; possible disulfiram-like reactions; may enhance hypoglycemic effects of sulfonylureas
β-Lactam[a]	Antibiotic-associated diarrhea, pseudomembranous colitis; genital moniliasis; hepatic dysfunction
Rifampin	Orange discoloration of body secretions; hepatotoxicity; should not be used as monotherapy; significant drug-drug interactions; increased requirement for anticoagulant drugs; may decrease contraceptive efficacy
Fluoroquinolones	Phototoxicity; tendon rupture; very rarely, arrhythmia; may cause disturbances in blood glucose levels and lower seizure threshold; should not be taken with antacids
Metronidazole	Peripheral neuropathy; ataxia; disulfiram-like reaction; caution with concurrent anticoagulant therapy
Fluconazole	Hepatotoxicity; prolongation of QT interval; drug-drug interactions

[a]For example, cephalexin, cefadroxil, dicloxacillin.
Modified from Sia IG, Berbari EF, Karchmer AW. Prosthetic joint infections. Infect Dis Clin North Am 2005;19:885–914, with permission.

now recommended to receive prophylactic antimicrobials.[46] It remains to be seen what future recommendations will hold for antimicrobial prophylaxis to prevent hematogenous prosthetic joint infection following dental, genitourinary, or gastroenterology procedures.

CONCLUSION

The diagnosis, treatment, and prevention of shoulder arthroplasty infection, and prosthetic joint infection in general, present a complex series of decisions that incorporate multiple disciplines. Future needs include better clinical trials to better define optimal medical and surgical strategies for these complex and potentially devastating infections.

REFERENCES

1. Patel R, Osmon DR, Hanssen AD. The diagnosis of prosthetic joint infection: current techniques and emerging technologies. *Clin Orthop Relat Res* 2005;437:55–58.
2. Powles JW, Spencer RF, Lovering AM. Gentamicin release from old cement during revision hip arthroplasty. *J Bone Joint Surg Br* 1998;80:607–610.
3. Seitz WH Jr, Damacen H. Staged exchange arthroplasty for shoulder sepsis. *J Arthroplasty* 2002;17:36–40.
4. Topolski MS, Chin PY, Sperling JW, et al. Revision shoulder arthroplasty with positive intraoperative cultures: the value of preoperative studies and intraoperative histology. *J Shoulder Elbow Surg* 2006;15:402–406.
5. Sperling JW, Kozak TK, Hanssen AD, et al. Infection after shoulder arthroplasty. *Clin Orthop Relat Res* 2001;382:206–216.
6. Bernard L, Lubbeke A, Stern R, et al. Value of preoperative investigations in diagnosing prosthetic joint infection: retrospective cohort study and literature review. *Scand J Infect Dis* 2004;36:410–416.
7. Brems JJ. Shoulder arthroplasty in the face of acute fracture: puzzle pieces. *J Arthroplasty* 2002;17:32–35.
8. Sia IG, Berbari EF, Karchmer AW. Prosthetic joint infections. *Infect Dis Clin North Am* 2005;19:885–914.
9. Codd TP, Yamaguchi K, Pollock RG, et al. Infected shoulder arthroplasties: treatment with staged reimplantations vs resection arthroplasty. American Academy of Orthopaedic Surgeons Scientific Program No. 59.
10. Parvizi J, Ghanem E, Menashe S, et al. Periprosthetic infection: what are the diagnostic challenges? *J Bone Joint Surg Am* 2006;88(suppl 4):138–147.
11. Trampuz A, Hanssen AD, Osmon DR, et al. Synovial fluid leukocyte count and differential for the diagnosis of prosthetic knee infection. *Am J Med* 2004;117:556–562.
12. Piper K, et al. Diagnosis and microbiology of prosthetic shoulder infection. Presented at 16th European Congress of Clinical Microbiology and Infectious Diseases; Nice, France; April 1–4, 2006.
13. Coste JS, Reig S, Trojani C, et al. The management of infection in arthroplasty of the shoulder. *J Bone Joint Surg Br* 2004;86:65–69.
14. Ince A, Seemann K, Frommelt L, et al. One-stage exchange shoulder arthroplasty for periprosthetic infection. *J Bone Joint Surg Br* 2005;87:814–818.
15. Ramsey ML, Fenlin JM Jr. Use of an antibiotic-impregnated bone cement block in the revision of an infected shoulder arthroplasty. *J Shoulder Elbow Surg* 1996;5:479–482.
16. Wirth MA, Rockwood CA Jr. Complications of total shoulder-replacement arthroplasty. *J Bone Joint Surg Am* 1996;78:603–616.
17. Trampuz A, Piper KE, Jacobson MJ, et al. Sonication of removed hip and knee prostheses for diagnosis of infection. *N Engl J Med* 2007;357:654–663.
18. Waldvogel FA. Ultrasound: now also for microbiologists? *N Engl J Med* 2007;357:705–706.
19. Bauer TW, Parvizi J, Kobayashi N, et al. Diagnosis of periprosthetic infection. *J Bone Joint Surg Am* 2006;88:869–882.
20. Lonner JH, Desai P, Dicesare PE, et al. The reliability of analysis of intraoperative frozen sections for identifying active infection during revision hip or knee arthroplasty. *J Bone Joint Surg Am* 1996;78:1553–1558.
21. Pace TB, Jeray KJ, Latham JT Jr. Synovial tissue examination by frozen section as an indicator of infection in hip and knee arthroplasty in community hospitals. *J Arthroplasty* 1997;12:64–69.
22. Wirth MA, Rockwood CA Jr. Complications of shoulder arthroplasty. *Clin Orthop Relat Res* 1994;307:47–69.
23. Drancourt M, Argenson JN, Tissot-Dupont H, et al. Psoriasis is a risk factor for hip-prosthesis infection. *Eur J Epidemiol* 1997;13:205–207.
24. Berbari EF, Hanssen AD, Duffy MC, et al. Risk factors for prosthetic joint infection: case-control study. *Clin Infect Dis* 1998;27:1247–1254.
25. Jover-Saenz A, Barcenilla-Gaite F, Torres-Puig-Gros J, et al. Risk factors for total prosthetic joint infection: case-control study. *Med Clin (Barc)* 2007;128:493–494.
26. Marculescu CE, Berbari EF, Hanssen AD, et al. Outcome of prosthetic joint infections treated with debridement and retention of components. *Clin Infect Dis* 2006;42:471–478.
27. Li JT, Markus PJ, Osmon DR, et al. Reduction of vancomycin use in orthopedic patients with a history of antibiotic allergy. *Mayo Clin Proc* 2000;75:902–906.
28. Jerosch J, Schneppenheim M. Management of infected shoulder replacement. *Arch Orthop Trauma Surg* 2003;123:209–214.
29. Mileti J, Sperling JW, Cofield RH. Reimplantation of a shoulder arthroplasty after a previous infected arthroplasty. *J Shoulder Elbow Surg* 2004;13:528–531.
30. Phelan DM, Osmon DR, Keating MR, et al. Delayed reimplantation arthroplasty for candidal prosthetic joint infection: a report of four cases and review of the literature. *Clin Infect Dis* 2002;34:930–938.
31. Meehan AM, Osmon DR, Duffy MC, et al. Outcome of penicillin-susceptible streptococcal prosthetic joint infection treated with debridement and retention of the prosthesis. *Clin Infect Dis* 2003;36:845–849.
32. Loebenberg MI, Zuckerman JD. An articulating interval spacer in the treatment of an infected total shoulder arthroplasty. *J Shoulder Elbow Surg* 2004;13:476–478.
33. Cui Q, Mihalko WM, Shields JS, et al. Antibiotic-impregnated cement spacers for the treatment of infection associated with total hip or knee arthroplasty. *J Bone Joint Surg Am* 2007;89:871–882.
34. Braman JP, Sprague M, Bishop J, et al. The outcome of resection shoulder arthroplasty for recalcitrant shoulder infections. *J Shoulder Elbow Surg* 2006;15:549–553.
35. Debeer P, Plasschaert H, Stuyck J. Resection arthroplasty of the infected shoulder: a salvage procedure for the elderly patient. *Acta Orthop Belg* 2006;72:126–130.
36. Tice AD, Rehm SJ, Dalovisio JR, et al. Practice guidelines for outpatient parenteral antimicrobial therapy: IDSA guidelines. *Clin Infect Dis* 2004;38:1651–1672.
37. Zimmerli W, Widmer AF, Blatter M, et al. Role of rifampin for treatment of orthopedic implant-related staphylococcal infections: a randomized controlled trial. *JAMA* 1998;279:1537–1541.
38. Zimmerli W, Trampuz A, Ochsner PE. Prosthetic-joint infections. *N Engl J Med* 2004;351:1645–1654.
39. Anguita-Alonso P, Hanssen AD, Osmon DR, et al. High rate of aminoglycoside resistance among staphylococci causing prosthetic joint infection. *Clin Orthop Relat Res* 2005;439:43–47.
40. Marculescu CE, Osmon DR. Antibiotic prophylaxis in orthopedic prosthetic surgery. *Infect Dis Clin North Am* 2005;19:931–946.
41. Bratzler DW, Houck PM. Antimicrobial prophylaxis for surgery: an advisory statement from the national surgical infection prevention project. *Clin Infect Dis* 2004;38:1706–1715.
42. Jiranek WA, Hanssen AD, Greenwald AS. Antibiotic-loaded bone cement for infection prophylaxis in total joint replacement. *J Bone Joint Surg Am* 2006;88:2487–2500.
43. American Dental Association, American Academy of Orthopedic Surgeons. Antibiotic prophylaxis for dental patients with total joint replacements. *J Am Dent Assoc* 2003;134:895–899.
44. American Urological Association, American Academy of Orthopaedic Surgeons. Antibiotic prophylaxis for urological patients with total joint replacements. *J Urol* 2003;169:1796–1797.
45. Hirota WK, Petersen K, Baron TH, et al. Guidelines for antibiotic prophylaxis for GI endoscopy. *Gastrointest Endosc* 2003;58:475–482.
46. Wilson W, Taubert KA, Gewitz M, et al. Prevention of infective endocarditis: guidelines from the American Heart Association—a guideline from the American Heart Association Rheumatic Fever, Endocarditis, and Kawasaki Disease Committee, Council on Cardiovascular Disease in the Young, and the Council on Clinical Cardiology, Council on Cardiovascular Surgery and Anesthesia, and the Quality of Care and Outcomes Research Interdisciplinary Working Group. *Circulation* 2007;115:1736–1754.

Joaquin Sanchez-Sotelo

Outcomes of Revision Surgery in Shoulder Arthroplasty

INTRODUCTION

The multiple modes of failure of primary shoulder arthroplasty have been well delineated in previous chapters of this book. The chapters following this one will describe in detail surgical techniques used in revision surgery and specific procedures performed for each particular indication. The present chapter reviews the outcomes of revision shoulder arthroplasty reported in studies published to date.

The literature on revision shoulder arthroplasty is somewhat difficult to analyze. Most articles report on the outcome of revision for specific indications, such as progressive glenoid erosion in hemiarthroplasty, glenoid component loosening, periprosthetic fractures, and so on. However, many patients included in most published studies had several problems addressed at the time of their revision surgery; a patient undergoing revision for glenoid loosening may also have associated instability and a large rotator cuff tear. The overall results often represent the outcome of a mixed combination of surgical procedures in varied patient populations. Reverse shoulder arthroplasty has emerged as one of the main prosthetic designs for revision surgery, but most studies combine in the same series primary and revision reverse prostheses implanted for multiple indications, further complicating analysis of the literature on revision shoulder arthroplasty.

One additional challenge in analyzing the published literature on revision shoulder arthroplasty lies in the difficulty diagnosing with certainty a deep infection. The relatively high prevalence of cultures positive for *Propionibacterium acnes* in revision cases with a negative preoperative evaluation for infection has been only recently recognized.[1] Revision shoulder arthroplasty is associated with a relatively high incidence of persistent pain, and it is difficult to ascertain whether some patients with a painful arthroplasty may have an underlying unrecognized low-grade infection.

The information available in the literature has been organized in this chapter according to the indication for the revision surgery—glenoid erosion or loosening, humeral loosening or periprosthetic fracture, infection, instability, and rotator cuff tear. A separate section is dedicated to the outcome of reverse shoulder arthroplasty in the revision setting.

GLENOID COMPONENT LOOSENING

Radiographic loosening of the glenoid component has been noted to develop in a relatively high number of total shoulder arthroplasties[2] (Fig. 6.1). However, there is limited published information on revision surgery for glenoid loosening. After removal of a loose glenoid component, a new glenoid component may be implanted in patients with sufficient remaining bone stock; otherwise, the glenoid may be reamed or bone grafted, revising the total shoulder to a hemiarthroplasty. Polyethylene liner exchange is an option for patients with wear of a metal-backed modular glenoid components, rarely used at the present time. In general, revision for glenoid component loosening seems to be associated with a better outcome than revision for soft tissue reconstructions.[3]

The Mayo Clinic experience with glenoid revision surgery after total shoulder arthroplasty was first reviewed by Antuna et al.[4] The authors reported on 48 shoulders reviewed a mean of 4.9 years after glenoid revision for implant mechanical failure (43 shoulders) or instability secondary to malposition and wear (5 shoulders). The majority of cases had additional problems leading to revision surgery, including instability (17 shoulders), humeral component loosening (12 shoulders), malposition (4 shoulders), and stiffness (4 shoulders). In 18 shoulders the severity of glenoid bone loss after removal of the component was so severe that a reimplantation of a new component was not possible. In five shoulders, the worn polyethylene liner of a well-fixed metal-backed component was replaced. In the remaining 25 shoulders, the glenoid component was revised to an uncemented metal-backed component (8 shoulders) or a cemented component (17 shoulders).

Overall, revision surgery was associated with substantial improvements in pain, motion, and function. Satisfactory pain relief was achieved in 86% of patients with a new glenoid component and 66% of the patients with component removal. Additional surgery was performed in approximately 25% of the shoulders to treat instability (3 shoulders), painful glenoid arthritis (3 shoulders), glenoid loosening (2 shoulders), periprosthetic fracture (2 shoulders), and resection for deep infection (1 shoulder). Glenoid periprosthetic lucency was present in 42% of the shoulders that underwent

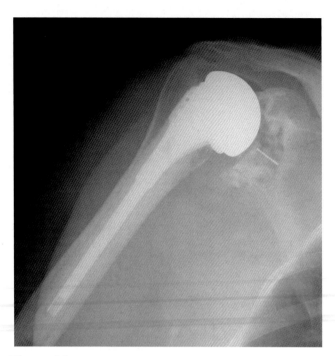

Figure 6.1.   Aseptic loosening of an all-polyethylene cemented glenoid component. The component has shifted in position, and there is substantial glenoid bone loss. Note also the humeral component malpositioning.

implantation of a new glenoid component, but it was incomplete in most.

More recently, three separate studies from the Mayo Clinic analyzed in more detail the outcome of polyethylene exchange for wear, revision or removal for glenoid aseptic loosening, and implantation of a glenoid component in patients with previous component removal and bone grafting.

Cheung et al[5] reported on 12 shoulders that underwent revision surgery to exchange the polyethylene liner of a well-fixed metal-backed modular glenoid component. Eight shoulders had associated instability. The humeral component was also revised in seven shoulders. Results were rated as satisfactory in only four cases; better results were obtained in patients with an intact rotator cuff and no instability.

Cheung et al[5] also analyzed the results of 68 shoulders revised for glenoid aseptic loosening with either placement of a new glenoid component (33 shoulders) or component removal and bone grafting (35 shoulders). Eight of the revision glenoid components were uncemented, and the remaining 25 were cemented. In the group treated with revision a reoperation was required in 14 cases: removal of a loose glenoid component (1), polyethylene exchange (1), resection for instability (2), rotator cuff repair (2), and periprosthetic fracture (1). Nineteen additional patients had an unsatisfactory result secondary to persistent pain (3), limited motion (12), or both (4). There were radiolucent glenoid lines in 13 shoulders, mostly incomplete, and a change in component position in 2 shoulders. In the group treated with removal, seven shoulders had a reoperation for ongoing pain: six had replacement of a new glenoid component, and one had a resection arthroplasty. Twenty-five additional shoulders were rated as unsatisfactory because of ongoing pain (2), lack of motion (16), or both (7).

Revision was associated with better survival free of reoperation at 5 years compared to component removal.

Phipatanakul and Norris[6] reported better pain relief with removal of the glenoid component and bone grafting in a consecutive series of 24 patients with glenoid loosening and osteolysis. Satisfactory pain relief was reported in 75% of the patients, although motion remained largely unchanged. Neyton et al[7] reported approximately 50% pain relief with removal of a loose glenoid component and reconstruction using corticocancellous bone grafting in a consecutive series including only 9 patients.

A novel approach for the treatment of glenoid loosening after shoulder arthroplasty consists of removing the component arthroscopically. O'Driscoll et al[8] reported on five cases in which complete removal of the loose component and cement was achieved arthroscopically, providing complete relief in three patients and partial pain relief in two patients.

The outcome of replacing a new glenoid component in patients with ongoing pain after component removal has been documented to be satisfactory in terms of pain relief but not in terms of improved motion.[6,9,10]

GLENOID ARTHRITIS

Pain originating on the unresurfaced glenoid is one of the main modes of failure of shoulder hemiarthroplasty (Fig. 6.2). Reoperation to implant a new glenoid component is one of the most successful revision procedures.[3]

The Mayo Clinic experience with conversion of a painful hemiarthroplasty to a total shoulder arthroplasty was reviewed by Sperling and Cofield.[11] Eighteen hemiarthroplasties revised for painful glenoid erosion were evaluated at an average follow-up time of 5.5 years. The glenoid component was fixed with cement in ten shoulders, and a porous-coated component was used in the remaining eight. The humeral component was revised in all but one case. Revision to a total shoulder arthroplasty was significantly associated with pain relief. However, seven shoulders were rated as unsatisfactory secondary to the need for additional surgery in two cases (resection for deep infection and revision for instability) and limited motion in five cases.

Carroll et al[12] reviewed the outcome of 16 consecutive patients who underwent revision surgery for a failed hemiarthroplasty. A cemented all-polyethylene component was used in 15 cases and a metal-backed cemented component in one case. Approximately 30% of the patients had humeral component malposition, and 50% of the humeral components were revised. At a mean follow-up of 5.5 years, the results were graded as excellent or satisfactory in 53% of the patients. Five patients underwent additional surgery for glenoid component loosening (2), deep infection (2), and acromioplasty (1). Revision surgery was associated with improvement in pain, but it was somewhat unpredictable. In this paper, the authors pointed out the complexity of revising a failed hemiarthroplasty to a total shoulder arthroplasty.

HUMERAL LOOSENING

Radiographic loosening of the humeral component has been noted to occur mostly with press-fit humeral components.[13] Revision of the humeral component is reported in many

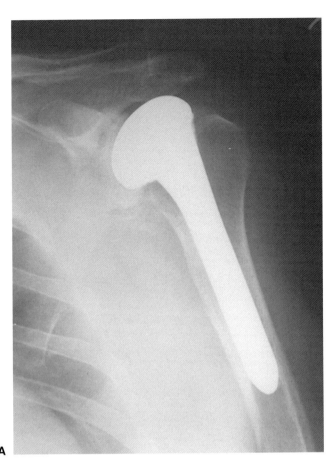

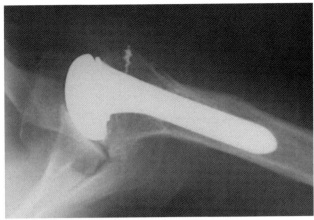

Figure 6.2. Progressive painful glenoid erosion after hemiarthroplasty for osteoarthritis.

patients undergoing revision shoulder arthroplasty for glenoid loosening or erosion, instability, and other reasons. However, there is limited information about the outcome of revision surgery performed for aseptic loosening of the humeral component, except for isolated case reports.[14,15]

The Mayo Clinic experience with revision shoulder arthroplasty for humeral aseptic loosening was recently reviewed (Fig. 6.3). Thirty-eight consecutive humeral revisions performed for aseptic loosening were reviewed at a mean follow-up time of 7 years. The initial surgery had been a total shoulder arthroplasty in 37 cases and a hemiarthroplasty in one case. The glenoid component was removed in 25 shoulders, revised in 10 shoulders, and left unrevised in 2 shoulders; a new glenoid component was implanted at the time of revision of the only hemiarthroplasty. Standard-length stems were used in 19 shoulders and longer revision stems in 17 shoulders; cement fixation was used in 29. An associated rotator cuff tear was repaired in five shoulders and humeral bone graft was required in 11 shoulders.

Revision surgery was significantly associated with improved pain and motion; both were better in those cases in which a glenoid component could be implanted. At most recent follow-up, five revision glenoid components and four revision humeral components were considered to be radiographically loose; shoulder instability was identified in 13 shoulders, of which seven had instability before revision surgery. Complications included six periprosthetic fractures and one deep infection requiring resection. Two additional patients required reoperation to bone graft or revise the glenoid. Survival free of reoperation, humeral

revision, or removal and radiographic humeral loosening at 10 years was, respectively, 89%, 95%, and 91%. The data from this study show that revision of the humeral component is associated with a relatively low rate of mechanical failure and that the overall clinical results depend mostly on the ability to implant a glenoid component and restore motion and stability.

PERIPROSTHETIC HUMERAL FRACTURES

The evaluation and treatment of periprosthetic humeral fractures has been the topic of several published studies.[16–19] The outcome of revision surgery for the treatment of periprosthetic humeral fractures depends on the type of fracture being treated (Fig. 6.4). The Mayo Clinic classification divides periprosthetic humeral fractures into types A (at the tip of the humeral component with proximal extension), B (at the tip of the humeral component with distal extension), and C (distal to the tip of the humeral component). In contradistinction to periprosthetic fractures of the lower extremity, some humeral periprosthetic fractures may be satisfactorily treated without surgery (type C and type A with a well-fixed humeral component).

Campbell et al[16] reported the outcome of 21 periprosthetic humeral fractures followed for a mean of 2 years. Cast or brace immobilization provided a good outcome for type C fractures. On the contrary, type B fractures did well only when treated surgically with revision to a long-stemmed humeral component and internal fixation. Worland et al[18] published the outcome on a

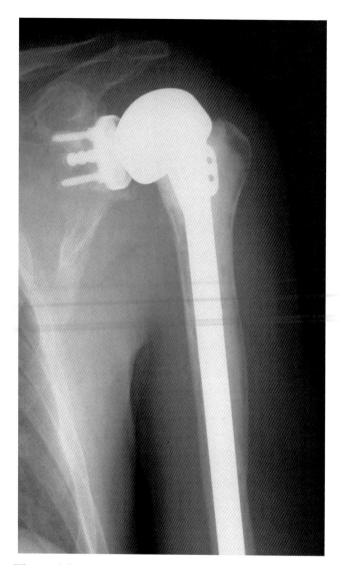

Figure 6.3.   Successful revision for humeral aseptic loosening using a long-stemmed cemented humeral component.

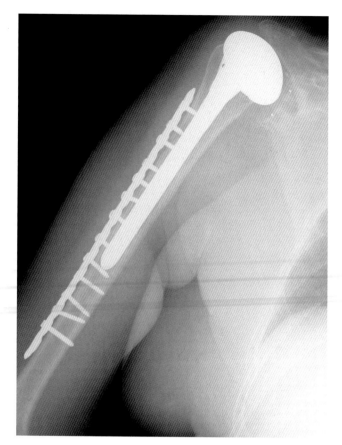

Figure 6.4.   Humeral periprosthetic fractures may be treated nonoperatively, with fixation, or revision surgery depending on fracture location and component fixation.

smaller series of six periprosthetic fractures; surgery was required in five and union was obtained in all. Four of the fractures were treated with revision to a long-stemmed humeral component.

The initial Mayo Clinic experience was published by Wright and Cofield.[19] Union was obtained with nonoperative treatment in long oblique and spiral fractures distal to the tip of the prosthesis, but surgery was required either initially or after failed nonoperative treatment in four of the nine shoulders. More recently, Kumar et al[17] reported 16 periprosthetic fractures after a total shoulder arthroplasty (10 shoulders) or a hemiarthroplasty (6 shoulders). Two shoulders had developed substantial osteolysis before the fracture. There were six type A fractures, six type B fractures, and three type C fractures; the remaining proximal fracture could not be classified with this system.

Nonoperative treatment led to fracture union in three type A, one type B, and two type C fractures; the average time to union was approximately 6 months. Nonoperative treatment failed in one type A and four type B fractures. Surgery was performed in these five shoulders after failed nonoperative treatment and five additional shoulders immediately after the fracture. Surgery

included open reduction and internal fixation when the component was well fixed (5 shoulders) and revision to a long-stemmed humeral component when the component was loose (5 shoulders), including revision to a tumor prothesis in one shoulder. The average time to union after surgery was approximately 9 months.

At an average follow-up of 5 years, average active elevation and external rotation were 107 degrees and 43 degrees, respectively. Radiographically, a complete radiolucent line surrounding the humeral component was found in two shoulders. Results were rated as excellent in three, satisfactory in four, and unsatisfactory in nine shoulders. Unsatisfactory results were secondary to persistent pain (1), poor motion (5), or both (3). One patient developed a deep periprosthetic infection, which responded to irrigation, debridement, and intravenous antibiotics.

INFECTION

Deep periprosthetic infection after shoulder arthroplasty probably is more common than reported. This is partly due to the difficulty in establishing a preoperative diagnosis of infection, because most preoperative tests tend to be negative in a high proportion of patients with positive intraoperative cultures.[1] The most commonly used options for treatment of this complication include antibiotic suppression, irrigation and debridement, implant removal, and one- or two-stage shoulder reimplantation.

Coste et al[20] reviewed the experience of the Aequalis shoulder group in a series of 42 deep infections (acute in 12, subacute in 6, and chronic in 24 shoulders) treated with antibiotic suppression, resection arthroplasty, irrigation and debridement, cement spacer, and one- or two-stage reimplantation. At a mean follow-up of 32 months, 71% of the patients were free of infection. The mean Constant score was 38 points, and the mean active elevation was 74 degrees.

Sperling et al[21] reviewed the outcome of 32 infected shoulder arthroplasties (23 total shoulder arthroplasties and 9 hemiarthroplasties) treated at the Mayo Clinic. The infection was considered acute in four, subacute in five, and chronic in 23 shoulders. The most common microorganisms were *Staphylococcus aureus* (13 shoulders), coagulase-negative *Staphylococcus* (9 shoulders), and *Propionibacterium acnes* (5 shoulders). Patients were treated with resection arthroplasty (20 shoulders), debridement (6 shoulders), one-stage reimplantation (2 shoulders), and two-stage reimplantation (3 shoulders). These two series and other published studies will be analyzed by treatment modality.

RESECTION ARTHROPLASTY

Resection arthroplasty successfully eliminated the infection in all 20 shoulders included in the Mayo Clinic series, although it required on average two debridement procedures.[21] Of the 11 patients followed longer than 2 years, 7 had no or slight pain, average active abduction was 69 degrees, and active external rotation was 31 degrees. Results were graded as successful in three shoulders. Eradication of infection was achieved in seven of the ten patients in the series reported on by Coste et al[20]; the Constant score increased to 30 points, mostly secondary to improvement in pain, but motion remained limited. Similar results were published by Braman et al[22] in a series of seven patients treated with resection-arthroplasty for a recalcitrant infection; infection was resolved, pain was mild or moderate, but function was limited, and none of the shoulders was rated as satisfactory.

DEBRIDEMENT

Debridement with implant retention was performed in six of the shoulders included in the Mayo Clinic series.[21] Three shoulders failed this treatment and underwent resection-arthroplasty. The result was rated as satisfactory in one of the other three shoulders, but none experienced recurrence of infection. In the series of Coste et al,[20] infection was eradicated in only two of the eight patients treated with open or arthroscopic debridement and function remained largely unchanged.

ONE-STAGE REIMPLANTATION

One-stage reimplantation was performed in two of the patients included in the study by Sperling et al.[21] Treatment failed in one patient, who required resection arthroplasty, and was successful in the second patient, who experienced complete pain relief and achieved good range of motion. One-stage reimplantation was very successful in the series by Coste et al[20]; the infection was eradicated in all three patients, who at most recent follow-up had the highest mobility score of all groups. A larger series of patients was reviewed by Ince et al.[23] Nine one-stage reimplantations were followed for a mean of 6 years; infection

was eradicated in all patients, and their mean Constant score was 33.6 points. Additional surgery was required in three shoulders for the treatment of a periprosthetic fracture, recurrent instability, and an acromion nonunion.

TWO-STAGE REIMPLANTATION

Two-stage reimplantation was attempted in three of the patients included in the initial Mayo Clinic series.[21] At a mean follow-up of 5 years, all patients had no or mild pain; their mean active elevation and external rotation were 100 degrees and 30 degrees, respectively; and none became reinfected. The Mayo Clinic experience was updated by Mileti et al[24] to a series of only four patients; at a mean follow-up of 7 years, there were no reinfections and the patients had approximately the same motion and pain relief as in the previous report. Two-stage reimplantation eradicated the infection in six of the ten patients included in the series by Coste et al[20]; their mean Constant score was 35 points, and their mobility score was 13 points. Seitz and Damacen[25] also reported on eight infected shoulder arthroplasties treated with implant removal, placement of an antibiotic-loaded cement spacer, intravenous antibiotics, and reimplantation of a total shoulder arthroplasty (3 shoulders) or hemiarthroplasty (5 shoulders). There were no reinfections, and all patients expressed pain relief, although overhead motion remained limited.

INSTABILITY

Instability is another relatively common indication for revision shoulder arthroplasty. Analysis of the outcome of revision for instability is difficult to perform because some reports include mixed populations of patients with anteroposterior instability and patients with anterosuperior escape secondary to massive cuff deficiency.

Moeckel et al[26] reported on seven cases of anterior instability and three of posterior instability. Revision surgery restored stability in nine shoulders, but two shoulders required two procedures before stability was achieved. Wirth and Rockwood[27] reported on 11 cases of posterior instability, six of anterior instability, and one of inferior instability and also achieved stability in all but one shoulder.

The Mayo Clinic experience has been less satisfactory (Fig. 6.5). Sanchez-Sotelo et al[28] reported on 33 shoulder arthroplasties (26 total shoulder arthroplasties and 7 hemiarthroplasties) reoperated for anterior (19 shoulders) or posterior (14 shoulders) instability. Intraoperatively, instability was attributed to soft-tissue deficiencies in 21 shoulders, isolated component malposition in 1 shoulder, and combined soft-tissue problems and component malposition in 11 shoulders. One shoulder was treated with resection arthroplasty and the remaining 32 with component repositioning and soft-tissue repair as needed.

Revision surgery restored stability only in nine of the 32 shoulders. Additional surgery to correct persistent stability was performed in 11 shoulders. At most recent follow-up, only 14 of the initial 33 shoulders were stable. Anterior instability was associated with a higher failure rate than posterior instability. Overall results were graded according to the Neer system as excellent in four, satisfactory in six, and unsatisfactory in 23 shoulders.

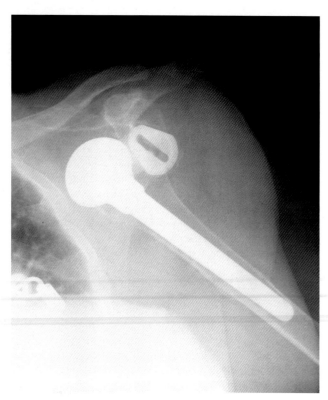

Figure 6.5. Revision surgery for instability seems to be associated with a high failure rate.

ROTATOR CUFF REPAIR

Rotator cuff tears are estimated to complicate between 2% and 3% of shoulder arthroplasties. Several authors have reported isolated cases of rotator cuff repair after arthroplasty.[29] However, there is only one study on the outcome of rotator cuff repair after shoulder arthroplasty. Hattrup et al[30] reported on 18 rotator cuff repairs performed in patients with a shoulder hemiarthroplasty (four shoulders) or total shoulder arthroplasty (14 shoulders). At the time of revision surgery, tears were classified as medium in five shoulders, large in 12 shoulders, and massive in one shoulder. The humeral component was revised in 10 shoulders and the glenoid component was revised in 9 shoulders.

Clinically satisfactory tendon healing was achieved in four shoulders. There were no differences in pain between patients with healed and unhealed repairs, but an intact rotator cuff was associated with better active motion and function. A second attempt to repair the rotator cuff was made in six shoulders; at the time of the second repair, the glenoid component was revised in three shoulders and removed in one shoulder. One additional patient was reoperated to implant a new glenoid component. Earlier surgery was not associated with an improved outcome.

REVISION TO A REVERSE PROSTHESIS

The use of a reverse prosthesis design in revision surgery has continued to increase in part because of the growing popularity of this design concept and in part because of the disappointing results of revision surgery in situations such as instability or cuff tears. Most published information on the outcome of reverse arthroplasty for revision surgery has been in series combining primary and revision cases. As it might be expected, the use of a reverse prosthesis in the revision setting seems to be associated with inferior clinical outcomes and a higher complication rate compared to those with primary arthroplasty.[31,32]

Boileau et al[31] reported on 18 revisions performed using the Delta 3 reverse prosthesis for failed bipolar hemiarthroplasties in patients with cuff tear arthropathy (2 shoulders), failed shoulder hemiarthroplasty for an acute proximal humeral fracture (12 shoulders), or two-stage reimplantation for a deep infection. Of interest, after revision surgery only 36% of the patients reported no or mild pain. At most recent follow-up, mean active elevation and external rotation were 113 degrees and 1 degree, respectively, and the average Constant score improved from 15 to 46 points. Reoperations included resection arthroplasty for deep infection in two shoulders, one-stage reimplantation for deep infection in one shoulder, revision for humeral aseptic loosening in one shoulder, and revision for a humeral periprosthetic fracture in one shoulder.

Wall et al[32] reported on 45 revision reverse prostheses followed for a minimum of 2 years. The Constant score improved from 20 points to 52 points. At most recent follow-up, mean active elevation and external rotation were 118 degrees and 9 degrees, respectively. An intraoperative fracture occurred at the time of revision in 24% of the cases. Additional complications included dislocation and infection. One humeral component developed radiographic aseptic loosening.

Werner et al[33] reviewed the outcome of revision of a failed hemiarthroplasty to a reverse prosthesis. Their study included 21 revisions for failed hemiarthroplasty (15 shoulders) or total shoulder arthroplasty (five shoulders) for acute proximal humerus fracture, and one failed hemiarthroplasty for osteoarthritis. Complications developed in 12 patients, and 38% of the patients required a reoperation. There were three hematomas, three dislocations, three deep infections, one nerve injury, one glenoid loosening, and two acromial fractures. Two patients required removal or revision of the prosthesis. At most recent follow-up, the mean Constant score was 55 points and mean active elevation was 96 degrees.

More recently, Levy et al[34,35] published two studies on the outcome of reverse shoulder arthroplasty for failed hemiarthroplasty in patients with cuff tear arthroplasty[34] and after a proximal humerus fracture.[35] In their first study, these authors reported on the outcome of 19 revisions of a failed hemiarthroplasty for cuff tear arthropathy[34]; after a minimum follow-up of 2 years, mean forward elevation improved by 26 degrees. The rate of prosthesis-related complications was 32%, and the risk of a complication was increased in patients with severe humeral or glenoid bone loss. In a separate study, they assessed the outcome of 29 revisions for failed hemiarthroplasty with tuberosity failure.[35] Surgery result was improved, with significant improvements in pain and function; at most recent follow-up, mean active elevation was 70 degrees. The overall complication rate was 28%.

OVERVIEW

Revision shoulder arthroplasty often represents a complex procedure aimed to solve combined modes of failure of the primary arthroplasty. Component loosening, instability, rotator cuff

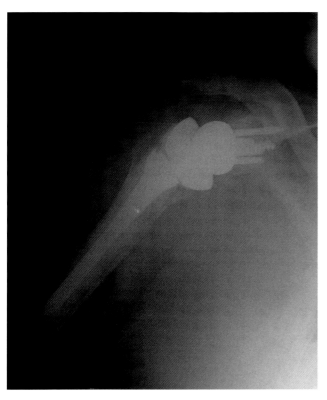

Figure 6.6. Revision to a reverse prosthesis represents a promising option for the more complicated cases with severe cuff insufficiency.

tearing, and progressive bone loss usually coexist. Procedures that could be considered successful in terms of component revision are often rated as unsuccessful secondary to persistent pain, lack of motion, or instability. Revision for deep infection may successfully eradicate the infection, but motion and functional gains are less predictable. A recent outcome analysis of a consecutive series of 78 shoulders that underwent revision for multiple reasons showed that revision or implantation of a glenoid component and internal fixation of periprosthetic fractures provided the best outcomes, whereas tuberosity and soft-tissue reconstructions and revision because of infection have poor outcomes.[3] Revision using a reverse prosthesis seems to be associated with better clinical outcomes for difficult situations in which there is not only a failed arthroplasty but also cuff insufficiency (Fig. 6.6). However, the outcome of reverse prostheses in the revision setting does not parallel the outcome in primary surgery and is associated with a substantial complication and reoperation rate.

REFERENCES

1. Topolski MS, Chin PY, Sperling JW, et al. Revision shoulder arthroplasty with positive intraoperative cultures: the value of preoperative studies and intraoperative histology. *J Shoulder Elbow Surg* 2006;15:402–406.
2. Torchia ME, Cofield RH, Settergren CR. Total shoulder arthroplasty with the Neer prosthesis: long-term results. *J Shoulder Elbow Surg* 1997;6:495–505.
3. Dines JS, Fealy S, Strauss EJ, et al. Outcomes analysis of revision total shoulder replacement. *J Bone Joint Surg Am* 2006;88:1494–1500.
4. Antuna SA, Sperling JW, Cofield RH, et al. Glenoid revision surgery after total shoulder arthroplasty. *J Shoulder Elbow Surg* 2001;10:217–224.
5. Cheung EV, Sperling JW, Cofield RH. Polyethylene insert exchange for wear after total shoulder arthroplasty. *J Shoulder Elbow Surg* 2007;16:574–578. E-pub.
6. Phipatanakul WP, Norris TR. Treatment of glenoid loosening and bone loss due to osteolysis with glenoid bone grafting. *J Shoulder Elbow Surg* 2006;15:84–87.
7. Neyton L, Walch G, Nove-Josserand L, et al. Glenoid corticocancellous bone grafting after glenoid component removal in the treatment of glenoid loosening. *J Shoulder Elbow Surg* 2006;15:173–179.
8. O'Driscoll SW, Petrie RS, Torchia ME. Arthroscopic removal of the glenoid component for failed total shoulder arthroplasty: a report of five cases. *J Bone Joint Surg Am* 2005;87:858–863.
9. Antuna S, Sperling JW, Cofield RH. Reimplantation of a glenoid component after component removal and allograft bone grafting: a report of 3 cases. *J Shoulder Elbow Surg* 2002;11:637–641.
10. Cheung EV, Sperling JW, Cofield RH. Reimplantation of a glenoid component following component removal and allogenic bone grafting. *J Bone Joint Surg Am* 2007;89:1777–1783.
11. Sperling JW, Cofield RH. Revision total shoulder arthroplasty for the treatment of glenoid arthrosis. *J Bone Joint Surg Am* 1998;80:860–867.
12. Carroll RM, Izquierdo R, Vazquez M, et al. Conversion of painful hemiarthroplasty to total shoulder arthroplasty: long-term results. *J Shoulder Elbow Surg* 2004;13:599–603.
13. Sanchez-Sotelo J, Wright TW, O'Driscoll SW, et al. Radiographic assessment of uncemented humeral components in total shoulder arthroplasty. *J Arthroplasty* 2001;16:180–187.
14. Klimkiewicz JJ, Iannotti JP, Rubash HE, et al. Aseptic loosening of the humeral component in total shoulder arthroplasty. *J Shoulder Elbow Surg* 1998;7:422–426.
15. Nystuen CM, Leopold SS, Warme WJ, et al. Cancellous impaction and cortical strut allografting for revision shoulder arthroplasty: a case report. *J Shoulder Elbow Surg* 2006;15:244–248.
16. Campbell JT, Moore RS, Iannotti JP, et al. Periprosthetic humeral fractures: mechanisms of fracture and treatment options. *J Shoulder Elbow Surg* 1998;7:406–413.
17. Kumar S, Sperling JW, Haidukewych GH, et al. Periprosthetic humeral fractures after shoulder arthroplasty. *J Bone Joint Surg Am* 2004;86:680–689.
18. Worland RL, Kim DY, Arredondo J. Periprosthetic humeral fractures: management and classification. *J Shoulder Elbow Surg* 1999;8:590–594.
19. Wright TW, Cofield RH. Humeral fractures after shoulder arthroplasty. *J Bone Joint Surg Am* 1995;77:1340–1346.
20. Coste JS, Reig S, Trojani C, et al. The management of infection in arthroplasty of the shoulder. *J Bone Joint Surg Br* 2004;86:65–69.
21. Sperling JW, Kozak TK, Hanssen AD, et al. Infection after shoulder arthroplasty. *Clin Orthop Relat Res* 2001;382:206–216.
22. Braman JP, Sprague M, Bishop J, et al. The outcome of resection shoulder arthroplasty for recalcitrant shoulder infections. *J Shoulder Elbow Surg* 2006;15:549–553.
23. Ince A, Seemann K, Frommelt L, et al. One-stage exchange shoulder arthroplasty for periprosthetic infection. *J Bone Joint Surg Br* 2005;87:814–818.
24. Mileti J, Sperling JW, Cofield RH. Reimplantation of a shoulder arthroplasty after a previous infected arthroplasty. *J Shoulder Elbow Surg* 2004;13:528–531.
25. Seitz WH, Jr, Damacen H. Staged exchange arthroplasty for shoulder sepsis. *J Arthroplasty* 2002;17(4 suppl 1):36–40.
26. Moeckel BH, Altchek DW, Warren RF, et al. Instability of the shoulder after arthroplasty. *J Bone Joint Surg Am* 1993;75:492–497.
27. Wirth M, Rockwood C. Glenohumeral instability following shoulder arthroplasty. *Orthop Trans* 1995;19:459.
28. Sanchez-Sotelo J, Sperling JW, Rowland CM, et al. Instability after shoulder arthroplasty: results of surgical treatment. *J Bone Joint Surg Am* 2003;85:622–631.
29. Gartsman GM, Russell JA, Gaenslen E. Modular shoulder arthroplasty. *J Shoulder Elbow Surg* 1997;6:333–339.
30. Hattrup SJ, Cofield RH, Cha SS. Rotator cuff repair after shoulder replacement. *J Shoulder Elbow Surg* 2006;15:78–83.
31. Boileau P, Watkinson D, Hatzidakis AM, et al. Neer Award 2005: the Grammont reverse shoulder prosthesis—results in cuff tear arthritis, fracture sequelae, and revision arthroplasty. *J Shoulder Elbow Surg* 2006;15:527–540.
32. Wall B, Nove-Josserand L, O'Connor DP, et al. Reverse total shoulder arthroplasty: a review of results according to etiology. *J Bone Joint Surg Am* 2007;89:1476–1485.
33. Werner CM, Steinmann PA, Gilbart M, et al. Treatment of painful pseudoparesis due to irreparable rotator cuff dysfunction with the Delta III reverse-ball-and-socket total shoulder prosthesis. *J Bone Joint Surg Am* 2005;87:1476–1486.
34. Levy JC, Virani N, Pupello D, et al. Use of the reverse shoulder prosthesis for the treatment of failed hemiarthroplasty in patients with glenohumeral arthritis and rotator cuff deficiency. *J Bone Joint Surg Br* 2007;89:189–195.
35. Levy J, Frankle M, Mighell M, et al. The use of the reverse shoulder prosthesis for the treatment of failed hemiarthroplasty for proximal humeral fracture. *J Bone Joint Surg Am* 2007;89:292–300.

Techniques in Revision Shoulder Arthroplasty

Steve A. Petersen

Surgical Exposures

INTRODUCTION

Surgical exposure is everything when confronted with the challenges of revision and complex shoulder arthroplasty. Periarticular soft tissue scarring and insufficiency, rotator cuff pathology, proximal humeral or glenoid bone loss and deformity, and an assortment of prosthetic designs all require a versatile approach for shoulder arthroplasty. These techniques include the deltopectoral, anteromedial, and anterosuperior approaches to the shoulder.[1–3] The indications, advantages, and disadvantages of each surgical approach and their specific technique will be reviewed and illustrated.

PATIENT PREPARATION

Standard for all of the surgical approaches is patient positioning and preparation. Patients are positioned in a modified beach chair position using a standard or modified operating table that allows for flexion of approximately 45 degrees at the waist and 30 degrees of flexion at the knees to prevent the patient from sliding distally. Placement of pillows under the knees is a technique that is helpful to maintain the flexed position. The head and neck are secured on a well-padded head rest, with the cervical spine in a neutral position, and the entire arm is draped free. The patient's positioning requires extension of the humerus for the preparation of the humeral component, without interference from the operating table. For this reason the patient is often positioned toward the edge of the operating table, with the lateral border of the scapula supported and the thorax secured. Operating table extensions specifically designed for shoulder surgery usually include a padded head rest, an elevated back support, and the removal of a lateral portion of the table that leaves the shoulder girdle exposed for the requisite intraoperative shoulder positioning. The surgeon may rotate the operating table to face the anesthesiologist, allowing all of the surgical assistants to be on the operative side of the patient.

Anesthetic technique is discussed between the anesthesiologist and the patient. An anterior interscalene regional anesthesia combined with general anesthesia offers the benefit of satisfactory postoperative pain management with intraoperative relaxation of the shoulder girdle musculature that is necessary for the procedure.

DELTOPECTORAL APPROACH

The deltopectoral approach is considered the standard approach for total shoulder arthroplasty.[3–5] It allows for the preservation of the origin of the anterior deltoid and a predictable exposure to the proximal humerus and inferior glenoid. The deltopectoral approach is limited in patients with frail deltoids, severe osteopenia, advanced osseous deformities involving the proximal humerus, and repairable posterosuperior rotator cuff tears.[1] Neurological complications have also been associated with the deltopectoral approach.[6,7]

The surgical approach through the deltopectoral interval is facilitated by the use of an arm rest or Mayo stand, with the arm slightly abducted, reducing tension on the deltoid. The anterior skin incision begins approximately 1.5 cm medial to the acromioclavicular joint, extending distally and slightly lateral to the coracoid and ending medial to the anterior insertion of the deltoid (Fig. 7.1). Sharp dissection through the subcutaneous tissues extends to the deltoid fascia, and the cephalic vein is identified, preserved, and retracted medially, ligating or cauterizing the lateral branches from the deltoid muscle. The cephalic vein is identified proximally with elevation of a medial subcutaneous flap that exposes the infraclavicular triangle formed by the medial margin of the deltoid, lateral margin of the pectoralis major, and inferior margin of the clavicle (Fig. 7.2).

The deltopectoral fascia is released along the entire incision to the deltoid insertion.[3] Exposure may be improved with the release of the proximal centimeter of the pectoralis major insertion, ensuring protection of the underlying long head of the biceps by placing a flat retractor under the superior margin of the pectoralis tendon (Fig. 7.3). The acromial and deltoid branches of the thoracoacromial artery are cauterized proximally, and the clavipectoral fascia lateral to the short head of the biceps musculature is released from the coracoacromial ligament to the deltoid insertion. The coracoacromial ligament is preserved if there is associated thinning, fibrosis, or tearing of the rotator cuff. After release of the clavipectoral fascia, exposure of the subdeltoid and subacromial spaces is often facilitated by slight flexion of the arm and the axillary nerve is protected as it exits the quadrilateral space posteriorly. In patients with marked internal rotation contractures a more generous release of the pectoralis tendon and release of the

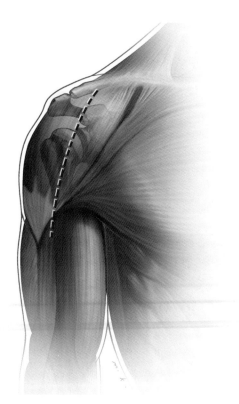

Figure 7.1. Deltopectoral approach. The shoulder and arm are draped free. The skin incision extends from the distal clavicle to the anterior insertion of the deltoid, passing lateral to the coracoid process.

latissimus dorsi tendon insertion may be necessary. An extended exposure of the deltopectoral approach can be obtained with elevation of the anterior deltoid insertion in continuity with its distal periosteum.[5] This maneuver should be done with caution because both the clavicular and anterior acromial origins of the deltoid insert into the anterior 20% of

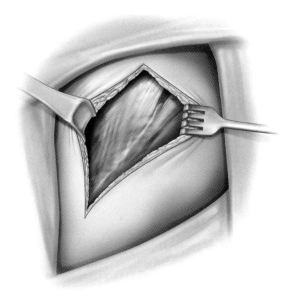

Figure 7.2. A limited medial soft tissue flap is developed proximally, exposing the cephalic vein and the deltopectoral interval.

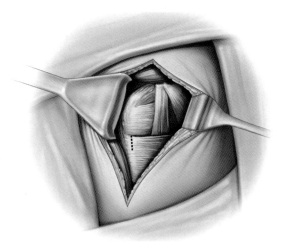

Figure 7.3. As the deltopectoral interval is developed distally, the deltoid is retracted laterally and the pectoralis major medially, the exposure is often aided with gentle external rotation. The superior border of the pectoralis tendon can be released to facilitate exposure, protecting the underlying long head of the biceps.

the deltoid tuberosity and a generous release could contribute to postoperative deltoid weakness.[8]

Palpation of the axillary nerve is necessary to ensure its protection throughout the procedure. Careful blunt dissection under the conjoined tendon develops the subcoracoid space and allows for palpation of the axillary nerve. The nerve is also palpated deep to the deltoid along its posterior course at the level of the superior margin of the pectoralis major tendon. The axillary nerve can be gently tugged anteriorly to ensure its continuity throughout the procedure.[9] The location of the axillary nerve also allows for estimation of the lower subscapular nerve, which is posterior or immediately lateral to the axillary nerve.[10] Knowledge of the lower subscapular nerve's location will limit dissection of the anterior surface of the subscapularis to an area lateral to the axillary nerve, avoiding denervation of the lower subscapularis during exposure and mobilization of the subscapularis tendon.

An arthrotomy through the subscapularis and anterior capsule is best accomplished with the shoulder placed in slight external rotation and adduction, limiting the lateral excursion of the axillary nerve.[11] Exposure is further improved with a subdeltoid retractor placed laterally and a medial retractor placed under the conjoined tendon. The brachial plexus lies within 2 cm of the anterior glenoid rim, and careful medial retraction is essential to avoid traction on the musculocutaneous nerve, which is closest in proximity to the retractor blade.[12] The incision for the arthrotomy extends vertically from the supraglenoid tubercle, medial to the long head of the biceps tendon, to the surgical neck of the humerus, requiring coagulation of the anterior circumflex vessels (Fig. 7.4). Placement of the arthrotomy incision can be variable and depends on the severity of the anterior soft tissue contractures as evidenced by the limitation in external rotation. An incision immediately medial to the intratubercle groove is recommended to maintain the length of the subscapularis tendon, allow for restoration of external rotation, and provide soft tissue balancing of the glenohumeral joint.

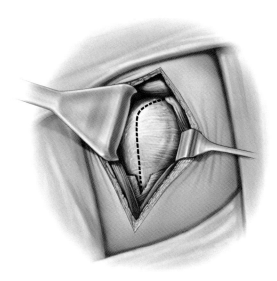

Figure 7.4. The arthrotomy incision extends from the superior aspect of the base of the coracoid process, just above the superior aspect of the subscapularis tendon, vertically along the lesser tuberosity, medial to the intertubercular groove, and ending inferiorly at the proximal humeral insertion of the inferior glenohumeral ligament. The incision may vary depending on limitation of external rotation from anterior soft tissue contractures.

Rarely, a severe internal rotation contracture may require a Z-lengthening of the subscapularis, provided that there is ample tissue thickness involving the subscapularis and anterior capsular complex. If the tissue quality is poor or thin, the length of the subscapularis tendon is preserved and later reattached medial to its anatomic insertion.

With external rotation, the inferior capsule is released from its articular and proximal humeral attachment. The inferior glenohumeral capsular attachment extends up to 2 cm distal to its articular insertion; its complete release is required for glenoid exposure.[13] A thin flat or Cobb retractor can be placed intra-articularly during the release of the inferior capsule to protect the axillary nerve. The final inferior capsular release extends from the 1 o'clock position to the 7 o'clock position for the exposure of a right shoulder (Fig. 7.5).

Resection of the proximal humerus is a technique dependent on the arthroplasty system used. The arm is removed from the Mayo stand and placed in extension for resection and preparation of the proximal humerus. A large, flat Darrach-type retractor is placed under the humeral head and with gentle external rotation and extension the humeral head is dislocated through the levering action of the retractor (Fig. 7.6). A small forked or flat retractor is placed anterior to the biceps before humeral head resection to protect the long head of the biceps and rotator cuff insertion. If there is marked biceps tendonosis identified at the time of proximal humeral preparation, a biceps release or tenodesis can be performed, depending on the surgeon's preference. Osteophytes are removed, and the humeral head is resected at the level of the rotator cuff insertion in the amount of retrotorsion dictated by the total shoulder system used.

Glenoid exposure requires that the arm be replaced on the padded Mayo stand in 70 to 90 degrees of abduction and slight flexion, relaxing the deltoid and decreasing tension on the brachial plexus. The humeral head is retracted posteroinferiorly, with a humeral head retractor placed over the posterior glenoid rim. Several retractors have been developed for retraction of the proximal humerus, including ring-type (Fukuda) retractors, humeral neck or cobra-type retractors, or Darrach-type elevators (Fig. 7.7). Regardless of surgeon preference, it is often useful to have more than one humeral head retractor available for glenoid exposure, anticipating situations that may favor a specific retractor design. Hypertrophic synovium, intra-articular scar, and the glenoid labrum are excised. The anterior capsular attachment is sharply released from the anterior glenoid rim, and a forked or flat retractor is placed deep to the capsule, exposing the anterior glenoid neck (Fig. 7.8). The degree of periarticular soft tissue contracture can limit glenoid exposure, and additional capsular releases may be required (Fig. 7.9).

Soft tissue closure requires the secure repair of the subscapularis-anterior capsular complex, the assessment of axillary nerve integrity, and a routine subcutaneous and skin closure. The subscapularis can be reattached to its tendinous stump or sutured to bone through transosseous tunnels similar to techniques used for an open rotator cuff repair. Transosseous suture placement can occur through the osteotomy site or through bone tunnels placed within the lesser tuberosity by a large trocar needle, curved awls, or a needle-tipped burr. Medial attachment of the subscapularis insertion or Z-lengthening of the subscapularis tendon may be indicated when severe preoperative anterior soft tissue contracture prevents the restoration of external rotation.

Postoperative immobilization and rehabilitation are dependent on soft tissue quality, glenohumeral joint stability, and associated rotator cuff repairs. Patients free of soft tissue insufficiency, shoulder instability, or rotator cuff tearing are protected in a sling immobilizer for 6 weeks, allowing a protected passive range of motion determined at the time of surgery. Full active range of motion can be initiated at 8 weeks and resistive strengthening starting at 10 to 12 weeks. Soft tissue, rotator cuff, and shoulder instability concerns usually require a longer period of immobilization with or without the addition of abduction or external rotation bracing. Shoulder motion is delayed with the advancement to active motion and strengthening exercises dictated by soft tissue healing. Caution is always exercised with compromised soft tissues, and sling immobilization with protected motion for approximately 12 weeks is usually required.

Neurological complications after shoulder arthroplasty have an incidence ranging from 0.6% to 4.3%.[7] A series from the Mayo Clinic reported a 4.3% incidence of neurological injury occurring after total shoulder arthroplasty.[6] The use of methotrexate for rheumatoid arthritis, a deltopectoral approach, and shorter operating times were associated with postoperative nerve injury related to total shoulder arthroplasty.

The incidence of intraoperative nerve dysfunction using a deltopectoral approach for total shoulder arthroplasty has been prospectively evaluated.[7] Peripheral nerve function was monitored with both transcranial electrical motor evoked potentials as well as electromyography (EMG). Of the patients in the study, 57% had episodes of nerve dysfunction intraoperatively, thought to be related to a traction neuropraxia, of which none returned to normal baseline function with removal of the retractor alone. Repositioning the arm to a neutral

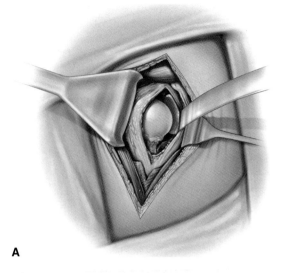

A

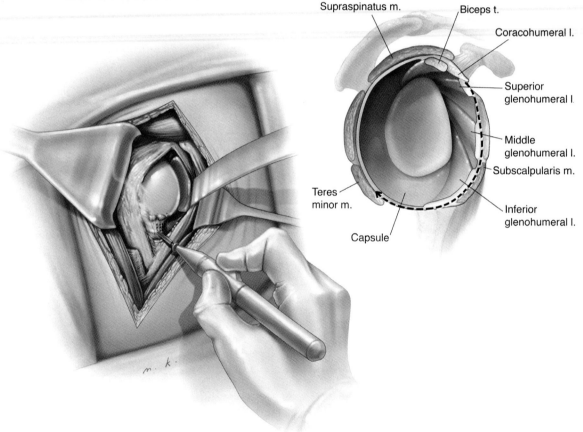

B

Figure 7.5.   **(A,B)** By carefully externally rotating the shoulder, the inferior glenohumeral ligament is released from its humeral insertion. This maneuver permits ample exposure to the proximal humerus and glenoid.

Supraspinatus m.   Biceps t.

Coracohumeral l.

Superior glenohumeral l.

Middle glenohumeral l.

Subscalpularis m.

Inferior glenohumeral l.

Teres minor m.

Capsule

position allowed for 77% of the patients to have return of their nerve function. Overall, 5 of 30 (16.7%) patients had permanent EMG changes following surgery that involved the axillary nerve on three occasions and the lower trunk on one occasion. One patient had objective weakness but refused a postoperative EMG study to determine the location of the neurological injury. Abnormalities in nerve function were related to shoulder positioning in abduction, external rotation, and extension in 50% of the nerve dysfunction episodes. Adduction, external rotation and extension, and abduction with at least 90% elbow

flexion were other arm positions that resulted in nerve dysfunction. Decreased external rotation and arm extension reduced or eliminated nerve compromise, with nerve function returning within 5 minutes. Patients who had less then 10 degrees of passive preoperative external rotation at the side and had prior open surgery had the greatest risk factor for developing nerve dysfunction during surgery. Operative time was not a factor in the development of nerve dysfunction during surgery. Nerve dysfunction occurred most often during humeral (33%) and glenoid preparation (50%). Shoulder positioning should be

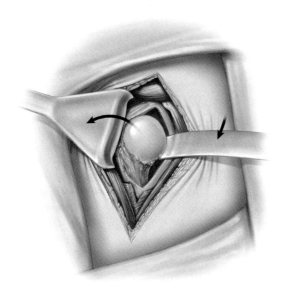

Figure 7.6. The humeral head is exposed by gentle shoulder extension and external rotation, aided by the levering action of a Darrach-type retractor.

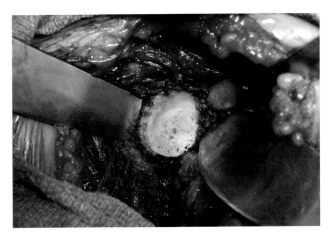

Figure 7.8. Glenoid exposure. A cobra retractor retracts the humeral head posteriorly, a forked retractor retracts the anterior capsule and subscapularis anteriorly, and small Hohmann retractor protects the biceps insertion posterosuperiorly.

carefully monitored during the exposure of the proximal humerus and glenoid, particularly in patients who have had prior surgery with limited external rotation.

Subscapularis dysfunction following total shoulder arthroplasty has been associated with the subscapularis tenotomy that is required for the deltopectoral approach.[14,15] Postoperative ultrasound studies have estimated the incidence of subscapularis tendon detachment to be 13%. Of interest, outcomes measures have not been consistently different among patients with or without subscapularis detachment, although patients may have difficulty tucking in their shirt with subscapularis insufficiency. Lesser tuberosity osteotomy techniques have been developed to minimize postoperative subscapularis insufficiency and maximize healing (Fig. 7.10). Despite predictable osteotomy healing and satisfactory postoperative subscapularis function, computed tomography studies have demonstrated a

progression of fatty infiltration of the subscapularis in 44% of the shoulders that had a healed osteotomy.[16] At the present time the advantages of a lesser tuberosity osteotomy over standard techniques remains a work in progress.

ANTEROMEDIAL APPROACH

The anteromedial approach was described by Neer[17,18] as a short deltopectoral approach with detachment of the anterior portion of the deltoid from the clavicle and anterior acromion. This approach was initially favored for total shoulder arthroplasty but was later discontinued because of concerns related to

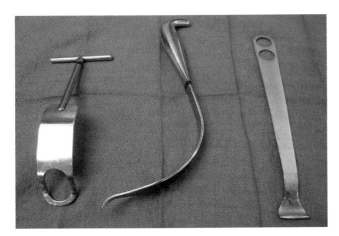

Figure 7.7. An assortment of glenoid retractors is helpful for glenoid exposure. From *left* to *right* are a ring (Fukuta) retractor, cobra retractor, and a humeral neck retractor.

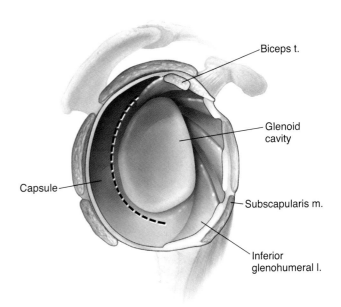

Biceps t.

Glenoid cavity

Capsule

Subscapularis m.

Inferior glenohumeral l.

Figure 7.9. The posterior capsular release for glenoid exposure.

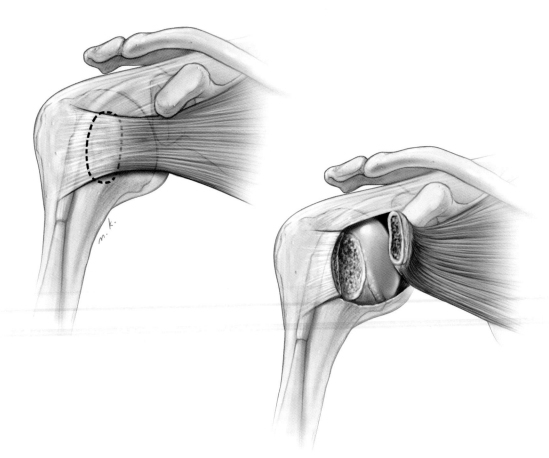

Figure 7.10. The lesser tuberosity osteotomy as an alternative approach to the glenohumeral joint.

the detachment of the anterior deltoid origin, resulting in deltoid weakness.[3]

Contemporary indications for the anteromedial approach have evolved, accounting for 5.9% of approaches used for shoulder arthroplasty in a study evaluating its effect on patient outcomes.[1] The anteromedial approach is indicated in patients with frail or fibrotic deltoids that will not tolerate or permit retraction, severe osteopenia that places the humerus at risk for fracture during rotation and preparation of the humerus, severe proximal humeral bony deformities that require extensive exposure, and posterosuperior rotator cuff tearing that is amenable to repair. The anteromedial approach for total shoulder arthroplasty can also be considered for patients at risk for neurological injury. With careful repair of the deltoid, preservation of deltoid strength can be predictably achieved.

The incision for the anteromedial exposure is identical to that for the extended deltopectoral approach. The deltopectoral fascia is released from superior to inferior, the cephalic vein is mobilized medially, and the subdeltoid, subacromial, and subcoracoid regions are carefully freed of adhesions after the clavipectoral fascia is excised.[19] Retractors are carefully placed deep to the deltoid and conjoined tendon, and the proximal centimeter of the pectoralis may require release for improved exposure. The clavicular and acromial origin of the anterior deltoid are identified, and the fascia is incised over the lateral clavicle between the deltoid and trapezial musculature, continued laterally over the mid-superior aspect of the acromioclavicular

joint capsule and along the anterior acromion, carefully elevating the deltoid from bone (Fig. 7.11). Traction sutures or atraumatic clamps are placed along the edge of the incised deltoid origin that is reflected laterally. The subacromial and subdeltoid spaces may require further release of adhesions caused by previous trauma or bursal inflammation. Extension and internal rotation will allow the visualization of the posterior portion of the supraspinatus, infraspinatus, and teres minor for repair, if necessary. The remainder of the anteromedial approach is identical to that described for the extended deltopectoral technique for proximal humeral and glenoid preparation and exposure.

Although the anteromedial approach allows for excellent exposure, the release of the anterior deltoid origin raises concerns of preserved deltoid function. Attention to meticulous technique is necessary for repair of the anterior deltoid at the conclusion of the procedure. A no. 2 or 3 braided nonabsorbable suture may be preferred for repair of the deltoid, the repair proceeding from lateral to medial. Transosseous repair through the anterior acromion uses either a needle-tip burr or a trocar needle, securing the detached muscle origin to its acromial detachment. Simple sutures have proved to be adequate, and the closure proceeds medially through the acromioclavicular joint capsule, repairing the released trapezial fascia. A needle-tip burr or small drill bit is used for the repair of the deltoid to its clavicular origin (Fig. 7.12).

Postoperative rehabilitation requires the cautious advancement of motion guided by the intraoperative assessment of tissue quality and the limits imposed by rotator cuff repairs. An

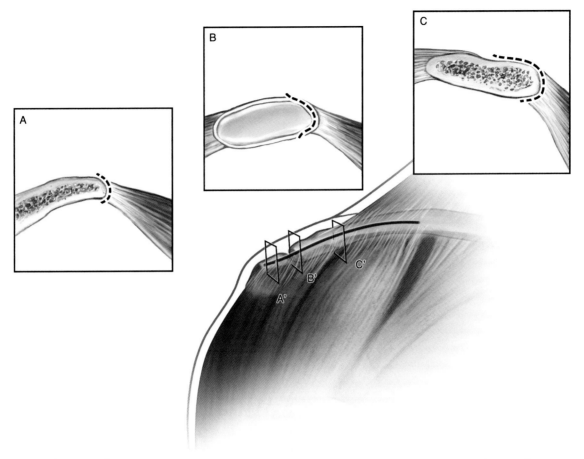

Figure 7.11. Anteromedial approach. The skin incision is the same used for the deltopectoral approach. The deep incision, after developing the deltopectoral interval, incises the anterior deltoid from the bone on the anterior aspect of the acromion process (**A**), through a portion of the acromioclavicular joint capsule (**B**) and from the bone of the clavicle (**C**).

immobilizer or abduction brace is used for the first 4 to 6 weeks, with passive range of motion performed as determined intraoperatively. Therapy is advanced in a manner similar to that discussed for the deltopectoral approach.

Successful outcomes following an anteromedial approach are dependent on satisfactory preoperative and postoperative anterior deltoid strength, the integrity of the rotator cuff, and the preoperative diagnosis. Patients with rheumatoid arthritis can be weaker than those with osteoarthritis or posttraumatic arthritis.[1]

ANTEROSUPERIOR APPROACH

The anterosuperior approach has been favored by some because of its improved access to the posterosuperior tendons of the rotator cuff and direct approach to the glenoid through the rotator interval.[2,20] Its disadvantages include a limited exposure to the proximal humerus and inferior glenoid and the potential for anterior deltoid weakness.

The incision for the anterosuperior approach can be variable. Either a saber-type incision over the anterolateral acromion directed lateral to the acromioclavicular joint toward the anterior axillary fold or a lateral incision from posterior to the acromioclavicular joint to the mid-aspect of the deltoid

musculature can be used (Fig. 7.13). Sharp dissection through the subcutaneous tissue proceeds to the superficial fascia of the anterior deltoid. Medial and lateral subcutaneous flaps are developed, and the deltoid is released from its anterior acromion origin. The approach can be extended medially if distal clavicular resection for symptomatic acromioclavicular joint arthritis is required.

The deltoid is split along its fibers immediately lateral to the acromioclavicular joint for a distance of 4 cm (Fig. 7.14). A stay suture is placed at the distal margin of the split to avoid its propagation and potential injury to the axillary nerve. Careful retraction of the anterior deltoid and the release of subacromial and subdeltoid soft tissue adhesions are preceded by the incision of the clavipectoral fascia. Tenotomy of the upper subscapularis and exposure and preparation of the proximal humerus and glenoid proceed in the same manner as with the deltopectoral and anteromedial approaches. Arm positions necessary to accommodate the steps of the exposure are the same as previously discussed. Repair of the deltoid to the acromion and distal clavicle requires the same meticulous attention as that for the anteromedial approach. Postoperative rehabilitation is similar to that described for the anteromedial approach by providing the protection necessary for the repaired anterior deltoid origin.

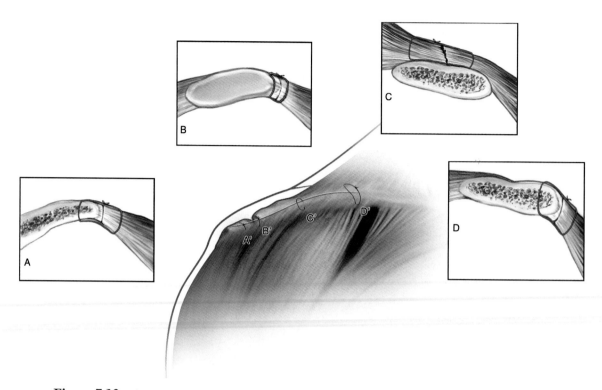

Figure 7.12. Anteromedial approach. The deltoid with acromioclavicular joint capsule and the limited amount of deltoid fascia are meticulously repaired to bone or soft tissue. **(A)** Repair through bone to the anterior aspect of the acromion process. **(B)** Repair to the acromioclavicular joint capsule. **(C)** Repair to the trapezius muscle and fascia. **(D)** Repair through burr holes to the clavicle.

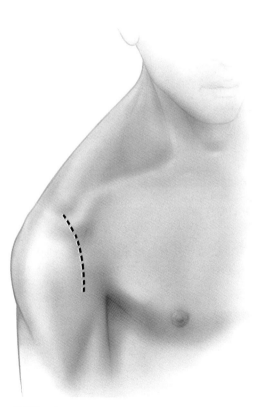

Figure 7.13. Anterosuperior approach, saber-type incision. A more lateral incision is another option.

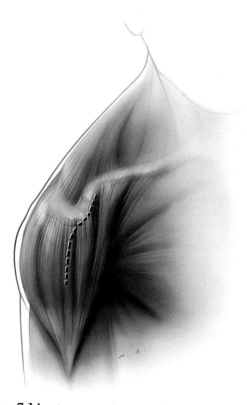

Figure 7.14. Anterosuperior approach. The anterior deltoid is elevated from the anterolateral acromion, with an anterior deltoid split extending 4 cm distally—either from the acromioclavicular joint or the anterolateral corner of the acromion.

The advent of reverse shoulder arthroplasty for shoulders with irreparable rotator cuff tearing and associated arthritis has popularized the anterosuperior approach.[21] If there is marked superior or anterosuperior humeral subluxation, the anterosuperior approach takes advantage of the absent rotator cuff, allowing the procedure to be performed by preserving the majority of the subscapularis insertion and decreasing the risk of postoperative instability. Potential anterior deltoid compromise resulting from deltoid origin release or axillary nerve injury from the deltoid split is a concern given that the anterior deltoid provides the primary motor function for the reverse arthroplasty design.

The anterosuperior approach places the axillary nerve at risk with its deltoid split. The safe area for the axillary nerve after a deltoid split varies.[11–23] The minimum distance from the axillary nerve to the anterior acromion has been measured at 2 to 2.5 centimeters, with 25% of cadaveric shoulders having less than a 4-cm distance between the nerve and the anterior acromion. Arm positioning during the anterosuperior approach is also important because abduction shortens the distance between the axillary nerve and anterior acromion by up to 30%.[10]

SUMMARY

Although the deltopectoral approach remains the standard for most shoulder arthroplasty procedures, having knowledge of other surgical approaches for specific indications is desirable. The deltopectoral exposure has limitations in conditions with a frail or fibrotic deltoid, severe osteopenia, proximal humeral deformity, or a potential for neurological compromise. The anteromedial and anterosuperior approaches may be favored in these circumstances and have proven their value and versatility. Alternative surgical approaches for shoulder arthroplasty have been described and represent modifications of the three commonly used procedures discussed in this chapter, without additional advantages.[24]

The shoulder surgeon is encouraged to be familiar with several exposures to the shoulder that will allow adjustments to the challenges of revision and complex shoulder arthroplasty.

REFERENCES

1. Gill DR, Cofield RH, Rowland C. The anteromedial approach for shoulder arthroplasty: the importance of the anterior deltoid. *J Shoulder Elbow Surg* 2004;13:532–537.
2. MacKenzie DB. The anterosuperior exposure for total shoulder replacement. *Orthop Traumatology* 1993;2:71–77.
3. Neer CS II, Watson KC, Stanton FJ. Recent experiences in total shoulder replacement. *J Bone Joint Surg Am* 1982;64:319–337.
4. Boileau P, Watkinson D, Hatzidakis AM, et al. The Grammont reverse shoulder prosthesis: results in cuff tear arthritis, fracture sequelae, and revision arthroplasty. *J Shoulder Elbow Surg* 2006;15:527–540.
5. Cofield RH. Total shoulder replacement: managing bone deficiencies. In: Craig EV, ed. *Master Techniques in Orthopaedic Surgery: The Shoulder.* 2nd ed. Baltimore: Lippincott Williams & Wilkins; 2004:549–575.
6. Lynch NM, Cofield RH, Sibert PL, et al. Neurologic complications after total shoulder arthroplasty. *J Shoulder Elbow Surg* 1996;5:53–61.
7. Nagda SH, Rogers KJ, Sestokas AK, et al. Peripheral nerve function during shoulder arthroplasty using intraoperative nerve monitoring. *J Shoulder Elbow Surg* 2007;16(3 suppl): 2S–8S.
8. Klepps S, Auerbach J, Calhan D, et al. A cadaveric study on the anatomy of the deltoid insertion and its relationship to the deltopectoral approach to the proximal humerus. *J Shoulder Elbow Surg* 2004;13:322–327.
9. Flatow EL, Bigliani LU. Locating and protecting the axillary nerve in shoulder surgery. *Orthop Rev* 1992;21:503–505.
10. Yung S-W, Lazarus MD, Harryman DT II. Practical guidelines to safe surgery about the subscapularis. *J Shoulder Elbow Surg* 1996;5:467–470.
11. Burkhead WZ Jr, Scheinberg RR, Box G. Surgical Anatomy of the axillary nerve. *J Shoulder Elbow Surg* 1992;1:31–36.
12. McFarland EG, Caicedo JC, Guitterez MI, et al. An anatomic relationship of the brachial plexus and axillary artery to the glenoid: implications for anterior shoulder surgery. *Am Sports Med* 2001;29:726–733.
13. Sugalski MT, Wiater JM, Levine WN, et al. An anatomic study of the humeral insertion of the inferior glenohumeral capsule. *J Shoulder Elbow Surg* 2005;14:91–95.
14. Armstrong A, Lashgari C, Teefey S, et al. Ultrasound evaluation and clinical correlation of subscapularis repair after total shoulder arthropathy. *J Shoulder Elbow Surg* 2006;15: 541–548.
15. Miller SL, Hazrati Y, Klepps S, et al. Loss of subscapularis function after total shoulder replacement: a seldom recognized problem. *J Surg Elbow Surg* 2003;12:29–34.
16. Gerber C, Yian EH, Priffman AW, et al. Subscapularis muscle function and structure after total shoulder replacement with lesser tuberosity osteotomy and repair. *J Bone Joint Surg Am* 2005;87:1739–1745.
17. Neer CS II. Articular replacement for the humeral head. *J Bone Joint Surg Am* 1955; 37:215–228.
18. Neer CS II. Replacement arthroplasty for glenohumeral osteoarthritis. *J Bone Joint Surg Am* 1974;56:1–13.
19. Cooper DE, O'Brien SJ, Warren RF. The supporting layers of the glenohumeral joint: an anatomic study. *Clin Orthop* 1993;289:144–155.
20. Levy O, Copeland SA. Cementless surface replacement arthroplasty of the shoulder. *J Bone Joint Surg Br* 2001;83:213–221.
21. Sirveaux F, Favard L, Oudet D, et al. Grammont inverted total shoulder arthroplasty in the treatment of glenohumeral osteoarthritis with massive rupture of the cuff. *J Bone Joint Surg Br* 2004;86:388–395.
22. Cetik D, Uslu M, Acar HI, et al. Is there a safe area for the axillary nerve in the deltoid muscle? A cadaveric study. *J Bone Joint Surg Am* 2006;88:2395–2399.
23. Kontakis GM, Steriopoulos K, Damilakis J, et al, The position of the axillary nerve in the deltoid muscle: a cadaveric study. *Acta Orthop Scand* 1999;70:9–11.
24. Kuz JE, Pierce TD, Braunohler WM. Coronal transacromial osteotomy surgical approach for shoulder arthroplasty. *Orthopaedics* 1998;21:155–162.

Revision Shoulder Arthroplasty: Understanding Implant Options

INTRODUCTION

The complex problems of revision shoulder arthroplasty demand a wide armamentarium of implants and techniques. The prostheses available vary from country to country, and their commercial names also vary. This review discusses implant features rather than specific commercially available prostheses. Although theoretical considerations are important, surgeons also need to be familiar with and comfortable with the prostheses they use and theoretical solutions should be tempered with the individual surgeon's comfort with the available prostheses.

It is essential in revision cases to ensure that the appropriate prostheses are available in the operating room. This may mean several different options being preordered. Preoperative planning is essential, and if the operating surgeon was not responsible for the index procedure, preliminary confirmation of the details of the primary implant should be sought well in advance. The surgeon should keep potential complications in mind when preordering prostheses. An intraoperative humeral shaft fracture is relatively easily attended to if a long-stemmed prosthesis is available, but can otherwise present major logistic difficulties. If a glenoid revision proves technically impossible, having allograft bone available may save the day. Similarly, having a range of large humeral head prostheses available is essential. There is no substitute for careful preoperative planning and precautions.

Each revision case presents its own problems. Here we approach the problems from an anatomic viewpoint, discussing which implant features are relevant to each particular issue (Fig. 8.1 and Table 8.1). Examples will be given to illustrate particular points rather than to endorse specific products. On rare occasions, available prostheses may not meet case-specific requirements. Some prosthesis manufacturers offer a CAD CAM (computer-assisted design, computer-assisted manufacturing) facility for custom-made prostheses, and the surgeon may wish to consider these options in advance. This service enables changes to stem diameter, length, offset, or glenoid component geometry and can be especially useful in the setting of dysplasia. Recent advances in the design (Table 8.2) and application of

reverse prostheses have introduced a new era in revision arthroplasty, allowing functional results to be achieved in cases previously doomed to flail shoulders or salvage arthrodeses. The reverse arthroplasty options will be reviewed independently, in the second part of this chapter.

REVISION ARTHROPLASTY IN CASES WITH FUNCTIONAL ROTATOR CUFFS

HUMERAL PROSTHESIS REVISION

Humeral Head Issues

Humeral stem revision is not always necessary. When modular humeral stems are in situ, and their version is appropriate, removal of the prosthetic head often allows adequate glenoid access without removal of a well-fixed humeral stem. After glenoid revision, the humeral head size may need to be altered. Appropriate tissue tensioning and subacromial clearance for the tuberosity may require larger or smaller heads. If eccentric humeral heads are available to match the existing stem, eccentricity may be helpful in achieving appropriate tissue tension and prosthetic stability. For example, increased anterior eccentricity may be used to provide some posterior capsular tightening, a somewhat counterintuitive but effective maneuver (Fig. 8.2).

Although there are some theoretical concerns regarding the "reuse" of Morse taper fittings, this does not appear to be a clinical problem.

Metaphyseal Issues

Revision arthroplasty may be required for tuberosity fracture, nonunion, or malunion after hemiarthroplasty. Lesser tuberosity osteotomy for subscapularis mobilization in a primary procedure may have failed to unite. Prosthesis removal may have caused fractures of either or both tuberosities. In these situations, analogous to fresh three- and four-part fractures, a fracture prosthesis (with a thin metaphysis and multiple suture

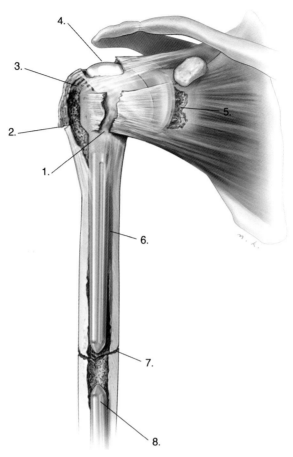

Figure 8.1. Common problems in revision shoulder arthroplasty.
(See Table 8.1. for potential solutions to each numbered problem.)

TABLE 8.1	Potential Solutions to Common Problems*

1. Failure of subscapularis
   Tendon transfer (pectoralis major)
   Tendon allograft
   Revision prosthesis
2. Loss of metaphyseal bone
   Impaction grafting
   Tumor prosthesis
   Allograft
3. Tuberosity malunion (after fracture)
   Fracture prosthesis
   Stem with metaphyseal in-growth/on-growth surface
   Features that provide the ability to hold graft—for example,
      suture holes, multiple fins
4. Loss of rotator cuff
   Tendon transfer (latissimus dorsi ± teres major)
   Cuff allograft
   Cuff tear arthropathy head
   Revision prosthesis
   Epoca Reco glenoid prosthesis
5. Glenoid issues
   Abnormal glenoid version
      Metal-backed/graft friendly prosthesis
   Glenoid loosening and bone loss
      Bone graft
      Glenoid prostheses of variable keel/peg size and length
      Metal-backed glenoid component
      Auxiliary glenoid fixation—for example, plate attachment

6. Humeral malposition
   Stems of variable thickness—for example, fracture stem or
      standard
7. Humeral shaft fracture, bone loss or cortical window
   Long stem prosthesis
   Centering device
   Allograft struts with cabling
8. Presence of total elbow arthroplasty
   Prostheses with variety of stem lengths

Unnumbered problems (in reference to Fig. 8.1)
   Infection
      Pre-made antibiotic-impregnated PMMA spacers
   Failed reverse prosthesis
      Eccentric glenosphere
      Salvage head
   Instability secondary to soft tissue loss
      Muscle-tendon transfers
      Allograft tendon
      Reverse implant

*Refer to problems numbered in Figure 8.1.

TABLE 8.2	Design Considerations in Revision Shoulder Arthroplasty	
Glenoid Side		**Humeral Side**

Glenoid Side

- Variable glenoid size (radius)
- Variable poly thickness
- Variety of peg/keel configurations to fill a glenoid defect
- All poly and metal-backed options
- Modularity
- Surface coatings to improve bone in-growth/on-growth
- Variable screw angle and position, ideally with locking option
- Features to allow screw fixation to bone-deficient glenoid
- Option to convert baseplate to reverse option without revision if stable

ADDITIONAL REVERSE SPECIFIC CONSIDERATIONS
- Eccentric glenosphere
- Variable peg length
- Variable peg diameter

Humeral Side

- Variable head sizes
- Variable head offsets
- Variable head eccentricity
- Variable stem diameter
- Variable stem length
- Cemented and uncemented options
- Bone in-growth for uncemented option
- Modular metaphysis
- Suture holes in the metaphysis
- Soft tissue spacer
- Cuff tear arthropathy head options
- Convertible from standard to reverse without stem change

- Variable metaphyseal height
- Variable metaphyseal offset
- Retentive and nonretentive liners
- Variable polyethylene thickness
- Salvage heads

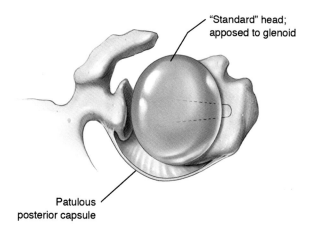

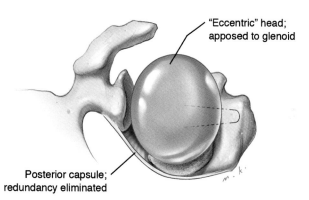

Figure 8.2.   Tightening of posterior capsule by use of an eccentric modular head.

holes in the fins) is sometimes useful. Tuberosity reconstruction is certainly facilitated by these features, and having a suture hole on the medial aspect of the humeral neck is almost a prerequisite for secure cerclage repair of the tuberosities. If necessary, this can be combined with local bone graft to help restore anatomic normality. There is a certain attraction to securing shell-like tuberosities over bone graft rather than over underlying cement or metal. Many fracture prostheses have on-growth or in-growth features on their metaphyseal surfaces to facilitate this (Fig. 8.3).

Extensive loss of metaphyseal cancellous bone in the presence of intact or near intact cortical bone lends itself to cementing or bone grafting. Very occasionally, the loss of metaphyseal cortical bone may be so extensive as to warrant the use of a tumor prosthesis, with a prosthetic metaphyseal component. This rare situation requires careful preoperative assessment because the necessary prostheses may need to be preordered or even custom made. In these situations, rotator cuff (re)attachment is often problematic and such cases may be better treated with a reverse prosthesis.

Diaphyseal Issues

Although cement removal is clearly desirable, revision humeral stem replacement is not entirely analogous to femoral prosthesis revision in hip surgery. Complete cement removal is sometimes neither possible nor desirable, and there may be occasions in which a revision prosthesis is cemented inside an existing cement mantle. If this is anticipated, the diameter of the new prosthesis clearly needs to be less than that of the primary and preplanning is essential. On other occasions, cement removal may leave a capacious diaphysis, in which impaction grafting can be employed. If this is considered, not only do the appropriate prostheses need to be arranged but also impaction broaches and other instruments. The use of allograft bone in humeral impaction grafting

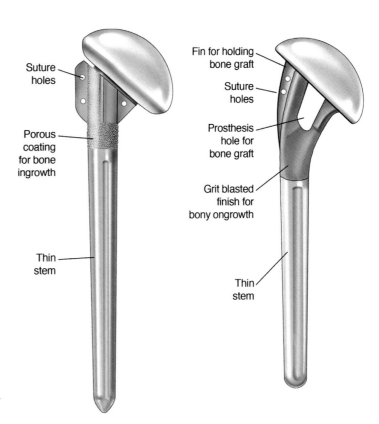

Figure 8.3. Metaphyseal design features and surfaces to enhance tuberosity offset and bony in-growth and on-growth.

is contentious and beyond the scope of this discussion. Pressurization of cement is hazardous in revision shoulder replacement because cement can escape through cracks or vascular foramina and burn adjacent structures. The radial nerve is particularly at risk in this setting, and the use of cement restrictors should be cautious. Stem-centering devices, however, may be helpful.

Whenever prosthetic stems need to be removed, the possibility of humeral shaft fracture must be anticipated. Long-stemmed prostheses should be available. Even if the primary stem is removed without humeral fracture, there is often a residual thinning and weakening of the cortex at the level of the tip of the primary prosthesis. The revision prosthesis should extend beyond this stress riser by a minimum of two diaphyseal diameters to reduce the risk of subsequent periprosthetic fracture. Most current designs offer a range of stem lengths for this purpose. Consideration may also be given to the use of diaphyseal cabled allograft bone struts to improve bone stock and construct strength. Again, preoperative planning is essential.

It is not uncommon in rheumatoid arthritis to find elbow and shoulder replacements in the same arm. The closer the prosthetic tips are to each other, the greater the risk of fracture. These issues need to be considered when planning prosthetic length.

Infection: Temporary Prostheses for Use in Infected Revision Surgery

Revision in the presence of (or because of) sepsis presents particular problems. These are discussed in detail elsewhere in this monograph. The commercial availability of antibiotic-impregnated polymethylmethacrylate (PMMA) temporary prostheses, however, warrants mention here.

These devices can be implanted as the first stage of a two-stage revision for sepsis. A range of stem widths and head sizes allows for maintenance of space for a subsequent definitive prosthesis. The local release of antibiotics (usually gentamicin) helps counter infection, and the smooth articulating surface allows at least some movement with relative comfort while awaiting definitive revision. Whether these preprepared temporary prostheses produce better ultimate outcomes than the less expensive temporary spacers hand-made intraoperatively is unclear.

GLENOID REVISION

Glenoid prosthetic loosening is possibly the most common indication for revision shoulder arthroplasty. Preliminary computed tomography (CT) scanning is invaluable (and virtually mandatory). The extent of glenoid bone stock loss determines the revision procedure. Contained and uncontained defects present different problems.

In cases of simple dissociation or excessive wear of the polyethylene liner of a metal-backed glenoid, simple exchange (replacement) of the polyethylene is sometimes an option. If this possibility exists, there is a degree of urgency to the revision, which should be performed before metal-on-metal contact destroys the glenoid-locking mechanism. The prosthesis being revised may be outdated and no longer in regular use, but most manufacturers carry components for at least 20 years. Preordering is obviously essential. If the cause of a liner dissociation is apparent at surgery, that too should be corrected (minor posterior instability may loosen or eccentrically wear the polyethylene).

When the glenoid defect is contained (i.e., there is intact or virtually intact circumferential cortical bone), the extent of cancellous bone loss determines technique and prosthesis. If the primary prosthesis can be removed while leaving a significant amount of cancellous bone, recementing a standard glenoid prosthesis may be possible. If extensive bone grafting (autograft, allograft, or bone substitute) is required, a decision needs to be made whether to replace the glenoid at the time of surgery or to plan a staged revision at some later date, when the graft has consolidated.

Contained Defects

The principles of impaction grafting with cementation can be applied to the glenoid in the setting of a contained glenoid defect. These authors have no experience with this technique, but it has been described. Solid packing, underimpaction, of a contained glenoid defect allows the use of a cemented glenoid prosthesis. In this situation, it is ideal if the prosthesis can rest on the cortical rim of the glenoid to maintain compaction and preserve stability. This scenario may lend itself to metal-backed prostheses (Fig. 8.4). When there is a cortical rim on which to sit a metal back, the baseplate can be used to maintain graft integrity and prevent graft "leakage." Fixation screws can be employed to cross the graft and take hold on native bone, preferably including cortex. Although it is widely believed that metal-backed glenoids have a shorter lifespan than all-polyethylene prostheses, the one-stage insertion of a metal-backed prosthesis may be preferable to the two-stage use of a polyethylene prosthesis preceded by first-stage grafting. Some metal-backed prostheses also allow the surgeon to employ variable glenoid prosthetic thicknesses, which may assist in tissue tensioning and the restoration of normal biomechanics. Thicker polyethylene inserts, however, are more likely to dissociate from the underlying baseplate (same underlying fixation system and strength, but altered forces with differing polyethylene insert thickness). When the removal of a primary glenoid prosthesis leaves a medium-sized contained defect, a metal-backed glenoid with a larger keel or central peg may reduce or eliminate the need for bone grafting, the keel or peg occupying a greater space than the initial polyethylene prosthesis.

The use of metal-backed glenoids is controversial. Careful consideration of preoperative CT scanning is important in this setting. Some metal-backed prostheses also come with an anterior glenoid plate that can be screwed onto the anterior glenoid cortex, allowing additional stability, an attractive feature in the revision setting (e.g., the Arrow prosthesis and some SMR options). This particular feature is more widely used in reverse prostheses, discussed below.

Glenoid Version

Problems of glenoid version have previously been addressed with the use of augmented and wedged prostheses, but these have fallen into relative disfavor, having been associated with early loosening. Correction of glenoid version with bone grafting is a technically demanding procedure. When this is under-

Antero-posterior view

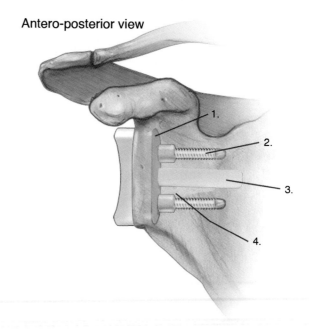

Axillary view

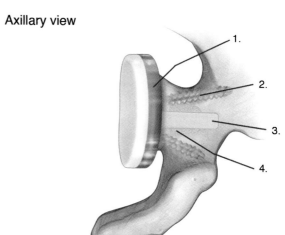

Figure 8.4. Use of a metal-backed prosthesis to enclose a bone-grafted, contained glenoid defect.

1. Metal baseplate overlaps and rests on cortical rim, for stability and to maintain compaction/retention of bone graft.
2. Defect/void filled with compacted bone graft.
3. Fixation screws across graft to engage native bone, ideally passing through cortex to provide compression.
4. Large peg/stem helps fill void, reducing required graft volume.

taken, it is desirable to fix the glenoid prosthesis in native, nongraft bone. This may demand the use of a very thin central peg or keel, a smaller than usual prosthesis, or slight repositioning, usually anteriorly, of the glenoid prosthesis, so that the fin or keel is entirely within nongraft bone. This arrangement generally precludes the use of a multipegged prosthesis.

UNCONTAINED GLENOID DEFECTS

The first consideration in this setting is to produce a contained glenoid, preferably with good bone stock between the cortices as well. Each case presents its own problems. Cortical, bicortical, or tricortical bone grafting is usually employed, with or without internal fixation. In this setting, it is not uncommon for the surgeon to replace the humeral head with a larger than usual prosthesis, to await glenoid bone consolidation, and to then return to the shoulder as a staged procedure, inserting a glenoid prosthesis and usually reducing the size of the humeral head. Surgeons should allow for both possibilities when arranging prostheses for such cases. The pain relief gained from bone grafting alone is often such that patients are not unhappy with the status quo, and glenoid resurfacing is not always necessary. If per chance a stable construct can be obtained at the index revision procedure, the considerations discussed previously for contained defects apply, and the glenoid may be resurfaced at the first revision procedure. Again, "prosthetic provision" needs to be arranged preoperatively.

Hybrid Prostheses

If only one side of a prosthesis requires revision, surgeons need not fear a hybrid prosthesis (i.e., glenoid from prosthesis "A" and humerus from prosthesis "B"). There is no universal agreement regarding optimal "diametral mismatch" between humerus and glenoid. Revision surgery often demands compromise, and any diametral mismatch between 0 and 6 mm may be contemplated (with the humeral diameter obviously never greater than that of the glenoid). This "mix and match" approach is often preferable to the unnecessary removal and replacement of a well-fixed component.

CUFF DEFICIENT SHOULDERS REQUIRING REVISION ARTHROPLASTY

When an unconstrained total shoulder arthroplasty is used, it is important that the humeral head is centered on the glenoid. Otherwise, eccentric forces on the top of the glenoid prosthesis produce rapid loosening, the so-called rocking horse phenomenon. In the absence of an intact rotator cuff or a small balanced cuff tear, standard unconstrained glenoid prostheses should not be used. Recently, the reverse prosthesis has gained favor in this setting.

Other options include the use of a large humeral head that rests on the undersurface of the acromion. The so-called cuff tear arthropathy head, which does not have a prominent greater tuberosity, and thus avoids one aspect of subacromial impingement, is favored by some surgeons. Although cuff tear arthropathy heads may slightly improve the mechanical advantage (lever arm) of the deltoid, any inability to flex or abduct against gravity preoperatively is likely to persist after revision.

Another nonreverse option is the use of a reconstruction glenoid-support prosthesis, which lowers the humeral head by interposing an extended glenoid prosthesis between the head and the acromion. These prostheses, such as the Epoca prosthesis (Fig. 8.5), aim to provide a more normally positioned articulating glenoid surface and restore the lever arm of the deltoid to improve its efficiency. Unlike earlier unconstrained glenoid prostheses, such as the Plus 400 and Plus 800 all-polyethylene glenoids, these glenoid prostheses are in physical contact with the acromion and coracoid and thus much less likely to loosen.

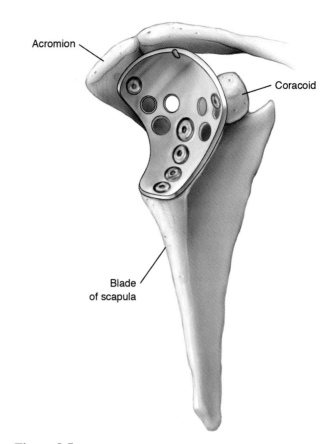

Figure 8.5. Diagrams based on the Epoca glenoid prosthesis for the rotator cuff deficient shoulder.

Experience with these prostheses is relatively limited to date, and to the best of these authors' knowledge, no long-term results have been reported.

REVERSE PROSTHESES FOR CUFF DEFICIENT SHOULDERS

Recent advances in "reverse prostheses" have resulted in good early and medium-term results. The principles of medialization of the center of rotation and enhancement of the deltoid muscle length have meant that patients without rotator cuffs have been able to regain antigravity flexion and abduction. (A good deltoid is an absolute prerequisite.) If some external rotators remain, external rotation may be retained. Frequently, however, the procedure is used in the absence of active external rotator muscle units. Surgical transfer of the latissimus dorsi and teres major tendons can be employed to restore antigravity external rotation and significantly enhance function. The pectoralis major is usually adequate for active internal rotation, even in the absence of subscapularis.

Humeral Prosthesis (Reverse)

METAPHYSEAL CONSIDERATIONS. On the humeral side, considerations in prosthesis choice are similar to those discussed previously in the unconstrained prosthesis review. Both cemented and uncemented stems are available. In the revision situation, cancellous bone is often deficient and cemented prostheses are generally indicated. In cases of significant metaphyseal bone loss, some prosthesis systems provide modular metaphyseal extensions that can be used to optimize humeral length and offset and thereby deltoid tension. Variable polyethylene thicknesses also add to the available permutations and allow fine-tuning of soft tissue tension. Lateralized and "retentive" polyethylene liners allow even further fine-tuning of soft tissue tensioning. The surgeon needs to consider these aspects when choosing a prosthesis. In particular, cases with deficient metaphyseal bone require prostheses with extensive inventory options. Recently, some manufacturers (e.g., SMR) have designed prostheses in which the same modular humeral stems can fit the metaphyseal components of both standard (unconstrained) and reverse prostheses, allowing interchangeability without humeral stem revision. These prostheses are not yet widely used, but this may be the direction for the future.

If the greater tuberosity is totally lacking in a revision scenario (e.g., in a failed hemiarthroplasty for fracture), a proximal humeral allograft may help. The allograft greater tuberosity not only provides lateral support for the new prosthesis but also may, by displacement, lateralize the line of action of the deltoid, improving (or restoring) its mechanical advantage. The choice of a prosthesis with a relatively thin metaphysis may facilitate the fitting of such an allograft.

If the patient does not have antigravity external rotators before revision surgery, the surgeon may consider combined latissimus and teres major transfer. This commits the surgeon to a deltopectoral approach (which is usual for revision surgery). The prosthesis used should have appropriate soft tissue fixation features in the metaphyseal portion of the prosthesis. In the future, soft tissue on-growth surfaces may also be available.

DIAPHYSEAL CONSIDERATIONS. The stem length considerations and the choices of stem width, cemented and uncemented, discussed in the preceding section on unconstrained prostheses, apply to the reverse prostheses as well. When a humeral stem is to be removed, the risk of humeral fracture needs to be considered and long-stemmed prostheses should be available in the operating room. If cement removal is incomplete, narrow-stemmed prostheses need to be available.

Choice of Glenospheres (Reverse)

The technical considerations discussed in the first section of this chapter again apply. Contained glenoid defects can usually be grafted sufficiently to allow one-stage revision arthroplasty. The use of a glenosphere baseplate with variable screw angulation facilitates this because it allows fixation screws to be directed toward solid native bone stock. Glenosphere baseplates with long central pegs are intrinsically more stable, and when fixation appears tenuous, these options should be considered. Similarly, locking techniques available with some newer prostheses enhance the stability of the variable angle fixation screws. Recently released prostheses employing locking screws for baseplate fixation are at least theoretically more stable and may be particularly applicable to the revision setting. Similarly, the ability to use wide-threaded screws may help fixation in porotic bone.

In seeking glenosphere stability, convex baseplates are at least theoretically preferable to earlier flat-based plates and this aspect warrants consideration. Other systems increase glenosphere stability by the use of an anterior plate screwed onto the glenoid neck. It is clearly desirable for glenosphere fixation to be through native bone. In the revision situation, the best bone may be away from the center of the glenoid. In this situation, a system with an eccentric glenosphere option may be useful, with the central peg of the baseplate being placed away from the center of the glenoid but with the center of the glenosphere still being located in a biomechanically desirable position. This option of an "eccentric glenosphere" may be particularly attractive in the revision of a glenosphere in which impingement may have notched the lower pole of the bony glenoid, necessitating a more proximal central peg in the revision procedure (Fig. 8.6).

At least theoretically, the closer the center of rotation of the glenosphere is to the native glenoid, the less loosening forces are on it. With this in mind, a reverse prosthesis that lateralizes the center of rotation of the glenosphere may not be as mechanically sound as others, even though it may improve external rotation strength.

In the same way that humeral stems are now being made to be interchangeable between unconstrained and reverse prostheses, metal glenoid baseplates are available that can be used for both unconstrained glenoids and reverse glenospheres. Using such baseplates for primary prostheses carries the possible disadvantages of a metal-backed prosthesis, such as a potentially reduced prosthetic lifespan, but may be indicated in patients with weak or failing rotator cuffs or other

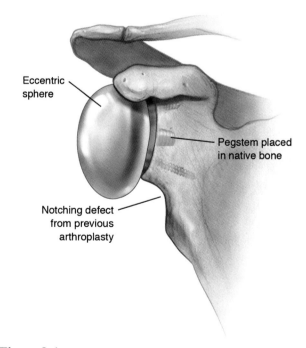

Figure 8.6. Use of an eccentric glenosphere in the setting of a notched glenoid neck. Ideally, the glenosphere should be inclined downward 5 to 10 degrees and extend beyond the lower pole at the glenoid.

TABLE 8.3	Specific Design Features Valuable in Revision Shoulder Arthroplasty (Selected Available Implants)	
Design/Company	*Glenoid*	*Humerus*
STANDARD IMPLANTS		
SMR (Orthotech)	• Metal-backed glenoid • Titanium + HA coating • Press-fit central corrugated peg • Four baseplate sizes • Three-pegged all-polyethylene glenoid	• Cemented or uncemented stems • Modular metaphysis that can be exchanged in situ and version altered • Trauma or elective body • Convertible to reverse without need for stem removal • Eccentric heads • Cuff tear arthropathy head
Global (Depuy)	• Five-pegged or anchor-pegged or keeled all-polyethylene glenoid	• Uncemented stem—can be cemented • Smaller fracture stem available • Reverse Morse taper enabling glenoid access without stem removal • Cuff tear arthropathy head
Bigliani/Flatow (Zimmer)	• Biconcave shaped glenoid • Three-pegged or keeled all-polyethylene glenoid	
Trabecular metal (Zimmer)		• Uncemented stem—can be cemented • Tantalum porous coating over the metaphysis • Two different neck angles per stem • Smaller fracture stem available • Extra large heads for cuff tear arthropathy
Aequalis (Tornier)	• Four-pegged or keeled all-polyethylene glenoid	• Uncemented stem—can be cemented • Smaller fracture stem available
Cofield 2 (Smith + Nephew)	• Keeled all-polyethylene glenoid • In-line pegged all-polyethylene glenoid • Metal-backed in-growth component with supplemental screw fixation	• Cemented stem—can be uncemented • Chrome-cobalt stem • Relatively thin metaphysis • Sintered beads over metaphysis for bony ingrowth • Large unipolar head for cuff tear arthropathy
PROMOS (Smith + Nephew)	• Four-pegged all-polyethylene glenoid	• Uncemented stem • Modular metaphysis • Rectangular metaphyseal body • Inclination set allows neck angle variation
Solar (Stryker)	• Two or four divergent pegged or keeled all-polyethylene glenoid	• Cemented or uncemented stems
Biomodular (Biomet)	• Three-pegged all-polyethylene glenoid	
Nottingham 1 (Biomet)	• Metal-backed glenoid • Plasma-sprayed HA-coated porous finish	• Cemented or uncemented stems • Cobalt-chrome stem • Reverse Morse taper enabling glenoid access without stem removal
Mosaic stem (Biomet)		• Cemented stem • Three-piece modular humeral stem for complex revision or salvage/oncology situations • Modular metaphysis

• All except Nottingham 1 have an all-polyethylene glenoid.
• All have stems of variable lengths and diameters.
• All have titanium stems, except for Cofield 2 and Nottingham 1.
• All standard stems have metaphyseal suture holes.
• All systems have eccentric head options, except Nottingham 1.

(continued)

TABLE 8.3	Specific Design Features Valuable in Revision Shoulder Arthroplasty (Selected Available Implants) *(continued)*	
Design/Company	*Glenoid*	*Humerus*
REVERSE IMPLANTS		
SMR (Orthotech)	• Poro-titanium + HA coating • Variable peg diameter • Two baseplate sizes • Two screw holes with variable angle • 36-mm glenosphere only • Eccentric glenosphere available	• Modular metaphysis • Cuff tear arthropathy head
Delta Extend (Depuy)	• HA coating • Four screw holes with variable angle • Locking cannulated screws • 38- or 42-mm glenospheres • Eccentric glenosphere available • Revision glenoid bearing tray with four-hole anterior plate available	• Modular uncemented stem • Monoblock cemented fracture stem • +3-, +6-, and +9-mm offsets • Cuff tear arthropathy head
Trabecular metal reverse (Zimmer)	• Tantalum coating • Variable peg length • Two screw holes with variable angle • Locking screw cap • No central hole on glenosphere • 36- or 40-mm glenospheres	• Monoblock metaphysis • 0-, +3-, and +6-mm offsets
Aequalis reverse (Tornier)	• HA coating • Four screw holes with variable angle • Locking head screws • Hemispherical heads for compression • 36- or 42-mm glenospheres	• Modular metaphysis • +6-, +9-, and +12-mm offsets
TESS (Biomet)	• Poro-titanium + HA coating • Four baseplate sizes • Four screw holes • 36- or 41-mm glenospheres	• Modular metaphysis • +6- and +8-mm offsets

• All have metal-backed titanium base plates.
• All have cemented and uncemented stems.
• All have metaphyseal suture holes, except TESS.
• All have metaphyseal extension to increase length, except TESS.
• All convertible to hemiarthroplasty, except TESS.

HA, hydroxyapatite.

biological issues that make ultimate revision to a reverse prosthesis likely.

CONCLUSION

Prosthesis selection is critical in revision shoulder arthroplasty. Most commercially available implants have similar basic features, but some prostheses have design features especially suited to certain scenarios, particularly for revision arthroplasty (Table 8.3). There is no one ideal implant that meets all possible challenges,

and the surgeon should balance the theoretical benefits of a new prosthesis with the benefits of familiarity with his or her "usual" prosthesis.

Reverse prostheses address not only the rotator cuff deficient shoulder in a primary setting but also a number of problems faced in revision total shoulder arthroplasty. As we become more familiar with these prostheses and as their designs become more refined, the role of these prostheses in revision surgery will almost certainly increase. Whether computer-assisted surgery (navigation) is to find a place in revision shoulder arthroplasty remains to be seen.

Christopher M. Jobe
Wesley P. Phipatanakul
John G. Bowsher

Component Fixation

INTRODUCTION

The term "fixation" suggests an unchanging relationship between what is prosthetic and what is biological. Permanence would seem unobtainable where one side is subjected to large, variable forces, chemical corrosion, and fatigue and the other side to biological remodeling and the effects of aging and inflammation. Yet, painless fixation of prostheses to bone has been shown to be successful in some cases for 20 to 30 years and even longer.

The aim of design and surgery is to place an implant that is mechanically sound and durable on the prosthetic side and create a micromechanical environment on the bony side that stimulates local tissues to maintain fixation. This micromechanical environment can be affected by joint stability and mechanics. In addition, attention must be paid to the patient's ability to respond to the micromechanical environment with bone maintenance and turnover. We will review the relevant information gathered in the study of this living relationship between bones and implants in all anatomic regions, including dental implants. We begin with the principles of fixation in general and move on to specific primary techniques, the anatomic peculiarities of the shoulder, removal techniques, and mechanisms of failure of primary fixation and then suggest how the principles gathered from these areas might be applied to revision and complex shoulder arthroplasty.

FIXATION OVERVIEW

The purposes of fixation are the effective painless transmission of force between the prosthesis and bone and maintenance of a fixed position of the prosthesis relative to the bone. Because of the differences in stiffness between bone and prosthesis there will always be some micromotion between bone and prosthesis. The goal of surgery and prosthetic design is to see that this relative motion is minimized, that is, kept less than 40 to 70 microns.[1]

Studies of the interface between bone and prosthetic material have shown that there is always an interposing layer and that this layer is thinnest, almost acellular, in the best fixation and thicker where there is greater motion between prosthesis and bone.

The material of the interposing layer performs best when it is loaded in compression and the stress (force per unit area) is kept low. These two elements are the most important in strategy of fixation (Fig. 9.1). The stress on the interface both immediately postoperatively and more remote in time should be compressive in direction, relatively low, and evenly distributed.

A thick interface layer is undesirable because it has poor transmission of forces from the prosthesis to the bone and allows greater relative motion. This leads to uneven distribution of stresses, which can produce additional motion and greater loosening, migration, and pain.

Both macroscopically and microscopically the contours of the interfaces should be such that they convert shear and tensile stresses to compressive stresses.

The life of a prosthetic fixation may be divided into three phases: an initial healing phase, a maintenance phase and a late or failing phase. Each of these phases has its own set of influencing factors.

GENERAL CHRONOLOGY

Immediately after surgery there is, secondary to the trauma of surgery, a zone of bone death in contact with the prosthetic or cement surface.[1] There is an intervening conversion film of glycoproteins that is immediately applied to the surface. Even in the immediate postoperative period there will be motion between prosthesis and bone, because of the variable stiffness of the biological and prosthetic materials. It is the goal of the surgeon and the prosthesis designer to minimize these motions and minimize and direct the loads because these direct the maturation of the healing zone. Low motion and low loads of a mainly compressive nature lead to the thinnest intervening layer between the prosthesis and the bone—a tight attachment called osseointegration. In dental implantology, this low-motion, low-load state can be achieved by not applying load to the implant for a period of 6 to 12 weeks to allow the healing zone to mature. In orthopaedic surgery we do not have this luxury. The aim then of the design of the prosthesis and the design for the insertion procedure is to do as little damage to the bone as possible and provide as broad a surface as possible for low and compressive loads.

The prosthesis is initially against a layer of injured and dead bone, and thus the ability of the patient to apply bone over injured trabeculae and later to turn over bone and replace dead bone with living bone is important. It is helpful to

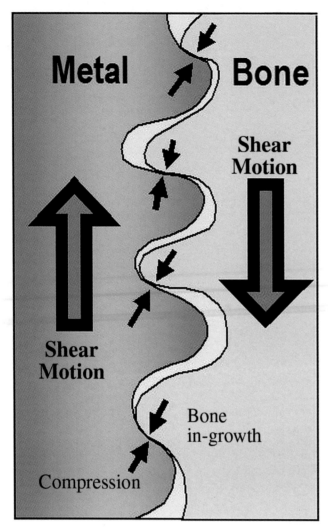

Figure 9.1. Illustration demonstrates the importance of converting shear to compression forces needed to allow for bony in-growth. The interposing layer between bone and prosthetic material should be thin for better fixation.

have the implant against a dense cancellous bone to diffuse loads over greater amounts of cancellous bone, thereby decreasing the stress on any particular trabecula of bone. The density of the patient's bone and the patient's ability to heal and turn over bone has an early and important effect on the success of fixation.

The immediate goal is to create a macrointerlock to minimize any motion between prosthesis and bone. As the bone heals, new layers of bone are laid down on the old trabeculae. This healing or maturation phase takes approximately 3 months to complete to achieve the most rigid attachment possible. The stiffness of the mature interposed layer is less than that of cancellous bone. It resists shear and tension poorly but will increase in stiffness with increasing compression loads. It is to be hoped that in the continued remodeling of the bone the micromechanical environment is such that the bone continues to replace itself and remodel against the uneven surfaces of the prosthesis, thereby creating a constancy of fixation to what is a constantly changing tissue.

Maintenance Phase

In the maintenance phase, prosthesis and bone have a stable geometric relationship. Ideally there is no migration of the prosthesis relative to the bone. We must assume that several things are taking place. The first is that bone remodeling is sufficient and the material properties and the health of the bone are being maintained so that the bone portion of the microinterlock is maintained. Second, that there is no fatigue failure of prosthetic materials such as cement or metal that are interdigitated with the bone. Third, a sufficiently low rate of wear of the prosthetic materials is occurring so that inflammatory osteolysis is not produced from wear products.[2] Finally, the overall loads on the joint have maintained a similar magnitude and a similar vector of application. With these four conditions prevailing, the micromechanical environment is sufficient to maintain the microinterlock.

Late or Failing Phase

In the late phase of attachment, which may last for several years, the degree of attachment between prosthetic material and bone breaks down. Several factors may contribute to this: fatigue failure of materials in the interlock, a change in the joint reaction vector such as a failure of a large portion of the rotator cuff, or a change in bone remodeling secondary to illness, medication, or aging. We must assume that in most cases fixation failure begins with a partial loss of attachment resulting in increased stress on the remaining healthy attachment. In areas of increased motion between prosthetic material and bone, the interface tissue becomes thicker (millimeters) and less mechanically stiff. At this point it may be possible to see it on the radiograph as a radiolucent line.[3–5] Where the radiolucent lines exist, there is no efficient transfer of stress between prosthetic material and bone (Fig. 9.2). We can also assume that this process repeats itself, causing the line to progress. Finally the prosthesis may migrate within the bone even before the loss of fixation becomes painful. At the hip and knee it is estimated that about 4 mm of migration occurs before pain ensues.

The phases described here are an idealization of clinical experience and do not occur in every patient. As it has been shown that a country can go "from barbarism to decadence without the usual intervening period of civilization," so a prosthetic fixation may pass from the early healing phase to failure without passing through the period of maintenance. Conversely, it is the hope of every surgeon that the patient's prosthesis fixation will enter into a sufficiently long maintenance phase so that the failing phase will not be reached during the patient's lifetime.

STRATEGIES FOR FIXATION

CONFORMING THE PROSTHESIS TO THE BONE

Cementation

The aim of cementation is to interdigitate the prosthetic material into the interstices of the trabecular bone. The surgeon produces an immediate interdigitation between materials that are prosthetic and those that are trabecular bone. There are several important considerations in cementation strategy. A basic

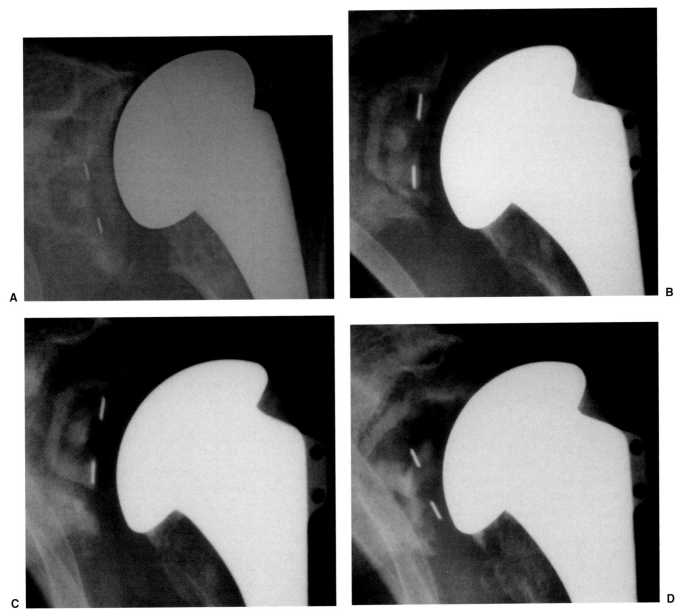

Figure 9.2. Anteroposterior radiograph **(A)** demonstrates excellent cement interdigitation with native bone. In contrast, this 6-week follow-up anteroposterior radiograph **(B)** demonstrates a radiolucent line that indicates poor transfer of stress between the prosthesis and bone. This 7.5-month radiograph **(C)** shows progression of the radiolucent zone with eventual glenoid component cutout **(D).**

requirement is to have a bony surface that is on the one hand porous, that is, capable of interdigitation, yet on the other hand is not so porotic that individual trabeculae are overloaded. The extremes that must be avoided are (a) complete removal of cancellous bone so that the cement is placed against cortical bone and (b) cementation to very osteoporotic bone in which there are very few trabeculae. In the first situation, cementing against cortical bone, the density of the bone is sufficient, but because of the regularity of the surface there is little interdigitation with the cement. In the second situation, too few trabeculae would result in voids, with no bone cement contact. In those few bony trabeculae that are in contact with cement, there would be an increased stress that one would prefer be diffused over a greater number of trabeculae.

A common strategy for ensuring that there is sufficient cancellous bone is impaction grafting to fill the void with dense yet trabecular bone and then cementing to the grafted bone, which, in the healing phase, will be incorporated into the recipient bone.[6] To a certain extent, in all cemented prostheses there is some impaction grafting, although in primary fixation, impacted bone is host bone that maintains within it living cells.

Because most histology studies are performed on failed cemented prostheses, many surgeons assume that osseointegration against methacrylate cannot be achieved and that methacrylate almost always causes a thicker fibrous interposition layer. This has proved not to be true in studies done on total joints that were successful for long periods and the interface was studied after the patient died of some other illness.[7]

Osseointegration against cement is possible. The determining factor is not the material but rather the micromechanical environment and the patient's bone.

IMPLICATIONS FOR THE CEMENT TECHNIQUE. The requirements for good cementation are abundant trabecular bone with clean interstices, which can be achieved through lavage or pressurized carbon dioxide.[4] A textured backside to polyethylene improves fixation.[8,9] The bone can be reinforced through impaction grafting. We want to use cement of normal viscosity because low-viscosity cement does not completely push blood and fat out of the interstices.[10] Secondly, we need to create a pressure differential. Cement is applied with pressure, particularly in the glenoid, where the demands on the cement are so high. This pressure differential can be augmented by a weep hole with suction via the coracoid from the deep vault of the glenoid.[11] Through the weep hole technique, there can be a continuous removal of blood, fat, and other liquid from the vault of the glenoid as the cement is being advanced into the glenoid. A combination of these two techniques, weep hole and applied pressure, has been shown to be very effective in preventing radiolucent lines in the initial postoperative period.[11]

IMPLICATIONS FOR DESIGN: CEMENT. The aim of the designer is to achieve an interface that is loaded in compression with an even dispersal of the loading force over a large area of bone. On the glenoid side this is achieved by keels or pegs. In both designs the articular portion of the glenoid prosthesis is supported by hard subchondral bone. With reasonable joint mechanics the interface between the articular portion of the prosthesis and subchondral bone is loaded in compression. The keel or pegs are to convert shear and other loads into compression on the interface.

The advantage of the keel over the pegs is the large interface area over which the load is spread. The disadvantage of the keel is the technical difficulty in achieving a good cement interdigitation free of radiolucent lines.

The advantage of the peg design is the ability to pressurize the small holes that receive the pegs. Pegs also have the advantage of being dispersed around the glenoid, giving them an attachment away from the center of the glenoid.

Fixation problems are unusual in the humerus, probably because of a combination of reasons. Glenohumeral loads are lower than those seen at other joints. The humeral bone–prosthetic interface has a larger interface than the glenoid has over which to disperse the loads, and the long stem gives a mechanical advantage for resisting rotational loads in the coronal and sagittal planes. The surgeon may elect to cement the entire stem or just the proximal end and let the stem or a split stem control the diaphysis.

Press Fit

In press fit without in-growth, the original humerus fixation method, the prosthesis must be mechanically stable at the time of surgery. There must be a macrointerlock between the prosthesis and the host bone. This means that there must be sufficient bone in all areas to bear the stresses. This often requires impaction grafting of the cancellous bone, particularly osteoporotic bone, as opposed to rasping or curetting. A more flexible metal should be used so as to decrease the relative motion between bone and metal and stress shielding. Titanium alloys are currently preferred for this. The distribution of the forces should be such that stress-guided remodeling does not alter the bone significantly with time. The anteroposterior design of the humeral implant should be a taper rather than a cylinder to resist settling forces to steady the prosthesis against the denser cancellous bone closer to the cortical bone.[12] In the healing phase it is to be hoped that the bone will grow very close to the metal with a minimal interpositional layer.

Over a long period, a press fit prosthesis tends to settle, and smooth surfaces provide very little barrier to the migration of wear particles. Osteoporotic bone offers fewer trabeculae against the metal for force transmittal, making it more likely to fail during remodeling. This interface is more likely to mature into a fibrous layer, leading to a progressive settling or loosening process.

Bony In-Growth onto or into the Prosthesis: Roughened Metal, Porous Metal, Metal on Carbon Mesh, and Magic Peg

To create bony in-growth into or onto an in-growth surface, an optimal micromechanical environment has to be provided. This also has implications for the designer and the surgeon. For the designer, a rigid macrointerlock must be achievable at surgery so that there is minimal motion of the metal in-growth surface relative to the bony surface. The designer will choose a less stiff material such as titanium as opposed to cobalt chromium (Co-Cr). Applying metal to a carbon mesh can create a material with properties nearly identical to those of cancellous bone.[13,14] The same shaping requirements described for press fit also apply to bony in-growth. The prosthesis should avoid linear and rotational translation relative to the bone. Shear and tensile forces on the surface should be resisted by compressive stresses elsewhere to prevent loosening. This may necessitate a larger size selection so that the prosthesis will be appropriate for the bone into which it is being inserted. Delicate surgical technique is needed out so that the bone against which the material is applied is in the best shape and contains the greatest number of living elements. Impaction grafting will be helpful here as well.[15,16]

For metallic surfaces the optimum pore size is in the range of 100 to 400 microns and the allowable micromotion has to be less, at 150 microns.[1] There is an upper limit to the porosity of the metal because the metal may become the weak link and be subjected to fatigue failure of small bits of metal. This relationship of the appropriate amount of bone to metal is similar to the desired ratio of bone to cement in cement fixation.

One hundred percent bony in-growth is rarely achieved, but a certain percentage is desirable to achieve the right micromechanical environment for the bone surface for now and for the long term. The rough or porous metal is placed on the prosthesis on the interface closest to the articular attachment. This is done to mimic the normal stress loading of the bone to create as near normal bone remodeling as possible. It is also done to facilitate later removal should that become necessary.

An additional advantage of the in-growth prostheses is that the combination of bone and soft tissue in-growth inhibits the migration of microscopic wear particles into the bone prosthesis interface.

Compression Loading of the In-Growth Interface

The "compress" technique is a variation on bony in-growth largely used in tumor surgery to attach prostheses to diaphyseal bone.[17] It succeeds because of the compressive micromechanical environment of the interface. In this technique, the bony in-growth surface is applied directly to the cut cortical surface of the shaft of a bone, usually following a tumor resection or a resection of a large amount of bone for infection. The compress mechanism produces a high compression load via a spring that is attached to the intramedullary surface of the bone by cross pinning.[17] Because of the high compression load, bending forces do not create distraction at the interface but instead merely a decrease in the compression load in what would ordinarily be the tension side of the attachment. In this fashion, with bony in-growth and stability, the prosthesis becomes a more natural prosthetic extension of the bone. The interface of the glenoid side of reverse prostheses may succeed via a similar mechanism. By compression loading, shear and bending loads produce less micromotion, thereby allowing in-growth.

Trabecular Shaped Material

A novel approach to bone in-growth is to create a combination material with similar material properties to trabecular bone, a similar internal structure, and a surface chemistry conducive to bone in-growth.[18,19] The first of these is "trabecular metal" (Zimmer). The trabecular framework is made of graphite, which creates the structure and mechanical properties similar to bone. Tantalum provides the surface onto which the bone can grow.

The design constraints will be similar to what was discussed previously—avoidance of stress risers, initial macrointerlock, compression loading, and dispersed loading.

Long-term success will depend on several factors mentioned previously. Most important will be the material's resistance to fatigue, its attachment to the prosthesis, and the patient's bone metabolism.

Fluted Peg

The fluted peg is a variation on bony in-growth but using polyethylene.[20] In this technique a peg that has horizontal flaps attached in a circular fashion is inserted into the bone; the flaps resist the peg pulling out of the bone to create a stable micromechanical environment. With time, bone is anticipated to grow into the spaces between the flaps to create a bony fixation for the polyethylene. Concerns about the magic peg technique include back-sided wear of the polyethylene, failure of bone in-growth to occur, and fatigue of the plastic.

MECHANICS OF THE SHOULDER

To predict the micromechanical environment, we need to know the direction and magnitude of the loads that are applied to the articular surfaces and the bone. This information is used to design and insert prostheses so that the interface has a load that is as low as possible and that this decreased load is compressive.

The load on a joint, in a stable situation, must pass from bone to bone. The magnitude with the arm in 90 degrees of abduction is roughly one body weight. With more vigorous activities or with a weight held in the hand, the forces could be quite large.

The load on the humeral side is applied on the "ball" and is directed toward the center of the head. Loads not directed to the center of the head will lead to instability.

On the glenoid side the load is directed toward the socket, as shown by Poppen and Walker.[21] Soslowsky et al[22] demonstrated the areas of contact in different positions. These indicate the area where the force is applied. Initial load is on the anterior inferior glenoid and proceeds to anterosuperior (60 degrees), then a little less anterior (120 degrees), and back to the center of the inferior glenoid (180 degrees). Internal rotation alters the pattern, but it still overlies the socket.

In the arthritic shoulder, abnormal loading patterns are frequent if not the rule (Fig. 9.3). For example, very frequently arthritic shoulders have developed a posterior glenoid loading pattern as evidenced by a posterior subluxation and an uneven wear of the glenoid. Conversely, patients with a large rotator cuff tear may develop anterosuperior migration of the head, leading to an abnormal loading pattern. Another abnormal loading pattern is anterior instability. Each of these might lead to incongruent loading of a total joint arthroplasty. Prosthesis loosening rarely occurs in isolation without a contributing mechanical situation such as instability.[23]

IMMEDIATE AND SHORT-TERM FIXATION OF HUMERAL AND GLENOID PROSTHESES

Let us examine some of the strategies to achieve early macrointerlock between prosthesis and bone and a long-term stable loading pattern.

In the humerus, surface replacement is an obvious solution. If we attach a metallic surface replacement to the humeral head in the optimum anatomic position, the load across the glenohumeral joint will be spread out over a large surface area. In addition, the direction of this load will almost always be compressive. The surgeon determines the optimum radius of curvature to be replaced and removes osteophytes and just enough host bone that the surface replacement fits in the anatomic position. In addition, the surgeon tries to maximize the contact between living bone and the bony in-growth undersurface of the surface replacement.

In many situations, a surface replacement is not desirable or cannot be achieved. In these conditions the humeral head prosthesis is attached to a stem inserted in the bone. There has been considerable development in stem design over the years. These prostheses use the diaphyseal portion of the bone to determine 4 of the 6 degrees of freedom—rotation and translation about the anteroposterior axis and rotation and translation about the medial lateral axis.[24,25] The only variations left to the surgeon are the height of the cut and the rotation of the cut. Additionally, the surgeon may offset the head to match offsets in the patient's anatomy.

Early in the development of fixation, cementless fixation did not prove satisfactory. There was a tendency for the prosthesis to fall into varus and settle, particularly in osteoporotic bone and inflammatory arthritis. Current designs modify the upper portion of the prosthesis so that it has a more medial extension and is more wedge-shaped.[26] This prevents the prosthesis settling into varus or down the shaft. An additional strategy is to conceal

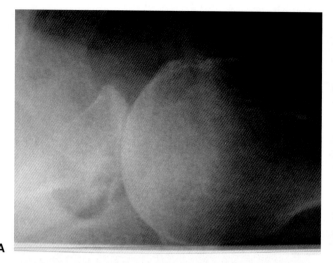

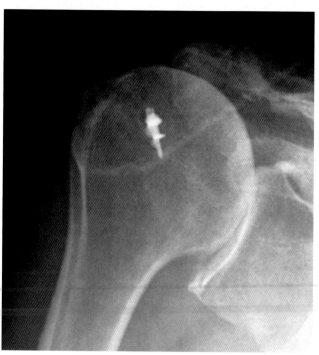

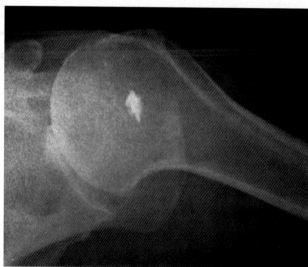

Figure 9.3. Axillary radiograph (**A**) shows typical abnormal loading pattern in osteoarthritis with development of posterior subluxation. A different loading pattern is seen in the cuff deficient patient, anterior/superior instability (**B** and **C**).

the collar of the prosthesis below the level of the osteotomy. This places the collar where it does not become part of the articulation yet it is still useful to limit settling of the prosthesis into varus or distally. The lower part of the stem can be made slotted so that it is somewhat compressible, allowing for application of the forces of the prosthesis against a larger area of bone. Manufacturing the prosthesis out of titanium makes it more flexible with respect to the bone, producing less motion between bone and prosthesis and less load transfer distally.

Glenoid

The glenoid side is almost always a surface replacement, with the exception of the inverse prostheses. The ideal replacement surface is about 4 mm of polyethylene resting on a layer of subchondral bone that is congruent with the nonarticular side of the prosthesis. Extending the prosthesis beyond the limits of the bony glenoid is not useful. It is in the backside attachment to the glenoid where the prostheses' designs differ most.

The backside can be made flat or round. The flat back has a rotational orientation in space and is therefore more liable to malalignment, whereas congruent, yet round, surfaces can have slight differences in rotation but still have the ultrahigh

molecular weight polyethylene applied to supporting subchondral bone.

The next controversy is between using a peg or a keel. The advantages of the pegs is that they seem to have better cementation and resistance to torque stresses because the pegs are farther from the center of the glenoid. Better cementation probably stems from a higher pressure achieved at the time of cementation when pegs are inserted into relatively small defects in the glenoid. This high pressure results in a better interdigitation of the cement. The disadvantage of the pegs stems from them being further from the center of the glenoid and may result in some drill through in trying to place this on the glenoid. Use of the keel has been somewhat problematic in the past because of the occurrence of a great number of radiolucent lines immediately postoperatively.[27] This has been attributed to the difficulty in clearing out blood from behind the cement at the moment of insertion.

There have been other changes in design to achieve better fixation. A keel that is offset somewhat more anteriorly will be in a more physiological area for bone loading.[28] A more anatomic shape of the articular surface as opposed to a standard oval provides for less edge loading and contributes to prosthesis longevity.

The degree of conformity between the two articular surfaces may have an adverse effect on the longevity of the prosthesis. A totally conforming prosthesis has increased joint stability, but also may have increased edge loading if there is obligatory translation of the head on that surface. On the other hand, a degree of nonconformity may decrease the area of contact between humerus and glenoid and lead to an initial increased wear rate. In the future, the choice of the surgeon may be determined by what the postoperative mechanics of the shoulder will be. For example, if the rotator cuff is intact and the head seems to be relatively well centered, the surgeon may choose a more conforming glenoid, whereas if there is obligatory translation, a less conforming articular surface may be chosen.

With regard to technique, defects in the bone cannot be made up with cement but need to be made up with bone. Perfect seating of the prosthesis is needed to achieve a uniform cement mantle on pegs or keel. Bone preparation should be neat and as atraumatic as possible, with a thought to the macrointerlock that is to be achieved. Fat should be removed from the bone surface by gas or saline, and the cement should be applied with a pressure differential that is achieved either by very high injection pressure or a weep hole to suction through the coracoid.[11] Finally, we want to insert enough cement so that there is good application of the pegs or keel but to avoid thin cement on the backside of the glenoid because this is subject to mechanical failure. We should also avoid angular malalignment relative to the joint reaction force.

FILLING THE GLENOID VOID WITH CANCELLOUS IMPACTION GRAFTING. The deeper portion of the glenoid is often filled with fat, especially in the elderly. This void can be filled by impaction grafting with cancellous bone. This enables the cement to make use of all of the increased area of the keel.

Glenoid Fixation Considerations in Reverse Shoulder

An alternative design for glenoid fixation involves bony ingrowth on a metallic surface as in the reverse prostheses (Fig. 9.4). Inverse prostheses are designed so that the glenoid might act as the fixed fulcrum. The convex articular surface is placed on the glenoid and the concave on the humerus. The original fixed fulcra prostheses have a long track record of failure, which seems to have been overcome by making the articular surface larger and looking to the biomechanics of the shoulder so that the interface between sphere and glenoid bone is always loaded in compression. A wide application surface is achieved by applying these prostheses over the entire surface of the lower portion of the glenoid. In addition to the joint reaction vector, attention is paid in the application of the prosthesis to avoid edge loading. One of the most frequent complications (Fig. 9.5) in the inverse prosthesis is contact between the inferior medial portion of the humeral socket against the bony neck of the glenoid, resulting in accelerated polyethylene wear and contact erosion of the glenoid neck, with subsequent osteolysis behind the prostheses from the plastic fragments.[29,30] This must be avoided by design elements and surgical maneuvers so that this glenoid neck contact does not occur.

ADVERSE LONG-TERM INFLUENCES ON THE PRIMARY PROSTHESIS. It is to be hoped that the micromechanical environment and patient well-being will lead to a long-term

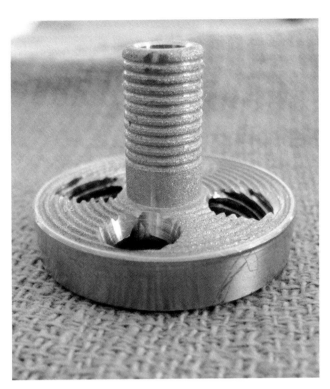

Figure 9.4. Photograph of a reverse prosthesis glenoid baseplate component. The central post is fluted with a grit blasted surface designed to promote bony on-growth.

maintenance of the prosthesis-bone relationship, but this is not always the case. Press-fit prostheses without bony ingrowth settled frequently, particularly in long-term patients and patients with rheumatoid arthritis. This has also been noted in fully cemented glenoids. Some migration of the prosthesis has been described even before pain occurs.

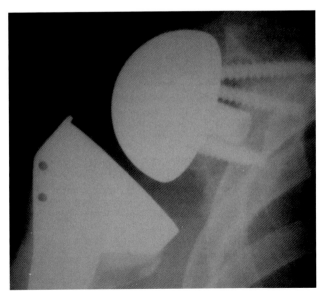

Figure 9.5. Anteroposterior radiograph demonstrating scapular notching phenomena in a reverse prosthesis that results from mechanical contact between the humeral component and scapula.

WEAR AND OSTEOLYSIS

CLINICAL GLENOID WEAR

Normal function of the shoulder joint causes repetitive eccentric loading of the polyethylene glenoid component, leading to significant deformation, wear, increased conformity, increased tensile stresses, and subsequent loosening.[31,32] Wear particle–induced osteolysis may also play a role in glenoid loosening similar to that experienced by hip and knee replacements.[2,33] It has been estimated that up to 60% of all total shoulder revisions are a result of loosening from wear and cold-flow deformation.[32,34]

Studies of retrieved glenoid components show common features, such as rim erosion, surface irregularities, component fracture, cracking, and gross wear.[35,36] Ultimately this damage and wear of the glenoid limits the long-term survivorship for most patients and needs to be improved to meet the increasing demands of modern patients.

The most prevalent wear mechanisms of polyethylene glenoids include adhesion, abrasion from third-bodies, burnishing, pitting, and delamination (fatigue wear).[35,36] Most glenoids exhibit more than just one of these wear mechanisms as they experience both conforming and nonconforming wear episodes under sliding and rolling.[31,32,37] The quantity of wear from glenoids is typically much higher compared to that in hip and knee replacements, and completely worn glenoids are seen more often than completely worn hips or knees.[31,32] Typical wear of glenoids at revision has been estimated at 25% loss of the original polyethylene surface.[38]

IN-VITRO GLENOID WEAR

Although total shoulder arthroplasty has been performed for over 25 years, to date there have been few attempts to simulate the in vivo wear of polyethylene glenoids in the laboratory. Therefore the effects of many current design parameters on wear and deformation of glenoids have yet to be proved experimentally.[39] Van der Pijl et al[39] were the first to build an in vitro shoulder prosthesis wear simulator consisting of one pneumatic test station. Although this novel glenoid simulator proved effective in reproducing correct physiological joint conditions, comparative wear data from various designs have yet to be published. Further developments in this area are imperative to begin evaluating new designs and materials, especially glenoid thickness, conformity of the articular surfaces, and polyethylene type (sterilization).

WEAR PARTICLE-INDUCED OSTEOLYSIS

Like hip and knee replacements, osteolysis (aseptic loosening) of the shoulder is linked with the release of polyethylene wear particles generated at the articular surfaces.[2,33,40,41] Although this mechanism is extremely complex, it is believed that wear particle size, morphology, and concentration of particles play a significant role.[42,43] A concentration of 1×10^{10} particles per gram of tissue was found in areas of osteolysis of the hip; however, such concentrations have yet to be reported for the shoulder. Such a large number of particles overload the phagocytic system, causing increased macrophage migration, leading to resorption of the trabecular bone at the bone-implant surface. It has also been reported that the most bioactive polyethylene wear particles are between 0.1 and 10 microns in size,[42] which unfortunately matches the typical size of polyethylene particles produced by all total joint procedures.

The volume of polyethylene wear that triggers osteolysis in the shoulder is unknown at this time and certainly requires further research to facilitate long-term predictions of survivorship. Clinical studies of the hip have suggested that wear rates greater than 160 mm³ per year resulted in an unacceptable incidence of osteolysis and revision within 10 years.[44,45] Thus wear rates of 10 to 80 mm³ per year were more clinically desirable, and it is generally believed that wear rates less than 5 mm³ per year could minimize the risk of osteolysis. There have been no quantitative reports of wear rates from failed glenoids in the literature, so it is not currently possible to associate a particular rate of glenoid wear and osteolysis.

The wear particles generated from polyethylene glenoids have been reported to be larger than those found from total hip procedures and similar to those from total knee procedures. Studies by Wirth et al[2] and Mabrey et al[45] reported average particle sizes of 1.04 and 1.18 microns from the shoulder, almost twice the size of those in the hip (0.62 microns).[2,46] Shoulder particles also demonstrated twice the elongation compared to hip particles, thus consisting of more fibrillar shaped particles. Although it is likely that shoulder particles are larger than those from the hip joint because of differences in loading and motion, the mean particle sizes reported by Wirth et al[2] and Mabrey et al may not accurately reflect the true size distribution of shoulder particles. Particle size distributions are non-normally distributed[45]; therefore the average particle size will be an overestimation of the most common particle size (Fig. 9.6). Thus it is possible that the median size of shoulder particles is submicron and thus more bioactive. Nevertheless, shoulder particles, whether submicron or micron sized, are still within the bioactive range for osteolysis (0.1 to 10 microns), explaining why many glenoids show radiolucent lines and aseptic loosening.[2,42]

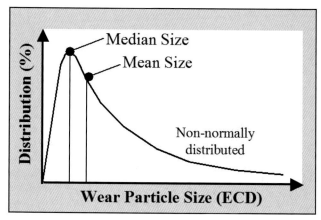

Figure 9.6. This graph illustrates the non-normally distributed size of wear particles. Note how the average particle size (mean) is larger than the most common particle size (median).

PREDICTIONS OF FUNCTIONAL BIOLOGICAL ACTIVITY

Osteolysis is a function of both volume concentration and sizes of polyethylene wear particles, so it may be possible to predict long-term biological responses, that is, estimate the functional biological activity of known polyethylene materials. Using data derived from cell culture studies of primary human macrophages, Fisher et al[46] and Endo et al[47] proposed a novel series of equations and constants that can be used to estimate biological activity. The functional biological activity (FBA) was given by FBA = V_{WR} × SBA, where V_{WR} was the volumetric wear rate (mm^3/Mc) and SBA (Specific Biological Activity = $\sum C(r) \times B(r)$, where C(r) was volume concentration for each particle size and B(r) is the biological activity constants. The biological activity constants range from 1 for the most bioactive particles (<1 μm) to 0.2 for lower active particles (>10 μm). The success of such FBA calculations in terms of predicting clinical outcomes is unknown at the time; however, such laboratory predictions should be closely followed and scrupulously tested when the data become available.

ALTERNATIVE MATERIALS

New Generation Cross-Linked Polyethylenes

There is no doubt that the wear and damage resistance of polyethylene glenoids needs to be improved. Development of material for glenoids is lagging behind that for the hip and knee. Hip and knee replacements are already using second-generation cross-linked polyethylenes, whereas first-generation cross-linked polyethylene and conventional non–cross-linked polyethylene are still being used in total shoulder replacement. It may be possible to learn from mistakes in the hip and knee to make developments in the shoulder. However, the question whether second-generation cross-linked polyethylenes are suitable for shoulder replacements is far from clear.

The hypothesis that decreased polyethylene wear equals increased clinical success may not be true for highly cross-linked polyethylenes (HXLPE).[48] A recent study reported a 20% increase in the FBA index for HXLPE compared to standard ultrahigh molecular weight polyethylenes (UHMWPE) in the hip.[46] Although the wear rate of HXLPE was 50% less compared to standard UHMWPE, the HXPLE generated 30% smaller wear particles that overall created a greater potential in FBA. This demonstrates that small change in wear particles sizes may have large changes in macrophage response.[48] How cross-linking influences wear particles from shoulder glenoids is currently unknown.

Contemporary HXLPEs have demonstrated improved wear resistance in laboratory studies but also raised some issues regarding remaining free radicals left by the annealing process causing oxidation and a significant decrease in resistance to crack propagation using the remelted process.[49–51] To overcome these perceived risks, polyethylene developments have focused on enhancing the cross-linking effect and oxidation resistance while maintaining mechanical properties.[52] The three types of second-generation HXLPE now available include sequentially enhanced, mechanically enhanced, and vitamin E–enhanced polyethylenes.[50,53] To date, none of these materials have been considered for glenoid use. Although these second-generation HXLPEs show great clinical promise in the hip and knee, little is known about the variables that can lead to high wear in these new materials in the shoulder, particularly synergistic effects of deformation and surface roughness.

Recent reports have also shown that HXLPE can be two times more sensitive to surface roughness than standard UHMWPE, negating any wear improvements under pristine conditions.[54] This is important to note because many glenoid components see gross damage during use. Thus it is only with sound experimental wear simulations under a variety of conditions that one can decide weather HXLPE offers any advantage over the polyethylenes already in use in the shoulder. Or will glenoid designers make mistakes similar to those in the hip with Hylamer cups?

Ceramics and Metals

To date there has been no clinical use of ceramic shoulder components. Ceramics are much harder than Co-Cr alloys (20 GPa versus 4 GPa) and subsequently do not become much rougher with use.[55,56] In the hip, both clinical and laboratory studies have reported 50% less wear for UHMWPE liners articulating against ceramic femoral heads compared to findings with Co-Cr heads.[55,56] Because many Co-Cr humeral components undergo sizeable damage, the use of ceramics may help to reduce poly glenoid wear. A disadvantage of ceramics components is that they can fracture; however, these fractures have been associated with smaller femoral heads and poor designs.[57,58] Therefore, with larger, thicker humeral components, the risks for fracture are drastically reduced. Successful ceramics in total hip and knee procedures include Biolox forte and the newer Biolox delta, which is an alumina-zirconia composite and is a much stronger ceramic.[59] A possible alternative ceramic is silicon nitride. Silicon nitride offers a hardness equal to that of Biolox forte but has a much improved flexural strength and fracture toughness (900 MPa versus 580 MPa).[60]

Possible improvements to Co-Cr humeral components include ion implantation and surface coatings. The potential benefits of N2-ion implantation as a surface modification to chromium-bearing components include a 30% to 50% increase in hardness, reduced friction, and increase in wettability. Currently, the use of ion-implanted Co-Cr femoral heads has been suggested to reduce clinical wear rates of polyethylene cups by 20%[61] and increase resistance of metallic surfaces against PMMA abrasion and corrosion.[62,63] However, to date there have been no ion-implanted Co-Cr shoulder components investigated.

INFLUENCE OF DESIGN ON WEAR

The most important surface considerations are conformity and load. In the highly conforming total hip procedure we see smaller particles. In the shoulder and knee procedures we see larger particles. The next design element is metal backing of the polyethylene. In design, metal backing, particularly on the glenoid, makes the polyethylene very thin over certain portions of the metal and subject to increased stress and a higher failure rate.[3] This may lead to early failure of the attachment of the metal, or it may produce a higher wear out rate and earlier osteolysis.[3] In the reverse prosthesis there is ample thickness to the polyethylene, but a design may bring the polyethylene into a high stress relationship with bone, the inferior neck of the glenoid, producing an increased rate of polyethylene destruction.

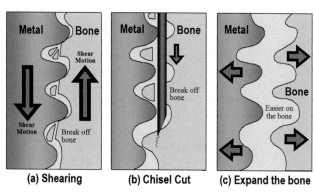

(a) Shearing   **(b) Chisel Cut**   **(c) Expand the bone**

Figure 9.7.   Illustration of disrupting the osseointegrated interface needed for prosthesis removal. **(A)** Straight shear force from an axial load. **(B)** An osteotome can be used to manually break off bone. **(C)** Performing an episiotomy relieves hoop stresses through bone expansion allows application of tension directly to the interface without excessive bone destruction.

REMOVAL TECHNIQUES

It is necessary from time to time to remove a component for reasons other than loosening. In these cases, what we know about fixation can be applied to facilitate removal. The surgeon will also ask in most cases how the removal technique will facilitate or at least not adversely affect attachment of a new component.

In disrupting an osseointegrated interface, our choices would seem to be between applying a shear force and applying a tensile force to the interface. Because of our desire to retain the shell of cortical bone, shear is the usual option, applying an axial load on the fixed component (Fig. 9.7A). When successful, this allows retention of the cortical bone but with an obvious tendency to smooth the inside surface of the bone. This smoothing effect is often compounded by the use of osteotomes (Fig. 9.7B) and other instruments to pull the cement away from the bone.

Episiotomy of the bone (Fig. 9.7C) allows tension to be applied directly to the interface without destruction of a lot of cancellous bone. The split bone will need reinforcing and decreased stress to allow healing. Following removal by either technique, the inner surface of the bone does not provide as desirable a surface for attachment as in the primary situation.

REVISION TECHNIQUES

How may we apply what has been learned from the study of primary prostheses to the application of a revision? Or, how may we apply this knowledge in a primary fixation in a complex situation in which there is missing bone or abnormal mechanical forces? We must assume that our revision techniques and subsequent interfaces are subject to the same influences as our primary techniques.

BONE DEFECTS: CONTAINED CANCELLOUS DEFECTS

Contained defects in the cancellous bone sheltered by a vault of cortical bone are often the result of osteolysis or the migration of a loose prosthesis. This type of defect has been shown to

be best treated with impaction grafting, which can be done either with the patient's own bone or by a radiated graft that has been augmented with the patient's own bone marrow as an aspirate.[64] Impaction grafting provides a very good, mechanically solid layer of cancellous bone between cement and cortical bone and has been shown in the optimal mechanical environment to fully incorporate. The bone, or remodeling bone, will grow right up to the layer of cement, providing a minimal layer of interface material and recreating an optimal relationship between bone and prosthetic material. Cartilage bits will not incorporate, so care in preparation of the graft is required.

BULK ALLOGRAFT: MAINLY CANCELLOUS

The mainly cancellous bulk allograft technique has been used on a limited basis in the shoulder but more frequently in the hip. A humeral head or other cortical cancellous combination graft is put in place to reconstruct a defect, for example, the edge of an articular surface. This type of graft has been shown to soften and collapse over time in the acetabulum. This occurs as the bone remodels and is revascularized. The resultant bone, however, is good-quality bone for a second revision. In some situations in which the graft is protected by metal or other mechanical construct, as in some knee revisions, allograft can be well incorporated without collapse. The successful knee revision probably avoids shear bending and tension on the graft.

BULK GRAFTS: MAINLY CORTICAL

The mainly cortical bulk graft can be used to replace the upper end of the humerus. This bone will partially heal to the host bone at the attachment site to the host humerus, but there is limited healing of tendons to this bone. In terms of long-term mechanical function it is best if this bone is minimally revascularized. If there is vigorous revascularization of this cortical graft, it is not remodeled to a similar cortical bone. In fact, the bone prosthesis combination disintegrates in the area of the cortical allograft. Because of its limited biological future, we need to think of this bulk allograft as part of the prosthesis, and thus both the prosthesis and this bone have to be fairly rigidly fixed to the host diaphysis.

BULK AUTOGRAFTING: MAINLY CORTICOCANCELLOUS

An example of bulk autografting would be attaching a prosthesis to the iliac crest and then transferring the prosthesis with its attached iliac crest to the host site. We can assume that because of the living cells within the graft and histocompatibility that this would have a faster rate of healing than bulk allograft and is hopefully less susceptible to collapse. The mechanical structure of the construct, that is, immediate fixation, must be sufficient to allow healing. Autograft with the patient's own bone, for example, the humeral head, if protected by the construct, does not collapse, but if unprotected by prosthesis, it will wear away or settle.

MASSIVE ROTATOR CUFF TEAR

A massive rotator cuff tear will change, in a grosser fashion, the direction of the joint reaction vector, leading to edge loading, possible early loosening, and certainly earlier wear of the glenoid prosthesis. In these conditions the revision surgeon will take into account the altered mechanics and design in such a fashion that bone-prosthesis interfaces will be loaded in compression after implantation (see discussion of compression).

MODIFICATION OF BONE METABOLISM

A major cause in loss of fixation of prosthesis may be the patient's own bone. The bone may be osteoporotic on the basis of age, medication, or disease. The bone may be unable, through its remodeling process, to erase fatigue deficits within itself. In the revision situation we want to correct the bone mineral metabolism as much as possible to ensure the longevity of the fixation. This may require surgical augmentation of the bone as is seen in impaction grafting, but some manipulation of the bone metabolism may be necessary as well. This has several implications for the surgeon and subsequent treating doctors. Medications that may lead to osteoporosis should be avoided if possible. One may have a preference for one nonsteroidal antiinflammatory drug over another based on a demonstrated lack of a tendency to produce osteoporosis. Some have suggested that bisphosphonate treatment adds to the endurance of a cemented fixation.[65] There has been some suggestion as well that parathormone treatment increases the rate of incorporation of bony in-growth fixation.[66]

AVOIDANCE OF FUTURE WEAR

Osteolysis is likely to be the biggest problem in the future, and we need prostheses that last longer in more active people. We need to do as much as possible to decrease the rate of wear. This will be done through prosthesis design and choice of materials to obtain somewhat even loading of the articular surface and the production of particles with less biological activity.

SUMMARY

Fixation is a long-term relationship between prosthesis and bone. Success depends on engineering of the prosthesis and performing the surgery to create an optimal micromechanical environment to maintain the arrangement. Maintaining the bony health of the patient is of long-term importance. Reverse situations require application of the same principles in a somewhat more creative fashion.

REFERENCES

1. Ling RS. Observations on the fixation of implants to the bony skeleton. *Clin Orthop Relat Res* 1986;210:80–96.
2. Wirth MA, Agrawal CM, Mabrey JD, et al. Isolation and characterization of polyethylene wear debris associated with osteolysis following total shoulder arthroplasty. *J Bone Joint Surg Am* 1999;81:29–37.
3. Boileau P, Avidor C, Krishnan SG, et al. Cemented polyethylene versus uncemented metal-backed glenoid components in total shoulder arthroplasty: a prospective, double-blind, randomized study. *J Shoulder Elbow Surg* 2002;11:351–359.
4. Edwards TB, Sabonghy EP, Elkousy H, et al. Glenoid component insertion in total shoulder arthroplasty: comparison of three techniques for drying the glenoid before cementation. *J Shoulder Elbow Surg* 2007;16:S107–S110.
5. Gartsman GM, Elkousy HA, Warnock KM, et al. Radiographic comparison of pegged and keeled glenoid components. *J Shoulder Elbow Surg* 2005;14:252–257.
6. Szabo I, Buscayret F, Edwards TB, et al. Radiographic comparison of two glenoid preparation techniques in total shoulder arthroplasty. *Clin Orthop Relat Res* 2005;431:104–110.
7. Maloney WJ, Jasty M, Burke DW, et al. Biomechanical and histologic investigation of cemented total hip arthroplasties: a study of autopsy-retrieved femurs after in vivo cycling. *Clin Orthop Relat Res* 1989;249:129–140.
8. Anglin C, Wyss UP, Pichora DR. Mechanical testing of shoulder prostheses and recommendations for glenoid design. *J Shoulder Elbow Surg* 2000;9:323–331.
9. Szabo I, Buscayret F, Edwards TB, et al. Radiographic comparison of flat-back and convex-back glenoid components in total shoulder arthroplasty. *J Shoulder Elbow Surg* 2005;14:636–642.
10. Miller MA, Race A, Gupta S, et al. The role of cement viscosity on cement-bone apposition and strength: an in vitro model with medullary bleeding. *J Arthroplasty* 2007;22:109–116.
11. Gross RM, McCarthy JA, Lomenth CS. The "weep hole" technique for improved glenoid fixation. *Tech Shoulder Elbow Surg* 2004;5:37–43.
12. Matsen FA 3rd, Iannotti JP, Rockwood CA Jr. Humeral fixation by press-fitting of a tapered metaphyseal stem: a prospective radiographic study. *J Bone Joint Surg Am* 2003;85:304–308.
13. Schildhauer TA, Peter E, Muhr G, et al. Activation of human leukocytes on tantalum trabecular metal in comparison to commonly used orthopedic metal implant materials. *J Biomed Mater Res A*, 2008. E-pub ahead of print.
14. Welldon KJ, Atkins GJ, Howie DW, et al. Primary human osteoblasts grow into porous tantalum and maintain an osteoblastic phenotype. *J Biomed Mater Res A* 2008;84:691–701.
15. Hacker SA, Boorman RS, Lippitt SB, et al. Impaction grafting improves the fit of uncemented humeral arthroplasty. *J Shoulder Elbow Surg* 2003;12:431–435.
16. Wirth MA, Lim MS, Southworth C, et al. Compaction bone-grafting in prosthetic shoulder arthroplasty. *J Bone Joint Surg Am* 2007;89:49–57.
17. Bhangu AA, Kramer MJ, Grimer RJ, et al. Early distal femoral endoprosthetic survival: cemented stems versus the Compress implant. *Int Orthop* 2006;30:465–472.
18. Meneghini RM, Lewallen DG, Hanssen AD. Use of porous tantalum metaphyseal cones for severe tibial bone loss during revision total knee replacement. *J Bone Joint Surg Am* 2008;90:78–84.
19. Spoerke ED, Murray NG, Li H, et al. A bioactive titanium foam scaffold for bone repair. *Acta Biomater* 2005;1:523–533.
20. Wirth MA, Korvick DL, Basamania CJ, et al. Radiologic, mechanical, and histologic evaluation of two glenoid prosthesis designs in a canine model. *J Shoulder Elbow Surg* 2001;10:140–148.
21. Poppen NK, Walker PS. Forces at the glenohumeral joint in abduction. *Clin Orthop Relat Res* 1978;135:165–170.
22. Soslowsky LJ, Flatow EL, Bigliani LU, et al. Quantitation of in situ contact areas at the glenohumeral joint: a biomechanical study. *J Orthop Res* 1992;10:524–534.
23. Antuna SA, Sperling JW, Cofield RH, et al. Glenoid revision surgery after total shoulder arthroplasty. *J Shoulder Elbow Surg* 2001;10:217–224.
24. Harris TE, Jobe CM, Dai QG. Fixation of proximal humeral prostheses and rotational micromotion. *J Shoulder Elbow Surg* 2000;9:205–210.
25. Peppers TA, Jobe CM, Dai QG, et al. Fixation of humeral prostheses and axial micromotion. *J Shoulder Elbow Surg* 1998;7:414–418.
26. Neer CS II, Watson KC, Stanton FJ. Recent experience in total shoulder replacement. *J Bone Joint Surg Am* 1982;64:319–337.
27. Murphy LA, Prendergast PJ, Resch H. Structural analysis of an offset-keel design glenoid component compared with a center-keel design. *J Shoulder Elbow Surg* 2001;10:568–579.
28. Simovitch RW, Zumstein MA, Lohri E, et al. Predictors of scapular notching in patients managed with the Delta III reverse total shoulder replacement. *J Bone Joint Surg Am* 2007;89:588–600.
29. Werner CM, Steinmann PA, Gilbart M, et al. Treatment of painful pseudoparesis due to irreparable rotator cuff dysfunction with the Delta III reverse-ball-and-socket total shoulder prosthesis. *J Bone Joint Surg Am* 2005;87:1476–1486.
30. Braman JP, Falicov A, Boorman R, et al. Alterations in surface geometry in retrieved polyethylene glenoid component. *J Orthop Res* 2006;24:1249–1260.
31. Scarlat MM, Matsen FA III. Observations on retrieved polyethylene glenoid components. *J Arthroplasty* 2001;16:795–801.
32. Amstutz HC, Campbell P, Kossovsky N, et al. Mechanism and clinical significance of wear debris-induced osteolysis. *Clin Orthop Relat Res* 1992;276:7–18.
33. Hasan SS, Leith JM, Campbell B, et al. Characteristics of unsatisfactory shoulder arthroplasties. *J Shoulder Elbow Surg* 2002;11:431–441.
34. Gunther SB, Graham J, Norris TR, et al. Retrieved glenoid components: a classification system for surface damage analysis. *J Arthroplasty* 2002;17:95–100.
35. Hertel R, Ballmer FT. Observations on retrieved glenoid components. *J Arthroplasty* 2003;18:361–366.
36. Swieszkowski W, Bednarz P, Prendergast PJ. Contact stresses in the glenoid component in total shoulder arthroplasty. *Proc Inst Mech Eng [H]* 2003;217:49–57.
37. Li S A. A retrieval analysis of polyethylene damage in total shoulder replacements. *J Bone Joint Surg B* 2004;86:418–419.
38. Bersee HEN, Van Der Pijl AJ, Swieszkowski W. Design of a wear simulator for in vitro shoulder prostheses testing. *Exper Tech* 2004;45–48.
39. Hirakawa K, Bauer TW, Stulberg BN, et al. Comparison and quantitation of wear debris of failed total hip and total knee arthroplasty. *J Biomed Mater Res* 1996;31:257–263.
40. McKellop HA, Campbell P, Park SH, et al. The origin of submicron polyethylene wear debris in total hip arthroplasty. *Clin Orthop Relat Res* 1995;311:3–20.
41. Green TR, Fisher J, Matthews JB, et al. Effect of size and dose on bone resorption activity of macrophages by in vitro clinically relevant ultra-high-molecular-weight polyethylene particles. *J Biomed Mater Res* 2000;53:490–497.
42. Shanbhag AS, Jacobs JJ, Black J, et al. Macrophage/particle interactions: effect of size, composition, and surface area. *J Biomed Mater Res* 1994;28:81–90.
43. Oparaugo PC, Clarke IC, Malchau H, et al. Correlation of wear debris-induced osteolysis and revision with volumetric wear-rates of polyethylene: a survey of eight reports in the literature. *Acta Orthop Scand* 2001;72:22–28.

44. Zichner LP, Willert HG. Comparison of alumina-polyethylene and metal-polyethylene in clinical trials. *Clin Orthop Relat Res* 1992;282:86–94.
45. Mabrey JD, Afsar-Keshmiri A, Engh GA, et al. Standardized analysis of UHMWPE wear particles from failed total joint arthroplasties. *J Biomed Mater Res (Appl Biomater)* 2002;63: 475–483, 2002.
46. Fisher J, Bell J, Barbour PS, et al. A novel method for the prediction of functional biological activity of polyethylene wear debris. *Proc Inst Mech Eng [H]* 2001;215:127–132.
47. Endo M, Tipper JL, Barton DC, et al. Comparison of wear, wear debris, and functional biological activity of moderately crosslinked and non-crosslinked polyethylenes in hip prostheses. *Proc Instn Mech Eng [H]* 2002;216:111–122.
48. Williams PA, Yamamoto K, Oonishi H, et al., Highly crosslinked polyethylenes in hip replacements: improved wear performance or paradox? *Tribol Trans* 2007;50:277–290.
49. Endo MM, Barbour PS, Barton DC, et al. Comparative wear and wear debris under three different counterface conditions of crosslinked and non-crosslinked ultra-high-molecular-weight polyethylene. *Biomed Mater Eng* 2001;11:23–35.
50. Kurtz SM, Mazzucco D, Rimnac CM, et al. Anisotropy and oxidative resistance of highly crosslinked UHMWPE after deformation processing by solid-state ram extrusion. *Biomaterials* 2006;27:24–34.
51. Muratoglu OK, Bragdon CR, O'Connor DO, et al. Unified wear model for highly crosslinked ultra-high-molecular-weight polyethylenes (UHMWPE). *Biomaterials* 1999;20:1463–1470.
52. Dumbleton JH, D'Antonio JA, Manley MT, et al. The basis for a second-generation highly crosslinked UHMWPE. Clin Orthop Relat Res 2006;453:265–271.
53. Essner A, Schmidt G, Herrera L, et al. Hip wear performance of a next generation crosslinked and annealed polyethylene. Fifty-first Orthopaedic Research Society 2005.
54. Bowsher JG, Williams PA, Clarke IC, et al. "Severe" wear challenge to 36-mm mechanically enhanced highly crosslinked polyethylene hip liners. *J Biomed Mater Res B Appl Biomater* 2008;86:253–263.
55. Clarke IC, Gustafson A. Clinical and hip simulator comparisons of ceramic-on-polyethylene and metal-on-polyethylene wear. *Clin Orthop Relat Res* 2000;379:34–40.
56. Semlitsch M, Willert HG. Clinical wear behavior of ultra-high-molecular-weight polyethylene cups paired with metal and ceramic ball heads in comparison to metal-on-metal pairings of hip joint replacements. *Proc Inst Mech Eng [H]* 1997;211:73–88.
57. Hannouche D, Nich C, Bizot P, et al. Fractures of ceramic bearings: history and present status. *Clin Orthop Relat Res* 2003;417:19–26.
58. Masonis JL, Bourne RB, Ries MD, et al. Zirconia femoral head fractures: a clinical and retrieval analysis. *J Arthroplasty* 2004;19:898–905.
59. Willmann G. New generation ceramics. In: Willmann G, ed. *Bioceramics in Hip Joint Replacement.* New York: Thieme; 2000.
60. Pfaff HG. A new ceramic material for orthopaedics. In Willmann G, ed. *Bioceramics in Hip Joint Replacement.* New York: Thieme; 2000.
61. Maruyama M, Capello WN, D'Antonio JA, et al. Effect of low-friction ion-treated femoral heads on polyethylene wear rates. *Clin Orthop Relat Res* 2000;379:183–191.
62. McKellop HA, Rostlund TV. The wear behavior of ion-implanted Ti-6A1-4V against UHMW polyethylene. *J Biomed Mater Res* 1990;24:1413–1425.
63. Rieu J, Pichat A, Rabbe LM, et al. Ion implantation effects on friction and wear of joint prosthesis materials. *Biomaterials* 1991;12:139–143.
64. Deakin DE, Bannister GC. Graft incorporation after acetabular and femoral impaction grafting with washed irradiated allograft and autologous marrow. *J Arthroplasty* 2007; 22:89–94.
65. Hilding M, Aspenberg P. Local peroperative treatment with a bisphosphonate improves the fixation of total knee prostheses: a randomized, double-blind, radiostereometric study of 50 patients. *Acta Orthop* 2007;78:795–799.
66. Tsiridis E, Gamie Z, Conaghan PG, et al. Biological options to enhance periprosthetic bone mass. *Injury* 2007;38:704–713.

Pierre Mansat
Michel Mansat

Morphology of the Arthritic Glenoid

THE NORMAL GLENOID

GENERAL ANATOMY

The scapula forms the posterior part of the shoulder girdle. It is a flat, triangular bone, with two surfaces, three borders, and three angles. The lateral angle is the thickest part of the bone and is sometimes called the head of the scapula. On it is the shallow pyriform, articular surface, the glenoid cavity, which is directed laterally and forward and articulates with the head of the humerus. It is broader below than above, and its vertical diameter is the longest. The surface is covered with cartilage in the fresh state. Its margins, slightly raised, give attachment to a fibrocartilaginous structure, the glenoidal labrum, which deepens the cavity.[1] Codman[2] in 1934 observed that the glenoid surface faces somewhat forward, upward and outward from the plane of the scapula. However, it was not until 1966, on the basis of radiographic studies conducted by Das et al[3] that measurements of the glenoid were performed. In 1971, using anteroposterior and axillary views of the shoulder, Saha[4] carefully defined these measurements. Since these first descriptions many studies have been performed to evaluate normal glenoid parameters (Table 10.1).

GLENOID SHAPE

The glenoid frequently has a pear-shaped aspect, with the superoinferior height greater than the anteroposterior width (Fig. 10.1); however, Checroun et al[5] found that 71% of specimens had a pear shape, whereas in 29% the shape appeared elliptical. Similar results were found by Prescher[6]; in 55% of the glenoids a notch was well expressed, with a pear-shaped appearance, and in 45% the notch was absent, resulting in an oval glenoid. In a cadaver study, Iannotti et al[7] measured 140 shoulders that were representative of a given population of patients. The average superoinferior dimension of the glenoid was 39 ± 3.7 mm (range 30–48 mm), and the average anteroposterior dimension of the lower half of the glenoid was 29 ± 3.1 mm (range 21–35 mm). The average anteroposterior dimension of the upper half of the glenoid at its midpoint was 23 ± 2.7 mm (range 18–30). The ratio of the anteroposterior measurement of the lower to the upper half of the glenoid was 1:08 ± 0.01; the ratio of the superoinferior to the anteroposterior measurement of the lower half was 1:07 ± 0.02; and the ratio of the superoinferior to the anteroposterior measurement of the top

half of the glenoid was 1:06 ± 0.06. For Checroun et al,[5] evaluating 412 skeletal scapulae that had intact glenoid surfaces, the mean maximum height was 37.9 mm (range 31.2–50.1, SD ± 2.7) and the mean maximum width was 29.3 mm (range 22.6–41.5, SD ± 2.4); glenoids from women were approximately 10% smaller than those from men; 85% of all measured glenoids ranged from 34 to 42 mm high and 24 to 32 mm wide; and the mean height-to-width ratio was 1.3 (±0.07). Churchill et al[8] confirmed that glenoid sizes were influenced by sex and race. The results of the literature are summarized in Table 10.1.

GLENOID VERSION

The earliest determinations of glenoid version in an adult population were performed on 50 macerated scapulae in 1966 by Das et al.[3] Thirty of these specimens demonstrated retroversion (average 4.6 degrees, range 2–12 degrees), and 20 demonstrated anteversion (average −4.2 degrees, range −2 to −10 degrees). The mean glenoid version for this group of 50 specimens was 1.1 degree of retroversion. Das et al[3] also reported that the mean glenoid version in ten normal subjects as determined by plain radiography was 4.9 degrees of retroversion. Eight of the shoulders had a retroverted glenoid, with a mean of 7.0 degrees, and two had an anteverted glenoid, with a mean version of −3.5 degrees. Saha[4] in 1971 studied 50 normal shoulders by plain radiography and found that 73.5% of his group demonstrated glenoid retroversion, with an average value of 7.4 degrees. The remaining 26.5% of this group demonstrated anteversion of the glenoid, with a range of 2 to 10 degrees. Cyprien et al[9] reported on glenoid version values in 50 normal men (100 shoulders) using measurements from frontal plain radiographs. Overall group mean glenoid version was 7.6 degrees of retroversion. Randelli and Gambrioli[10] first reported glenoid version in a normal group of 50 subjects by using data from computed tomography (CT) scans. They scanned 100 shoulders (20–48 years of age) using 5-mm slices through the glenoid fossa. They found that the glenoid exhibited a variable degree of retrotilt at different levels; in the upper portion of the glenoid, their subjects demonstrated version between 2 and 15 degrees of retroversion, with most of the values being close to 5 degrees. Slices through the middle of the fossa demonstrated version of 0 to 8 degrees, with the majority of shoulders being close to 2 degrees of glenoid retroversion; and slices through the lower aspect of the glenoid

TABLE 10.1 Parameters Describing the Normal Anatomy of the Glenoid

First Author	No.	Age (average years)	Methods of Measurement	Height (S/I) (mm)	Width (A/P) (mm)	Retroversion (degrees)	Inclination (degrees)	Radius Curvature (mm)	Cartilage Surface (cm²)	Depth (mm)
Testut[57]	–	–	–	35	25	–	–	–	–	–
Das[3]	50	–	Rx	–	–	1.1	–	–	–	–
Saha[4]	50	–	Rx	35	25	75% retroversion 25% anteversion	–	–	–	–
Cyprien[9]	100	37.2	Rx	–	–	7.6	–	–	–	–
Mallon[15]	110	–	Rx-CT	35	24	2 (RX) – 6 (CT)	–4	36.6	–	–
Tillmann[16]	–	–	–	35	25	–12 to +8	–	–	–	9 (S/I) – 2.5 (A/P)
Randelli[10]	100	–	CT	–	–	Upper: 2–15 Middle: 0–8 Lower: 2–15	–	–	–	–
Friedman[11]	63	–	CT	–	–	–2 ± 5	–	–	–	–
Iannotti[7]	140	–	MRI	39	Upper: 23 Lower: 29	–	–	–	–	–
Mintzer[56]	111	–	CT/MRI	–	–	3.4	–	–	–	–
Bicknell[51]	72	70	–	41	22.9	–	–	–	–	–
Couteau[28]	15	–	CT/FEA	–	–	8	–	–	–	–
Flatow[21]	–	–	–	–	–	–	–	–	5–6.3	–
Anetzberger[23]	–	–	–	–	–	–	–	–	7 ± 1.2	–
Bicos[52]	20	–	–	34.65	25.45	–	–	–	–	–
Churchill[8]	344	25.6	–	37.5 (M) 32.6 (F)	27.6 (M) 23.6 (F)	1.49 (M) 0.87 (F)	4 (M) 4.5 (F)	–	–	–
De Wilde[54]	49	18–25	CT	–	–	4.88 (M) 2.43 (F)	–	–	–	–
Gallino[17]	266	–	–	–	–	2.9	37 degrees S	–	–	–
Howell[55]	25	–	–	–	–	–	–	–	–	9 (S/I) 5 (A/P)
Jobe[19]	50	–	–	40	29	–	–	–	28% of the humeral head	–
Kwon[24]	12	–	3D-CT	37.8 (scapula) 39.1 (CT)	26.8 (scapula) 25.2 (CT)	1.6 (scapula) 1 (CT)	–	–	8.7	–
McPherson[18]	93	–	RX	33.9	28.6	–	–	32.6 (S/I) 40.6 (A/P)	–	5 (S/I) 2.9 (A/P)
Nyffeler[12]	100	–	Rx-CT	–	–	9 (Rx) 3 (CT)	–	–	–	–
Checroun[5]	412	58	–	37.9	29.3	–	–	–	–	–
Soslowsky[25]	32	72	Stereo	–	–	–	–	Cartilage: 26.37 (M) 23.62 (F) Bone: 34.46 (M) 30.28 (F)	5.79 (M) 4.68 (F)	–
Von Schroeder[58]	30	–	–	36	29	8	–	–	–	–
Aigner[22]	20	>60	–	–	–	–	–	–	6.03	–
De Wilde[53]	108	–	–	35.6	25.8	–	–	–	–	–
Kelkar[20]	9	50	–	–	–	–	–	27.2	–	–
Prescher[6]	–	–	–	–	–	4–8	–	–	6–8	–

CT, Computed tomography; MRI, magnetic resonance imaging; Rx, radiography; Stereo, stereophotogrammetry; A, anterior; I, inferior; P, posterior; S, superior; M, male; F, female.

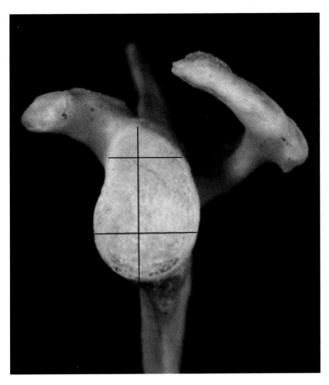

Figure 10.1. Pear-shaped appearance of the glenoid surface.

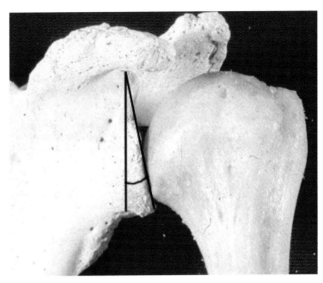

Figure 10.2. Measurement of the inclination of the glenoid in the coronal plane.

showed retroversion of 2 to 15 degrees, with most values near 7 degrees. Friedman et al[11] also used CT scans to determine glenoid version in 63 shoulders that did not show any radiographic evidence of disease. The mean age within the group was 57 years (range 20–87 years). In contradistinction to previous studies that demonstrated normal glenoid version to be retroverted, the mean glenoid version in this group was determined to be anteverted 2 ± 5 degrees (range 12 degrees of anteversion to 14 degrees of retroversion). In the literature on glenoid version, it appears that measurements made on plain radiographs of normal shoulders tend to yield readings with greater retroversion (7 degrees, 7.6 degrees) compared with specimen measurements (1.1 degrees) and CT and magnetic resonance imaging (MRI) measurements (2, 1, and 1.7 degrees in those older than 8 years). Plain radiography appears to overestimate retroversion when compared with specimens, CT, and MRI methodology.[12] This may be because plain radiographic axillary views of the glenoid superimpose levels of the glenoid that have different versions, as demonstrated in the CT work of Randelli and Gambrioli.[10] The results of the literature are summarized in Table 10.1.

INCLINATION

The angle of inclination of the glenoid is equivalent to the amount of glenoid tilt in the coronal plane and defines the position of the humeral head relative to the subacromial space (Fig. 10.2). Gouaze et al[13] described three types of inclination of the glenoid in healthy shoulders. Glenoid tilt in the coronal plane was ascendant in 45% of the shoulders (average angle 3 degrees, range 1–10 degrees), strictly vertical in 22%,

and descendant in 33% (average angle 4 degrees, range 1–12 degrees). Habermeyer[14] in a radiographic evaluation of 100 normal shoulders found that the glenoid was slightly directed downward, with an average inclination angle of −2.2 ± 4.1 degrees (range −12 to 7 degrees). Churchill et al[8] found the inclination to vary considerably. The mean inclination range was 3.6 ± 3.5 degrees to 5.3 ± 4.4 degrees (average 4.2 degrees), indicating a superiorly directed glenoid. In an effort to study the anatomic parameters of the scapula, Mallon et al[15] performed a radiographic analysis of 28 scapulae from cadavers, and 50 randomly selected posteroanterior chest radiographs were analyzed to measure what has been termed the upward rotation angle of the scapula, the angle of the lateral border of the scapula to a line perpendicular to the floor. The resting carrying angle of the glenoid fossa averaged −4 degrees (−13 to +8 degrees, ±3.7 degrees, + corresponding to a glenoid facing inferiorly). According to Tillmann and Petersen,[16] the glenoid is also tilted from superomedial to inferolateral an average of 15 degrees. Gallino et al,[17] through an anthropometric study of 266 scapulae belonging to the dynastic period of the Egyptian osteological collection of Turin, found 37 ± 12.5 degrees (10–68 degrees) of superior tilting of the glenoid. The results of the literature are summarized in Table 10.1.

RADIUS OF CURVATURE AND DEPTH

The glenoid is more curved superior to inferior (coronal plane) and relatively flatter in an anterior to posterior direction (sagittal plane). McPherson et al[18] found on radiographic examinations of 93 shoulders from embalmed cadavers that the glenoid radius of curvature measured 32.2 ± 7.6 mm in the anteroposterior view and 40.6 ± 14 mm in the axilolateral view. Glenoid depth was 5 ± 1.1 mm in the anteroposterior view and 2.9 ± 1 mm in the axilolateral view, again confirming that the glenoid is more curved superior to inferior. The glenoid arc of enclosure averaged 66 ± 12 degrees in the anteroposterior view but only 45.5 ± 15 degrees in the axilolateral view. The depth of cancellous bone behind the glenoid articular surface was similar in both views, measuring 20.9 and 19.2 mm. Jobe and Iannotti[19] reported that the average dimensions of the glenoid were 40 mm in the coronal plane, which was 96 degrees (±8 degrees) of coverage of the humeral head, and 29 mm in the transverse plane, which equaled 74 degrees (±6 degrees) of coverage. The result was 63 degrees (±10 degrees) of uncovered humeral head for motion in the coronal plane and 85 degrees (±12 degrees) of uncovered cartilage for motion in the transverse plane. The area of the glenoid is estimated to be approximately 28% of the area of the humeral head. Kelkar et al[20] confirmed this report, showing that the average radii of the humeral head and glenoid articular cartilage surfaces were 25.5 ± 1.5 mm and 27.2 ± 1.6 mm, respectively; the difference in the radii of curvature of the matching humeral head and glenoid cartilage surfaces was 1.7 ± 1.5 mm (range −1.2 to 3.8 mm); all glenoid subchondral bone surfaces had a larger radius of curvature than the matching humeral head bone surfaces (Fig. 10.3). The results of the literature are summarized in Table 10.1.

CARTILAGE SURFACE AREA

Statements from the literature regarding the average area of the glenoid surface vary among 5 and 6.3 cm^2,[21] 6.03 cm^2,[22] 7.1 ± 1.2 cm^2,[23] and 7.0 to 14.2 cm^2, with a mean of 8.7 ± 2.7 cm^2.[24] Glenoid vault volume varied widely depending on the overall size of the scapula (7.1–21.6 cm3). However, glenoid vault volume relative to glenoid surface area was more consistent, with a mean of 1.4 ± 0.2 cm^3/cm^2 (range 1.1–1.9 cm^3/cm^2).[24] Soslowsky et al[25] using a stereophotogrammetry method of measurement found a difference between the radius of curvature

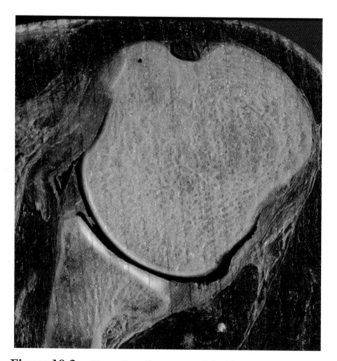

Figure 10.3. The radius of curvature of the glenoid cavity is greater than that of the humeral head.

glenoid when the cartilage was preserved (26.37 ± 2.42 [male] and 23.62 ± 1.56 [female]) or when only bone was present (34.56 ± 1.74 [male] and 30.28 ± 3.16 [female]). The glenoid cartilage surface area was evaluated to be 5.79 ± 1.69 cm^2 in males and 4.68 ± 0.93 cm^2 in females; glenoid cartilage thickness was estimated to be 2.16 ± 0.55 mm (range 3.81 ± 0.72 − 1.14 ± 0.6). The results of the literature are summarized in Table 10.1.

MINERALIZATION AND DENSITY

The orientation of the spongious bone close to the articular surface is functionally adapted to the strain. The spongious trabeculae are oriented vertical to the subchondral bone corresponding to the compressive stress acting in an axial direction. The compressive trabeculae are crossed cancellous right angles by tensional trabeculae, which are most prominent in the center of the glenoid cavity.[26] Mansat et al,[27] in a cadaveric study, analyzed the mechanical properties of the glenoid. Mechanical properties were found to be significantly higher at the center and posterior edge of the glenoid. Significant differences were also found in the three planes studied. The lateromedial Young's modulus (E1) was higher than the anteroposterior modulus (E2) and the superoinferior modulus (E3) (E1 = 372 ± 164 Mpa; E2 = 222 ± 79 Mpa; E3 = 198 ± 75 Mpa). The highest stiffness seems to be located at the central and posterior parts of the glenoid. These results have shown that the glenoid has anisotropic material properties.

Couteau et al[28] conducted a study to characterize in vivo glenoids with three different diagnoses by using CT and finite element analysis (Fig. 10.4A). Fifteen patients were analyzed in the normal group without osteoarthritis; the average age was 40 years (range 17–75). The glenoid from this group presented a central area in which the CT number variation was between 10 and 380 Hounsfield units (HU). At the periphery of this area, the CT number varied from 380 HU to 750 or 1,000 HU for only 2 or 3 mm. The CT number, as well as the density of the peripheral region, was greater in younger patients than in older patients (>50 years of age). The mean CT value was found to equal 278 (±101) HU (range 75–632). The greatest value on average was located at the center of the glenoid. Twenty-five percent of the glenoids presented a significant difference between the central level and the upper level. The greatest values were located at the lateral posterior region. Concerning the version angle, the mean value was 8 degrees of retroversion (range 2–17 degrees). Of the glenoids, 93% had a version angle of less than 15 degrees of retroversion (Fig. 10.4B). Frich et al[29] confirmed this, showing a higher mineralization and number of the subarticular trabeculae in the posterior glenoid that would indicate a more posterior stress distribution. Finally, Schultz et al,[26] studying 44 normal shoulder specimens, mean age 48 years (range 18–89 years), found a centrally accentuated pattern of mineral density distribution in only 18%, whereas a peripheral localization was present in 82%. Most frequently (68%) a bicentric distribution with opposing maximal values located close to the anterior and posterior glenoid rim was typical. The healthy shoulder, in spite of wide anatomic variability, has a constant stress distribution on the glenoid cavity that is not influenced by age or side.

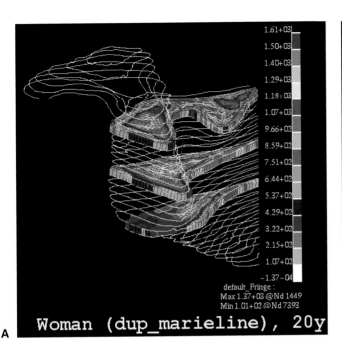

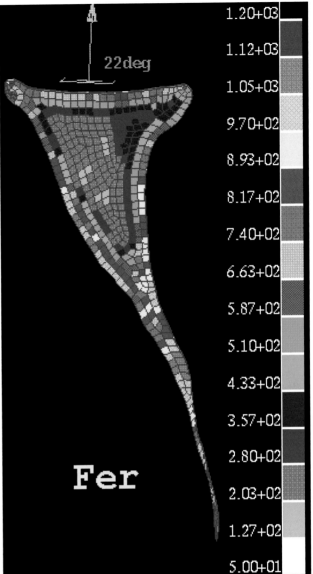

Figure 10.4. Three-dimensional computed tomography (CT) reconstruction of normal glenoid and finite element analysis of the all glenoid (**A**) and the principal midlevel slice (**B**). Note the homogeneous distribution of the bone properties from the periphery to the center of the glenoid. At the center of the glenoid there is a homogeneous area of low CT values. This area seems symmetrical to the central axis; however, there is a slight augmentation of the CT values close to the posterior surface. The cancellous area close to the subchondral surface is clearly seen.

SUMMARY

The glenoid is pear-shaped and slightly retroverted, with variable orientation in the sagittal plane. The cartilage surface area is 28% of the area of the humeral head. The radius of curvature is greater than that of the humeral head. Mechanical properties are significantly higher at the center and posterior edge of the glenoid.

GLENOID DYSPLASIA: VARIATION OF NORMAL

Brewer et al,[30] in 1983, identified the possibly of a congenital or developmental defect of the posterior part of the glenoid. There have been three reported cases of affected first-degree family members, and some authors believe an autosomal dominant inheritance pattern with low penetrance exists.[31] For Brewer et al,[30] the secondary centers of ossification of the scapula include one at the base of the coracoid process that appears in the 10th year and, if faulty, causes posterior rotation of the glenoid so that the articular surface faces backward; another ossification center, which is identified in the 15th year, is horseshoe-shaped and is in the midglenoid area; if it is faulty and hypoplastic, there is a flattening of the glenoid fossa. It has been concluded that these two defects—excessive retroversion of the glenoid and flattening of the glenoid fossa—are based on faulty development of the secondary centers of the scapula. However, osseous changes include both dysplasia of the glenoid and hypoplasia of the glenoid process with, in addition, cartilaginous changes with hypertrophy of both the articular cartilage and the glenoid labra.[32,33] This congenital defect of the glenoid is not common,[34] but Edelson,[35] examining 1,150 scapular bones, found a localized hypoplasia of the posteroinferior glenoid in 20% to 35% of the population studied. Patients usually show symptoms either in late adolescence or in the fifth or sixth decade, and many cases are detected as incidental findings on chest radiographs taken for other purposes. This implies that the true incidence may be significantly greater than the few reported cases would suggest.[36,37] The percentage of specimens exhibiting bilateral findings varied from 52% to 83%. The occurrence of mild degrees of arthritic changes in the glenoids was relatively common in specimens from older persons. Edelson[35] does not suggest that isolated posteroinferior glenoid hypoplasia is a causative factor in the development of shoulder joint arthritis. However, these two entities may coexist to produce the picture of exaggerated posterior wear that is sometimes seen at the time of total shoulder arthroplasty and may suggest the need for additional glenoid side surgery.[38] This picture, however, may simply be a combination of osteophytic change superimposed on a glenoid with posteroinferior hypoplasia.[39] The absence of posterior subluxation of the humeral head distinguishes dysplastic glenoid morphology from erosive biconcave glenoid morphology with posterior humeral subluxation, typically occurring in primary osteoarthritis.[40] The differential diagnosis of glenoid dysplasia includes birth injuries to the brachial plexus, with resultant hypoplasia of the shoulder girdle, avascular necrosis, multiple epiphyseal dysplasia, and deficiency of vitamin C or D. Brachial plexus injuries have associated neurological findings, and are most often unilateral. Avascular necrosis is also usually a unilateral abnormality. In cases associated with multiple epiphyseal dysplasia or avitaminoses, diffuse abnormalities are present. Wirth et al[37] categorized the glenoid dysplasia in three stages. "Mild grade" shoulders had a shallow, slightly irregular, and, in some instances, dentated glenoid fossa; although these shoulders were underdeveloped, some of the inferior aspect of the scapular neck and glenoid rim was present in all of them. In "Moderate grade," loss of the inferior part of the scapular neck and glenoid rim occurred and these glenoids were also characterized by a more irregular and elongated appearance compared with those with a milder grade of hypoplasia. "Severe grade" shoulders had extensive hypoplasia of the inferior part of the glenoid, which appeared confluent with the lateral scapular border; marked dysplasia of the humeral head; varus angulation of the humeral head; apparent joint incongruity; and associated scapular abnormalities, including an enlarged and inferiorly directed acromion, a prominent coracoid process, and hooking of the distal part of the clavicle.

THE ARTHRITIC GLENOID

Neer,[41] in 1961, was one of the first authors to describe primary degenerative lesions of the glenohumeral joint. He wrote: "*Although much attention has been given to the abnormalities of the soft-tissue structure of the shoulder joint, with but few exceptions the articular surfaces have been disregarded. There are several reasons for this: (1) Degeneration with true incongruity of the glenohumeral joint surfaces is much less frequent than in weight-bearing joints. (2) Lipping of the articular margins and narrowing of the joint space is observed at times as an incidental roentgen finding in a symptom-free patient. (3) Marginal osteophytes and excrescences around the head and in the floor of the bicipital groove are frequently associated with lesions of the soft tissues, for example, degenerative changes or tears of the supraspinatus tendon, bicipital tenosynovitis or rupture of the long head of the biceps, hyperplasia of the synovial membrane and subacromial bursa, all of which make it impossible to incriminate one single lesion as the source of pain.*" In a dissection study of 105 cadaver shoulders he observed: "*The articular surface of the glenoid is usually more severely involved than that of the humeral head, probably due to the smaller proportion of contact area of the larger humeral head and, therefore, less wear during joint motion.*"

In 1974,[42] in patients who underwent surgery for primary osteoarthritis with a shoulder arthroplasty, Neer found: "*The alteration at the end of the humerus occurred in a characteristic pattern. Thinning of the articular cartilage was most advanced in that area of the humeral head that is in contact with the glenoid when the arm is abducted between 60 and 100 degrees. This is the area of maximum joint reaction force and it was eburnated and sclerotic. Degenerative subarticular cysts occurred just superior to the mid-point of the articular surface. The largest osteophytes were located at the inferior margin of the joint, where they often covered the calcar... The articular surface of the glenoid was smooth but usually consisted of eburnated bone devoid of cartilage. Marginal osteophytes were often seen on roentgenograms. They could be palpated within the ligaments of the glenoid, especially inferiorly, but they were rarely visible at surgery.*"

Finally in 1982, Neer et al[43] reviewed their experience with 366 shoulder arthroplasties. Fifty-five patients (62 shoulders) had primary osteoarthritis. They found that: "*In advanced cases the glenoid becomes flattened and eroded posteriorly... The sloping glenoid may result in a posterior subluxation of the humeral head, which in extreme cases resembles an old posterior dislocation.*" At surgery he noted: "*Uneven wear of the glenoid in osteoarthritis or the arthritis of recurrent dislocation may result in the glenoid facing backward or forward, both situations requiring operative correction.*"

Although glenohumeral osteoarthritis is not common, Petersson,[44] evaluating 151 shoulders with an average age of 68 years, found alteration of the joint cartilage of the caput humeri and the glenoid cavity in 33% of cases. Cartilage degeneration was bilateral in 28 of 34 shoulders (82%); the degenerative changes were often more pronounced in the glenoid cavity. Kerr et al,[45] through a radiographic examination of 92 scapulae of cadaveric specimens and 50 consecutive patients 60 years of age or older, found the presence of osteophytes along the line of attachment of the labrum to the glenoid fossa in 73 (79%) of 92 specimens. Eburnation or central erosion of the glenoid fossa was evident in nine (10%) and 15 (16%), respectively. All 50 patients were men, with an average age of 68 years; moderate to severe degenerative-like changes of the glenohumeral joint were seen in only nine (14%) of the 65 shoulders and mild changes in six (9%). Joint space narrowing (<2 mm) was observed in six (67%) of nine shoulders with moderate to severe changes and in none with mild changes. In cadavers, eburnation and bony erosion predominated in the central part of the glenoid fossa of the scapula.

The common features of the arthritic glenoid are mainly an increase of the anteroposterior size because of osteophyte development and posterior wear causing glenoid retroversion. The results of literature are summarized in Table 10.2. Mullaji et al,[46] conducting CT evaluation of 45 arthritic shoulders, found that in osteoarthritis (OA), the maximum anteroposterior diameter of the glenoid was greater by 5 to 8 mm compared to normal (OA = upper part: 30.6 ± 7.4 mm; middle part: 33.3 ± 5.7 mm; lower part: 31.6 ± 6.9 mm. Normal = upper: 23.3 ± 3.9 mm; middle: 25.5 ± 3.5 mm; lower: 26.3 ± 3.4 mm.). All but one of the osteoarthritic glenoids were retroverted (mean 12.5 degrees), with a mean slope of 28.6 ± 10.8 degrees, significantly different from the mean normal retroversion of 3 degrees and slope of 39.9 ± 8.2 degrees. Medial displacement of the glenoid surface was greatest at the upper and middle levels; the surface was inclined superiorly rather than inferiorly. The best bone was in the anterior half at

TABLE 10.2			Parameters Describing the Anatomy of the Osteoarthritic Glenoid				
First Author	No.	Age (average) (years)	Methods of Measurement	Height (S/I) (mm)	Width (A/P) (mm)	Retroversion (degrees)	Depth (mm)
Friedman[11]	13	–	CT	–	–	11 ± 8	–
Walch[50]	113	–	CT	–	–	16	–
Mullaji[46]	45	–	CT	–	Upper: 30.6 ± 7.4 Middle: 33.3 ± 5.7 Lower: 31.6 ± 6.9	12.5	–
Habermeyer[14]	100	–	Rx	–	–	–	–
Karelse[47]	40	86	–	35.9 ± 3.6 27.2 ± 3	–	3.3	3.4 ± 1.2
Mansat[27]	38	60	CT	36.39	31	17.3	–
Couteau[28]	–	–	–	–	–	16	–

CT, Computed tomography; Rx, radiography; A, anterior; I, inferior; P, posterior; S, superior.

the upper and middle levels, with the remaining surface at these levels consisting of unsupported bone. The lower level was least affected. Karelse et al[47] found the same results evaluating 40 fresh-frozen human shoulders with signs of osteoarthritis. The measured glenoid orientation was 3.3 ± 2.7 degrees of retroversion (11 degrees of retroversion to 6 degrees of anteversion) and an inclination of 7.1 ± 3.5 degrees (range 1–16 degrees). The average dimensions of the glenoid in the superoinferior and anteroposterior directions were 35.9 ± 3.6 mm (range 30–44 mm) and 27.2 ± 3.0 mm (range 23–33 mm), respectively. Using CT scan evaluation, Friedman et al[11] showed that the osteoarthritic glenoid was more retroverted that in the control normal group, with an average of 11 ± 8 degrees of retroversion (range 2 degrees of anteversion to 32 degrees of retroversion). CT scans of the glenohumeral joint of the 13 patients revealed that the glenoid surface was often found to be diffusely worn; the wear sometimes extended down to the base of the coracoid process so that the humeral head was articulating with the coracoid. Glenoid erosion was generally more pronounced on the posterior aspect; the extent of the glenoid fossa was also changed by the presence of sharp osteophytes or hyperostosis anteriorly and posteriorly that distorted the normal anatomy and affected the glenoid version. As a result of uneven wear of the glenoid surface, mainly in a posterior direction, posterior subluxation of the humeral head was a common finding.[11]

It appears that a spectrum of glenoid wear exists. Edelson,[48] in 1995, examining 486 skeletons of subjects over the age of 60 years to study patterns of degenerative change in the glenohumeral joint, described three distinct types of glenohumeral joint involvement. In type I (29.6%) the glenoid had modest osteophytic formation circling the joint, with sclerotic changes mostly prominent in the posterosuperior portion. In type II (3.5%) the glenoid was augmented by osteophytes, principally around the lower half, but these changes were usually mild compared with those in the head. The sclerosis and wear pattern in advanced cases tended to localize on the posteroinferior aspect, but there was no evidence of exaggerated posterior wear leading to obvious architectural deficiency. In type III (4.7%) there was an extensive distortion of the glenoid. Based on a radiographic study, Nakagawa et al[49] classified primary gleno-

humeral osteoarthritis in three stages. The early stage (stage 1) was characterized by the presence of spur formation or bone sclerosis in the humeral head or glenoid. The advanced stage (stage 2) was characterized by the presence of spur formation or bone sclerosis in both the humeral head and the glenoid or by the presence of joint space narrowing. The end stage (stage 3) was characterized by the presence of spur formation, bone sclerosis, and joint space narrowing or the disappearance of the joint space. Sixteen patients (18 shoulders) were given the diagnosis of primary glenohumeral osteoarthritis (4.6% of all the patients with shoulder disease and 0.40% of all of the patients with orthopaedic conditions). There were two men and 14 women 60 to 86 years old (mean 71.9 years). Primary osteoarthritis was significantly more frequent in patients aged 60 years or older than in those younger than 60. There were stage 1 changes in 10, stage 2 in 5, and stage 3 in 3. Walch et al,[50] in 1999, was the first to classify the type of glenoid wear using CT scan evaluation. After serial CT scans of 113 osteoarthritic shoulders (average age 66.4 years), glenoid morphology was classified in three types according to the type of wear and the glenoid retroversion angle (Fig. 10.5). Mean glenoid retroversion was 16 degrees (range −12 to 50 degrees) for all series. In type A glenoid (59%) the humeral head is centered and the resultant forces are equally distributed against the surface of the glenoid. Glenoid retroversion averages 11.5 degrees (±8.8 degrees). The erosion may be minor (type A1 [43%]) or major (type A2 [16%]), marked by a central erosion that leads to a centered glenoid cupula. In advanced cases the humeral head protrudes into the glenoid cavity. In type B glenoid (32%) the humeral head is subluxated posteriorly and the distributed loads are asymmetrical. CT scan revealed numerous anatomic changes, more pronounced on the posterior margin of the glenoid; the retroversion averaged 18 degrees (±7.2 degrees). Two subgroups were identified—B1 (17%) showed narrowing of the posterior joint space, subchondral sclerosis, and osteophytes; and B2 (15%) demonstrated a posterior cupula that gave an unusual biconcave appearance to the glenoid. In type B2, there was excessive retroversion of the glenoid, but the value of the retroversion does not explain the biconcavity of the glenoid. In type C glenoid (9%) the morphology was defined by a glenoid retroversion of more than 25 degrees, regardless of the erosion.

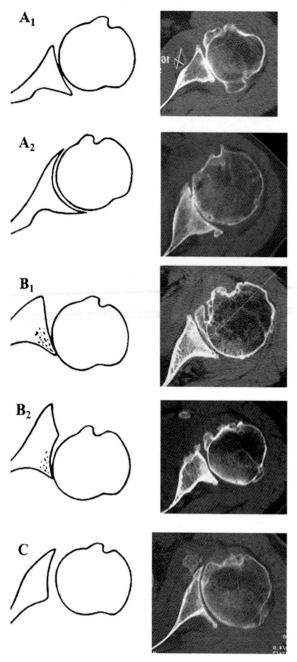

Figure 10.5. Classification of the osteoarthritic glenoid in the transverse plane according to Walch et al. (From Walch G, Badet R, Boulahia A, et al. Morphologic study of the glenoid in primary glenohumeral osteoarthritis. *J Arthroplasty* 1999;14:756–760, with permission.)

The retroversion was of dysplasic origin, and the humeral head was well centered or slightly subluxated posteriorly; the average retroversion was 35.7 degrees (±5.9 degrees). Mean patient age increased with the amount of the glenoid central erosion (A1, 62.3 years) and (A2, 71.3 years). In type B the posterior subluxation of the humerus head averaged 59% (56.8% to 61.7%) and seemed to be responsible for the posterior erosion that was minor in type B1 and important in type B2, with the typical biconcave appearance. Again the difference between the mean age, 63 years and 71 years, is statistically significant. The glenoid retroversion increased from type B1 (14.9 degrees) to type B2 (23.4 degrees) but does not explain the asymmetrical erosion

and posterior subluxation of the humeral head. The dysplastic type C (average age 61.4 years) represents another distinct mode of evolutionary phenomena because retroversion of more than 25 degrees is clearly congenital. The index of subluxation of the humeral head in type C varies and ranged from 35% to 75%, with an average value of 55%. The CT scan analysis of the glenoid morphology and the definition of different types of glenoid showed a wide range of polymorphism and evolution. Of primary glenohumeral osteoarthritis, 9% were associated with excessive retroversion as seen in dysplasic glenoid (type C) and must be differentiated from the osteoarthritis glenoid with an advanced posterior erosion as seen in type B2. We reviewed (nonpublished data) 36 patients (38 shoulders) with an average age of 60 years (range 53–78 years) in the context of preoperative planning for shoulder arthroplasty for primary osteoarthritis. Four radiographic views—anteroposterior views in neutral rotation, external rotation, and internal rotation, and an axillary view—were obtained and CT examination performed. Radiographs in neutral rotation showed joint narrowing, inferior humeral osteophytes, subchondral bone sclerosis in 90%, loose bodies in 10 cases, and bone cyst in 20 cases. According to the classification of Walch et al,[50] on CT scan evaluation we found the following: type A: 45% (A1 21% and A2 24%); type B: 52% (B1 18% and B2 34%); and type C: 4% (two cases). Glenoid retroversion was estimated to be 17.3 degrees on average (range 0–26 degrees). Glenoid slope (sagittal) described by Mullaji et al[46] was 23 degrees (range 10–43 degrees), the glenoid joint facing superiorly. Coronal slope of the glenoid was 12 degrees (range 0–30 degrees). Glenoid size was 31 mm, on average, from anterior to posterior (range 23–43 mm) and 36.39 mm, on average, from superior to inferior (range 30–45 mm).

However, Habermeyer et al[14] underlined that in osteoarthritis of the shoulder, the tilt of the glenoid surface undergoes an eccentric deformation not only in the anteroposterior but also in the superoinferior direction. In a radiographic evaluation of 100 shoulders with osteoarthritis, in the coronal plane on the anteroposterior view the inclination of the glenoid was measured. It was −12.6 ± 8.7 degrees in the osteoarthritic group compared to −2.2 ± 4.1 degrees in the control group. The mean inclination angle in patients with osteoarthritis was significantly lower than that in healthy patients. Four types of inclination have been described (Fig. 10.6): in type 0 the coracoid base line and the glenoid line run parallel; in type 1 the coracoid base line and the glenoid line intersect below the inferior glenoid rim; in type 2 the coracoid base line and the glenoid line intersect between the inferior glenoid rim and the center of the glenoid; in type 3 the coracoid base line intersects above the coracoid base. In the transverse plane, there were 20 A1, 26 A2, 28 B1, 25 B2, according to the classification of Walch et al.[50] Significantly more patients with osteoarthritis were found to have type 2 and 3 glenoids. Of patients with osteoarthritis, 47% showed both posterior and inferior glenoid wear. There was no correlation between the type of inclination and the type of glenoid morphology. Fifty-eight percent of patients with osteoarthritis had a static eccentric position of the humeral head in the coronal plane, which was correlated with the type of inclination; 49% of the patients showed a centered humeral head on both anteroposterior and axillary views. In osteoarthritis, eccentric inferior glenoid wear is frequent and independent from retroversion deformity of the glenoid. Normalization of the glenoid version in both transverse and coronal planes may reduce eccentric loading of the prosthetic glenoid, which has been associated with loosening.

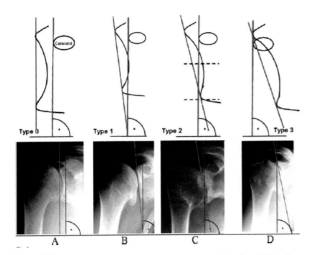

Figure 10.6. Classification of the osteoarthritic glenoid in the sagittal plane according to Habermeyer et al. (From Habermeyer P, Magosch P, Luz V, et al. Three-dimensional glenoid deformity in patients with osteoarthritis: a radiographic analysis. *J Bone Joint Surg Am* 2006;88:1301–1307, with permission.)

Habermeyer et al[14] advise normalizing type 2 and 3 glenoid inclination, as well as any angle of retroversion greater than 15 degrees, when glenoid replacement is performed in shoulder arthroplasty. Without normalization of the pathological glenoid tilt, a static uneven stress distribution onto the prosthetic glenoid may occur postoperatively.

Couteau et al[28] studied bone density in osteoarthritic shoulders using finite element analysis. They found the central area of low density was reduced compared to the normal glenoid because of increased values at the posterior margin of the glenoid, with thickening of the posterior region acting as a strengthening column to support the glenoid surface. This phenomenon was particularly apparent with greater uneven glenoid wear. The mean CT value was found to be 387 (±137) HU compared to 278 (±101) HU for normal shoulders. Ranges of CT variation were 72 to 987 HU. The greatest CT number was generally found at the three lowest levels; 70% of glenoids presented significant differences between the lower level and the upper level, with the greatest values located in the lateroposterior region. The version angle was 16 degrees of retroversion (range 0.2–50 degrees) (Fig. 10.7).

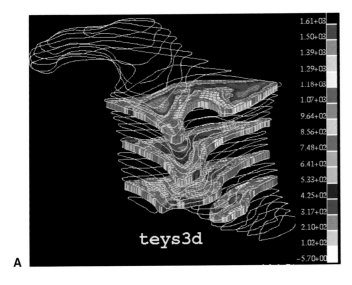

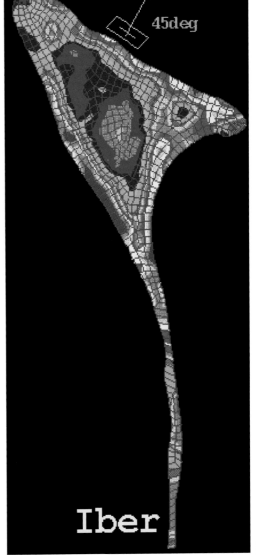

Figure 10.7. Three-dimensional computed tomography reconstruction of osteoarthritic glenoid and finite element analysis of the entire glenoid (**A**) and the principal midlevel slice (**B**). There is a flattening of the articular surface with overgrowth of the anterior and posterior margins of the glenoid corresponding to osteophytes. The humeral head tends to translate posteriorly, resulting in excessive load transferred to the posterior margin of the glenoid, leading to uneven glenoid response and wear. In terms of Hounsfield values, this phenomenon is represented by increased values at the posterior margin of the glenoid and is correlated to increased retroversion of the glenoid.

Osteoarthritic glenoids demonstrated alterations to the structure and geometry of the bones. It has been assumed that because of thickening of the anterior capsuloligamentous structures, the humeral head tends to translate posteriorly. This abnormal posterior translation results in excessive load transfer to the posterior margin of the glenoid, which may explain the reinforcement of the bone structure in this region. Moreover, the greatest CT densities were in the lower sections; asymmetrical wear of the glenoid fossa was the main characteristic of glenoids with primary osteoarthritis. An interesting finding is that the CT density reinforcement tended to be correlated with the version angle; visualization of the internal bone structure showed that the posterior aspect of the glenoid was undoubtedly the strongest area.

SUMMARY

The arthritic glenoid shows a larger size of the glenoid (greater width) and is more retroverted, showing centric or excentric wear. It is oriented superiorly. The mechanical properties are significantly higher at center and posterior edge of the glenoid.

REFERENCES

1. Gray H. The scapula (shoulder blade). In: Gray H. *Anatomy of the Human Body*. Philadelphia: Lea & Tebiger; 1918.
2. Codman EA. *The Shoulder: Rupture of the Supraspinatus Tendon and Other lesions in or about the Subacromial Bursa*. Boston: Thomas Todd; 1934.
3. Das SP, Ray GS, Saha AK. Observations on the tilt of the glenoid cavity of the scapula. *J Anat Soc India* 1966;15:114–118.
4. Saha AK. Dynamic stability of the glenohumeral joint. *Acta Orthop Scand* 1971;42:491.
5. Checroun AJ, Hawkins C, Kummer FJ, et al. Fit of current glenoid component designs: an anatomic cadaver study. *J Shoulder Elbow Surg* 2002;11:614–617.
6. Prescher A. Anatomical basics, variations, and degenerative changes of the shoulder joint and shoulder girdle. *Eur J Radiol* 2000;35:88–102.
7. Iannotti JP, Gabriel JP, Schneck SL, et al. The normal glenohumeral relationships. *J Bone Joint Surg Am* 1992;74:491–500.
8. Churchill RS, Brems JJ, Kotschi H. Glenoid size, inclination, and version: an anatomic study. *J Shoulder Elbow Surg* 2001;10:327–332.
9. Cyprien JM, Vasey HM, Burdet A, et al. Humeral retrotorsion and glenohumeral relationship in the normal shoulder and in recurrent anterior dislocation. *Clin Orthop* 1983;175: 8–17.
10. Randelli M, Gambrioli PL. Glenohumeral osteometry by computed tomography in normal and unstable shoulders. *Clin Orthop* 1986;208:151–156.
11. Friedman RJ, Hawthorne KB, Genez BM. The use of computerized tomography in the measurement of glenoid version. *J Bone Joint Surg Am* 1992;74:1032–1037.
12. Nyffeler RW, Jost B, Pfirrmann CWA, et al. Measurement of glenoid version: conventional radiographs versus computed tomography scans. *J Shoulder Elbow Surg* 2003;12:493–496.
13. Gouaze A, Castaing J, Soutoul JH, et al. Sur l'orientation de l'omoplate et de sa cavité glenoïde. [On the orientation of the scapula and of its glenoid cavity.] *Arch Anat Pathol* 1962;10:175–181.
14. Habermeyer P, Magosch P, Luz V, et al. Three-dimensional glenoid deformity in patients with osteoarthritis: a radiographic analysis. *J Bone Joint Surg Am* 2006;88:1301–1307.
15. Mallon WJ, Brown HR, Vogler JB 3rd, et al. Radiographic and geometric anatomy of the scapula. *Clin Orthop* 1992;277:142–154.
16. Tillmann B, Petersen W. Clinical anatomy. In Wülker N, Mansat M, Fu FH. *Shoulder Surgery*. London: Martin Dunitz; 2001:1–29.
17. Gallino M, Santamaria E, Doro T. Anthropometry of the scapula: clinical and surgical considerations. *J Shoulder Elbow Surg* 1998;7:284–291.
18. McPherson EJ, Friedman RJ, An YH, et al. Anthropometric study of normal glenohumeral relationships. *J Shoulder Elbow Surg* 1997;6:105–112.
19. Jobe CM, Iannotti JP. Limits imposed on glenohumeral motion by joint geometry. *J Shoulder Elbow Surg* 1995;4:281–285.
20. Kelkar R, Wang VM, Flatow EL, et al. Glenohumeral mechanics: a study of articular geometry, contact, and kinematics. *J Shoulder Elbow Surg* 2001;10:73–84.
21. Flatow EL, Soslowski LJ, Ateshian GA, et al. Shoulder joint anatomy and the effect of subluxations and size mismatch on patterns of glenohumeral contact. *Orthop Trans* 1991;15: 803–804.
22. Aigner F, Longato S, Fritsch H, et al. Anatomical considerations regarding the "bare spot" of the glenoid cavity. *Surg Radiol Anat* 2004;26:308–11.
23. Anetzberger H, Putz R. The scapula: principles of construction and stress. *Acta Anat* 1996;156:70–80.
24. Kwon YW, Powell KA, Yum JK, et al. Use of three-dimensional computed tomography for the analysis of the glenoid anatomy. *J Shoulder Elbow Surg* 2005;14:85–90.
25. Soslowsky LJ, Flatow EL, Bigliani LU, et al. Articular geometry of the glenohumeral joint. *Clin Orthop* 1992;285:181–190.
26. Schulz CU, Pfahler M, Anetzberger HM, et al. The mineralization patterns at the subchondral bone plate of the glenoid cavity in healthy shoulders. *J Shoulder Elbow Surg* 2002;11: 174–181.
27. Mansat P, Barea C, Hobatho MC, et al. Anatomic variation of the mechanical properties of the glenoid. *J Shoulder Elbow Surg* 1998;7:109–115.
28. Couteau B, Mansat P, Mansat M, et al. In vivo characterization of glenoid with use of computed tomography. *J Shoulder Elbow Surg* 2001;10:116–122.
29. Frich LH, Odgaard A, Dalstra M. Glenoid bone architecture. *J Shoulder Elbow Surg* 1998;7: 356–361.
30. Brewer BJ, Wubben RC, Carrera GF. Excessive retroversion of the glenoid cavity: a cause of non-traumatic posterior instability of the shoulder. *J Bone Joint Surg Am* 1986;68:724–731.
31. Fuhrman W, Koch F, Rauterberg K. Dominant erbliche hypoplasie und bewegungseinschrankung beider schultergelenke. *Zeitschr Orthop* 1968;104:584–588.
32. Collins JI, Colston WC, Swayne LC. MR findings in congenital glenoid dysplasia. *J Comput Assist Tomogr* 1995;19:819–821.
33. Manns RA, Davies AM: Glenoid hypoplasia: assessment by computed tomographic arthrography. *Clin Radiol* 1991;43:316–320.
34. Beluffi G, Fiori P, Rodino C. Bilateral glenoid hypoplasia. *Eur Radiol* 1998;8:986–988.
35. Edelson JG. Localized glenoid hypoplasia: an anatomic variation of possible clinical significance. *Clin Orthop* 1995;321:189–195.
36. Lintner DM, Sebastianelli WJ, Hanks GA, et al. Glenoid dysplasia: a case report and review of the literature. *Clin Orthop* 1992;283:145–148.
37. Wirth MA, Lyons FR, Rockwood CA Jr. Hypoplasia of the glenoid: a review of 16 patients. *J Bone Joint Surg Am* 1993;75:1175–1184.
38. Sperling JW, Cofield RH, Steinmann SP. Shoulder arthroplasty for osteoarthritis secondary to glenoid dysplasia. *J Bone Joint Surg Am* 2002;84:541–546.
39. Grignard F, De Maeseneer M, Scheerlinck T, et al. Glenoid dysplasia: radiographic and CT arthrographic findings. *J Belg Radiol* 1998;81:82–83.
40. Edwards TB, Boulahia A, Kempf JF, et al. Shoulder arthroplasty in patients with osteoarthritis and dysplastic glenoid morphology. *J Shoulder Elbow Surg* 2004;13:1–4.
41. Neer CS. Degenerative lesions of the proximal humeral articular surface. *Clin Orthop* 1961;20:116–125.
42. Neer CS. Replacement arthroplasty for glenohumeral osteoarthritis. *J Bone Joint Surg Am* 1974;56:1–13.
43. Neer CS, Watson KC, Stanton FJ. Recent experience in total shoulder replacement. *J Bone Joint Surg Am* 1982;64:319–337.
44. Petersson CJ. Degeneration of the glenohumeral joint. *Acta Orthop Scand* 1983;54:277–283.
45. Kerr R, Resnick D, Pineda C, et al. Osteoarthritis of the glenohumeral joint: a radiologic-pathologic study. *Am J Roentgenol* 1985;144:967–972.
46. Mullaji AB, Beddow FH, Lamb GHR. CT measurement of glenoid erosion in arthritis. *J Bone Joint Surg Br* 1994;76:384–388.
47. Karelse A, Kegels L, De Wilde L. The pillars of the scapula. *Clin Anat* 2007;92–99.
48. Edelson JG. Patterns of degenerative change in the glenohumeral joint. *J Bone Joint Surg Br* 1995;77:288–292.
49. Nakagawa Y, Hyakuna K, Otani S, et al. Epidemiologic study of glenohumeral osteoarthritis with plain radiography. *J Shoulder Elbow Surg* 1999;8:580–584.
50. Walch G, Badet R, Boulahia A, et al. Morphologic study of the glenoid in primary glenohumeral osteoarthritis. *J Arthroplasty* 1999;14:756–760.
51. Bicknell RT, Patterson SD, King GJ, et al. Glenoid vault endosteal dimensions: an anthropometric study with special interest in implant design. *J Shoulder Elbow Surg* 2007;16:96S–101S.
52. Bicos J, Mazzocca A, Romeo AA. The glenoid center line. *Orthopedics* 2005;28:581–585.
53. De Wilde LF, Berghs BM, Audenaert E, et al. About the variability of the shape of the glenoid cavity. *Surg Radiol Anat* 2004;26:54–59.
54. De Wilde LF, Berghs BM, VandeVyver F, et al. Glenohumeral relationship in the transverse plane of the body. *J Shoulder Elbow Surg* 2003;12:260–267.
55. Howell SM, Galinat BJ: The glenoid-labral socket: a constrained articular surface. *Clin Orthop* 1989;243:122–125.
56. Mintzer CM, Waters PM, Brown DJ. Glenoid version in children. *J Pediatr Orthop* 1996;16:563–566.
57. Testut L. Traité d'Anatomie Humaine. 7th ed. Tome 1: Ostéologie, Arthrologie, Myologie, Paris: Doin; 1921:503–504.
58. Von Schroeder HP, Kuiper SD, Botte MJ. Osseous anatomy of the scapula. *Clin Orthop* 2001;383:131–139.

Gilles Walch
Pascal Boileau
Lionel Neyton

Revision of the Glenoid Component

INTRODUCTION

Total shoulder arthroplasty has been reported to have better results than hemiarthroplasty at short- and long-terms follow-up in term of pain, activities of daily living, and range of motion. The glenoid side has been recognized as the weak part of the total shoulder arthroplasty.

Following Neer's introduction[1,2] in 1972, most of the glenoid components are the polyethylene keeled or pegged design used with cement.[3,4] Glenoid loosening has been reported to be the second most common complication in terms of frequency by Bohsali and Wirth,[5] with a rate of 5.3% in a metaanalysis of 2,540 cases. Radiographic evidence of loosening of a polyethylene component (complete radiolucent line wider than 2 mm in thickness, migration, tilt, or a shift of the component) was reported by Bohsali and Wirth[5] in 34% of 148 shoulders with more than 10 years of follow-up. Persistent concern regarding aseptic loosening of the cemented glenoid component has led to the use of metal-backed implants.[6–11] However, midterm follow-up results have demonstrated substantial issues related to progression of radiolucent lines, severe osteolysis, polyethylene wear, polyethylene–metal tray dissociation, glenoid tray fracture, and screw breakage. Although the use of an uncemented metal-backed component is now severely limited because of the number and varying types of complications, it may still be a choice for revisions.

Whereas the rate of glenoid complications seems to increase with mid- to long-term follow-up, the rate of revision for glenoid loosening is difficult to evaluate. Moreover, the causes for revision shoulder arthroplasty are often multifactorial. Problems such as prosthetic instability or rotator cuff tear may necessitate switching to a reverse system and revision of the glenoid even though it is not loose. Revision of the glenoid is influenced by several factors—whether it is loose, cemented or metal-backed, keeled or pegged, or anatomic nonconstrained or reverse semiconstrained and associated problems such as instability or rotator cuff tearing.

Glenoid revision should be thus considered a part of a more complex operation that may also necessitate humeral stem revision. The surgical options to revise a glenoid component sometimes depend more on the associated complications (instability, cuff) than the size of the glenoid defect. This chapter will discuss the problem of glenoid revision and focus on revision of nonconstrained types of glenoid components, both cemented and uncemented.

PREOPERATIVE PLANNING

High-quality standard anteroposterior radiographs obtained under fluoroscopic guidance, as well as an axillary profile view, are necessary to appreciate the glenoid component. Although plain radiographs are usually sufficient to evaluate radiolucent lines between the cement and the bone, shift, migration, or tilt of the component, computed tomography (CT) is helpful to better appreciate the anterior and posterior walls of the glenoid vault and to classify the defect as contained or noncontained when the anterior or posterior wall has been destroyed. Antuna et al[12] proposed a classification of glenoid bone stock. They categorized glenoid bone loss by location (central, peripheral, or combined) and severity (mild, moderate, severe).

The anteroposterior view in neutral rotation will detect a massive rotator cuff tear in the case of upward migration of the humeral head with decreased acromiohumeral distance. CT scan will show the state of the rotator cuff muscles and will detect cases with severe fatty infiltration, meaning complete loss of function and suggesting the use of a semiconstrained reverse-type implant as a revision prosthesis.

BIOLOGICAL EVALUATION

Laboratory tests, white blood cell count with differential, erythrocyte sedimentation rate, and C-reactive protein are systematically performed to rule out an infection. However, low-grade infection may be occult; cultures of intra-articular fluid may be necessary to detect a low-grade organism such as *Propionibacterium acnes,* necessitating 3 weeks of culture. In extreme cases of doubt about infection, three to five biopsies can be performed by diagnostic arthroscopy before the therapeutic decision.

Complete clinical observation, including review of the operative notes of the index procedure, are also part of the preoperative planning and must be taken into account to choose the best therapeutic option. Most of the time the type of treatment can be chosen preoperatively, leading to a precise choice of the instruments required, as well as the surgical approach(es), type of prosthesis, and type of graft (allograft, autograft, synthetic bone), including the need for iliac crest preparation (sterilization and draping).

TREATMENT OPTIONS

CONSERVATIVE TREATMENT

Radiographic evidence of glenoid component loosening with no functional impairment should be treated nonsurgically. Glenoid loosening is often a silent condition, well tolerated by the patient, and it is not rare for patients to have no pain until bone loss is very advanced. Poor general health status may also lead to conservative treatment including rest, adaptation in activities of daily living, pain medication, and nonsteroidal anti-inflammatory medications.

SIMPLE LOOSE GLENOID COMPONENT REMOVAL

When the patient is fragile and is not willing to accept a major procedure, the loose glenoid component is extracted and the joint debrided, including removal of the cement, with no additional procedure. This can be done through arthroscopy, as has been reported by O'Driscoll.[13] Loss of function following simple glenoid component removal is a biomechanical issue—medialization of the humeral head and wear of the remaining glenoid bone reduces the rotator cuff and deltoid moment arms and results in poor elevation of the extremity. Additionally, this progressive bone loss precludes future attempts at insertion of a glenoid component.

RESECTION ARTHROPLASTY

In the case of uncontrolled infection associated with glenoid loosening, resection arthroplasty, with or without bone graft reconstruction, may be performed. Although the objective results are poor, the patient may adapt well to the new situation and refuse secondary reimplantation.

IMPACTION BONE GRAFTING OF THE DEFECT WITHOUT REIMPLANTATION

The option of impaction bone grafting of the defect without reimplantation is proposed in the case of a massive defect to reconstruct the bone stock.

Impaction bone grafting is the treatment of choice when the patient is still young, the humeral component well cemented, and the rotator cuff sufficient to stabilize and center the humeral head. It may be also considered as the first step before reimplantation after healing of the graft. Although it is agreed that bone grafting of glenoid defects is effective, the type of graft employed remains debatable. Many options are available: morcellized or structural bone graft, allograft, autograft (iliac crest bone graft), or synthetic bone.

Antuna et al[12] packed morcellized cancellous allografts in the glenoid defect and noted subsequent mean medialization of the humeral head in relation to the glenoid of 7.5 mm. Despite this medialization, second-stage glenoid component implantation was possible in three cases; however, the remaining bone was not found to be equivalent to the amount of bone graft originally placed.[14]

Frankle et al[15] reported the results of 14 bulk allografts used in glenoid reconstruction during total shoulder revision surgery. Eleven patients were available for radiographic follow-up, four of whom demonstrated graft resorption and medialization of the humeral head.

Norris et al,[16] Hill et al,[17] and Humphrey et al[18] recommend mixing the allograft with demineralized bone matrix. Various forms of demineralized bone matrix can be used, for example, Allomatrix custom (Wright Medical Technology Inc., Memphis, Tennessee), Dynagraft (IsoTis OrthoBiologics US, Irvine, California), Grafton (Osteotech, Eatontown, New Jersey), and Opteform (Exactech, Gainsville, Florida). Results reported were satisfactory in terms of pain relief, but progressive graft subsidence was observed in a high percentage of cases. Thirteen percent of the cases underwent reoperation during the first 3 years for continuing pain and reimplantation of a nonconstrained glenoid component.

Our experience using cancellous allograft has been similar and resulted in severe compression and/or resorption of the bone graft, with medialization of the humeral head and loss of anterior elevation within 1 year after surgery (Fig. 11.1).

These findings prompted us to use iliac crest structural corticocancellous bone grafting, with the cortical surface apposed to the humeral head to provide some structural integrity and resist medialization.[19]

Technique

Surgery is performed using a combination of interscalene and general anaesthesia. Patients are placed in the modified beach chair position with the upper extremity and shoulder girdle draped free. Patients first undergo harvesting of an anterior iliac crest bone graft. A bicortical graft is harvested measuring 2 cm wide by 3 cm long by 1 cm deep. Underlying cancellous bone is then harvested using a curette, and the bone graft incision is closed in layers over a drain.

Attention is then turned to the shoulder. Exposure in revision surgery is dictated by the previous operation; therefore it is mandatory to have the previous operative report. In the majority of patients the deltopectoral approach was used during the primary procedure and will be used during the revision surgery. The previous scar is excised and any subcutaneous adhesions released. The deltoid and pectoralis major muscles are identified. The deltopectoral interval may be more easily found superiorly and medially with the arm placed in abduction. Initiating dissection of the deltopectoral interval proximally, one should stay in close contact to the muscular body of the pectoralis major to preserve the cephalic vein if present. A careful release of the acromiohumeral space must be performed. Identification of the lateral border of the conjoined tendon is performed. Scarring often makes the undersurface of the conjoined tendon adhere to the subscapularis. Dissection must proceed carefully to protect both tendon and muscle units and the musculocutaneous nerve. A Richardson retractor is placed deep to the conjoined tendon, retracting it medially. Identification of the axillary nerve should be performed and is facilitated by flexing the shoulder and elbow in adduction–neutral rotation to relax the conjoined tendon. The subscapularis tendon is then exposed and elevated from the lesser tuberosity by tenotomy. The glenohumeral ligaments and joint capsule are incised with the subscapularis, completing access to the glenohumeral joint. Multiple intra-articular biopsies are performed for culture.

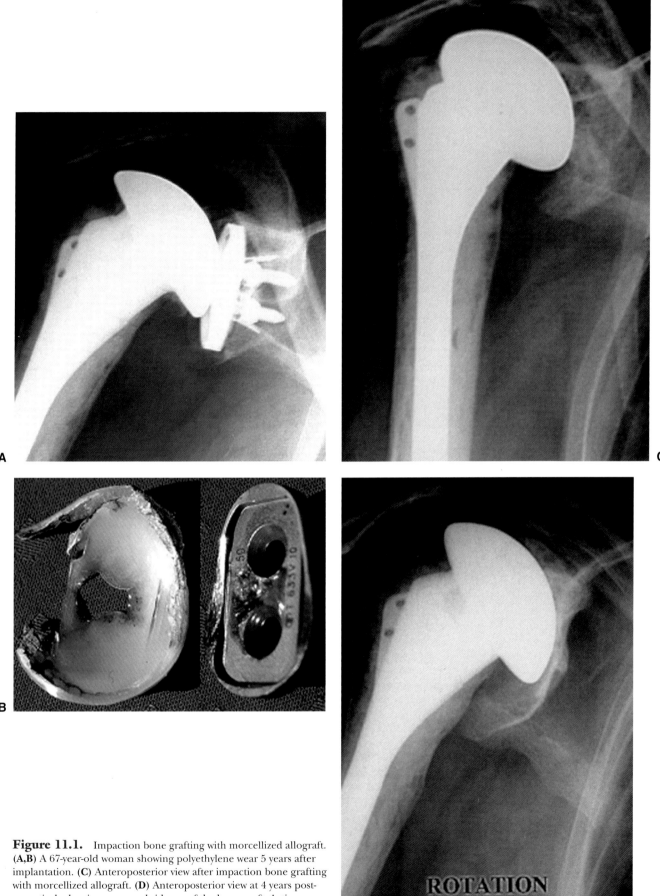

Figure 11.1. Impaction bone grafting with morcellized allograft. **(A,B)** A 67-year-old woman showing polyethylene wear 5 years after implantation. **(C)** Anteroposterior view after impaction bone grafting with morcellized allograft. **(D)** Anteroposterior view at 4 years post-operatively showing severe subsidence of the bone graft. Active forward elevation is 90 degrees, and pain is moderate.

In cases in which the previously placed humerus is modular, exposures may be accomplished by dissociating the humerus and removing the prosthetic humeral head. In cases in which it is necessary to remove the humeral stem, the deltopectoral approach can be easily extended into an anterolateral approach to the humerus, allowing humeral osteotomy for stem extraction.

Identification of the anterior and posterior aspects of the glenoid vault is critical. Once the anterior and posterior osseous glenoid is located, exposure is enhanced by placing glenoid rim retractors anterior and posterior to the glenoid. Hohman retractors are placed at the inferior and superior aspects of the glenoid. Loose glenoid implants are easily removed once exposure is adequate. Residual cement is removed, taking care to preserve as much bone as possible. In the case of metal-backed implants, any metal debris and metallosis are removed.

If the glenoid implant is not loose, mobilization is performed using thin osteotomes at the interface of the glenoid bone and the glenoid component. In some cases, we use a thin saw to cut off the well-cemented keel of the flange; progressive drilling of the keel with drill bits of increasing diameter is performed, allowing removal of the keel and the cement using small curettes. Once the implant and cement debris are removed, evaluation of the remaining glenoid bone stock is critical. Careful attention to the thickness of the anterior and posterior walls (if present) is necessary, as is determination of whether the defect is contained or uncontained.

In cases of an isolated central deficit, the bicortical bone graft is impacted into the central defect, with the cortical surface positioned laterally. Cancellous bone graft is then packed around and behind the bicortical graft. Graft fixation is a technical concern; during primary shoulder arthroplasty with glenoid bone deficiency, some authors recommend lateral to medial screw fixation of bone graft. Using this technique, the screw heads can potentially contact the humeral head and result in metallosis. Alternatively, bioabsorbable screws can be used. With isolated central defects we have not found it necessary to fixate the bone graft with screws. In this scenario, simple impaction of the graft provides adequate graft stability (Fig. 11.2). In cases of peripheral deficiency, we internally fixate the bone graft with screws placed in an anteroposterior direction to avoid contact with the prosthetic humeral head.

After surgery, the arm is placed in a sling for 1 month, with immediate pendulum exercises. During the second month, the sling is discontinued, activities of daily living are allowed as tolerated, and stretching exercises aiming toward complete recovery of active elevation are performed at least five times per day. No strengthening exercises are recommended. The stretching program is continued until 1 year postoperatively, at which time the range of motion can be considered as maximum (average 130 degrees of active forward elevation). We reported the results in the first cases at our institution, finding that bone grafting of glenoid defects with corticocancellous iliac crest graft resists medialization of the humerus, provided that the rotator cuff is intact and the humeral head well centered in the axial plane.[20] However, the functional gains were modest. Our experience has grown, and to date 30 procedures have been performed. Three of the patients underwent reoperation at an average of 18 months to implant a noncemented semiconstrained reverse prosthesis.

REIMPLANTATION OF CEMENTED POLYETHYLENE GLENOID WITH CEMENT AUGMENTATION

The results have proved to be significantly better than with simple removal,[12,19,21] but recurrent glenoid loosening is a major risk. The possibility exists to combine impaction glenoid bone grafting and a cemented polyethylene component at the same time; however, in our experience this option led to early migration of the glenoid component.

REIMPLANTATION OF AN UNCEMENTED IN-GROWTH COMPONENT FIXED WITH SCREWS WITH OR WITHOUT CANCELLOUS BONE GRAFT

This option of reimplantation of an uncemented in-growth component fixed with screws with or without cancellous bone graft is the most satisfying because it allows both restoration of the glenoid bone stock and reimplanting of the glenoid component, providing better pain relief.

Antuna et al[12] reported eight cases of revision with an uncemented in-growth nonconstrained glenoid component. Three were implanted without bone graft for a small contained defect, and five were implanted with cancellous bone graft. Although pain relief was satisfactory, 42% were observed to have a radiolucency at midterm follow-up. This option is possible only if the rotator cuff is intact. However, the use of a metal-backed glenoid implant with a nonconstrained prosthesis raises the question of the frequent possibility of rapid polyethylene wear.

Association of reverse prosthesis with glenoid bone grafting is a new option that was developed because of the success observed with the new semiconstrained prosthesis.[22,23] The metal-backed part of the glenoid allows at the same time bone grafting of the glenoid defect and fixation by means of the four peripheral screws.

In a minimal contained defect, morcellized cancellous iliac crest graft is impacted and a regular or extra-long pegged baseplate is selected. It is crucial that the central peg be anchored in the native glenoid bone rather than in the graft; we observed two that failed early because this rule was not followed. If anchorage of the baseplate is not strong enough to support the load of the humeral semiconstrained component, the sphere is screwed on the baseplate and 6 months later, the humeral component is inserted. Thus the glenosphere is loaded after healing of the glenoid graft. We have done that twice with excellent clinical and radiological midterm results (Fig. 11.3).

In a large cavitary or peripheral defect, it may be suitable to restore the glenoid bone stock with a structural corticocancellous iliac crest bone graft. This can be done either in two stages or in one stage, as proposed by Norris.[23] After reconstruction of the glenoid by a tricortical iliac crest bone graft, drilling and reaming of the graft to insert the baseplate is extremely difficult because of poor stability of the reconstruction. Norris recommended first harvesting the iliac crest with drilling and reaming, with implantation in situ of the baseplate with an extra-long peg. Then the iliac crest is osteotomized around the baseplate and the bone is shaped with a rongeur to fit the glenoid defect. A key point is to use a baseplate with an extra-long peg (25 mm or 30 mm instead of 15 mm) to anchor it in the native glenoid.

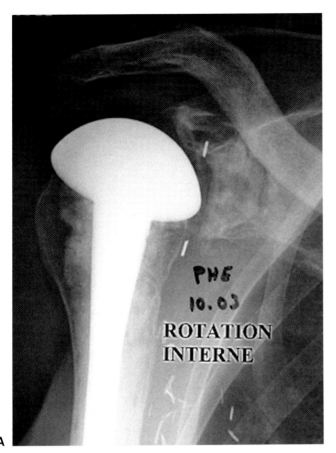

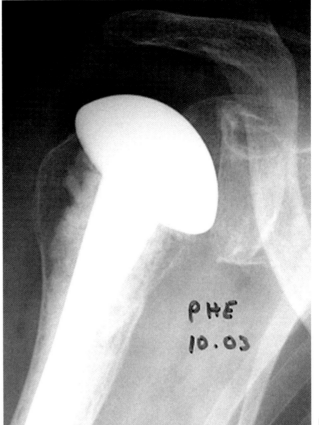

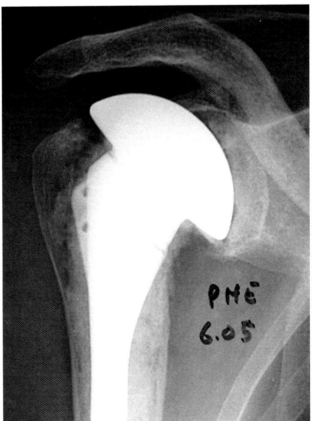

Figure 11.2. Structural corticocancellous iliac crest bone graft. **(A)** A 65-year-old woman showing polyethylene keel flat-backed glenoid component loose 11 years after implantation. **(B)** Postoperative anteroposterior view of structural corticocancellous iliac crest bone graft. **(C)** At 2-year follow-up, the graft is healed, with 3-mm medialization of the humeral head. Active forward elevation is 135 degrees, and no pain is reported.

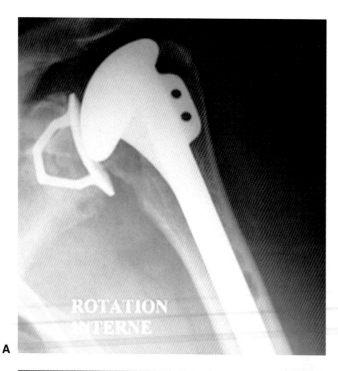

A

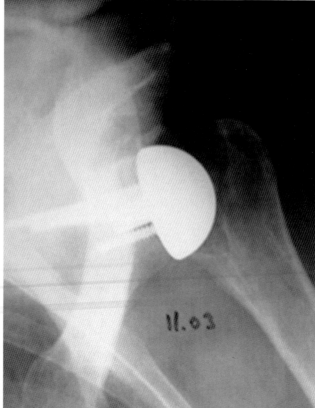

B

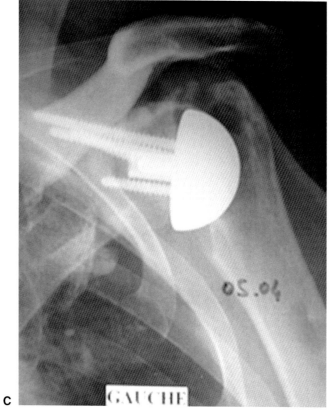

C

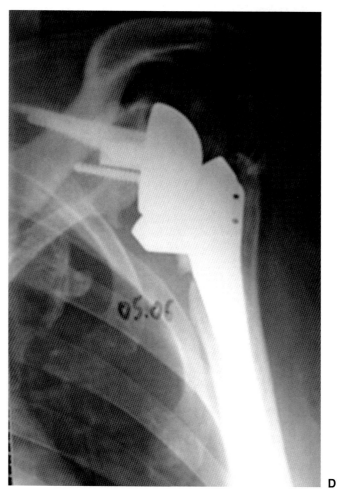

D

Figure 11.3. Two-stage revision with reverse prosthesis and bone grafting. **(A)** A 73-year-old man, 14 years after implantation of the total shoulder arthroplasty (Neer type metal-back glenoid), showing a supraspinatus tear and polyethylene wear. **(B,C)** Impaction bone grafting with morcellized cancellous iliac crest bone graft. To avoid loading an insufficiently stable construct, the humeral implantation was differed 6 months. **(D)** At 2 years after humeral implantation, active forward elevation is 150 degrees and no pain is reported.

110

Technique

The patient is positioned in the beach chair position, and the shoulder and iliac crest are prepped and draped.[23] The approach is the same as for impaction bone grafting as described above. Once the subscapularis is released, the humeral component is usually accessible and removed. Glenoid visualization is excellent when proximal humeral bone loss is present. The glenoid component and cement are removed. Larger defects, especially those with wall defects, are ideal cases for bone grafting with a tricortical iliac crest bone graft (TICBG). An incision is performed over the anterior iliac crest at least 2 cm lateral to the anterosuperior iliac spine. Dissection is carefully performed to avoid injuring the lateral femoral cutaneous nerve. The inner and outer tables of the crest are exposed. Then the glenoid baseplate is implanted onto the iliac crest. A pilot hole is placed at the top of the crest, taking aim between the two tables. A 7.9-mm-diameter, 25-mm-deep drill hole is placed, which frequently penetrates the outer and/or inner tables. The baseplate is then impacted into the crest. The baseplate is next cut out of the pelvis using an osteotome or saw. The TICBG with attached baseplate is removed. The wound is closed over a drain, and attention is turned again toward the shoulder. The TICBG is trimmed and shaped to fit the glenoid defect. The glenoid pilot hole is placed perpendicular to the axis of presumed native glenoid location. Placement of an accurate pilot hole is critical, and preoperative CT is useful for this step. Cannulated drills and reamers are used, so the direction of the hole can be established with a wire and modified if necessary,

before the actual pilot hole is placed. Care must be taken when reaming what remains of the native glenoid. If positioned correctly, the inferior border of the baseplate should be flush with the inferior border of the glenoid. Positioning the glenoid baseplate as low as possible on the glenoid results in less impingement of the humeral component onto the scapula. The TICBG and baseplate are implanted and fixed with screws. Once the screws have been placed, the baseplate is assessed for stability. If the construct is not sufficiently stable, the glenosphere may be placed without humeral implantation and the humeral implantation is deferred to a second stage, when the glenoid baseplate has had sufficient time to consolidate. Otherwise, if sufficient stability is achieved, the humeral side is implanted in standard fashion (Fig. 11.4). Soft tissue tensioning and selection of the polyethylene spacer is performed in standard fashion.

Postoperatively, the patients are restricted to pendulum exercises. Gentle aquatherapy is used when available. A sling is worn for 6 weeks. Physical therapy consists of passive range-of-motion exercises for at least 8 weeks, or until satisfactory bone healing is seen by radiograph. The optimal rehabilitation plan is individualized for each patient.

CONCLUSION

Success of glenoid revision is related largely to the remaining glenoid bone stock and the status of the rotator cuff. Careful

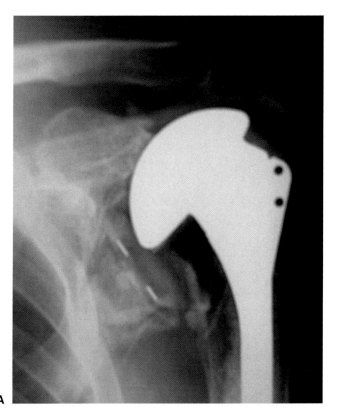

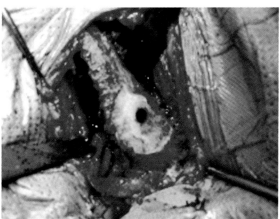

A   B

Figure 11.4.   One-stage tricortical iliac crest bone graft and reverse prosthesis (Norris technique) in a 75-year-old man **(A)** showing glenoid loosening 7 years after implantation. **(B)** The iliac crest is drilled and reamed in situ.

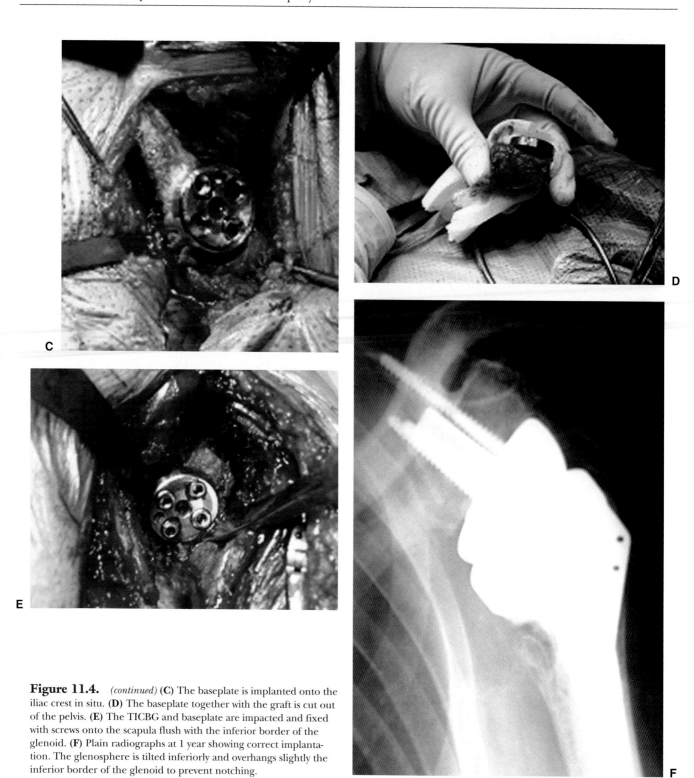

Figure 11.4. *(continued)* **(C)** The baseplate is implanted onto the iliac crest in situ. **(D)** The baseplate together with the graft is cut out of the pelvis. **(E)** The TICBG and baseplate are impacted and fixed with screws onto the scapula flush with the inferior border of the glenoid. **(F)** Plain radiographs at 1 year showing correct implantation. The glenosphere is tilted inferiorly and overhangs slightly the inferior border of the glenoid to prevent notching.

preoperative evaluation using CT arthrography helps to anticipate the surgical options to be used. Low-grade infection may be present and should be assessed preoperatively. Residual glenoid bone after component removal is often the determining factor in decision making for glenoid revisions options. In the younger population, the surgeon must keep in mind protecting or reconstructing the glenoid bone stock, whereas in the older patient, a more simple procedure to produce pain relief is the

main goal of revision surgery. The possibility to graft the glenoid defect and to solve the problem of a deficient rotator cuff in one stage by implanting a reverse prosthesis changed the prognosis of glenoid revisions. However, the type of graft to be used is still debatable. The complication rate following revision surgery for glenoid component loosening ranges from 11% to 25%. Additionally, multiple procedures increase the risk for infection of the shoulder.

Revision of loose glenoid implants, which was considered a "salvage procedure" or "limited-goal surgery," is now an ambitious challenge for the surgeon because restoration of reasonable function is possible

REFERENCES

1. Neer CS II. Replacement arthroplasty for glenohumeral osteoarthritis. *J Bone Joint Surg Am* 1974;56:1–13.
2. Neer CS, Watson KC, Stanton FJ. Recent experience in total shoulder replacement. *J Bone Joint Surg Am* 1982;64:319–337.
3. Gartsman GM, Elkousy HA, Warnock KM, et al. Radiographic comparison of pegged and keeled glenoid components. *J Shoulder Elbow Surg* 2005;14:252–257.
4. Lazarus MD, Jensen KL, Southworth C, et al. The radiographic evaluation of keeled and pegged glenoid component insertion. *J Bone Joint Surg Am* 2002;84:1174–1182.
5. Bohsali KI, Wirth MA, Rockwood CA. Complications of total shoulder arthroplasty: current concepts review. *J Bone Joint Surg Am* 2006;88:2279–2292.
6. Boileau P, Avidor C, Krishnan SG, et al. Cementless polyethylene versus uncemented metal backed glenoid components in total shoulder arthroplasty: a prospective, double-blind, randomized study. *J Shoulder Elbow Surg* 2002;11:351–359.
7. Burkhead W. Cementless shoulder arthroplasty. In: Friedman RJ, ed. *Arthroplasty of the Shoulder*. Stuttgart: Thieme; 1995:281–305.
8. Martin SD, Zurakowski D, Thornhill TS. Uncemented glenoid component in total shoulder arthroplasty: survivorship and outcomes. *J Bone Joint Surg Am* 2005;87:1284–1292.
9. Neer CS II, ed. *Shoulder Reconstruction*. Philadelphia: WB Saunders, 1990.
10. Sperling JW, Cofield RH, O'Driscoll SW, et al. Radiographic assessment of in-growth total shoulder arthroplasty. *J Shoulder Elbow Surg* 2002;9:507–513.
11. Wallace AL, Phillips RL, Mac Dougal GA, et al. Resurfacing of the glenoid in total shoulder arthroplasty: a comparison, at a mean of 5 years, of prostheses inserted with and without cement. *J Bone Joint Surg Am* 2005;81:510–518.
12. Antuna SA, Sperling JW, Cofield RH, et al. Glenoid revision surgery after total shoulder arthroplasty. *J Shoulder Elbow Surg* 2001;10:217–224.
13. O'Driscoll SW, Petrie RS, Torchia ME. Arthroscopic removal of the glenoid component for failed total shoulder arthroplasty: a report of five cases. *J Bone Joint Surg Am* 2005;87:858–863.
14. Antuna SA, Sperling JW, Cofield RH. Reimplantation of a glenoid component after component removal and allografts bone grafting: a report of three cases. *J Shoulder Elbow Surg* 2002;11:637–641.
15. Frankle MA, Long RA. Glenoid component failure treated with a bulk allograft for revision total surgery. Presented at the 18th Annual Meeting of the American Shoulder and Elbow Surgeons; October 24–27, 2001: Napa, Calif.
16. Norris TR, Phipatanakul WP. Treatment of glenoid loosening and bone loss due to osteolysis with glenoid bone grafting. *J Shoulder and Elbow Surg* 2006;15:84–87.
17. Hill JM, Norris TR. Long-term results of total shoulder arthroplasty following bone-grafting of the glenoid. *J Bone Joint Surg Am* 2001;83:877–883.
18. Humphrey CS, Kelly JD, Norris TR. Management of glenoid deficiency in reverse shoulder arthroplasty. In: Fealy S, Warren RF, Craig EV, et al. *Shoulder Arthroplasty*. New York: Thieme, 2006.
19. Neyton L, Sirveaux F, Roche O, et al. Résultats des reprises pour descellement glénoïdien: a propos d'une série multicentrique de 37 prothèses d'épaule [in French]. *Rev Chir Orthop* 2004;90:111–121.
20. Neyton L, Walch G, Nové-Josserand L, et al. Glenoid corticocancellous bone grafting after glenoid component removal in the treatment of glenoid loosening. *J Shoulder Elbow Surg* 2006;15:173–179.
21. Hawkins RJ, Greis PE, Bonutti PM. Treatment of symptomatic glenoid loosening following unconstrained shoulder arthroplasty. *Orthopedics* 1999;22:229–234.
22. Neyton L, Boileau P, Nové-Josserand L, et al. Glenoid bone grafting with a reverse design prosthesis. *J Shoulder Elbow Surg* 2007;16:71S–78S.
23. Norris TR, Kelly JD, Humphrey CS. Management of glenoid bone defects in revision shoulder arthroplasty: a new application of the reverse total shoulder prosthesis. *Tech Shoulder Elbow Surg* 2007;8:37–46.

Eiji Itoi
Hirotaka Sano

Muscle Contribution to Shoulder Stability

INTRODUCTION

Instability of the shoulder joint is an uncommon but well-recognized complication after unconstrained shoulder arthroplasty.[1-3] The incidence of instability after unconstrained shoulder arthroplasty ranges between 0% and 5%.[2,4,5] As Jahnke et al[2] described, both the degree and the direction of instability could be variable—it could be subluxation or dislocation to the superior, inferior, anterior, or posterior direction. Although the etiology of postoperative instability is multifactorial, dysfunction or deficiency of muscles is known to constitute one of the major pathogenetic factors for the instability.[1,3,5] To avoid instability after arthroplasties, surgeons should be aware of the biomechanical roles of shoulder muscles as stabilizers of the shoulder joint.

MECHANISM OF SHOULDER STABILIZATION BY MUSCLES

Shoulder musculature mainly acts as a dynamic stabilizer for the shoulder joint. There are four mechanisms to stabilize the shoulder by muscles: (a) passive tension from the bulk effect of the muscle itself, (b) concavity-compression effect, (c) joint motion that secondarily tightens the passive ligamentous constraints, and (d) the barrier effect of the contracted muscles.[6,7]

PASSIVE TENSION FROM THE BULK EFFECT OF THE MUSCLE

The passive role played by muscle bulk in joint stability is demonstrated by the increased passive arc of motion when the muscle is removed. Some authors reported that removal or release of muscles increased the translations of the humeral head in various directions.[8-10] However, contrary to those reports, Motzkin et al[11] demonstrated that removal of the deltoid with skin and subcutaneous tissue did not affect inferior translation of the humeral head as long as the intraarticular pressure was preserved. Itoi et al[12] also reported that the static contribution of the cuff muscles to the inferior stability of the shoulder is insignificant. Based on these studies, the bulk effect of muscles does not seem to play a major role in the stabilization of the shoulder joint.

CONCAVITY-COMPRESSION EFFECT

When the humeral head is compressed against the glenoid socket, a certain amount of force is necessary to translate the humeral head out of the glenoid. The greater the compressive force, the greater the translational force is. Lippitt et al[13] reported that the humeral head resisted translational forces of up to 60% of the compressive force in cadaveric shoulders with the labrum intact. This mechanism is called the concavity-compression effect and is considered one of the major stabilizing mechanisms. The great majority of compressive forces are generated by the rotator cuff muscles. The long head of the biceps (LHB), deltoid, and pectoral muscles also contribute to generate compressive force in certain positions.[13] In the prosthetic shoulders, this relationship was also confirmed by Fukuda et al,[14] who demonstrated that the subluxation resistance increased linearly with an increase in axial compressive force applied.

JOINT MOTION THAT SECONDARILY TIGHTENS THE PASSIVE LIGAMENTOUS CONSTRAINTS

It is known that external rotation of the humeral head tightens the inferior ligament and thus limits upward elevation. In strain gauge analysis using cadaveric shoulders, the inferior glenohumeral ligament was most tense in abduction, extension, and external rotation combined.[15] Thus the cuff musculature rotates the shoulder to a configuration rendered stable, at least in part, by tightening the ligament in the direction opposite the rotation.[16]

BARRIER EFFECT

The subscapularis muscle is important as an anterior barrier to resist anteroinferior displacement of the humeral head. When the subscapularis is lax or stretched, an anterior dislocation may occur. In prosthetic shoulders, it has been reported that a rupture of the repaired subscapularis tendon causes anterior instability.[3,5] Furthermore, the cross-sectional areas of the anterior (subscapularis) and posterior (infraspinatus and teres minor) rotators are approximately equal.[17] Thus the torques generated by these rotators are balanced and represent a force couple that resists both anterior and posterior translation of the humeral head.

DELTOID

The deltoid is a large bulky muscle, comprising approximately 20% of the shoulder muscles.[17,18] The most important function of the deltoid muscle is the elevation of the shoulder, and it has the largest moment arm as a shoulder elevator among shoulder muscles.[19] The deltoid muscle is divided into three portions—the anterior, middle, and posterior portions. The anterior deltoid takes its origin from the anterior and superior surfaces of the outer third of the clavicle and anterior acromion, the middle deltoid from the lateral margin of the acromion, and the posterior deltoid from the scapular spine. Thus the function of the deltoid could be different among these three portions in various arm positions.

Motzkin et al[11] investigated the static contribution of the deltoid muscle to inferior stability of the shoulder with the arm in adduction and abduction. The humeral head displacement did not change significantly after the removal of the deltoid; thus they concluded that the passive muscle tension of the deltoid was insignificant for the inferior stability. In the clinical setting, inferior subluxation immediately after shoulder arthroplasty may be caused by the weakness or inactivity of the deltoid muscle.[2] Such inferior subluxation recovers gradually as the patient starts to move the arm more actively. On the other hand, Michiels and Bodem[20] speculated that the anterior and posterior portions of the deltoid muscle contribute to the stabilization of the glenohumeral joint from electromyographic (EMG) analysis. Kronberg et al[21] also confirmed increased activity of the deltoid with an increased abduction angle (Fig. 12.1). Because the fiber direction of the deltoid is parallel to the humerus in this position, it adds to shoulder stability as a result

of the concavity-compression effect. Other investigators also reported the contribution of the deltoid to shoulder stability.[18,22] More recently, Kido et al[23] investigated the contribution of the three portions of the deltoid muscle to anterior stability in abduction and external rotation. Each of these three portions contributed equally to anterior stability under constant loading conditions, so they concluded that the deltoid muscle was an anterior stabilizer in this position.

Judging from these investigations, the main mechanism of the deltoid as a stabilizer seems to be the concavity-compression effect with the arm in abduction.

ROTATOR CUFF

PASSIVE MUSCLE TENSION

The subscapularis muscle has been thought to be important as an anterior barrier to resist anterior displacement of the humeral head. The subscapularis consistently tightens during both external rotation and abduction of the glenohumeral joint. Turkel et al[24] measured the change in external rotation after sectioning the subscapularis tendon and concluded that the passive tension of the subscapularis was the primary anterior stabilizer at 0 and 45 degrees of abduction. Ovensen and Nielsen[9] also reported that the subscapularis prevented anterior subluxation in lower angles of abduction. However, in higher angles of abduction, the inferior glenohumeral ligament acts as the primary stabilizer instead of the subscapularis.[9,24] One of the reasons why the subscapularis does not contribute greatly to anterior stability in higher angles of abduction might be the inequality of its material properties. Halder et al[25] reported that the inferior portion of the subscapularis tendon showed significantly lower ultimate load and stiffness than other portions of the tendon. Another important issue that may influence the stabilizing function of the subscapularis muscle is secondary changes of the muscle or tendon after recurrent dislocations or

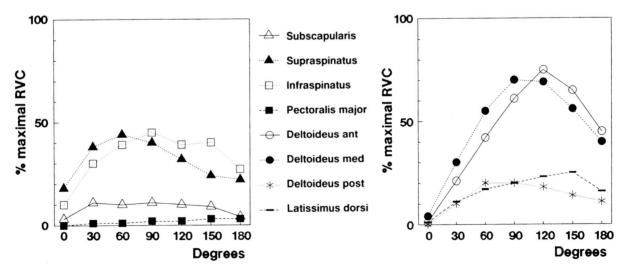

Figure 12.1. The normalized electromyographic activity during shoulder abduction. The anterior and middle parts of the deltoid were the most highly activated, at 90 to 120 degrees of abduction. (Reprinted from Kronberg M, Németh G, Broström L-Å. Muscle activity and coordination in the normal shoulder: an electromyographic study. *Clin Orthop* 1990;257:76–85, with permission.)

surgical interventions. Gamulin et al[26] found the presence of interstitial fibrosis and disuse atrophy in biopsy specimens of the subscapularis muscle with recurrent dislocations. Scheibel et al[27] demonstrated the presence of atrophy and fatty infiltration, particularly of the upper part of the subscapularis muscle, after an L-shaped tenotomy surgical approach. Using magnetic resonance imaging, Tuoheti et al[28] reported that the subscapularis tendon underwent an 18.7% decrease in thickness and a 29.1% decrease in cross-sectional area in shoulders with recurrent anterior dislocation. These changes should be taken into consideration when stabilizing function of the subscapularis muscle is discussed.

Posterior stability of the glenohumeral joint is also provided by passive tension of the rotator cuff muscles. Ovensen et al[10,29,30] demonstrated that the supraspinatus and infraspinatus/teres minor played important roles in stabilizing the shoulder posteriorly. Debski et al[31] also reported that passive tension of the rotator cuff muscles played a more significant role than other soft tissues, including the capsule, in posterior stability. Halder et al[32] measured the mechanical properties of four portions of the infraspinatus tendon. The peak stiffness in the midsuperior and inferior tendon sections may play a role in stabilizing the shoulder posteriorly, whereas the low ultimate failure load of the superior portion may explain the frequent extension of the rotator cuff tear into the infraspinatus tendon.

As for the inferior stability, Itoi et al[12,33] investigated the relationship between the passive tension of the cuff muscles and the inferior translation using cadaver shoulders. They elevated the supraspinatus and the other muscles in different orders and measured the displacement of the humeral head. Because no significant effects were observed after elevating the cuff muscles, they concluded that the contribution of passive tension of the rotator cuff muscles was insignificant.[12]

DYNAMIC CONTRACTION

It is generally accepted that the contraction of the rotator cuff muscles acts as a dynamic stabilizer for the glenohumeral joint. The stabilizing function of the cuff muscles depends on the force generated by each muscle and its anatomic relationship with the humeral head and the glenoid.

Historically, DePalma et al[34] emphasized that the subscapularis was the most important stabilizer among the rotator cuff muscles. Saha[35] introduced the concept of force couple provided by the anterior and posterior cuff muscles. The EMG studies showed that both the subscapularis and infraspinatus contracted to stabilize the shoulder in abduction.[21] Thus the combined contraction of the subscapularis and infraspinatus forms a force couple providing stability during midrange of elevation. Glousman et al[36] investigated the EMG activities of the shoulder muscles during the entire pitching sequence in the stable and unstable shoulders. The supraspinatus and the biceps demonstrated increased EMG activity in anteriorly unstable shoulders, which might be compensatory activity to stabilize the shoulder.[36]

Several in vitro studies have been carried out to clarify the stabilizing function of each of the rotator cuff muscles. Cain et al[37] found that the infraspinatus/teres minor was most effective in controlling external rotation of the humerus and reducing ligamentous strain, thereby playing an important role in anterior stability of the shoulder. Blasier et al[38] tested the

dynamic stabilizing function of the rotator cuff muscles in a displacement control study. According to their results, the supraspinatus, infraspinatus/teres minor, and subscapularis contributed equally to anterior stability of the abducted shoulder with the arm both in neutral and in external rotation. However, Lee et al[39] demonstrated that the contribution of each cuff muscle for dynamic stabilization of the shoulder was not equal and varied according to arm positions (Fig. 12.2).

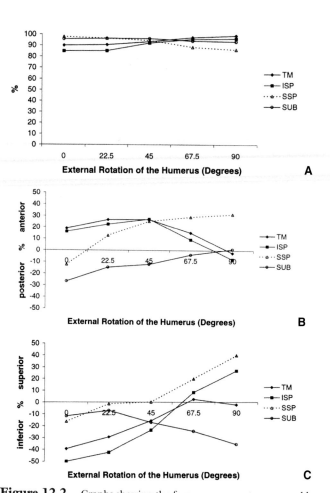

Figure 12.2. Graphs showing the force components generated by the rotator cuff muscles in the abducted and extended shoulder as the humerus was rotated from neutral to 90 degrees of external rotation in intervals of 22.5 degrees. The force components are expressed as percentages of the force applied to each muscle. **(A)** Compressive force components. The compressive force component of the posterior cuff muscles (the teres minor and the infraspinatus) increased significantly ($p < 0.05$) as the humerus was rotated to the end-range of motion. **(B)** Anterior to posterior shear force components. The direction and magnitude of the shear force changed significantly ($p < 0.05$) as the humerus was rotated to the end-range of motion. Positive values indicate anterior shear forces, and negative values indicate posterior shear forces. **(C)** Superior to inferior shear force components. The shear force changed significantly ($p < 0.05$) as the humerus was rotated to the end-range of motion. Positive values indicate superior shear forces, and negative values indicate inferior shear forces. TM, Teres minor; ISP, infraspinatus; SSP, supraspinatus; and SUB, subscapularis. (Reprinted from Lee S-B, Kim K-J, O'Driscoll, et al. Dynamic glenohumeral stability provided by the rotator cuff muscles in the mid-range and end-range of motion: a study in cadavera. *J Bone Joint Surg Am* 2000;82:849–857, with permission.)

The supraspinatus and subscapularis contributed more significantly as dynamic stabilizers than other muscles in the midrange of motion, whereas the subscapularis, infraspinatus, and teres minor contributed more significantly than the supraspinatus in the end range of motion, where the shoulder dislocation occurs. These studies suggest the clinical importance of strengthening the cuff muscles, especially the subscapularis, to prevent anterior instability of the shoulder. However, exercises of this muscle might not be adequate for all patients with anterior instability symptoms.[40,41]

INSTABILITY IN THE SHOULDER WITH ROTATOR CUFF TEAR

Anterior dislocation of the shoulder and rotator cuff tearing are often associated in the elderly population.[42,43] In such patients, recurrent anterior dislocation might be successfully stabilized by repairing the cuff tear.[42] These clinical findings suggest that the rotator cuff muscles can be important anterior stabilizers of the shoulder. Hsu et al[44] demonstrated biomechanically that both a large rotator cuff defect and a rotator interval tear affect joint stability.

INSTABILITY CAUSED BY FAILURE OF ROTATOR CUFF MUSCLES AFTER ARTHROPLASTY

In prosthetic shoulders, Moekel et al[5] reported that all the postoperative anterior instability was caused by rupture of the repaired subscapularis. Superior or anterosuperior instability is also known to be a common complication after shoulder arthroplasty.[2] Displacement in these directions is usually the result of dysfunction or failure of barrier effect of the rotator cuff resisting the superior shear force.[2,44] Recently, based on their finite element analysis, Hopkins et al[45] predicted that a shoulder with a dysfunctional supraspinatus might show an increased superior translation of the humeral head compared to the shoulder with an intact supraspinatus. According to these clinical and basic studies, rotator cuff tearing is one of the most important etiological factors for shoulder instability after arthroplasty.

REVERSE TOTAL SHOULDER ARTHROPLASTY

The treatment of irreparable rotator cuff tears associated with osteoarthritis of the glenohumeral joint is still challenging for shoulder surgeons, although the surgical outcome has been greatly improved by the development and introduction of reverse total shoulder arthroplasty. In this reverse ball-and-socket prosthesis, the center of rotation of the glenohumeral joint is medialized and the insertion of the deltoid muscle is moved distally, which increase both the lever arm and the pretension of the deltoid muscle.[46] However, controlling the tension of deltoid muscle is technically demanding. If the tension of the deltoid muscle is not sufficient, prosthetic instability may occur postoperatively.[47] Another unsolved problem after this procedure is failure to restore active external rotation, especially in patients who represent severe fatty infiltration of the teres minor muscle. It is unlikely that the restoration of active external rotation is possible by only the remnant deltoid muscle[47–49] (Table 12.1). On the basis of current design of the prosthesis, indication of reverse total shoulder arthroplasty should be carefully evaluated preoperatively.[47,50]

TABLE 12.1	Clinical Outcome after Reverse Shoulder Arthroplasty Stratified According to the Degree of Teres Minor Fatty Infiltration		
Clinical Outcome	*Group 1[a] (N = 30; Average Follow-Up 45 Months)*	*Group 2[b] (N = 12; Average Follow-Up 38 Months)*	*p Value*
Relative Constant score[c] (%)	83 ± 15.5 (26–100)	61 ± 12.6 (16–90)	<0.01
Absolute Constant score (*points*)			
Total activities of daily living	16 ± 4 (4–20)	12 ± 6.3 (5–19)	<0.01
Activity	7.6 ± 2.3 (3–10)	4.7 ± 2.1 (0–8)	0.060
Positioning	8.4 ± 2 (2–10)	7.3 ± 1.1 (2–10)	<0.01
Subjective shoulder value (% of normal shoulder)	72 ± 11.2 (20–100)	49 ± 13.8 (0–90)	<0.01
Force (kg)	5.4 ± 2.1 (2–8)	3.1 ± 1.4 (2–5)	0.154
Satisfaction	3.5 ± 2.4 (1–4)	2.8 ± 1.8 (1–4)	0.784
Postoperative external rotation (degrees)	28 ± 16.4 (0–70)	2 ± 18.7 (−50 to 30)	<0.001

Group 1 patients had Goutallier stage 0, 1, or 2 fatty infiltration of the teres minor; group 2 patients had stage 3 or 4 fatty infiltration.

[a]The values are given as the mean and standard deviation, with the range in parentheses.

[b]Calculated with the Mann-Whitney test, with a level of significance of <0.05.

[c]Adjusted for age and gender.

Reprinted from Simovitch RW, Helmy N, Zumstein MA, et al. Impact of fatty infiltration of the teres minor muscle on the outcome of reverse total shoulder arthroplasty. *J Bone Joint Surg Am* 2007;89:934–939, with permission.

BICEPS BRACHII

The biceps brachii is commonly considered to function as a flexor of the elbow and supinator of the forearm. Biomechanically, the LHB is a depressor of the humeral head.[51,52] In EMG studies, the contribution of the biceps brachii muscle during shoulder motion was controversial. Glousman et al[36] observed increased activity of the biceps in throwers with anterior shoulder instability, which suggested a possibility of the biceps as a stabilizer. In contrast, Yamaguchi et al[53] found no increase in activities of the LHB during most shoulder motions in patients with rotator cuff tears or volunteers with normal cuff tendons. They used a brace locked in neutral forearm rotation and 100 degrees of elbow flexion to minimize elbow-related biceps activity. However, because the elbow was flexed at 100 degrees, the biceps might be too shortened to be active during various shoulder motions. Also, they did not apply any load that might have made it difficult to detect a subtle activity of the muscle. Sakurai et al,[54] using a brace with the elbow in extension and forearm in neutral rotation, reported that both heads of the biceps muscle showed EMG activity during elevation and external rotation of the shoulder with a load equivalent to 30% of maximum abduction force. Kido et al[55] measured the EMG activity of the biceps in shoulders with and without rotator cuff tears. During arm elevation, 35% of patients with rotator cuff tears showed increased EMG activity of the biceps more than 10% maximum voluntary contraction (MCV), whereas none of the biceps in the normal shoulders exhibited more than 10%. In these patients, biceps activity increased with load application. Although the function of the biceps is still controversial, it is likely that the biceps has potential function as a mover or stabilizer of the shoulder joint, where these functions of all the other muscles may not be sufficient.

Rodosky et al[56] simulated a clinical entity known as a "superior labrum, anterior, and posterior" (SLAP) lesion by detaching the superior labrum with the LHB origin from the superior glenoid rim. They investigated the relation between the torsional rigidity and the LHB force and found that the torsional rigidity increased and the strain of the inferior glenohumeral ligament decreased with LHB loading. Judging from their results, the LHB seems to contribute to anterior stability of the shoulder by increasing torsional rigidity. Increased translation of the humeral head on the glenoid after creating a SLAP lesion was confirmed by other investigators.[57,58]

More direct observations of the stabilizing function of the LHB were carried out by Itoi et al.[59] They measured the displacement of the humeral head under constant translation force in various directions in the hanging arm position with and without loads to the LHB. The results showed that the LHB significantly stabilized the shoulder in the anterior, inferior, and posterior directions. Their further study revealed the LHB in combination with the short head of the biceps stabilizes the shoulder anteriorly with the arm in abduction and external rotation[60] (Fig. 12.3). Then they studied the stabilizing effects on the glenohumeral joint of each of the rotator cuff muscles and of the biceps with the arm in abduction and external rotation. Under physiological loading to each of these muscles, the biceps was found to be as efficient a stabilizer as the supraspinatus and infraspinatus/teres minor in stable shoulders. The biceps became more important than any of the cuff muscles when the shoulder was unstable. Based on these results, they

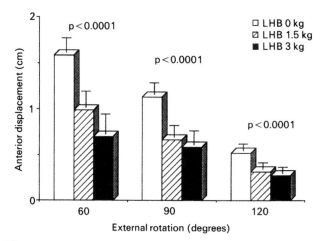

Figure 12.3. Displacements of the humeral head (mean ± SEM) with Bankart lesions related to LHB loadings. Displacement decreased significantly in all rotations ($p < 0.0001$ each). LHB, long head of the biceps. (Reprinted from Itoi E, Kuechle DK, Newman SR, et al. Stabilising function of the biceps in stable and unstable shoulders. *J Bone Joint Surg Br* 1993;75:546–550, with permission.)

recommended that strengthening of the biceps as well as rotator cuff muscles should be part of the rehabilitation program for anterior shoulder instability[61] (Fig. 12.4). Although Itoi et al[59,61] demonstrated that the LHB was a stabilizer in both the hanging and abducted positions, Pagnani et al[62] demonstrated that this stabilizing function of the LHB was most pronounced at middle and lower angles of elevation. Malicky et al[63] investigated the relationship between the stabilizing function of the biceps and the rotation of the shoulder. They found that the effectiveness of the biceps as an anterior stabilizer varied among rotations. The biceps was the most important stabilizer in neutral rotation, whereas it was the least important stabilizer in external rotation.

From the clinical point of view, it was reported that arthroscopic LHB tenotomy or tenodesis could reduce pain or dysfunction caused by an irreparable rotator cuff tear associated with LHB tendon lesion.[64,65] Although no studies dealt with stability of the glenohumeral joint after LHB tenotomy or tenodesis, Boileau et al[64] thought that LHB was unlikely to be an active humeral head depressor in shoulders with massive rotator cuff tears, because the reduction of acromiohumeral distance after these procedures was only 1.1 mm. Further studies with long-term follow-up would be necessary to clarify the clinical roles of the biceps muscle and the LHB tendon at the glenohumeral joint.

SCAPULAR ROTATOR MUSCLES

The scapular rotator muscles, including the trapezius, rhomboids, latissimus dorsi, serratus anterior, and levator scapulae, control the position of the scapula. The scapular inclination angle has a significant effect in prevention of inferior translation of the humeral head in the adducted position[33,66] (Fig. 12.5). Thus dysfunction of the scapular rotator muscles might be related to the development of inferior instability of the shoulder. Warner et al[67] found the dysfunction of axioscapular muscles (trapezius, serratus anterior, rhomboids, and levator scapulae) using moiré topological analysis in patients with anteroinferior

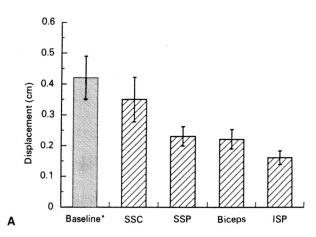

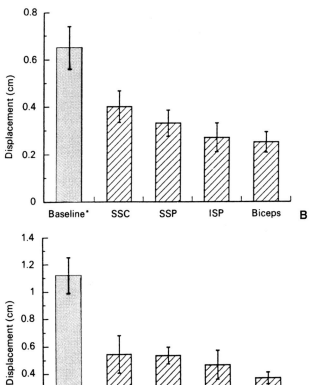

Figure 12.4. **(A)** Displacement of the center of the humeral head with the capsule intact and the humerus in 90 degrees of external rotation (mean ± SEM). The mean displacement with the SSC loaded was significantly larger than with the other muscles loaded ($p = 0.0009$). Baseline*, no load applied to the muscles. **(B)** Displacement of the center of the humeral head with the capsule vented (90 degrees of external rotation). The mean (±SEM) displacement with the biceps loaded was significantly smaller than with the SSC loaded ($p = 0.0052$). **(C)** Displacement of the center of the humeral head after creating an artificial Bankart lesion (90 degrees of external rotation). The mean (±SEM) displacement with the biceps loaded was significantly less than with the other muscles loaded ($p = 0.0132$). SSP, Supraspinatus; ISP, infraspinatus; SSC, subscapularis. (Reprinted from Itoi E, Newman SR, Kuechle DK, et al. Dynamic anterior stabilisers of the shoulder with the arm in abduction. *J Bone Joint Surg Br* 1994;76:834–836, with permission.)

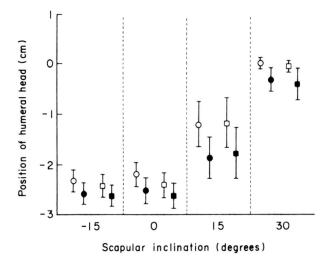

Figure 12.5. Position of the humeral head during sulcus test in fresh cadaver shoulders. There was a significant effect of scapular inclination on the loaded (*closed square*) and unloaded positions (*open square*) of the humeral head ($p < 0.0001$): the head position at −15 and 0 degrees was significantly lower than at 15 degrees, which was significantly lower than at 30 degrees. The position of the head before cuff removal (*closed circle*, loaded; *open circle*, unloaded) is also shown for comparison. Cuff removal had no significant effect on the position ($p < 0.74$) or displacement ($p < 0.65$) of the humeral head. The marks show the mean ± SEM. (Reprinted from Itoi E, Motzkin NE, Morrey BF, et al. Bulk effect of rotator cuff on inferior glenohumeral stability as function of scapular inclination angle: a cadaver study. *Tohoku J Exp Med* 1993;171:267–276, with permission.)

instability. From clinical experience, Pagnani and Warren[68] thought that scapular winging was associated with both anterior and posterior instability. Such observable alteration in the position of the scapula and the patterns of motion was defined as scapular dyskinesis by Kibler et al,[69,70] and appears to be a nonspecific response to a painful condition in the shoulder with glenohumeral pathologies. Scapular dyskinesis is successfully treated by physical therapy in most instances. In cases with structural problems in the glenohumeral joint, integrated scapular muscle rehabilitation should be started to reestablish muscle strength and activation patterns once the structural problems have been corrected surgically.[70]

REFERENCES

1. Cofield RH, Edgerton BC. Total shoulder arthroplasty: complications and revision surgery. *Instr Course Lect* 1990;39:449–462.
2. Jahnke AH Jr, Hawkins RJ. Instability after shoulder arthroplasty: causative factors and treatment options. *Semin Arthroplasty* 1995;6:289–299.
3. Sanchez-Sotelo J, Sperling JW, Rowland CM, et al. Instability after shoulder arthroplasty: results of surgical treatment. *J Bone Joint Surg Am* 2003;85:622–631.
4. Hennigan SP, Iannotti JP. Instability after prosthetic arthroplasty of the shoulder. *Orthop Clin North Am* 2001;32:649–659.
5. Moeckel BH, Altchek DW, Warren RF, et al. Instability of the shoulder after arthroplasty. *J Bone Joint Surg Am* 1993;75:492–497.
6. Itoi E, Hsu H-C, An K-N. Biomechanical investigation of the glenohumeral joint. *J Shoulder Elbow Surg* 1996;5:407–424.
7. Itoi E, Morrey BF, An K-N. Biomechanics of the shoulder. In: Rockwood CA Jr, Matsen FA III, Wirth MA, et al, eds. *The Shoulder.* 3rd ed. Philadelphia: WB Saunders; 2004:223–267.
8. Kumar VP, Balasubramaniam P. The role of atmospheric pressure in stabilizing the shoulder: an experimental study. *J Bone Joint Surg Br* 1985;67:719–721.
9. Ovensen J, Nielsen S. Stability of the shoulder joint: cadaver study of stabilizing structures. *Acta Orthop Scand* 1985;56:149–151.

10. Ovensen J, Nielsen S. Posterior instability of the shoulder: a cadaver study. *Acta Orthop Scand* 1986;57:436–439.

11. Motzkin NE, Itoi E, Morrey BF, et al. Contribution of passive bulk tissues and deltoid to static inferior glenohumeral stability. *J Shoulder Elbow Surg* 1994;3:313–319.

12. Itoi E, Motzkin NE, Morrey BF, et al. The static rotator cuff does not affect inferior translation of the humerus at the glenohumeral joint. *J Trauma* 1999;47:55–59.

13. Lippitt SB, Vanderhooft JE, Harris SL, et al. Glenohumeral stability from concavity-compression: a quantitative analysis. *J Shoulder Elbow Surg* 1993;2:27–35.

14. Fukuda K, Chen CM, Cofield RH, et al. Biomechanical analysis of stability and fixation strength of total shoulder prostheses. *Orthopedics* 1988;11:141–149.

15. Terry GC, Hammon D, France P, et al. The stabilizing function of passive shoulder restraints. *Am J Sports Med* 1991;19:26–34.

16. Dempster WT. Mechanisms of the shoulder joint. *Arch Phys Med Rehabil Am* 1965;46:49–70.

17. Bassett RW, Browne AO, Morrey BF, et al. Glenohumeral muscle force and moment mechanics in a position of shoulder instability. *J Biomech* 1990;23:405–415.

18. Lee S-B, An K-N. Dynamic glenohumeral stability provided by three heads of the deltoid muscle. *Clin Orthop* 2002;400:40–47.

19. Kuechle DK, Newman SR, Itoi E, et al. Shoulder muscle moment arms during horizontal flexion and elevation. *J Shoulder Elbow Surg* 1997;6:429–439.

20. Michiels I, Bodem F. The deltoid muscle: an electromyographical analysis of its activity in arm abduction in various body postures. *Int Orthop* 1992;16:268–271.

21. Kronberg M, Németh G, Broström L-Å. Muscle activity and coordination in the normal shoulder: an electromyographic study. *Clin Orthop* 1990;257:76–85.

22. Payne LZ, Deng X-H, Craig EV. The combined dynamic and static contributions to subacromial impingement: a biomechanical analysis. *Am J Sports Med* 1997;25:801–808.

23. Kido T, Itoi E, Lee S-K, et al. Dynamic stabilizing function of the deltoid muscle in shoulders with anterior instability. *Am J Sports Med* 2003;31:399–403.

24. Turkel SJ, Panio IMW, Marshall JL. Stabilizing mechanisms preventing anterior dislocation of the glenohumeral joint. *J Bone Joint Surg Am* 1981;63:1208–1217.

25. Halder A, Zobitz ME, Schultz F, et al. Structural properties of the subscapularis tendon. *J Orthop Res* 2000;18:829–834.

26. Gamulin A, Pizzolato G, Stern R, et al. Anterior shoulder instability: histomorphometric study of subscapularis and deltoid muscles. *Clin Orthop* 2002;398:121–126.

27. Scheibel M, Tsynman A, Magosch P, et al. Postoperative subscapularis muscle insufficiency after primary and revision shoulder stabilization. *Am J Sports Med* 2006;34:1586–1593.

28. Tuoheti Y, Itoi E, Minagawa H, et al. Quantitative assessment of thinning of the subscapularis tendon in recurrent anterior dislocation of the shoulder by use of magnetic resonance imaging. *J Shoulder Elbow Surg* 2005;14:11–15.

29. Ovensen J, Nielsen S. Anterior and posterior shoulder instability: a cadaver study. *Acta Orthop Scand* 1986;57:324–327.

30. Ovensen J, Søjbjerg JO. Posterior shoulder dislocation: muscle and capsular lesions in cadaver experiment. *Acta Orthop Scand* 1986;57:535–536.

31. Debski RE, Sakane M, Woo SL-Y, et al. Contribution of the passive properties of the rotator cuff to glenohumeral stability during anterior-posterior loading. *J Shoulder Elbow Surg* 1999;8:324–329.

32. Halder A, Zobitz ME, Schultz F, et al. Mechanical properties of the posterior rotator cuff. *Clin Biomech* 2000;15:456–462.

33. Itoi E, Motzkin NE, Morrey BF, et al. Bulk effect of rotator cuff on inferior glenohumeral stability as function of scapular inclination angle: a cadaver study. *Tohoku U Exp Med* 1993;171:267–276.

34. DePalma AF, Cooke AJ, Prabhakar M. The role of the subscapularis in recurrent anterior dislocations of the shoulder. *Clin Orthop* 1967;54:35–49.

35. Saha AK. Dynamic stability of the glenohumeral joint. Acta Orhop Scand 1971;42:491–505.

36. Glousman R, Jobe F, Tibone J, et al. Dynamic electromyographic analysis of the throwing shoulder with glenohumeral instability. J Bone Joint Surg Am 1988;70:220–226.

37. Cain PR, Mutschler TA, Fu FH. Anterior stability of the glenohumeral joint: a dynamic model. Am J Sports Med 1987;15:144–148.

38. Blasier RB, Guldberg RE, Rothman ED, et al. Anterior shoulder stability: contributions of rotator cuff forces and the capsular ligaments in a cadaver model. J Shoulder Elbow Surg 1992;1:140–150.

39. Lee S-B, Kim K-J, O'Driscoll, et al. Dynamic glenohumeral stability provided by the rotator cuff muscles in the mid-range and end-range of motion: a study in cadavera. J Bone Joint Surg Am 2000;82:849–857.

40. Burkhead WZ Jr, Rockwood CA Jr. Treatment of instability of the shoulder with an exercise program. J Bone Joint Surg Am 1992;74:890–896.

41. Werner CML, Favre P, Gerber C. The role of the subscapularis in preventing anterior glenohumeral subluxation in the abducted, externally rotated position of the arm. Clin Biomech 2007;22:495–501.

42. Itoi E, Tabata S. Rotator cuff tears in anterior dislocation of the shoulder. Int Orthop 1992;16:240–244.

43. Neviaser RJ, Neviaser TJ, Neviaser JS. Concurrent rupture of the rotator cuff and anterior dislocation of the shoulder in the older patient. J Bone Joint Surg Am 1988;70:1308–1311.

44. Hsu H-C, Boardman ND III, Luo Z-P, et al. Tendon-defect and muscle unloaded models for relating rotator cuff tear to glenohumeral stability. J Orthop Res 2000;18:952–958.

45. Hopkins AR, Hansen UN, Amis AA, et al. Glenohumeral kinematics following total shoulder arthroplasty: a finite element investigation. J Orhtop Res 2007;25:108–115.

46. Werner CML, Steinmann PA, Gilbart M, et al. Treatment of painful pseudoparesis due to irreparable rotator cuff dysfunction with the Delta-III reverse-ball-and-socket total shoulder prosthesis. J Bone joint Surg Am 2005;87:1476–1486.

47. Boileau P, Watkinson D, Hatzidakis AM, et al. The Grammont reverse shoulder prosthesis: results in cuff tear arthritis, fracture sequelae, and revision arthroplasty. J Shoulder Elbow Surg 2006;15:527–540.

48. Gerber C, Pennington SD, Lingenfelter EJ. Reverse Delta-III total shoulder replacement combined with latissimus dorsi transfer: a preliminary report. J Bone Joint Surg Am 2007;89: 940–947.

49. Simovitch RW, Helmy N, Zumstein MA, et al. Impact of fatty infiltration of the teres minor muscle on the outcome of reverse total shoulder arthroplasty. J Bone Joint Surg Am 2007;89: 934–939.

50. Rockwood CA Jr. The reverse total shoulder prosthesis: the new kid on the block. J Bone Joint Surg Am 2007;89:233–235.

51. Kumar VP, Satku K, Balasubramaniam P. The role of the long head of biceps brachii in the stabilization of the head of the humerus. Clin Orthop 1989;244:172–175.

52. Warner JJP, McMahon PJ. The role of the long head of the biceps brachii in superior stability of the glenohumeral joint. J Bone Joint Surg Am 1995;77:366–372.

53. Yamaguchi K, Riew KD, Galatz LM, et al. Biceps activity during shoulder motion: an electromyographic analysis. Clin Orthop 1997;336:122–129.

54. Sakurai G, Ozaki J, Tomita Y, et al. Electromyographic analysis of shoulder joint function of the biceps brachii muscle during isometric contraction. Clin Orthop 1998,354:123–131.

55. Kido T, Itoi E, Konno N, et al. Electromyographic activities of the biceps during arm elevation in shoulders with rotator cuff tears. Acta Orthop Scand 1998;69:575–579.

56. Rodosky MW, Harner CD, Fu FH. The role of the long head of the biceps muscle and superior glenoid labrum in anterior stability of the shoulder. Am J Sports Med 1994;22:121–130.

57. McMahon PJ, Burkart A, Musahl V, et al. Glenohumeral translations are increased after type II superior anterior-posterior lesion: a cadaveric study of severity of passive stabilizer injury. J Shoulder Elbow Surg 2004;13:39–44.

58. Pagnani MJ, Deng X-H, Warren RF, et al. Effect of lesions of superior portion of the glenoid labrum on glenohumeral translation. J Bone Joint Surg Am 1995;77:1003–1010.

59. Itoi E, Motzkin NE, Morrey BF, et al. Stabilizing function of the long head of the biceps: with the arm in hanging position. Orthop Trans 1992;16:775.

60. Itoi E, Kuechle DK, Newman SR, et al. Stabilizing function of the biceps in stable and unstable shoulders. J Bone Joint Surg Br 1993;75:546–550.

61. Itoi E, Newman SR, Kuechle DK, et al. Dynamic anterior stabilisers of the shoulder with the arm in abduction. J Bone Joint Surg Br 1994;76:834–836.

62. Pagnani MJ, Deng X-H, Warren RF, et al. Role of the long head of the biceps brachii in glenohumeral instability: a biomechanical study in cadavera. J Shoulder Elbow Surg 1996;5:255–262.

63. Malicky DM, Soslowsky LJ, Blasier RB, et al. Anterior glenohumeral stabilization factors: progressive effects in a biomechanical model. J Orthop Res 1996;14:282–288.

64. Boileau P, Baqué F, Valerio L, et al. Isolated arthroscopic biceps tenotomy or tenodesis improves symptoms in patients with massive irreparable rotator cuff tears. J Bone Joint Surg Am 2007;89:747–757.

65. Walch G, Edwards TB, Boulahia A, et al. Arthroscopic tenotomy of the long head of the biceps in the treatment of rotator cuff tears: clinical and radiographic results of 307 cases. J Shoulder Elbow Surg 2005;14:238–246.

66. Itoi E, Motzkin NE, Morrey BF, et al. Scapular inclination and inferior instability of the shoulder. J Shoulder Elbow Surg 1992;1:131–139.

67. Warner JJP, Micheli LJ, Arslanian LE. Scapulothoracic motion in normal shoulders and shoulders with glenohumeral instability and impingement syndrome: a study using moiré topologic analysis. Clin Orthop 1992;285:191–199.

68. Pagnani MJ, Warren RF. Stabilizers of the glenohumeral joint. J Shoulder Elbow Surg 1994;3: 173–190.

69. Kibler WB. The role of the scapula in athletic shoulder function. Am J Sports Med 1998;26: 325–337.

70. Kibler WB, McMullen J. Scapular dyskinesis and its relation to shoulder pain. J Am Acad Orthop Surg 2003;11:142–151.

Joseph D. Zuckerman
Jason L. Hurd

Managing Contractures and Deficiencies of the Shoulder Capsule and Rotator Cuff

INTRODUCTION

Soft tissue management is one of the most important aspects of revision total shoulder arthroplasty. It is a major determinate of both postoperative stability and range of motion. Successfully achieving soft tissue balance in the revision setting, however, can be challenging even for the most experienced shoulder surgeons. A broad spectrum of soft tissue disorders may be encountered, ranging from fibrosis to deficiency. Appropriate release of contractures, lengthening of shortened structures, and concentric balancing of the soft tissues will help maximize motion while maintaining stability. This chapter provides an overview of various soft tissue conditions that may complicate revision total shoulder arthroplasty, as well as our approach to the treatment of these complex problems.

STIFFNESS

Stiffness has been reported as the leading cause of failure and patient dissatisfaction after primary total shoulder arthroplasty.[1] During revision arthroplasty, scarred and contracted tissues must be mobilized. Often, this requires extensive releases to define soft tissue planes and reestablish motion. In some cases, lengthening procedures may be required.

Most often the previous surgery was performed through a deltopectoral approach. Whenever possible, the previous incision should be used; however, the shoulder is well vascularized and crossing incisions do not usually pose a problem. Extending the original incision proximally or distally in tight shoulders is often helpful. Full-thickness skin flaps are then developed medially and laterally to expose the deltopectoral interval. Commonly, the cephalic vein cannot be identified. In this instance the coracoid process serves as a useful landmark for identification of the proximal portion of the deltopectoral interval.

The deltopectoral interval, once identified, is developed. With severe scarring, electrocautery may be required to open this interval. Dissection should start at the coracoid process and proceed distally in line with the muscle fibers to the deltoid

insertion. Deeper dissection is then performed bluntly to expose the remnant of the clavipectoral fascia. In most revisions the true clavipectoral fascia is absent and is replaced by a layer of fibrotic tissue. All dissection must remain lateral to the coracoid process and conjoined tendon to avoid injury to neurovascular structures.

Once deeper fascial layer is exposed, the subacromial and subdeltoid spaces are mobilized by freeing adhesions. This is accomplished by first dividing the clavipectoral fascia layer along the lateral aspect of the conjoined tendon up to the coracoacromial ligament. We preserve the coracoacromial ligament whenever possible because of its contribution to the coracoacromial arch. The space directly under the coracoacromial ligament is then opened sharply with Mayo scissors or electrocautery. It is important to stay above the level of the rotator cuff tendons to avoid injury to these structures. Abundant scar tissue must occasionally be excised to allow entry into the subacromial space. Once sufficient space is created, a Darrach elevator is inserted and used to bluntly release adhesions between the supraspinatus and infraspinatus muscles and the overlying acromion. A combination of blunt and sharp dissections is then used to free the undersurface of the deltoid from adhesions starting proximally and progressing distally. Care must be taken to stay directly on the proximal humerus to avoid injuring the axillary nerve, which runs just superficial to the fascia on the undersurface of the deltoid. The subdeltoid space should be mobilized in a proximal to distal direction to its insertion; it should also be mobilized anteriorly to posteriorly, facilitated by rotation of the humerus. Following adequate release of scar tissue, the subacromial and subdeltoid spaces should be free of all adhesions and there should be continuity between the subacromial and subdeltoid spaces. The pectoralis major should be dissected off the underlying conjoined tendon muscles to complete mobilization of the deltopectoral layer. In some cases, severe scarring between the pectoralis major and the conjoined tendons makes it very difficult and somewhat risky to reestablish these layers. In this uncommon situation, we choose to mobilize the pectoralis major and conjoined tendon muscles as a single layer, focusing primarily on freeing adhesions to the underlying subscapularis.

The space under the conjoined tendon is then developed to expose the subscapularis tendon. By starting dissection just deep to the tip of the coracoid, the correct interval between the conjoined tendon and subscapularis tendon is more easily identified. Mobilization of the conjoined tendon off the underlying tissues can be difficult because of the dense adhesions. We have found that using the electrocautery to release the most lateral edge will allow entry into this interval. Blunt digital dissection combined with judicious use of the electrocautery can be used to complete the mobilization. The location of the neurovascular structures at the anteroinferior edge of the subscapularis requires careful dissection in this area. As a result we avoid sharp dissection in this area.

With the layers mobilized, a self-retaining retractor with variable depth blades can be placed to expose the deeper layers. If necessary, the proximal 1 cm of the pectoralis major insertion can be released to facilitate exposure. If the biceps tendon is intact, a tenodesis should be performed at this point by securing it to the lateral edge of the pectoralis major insertion with no. 2 nonabsorbable sutures. The tendon is then divided just proximal to the site of the tenodesis. The remaining proximal portion of the tendon can be resected later in the procedure when the glenonumeral joint is exposed.

For patients with external rotation beyond neutral, the subscapularis tendon is tenotomized 1 cm medial to its insertion. The incision starts at the rotator cuff interval and is carried distally. The subscapularis tendon and the underlying capsule are released from the humeral neck. A small Darrach retractor is then placed inside the inferior capsule. This maneuver places the inferior capsule on stretch while protecting the axillary nerve located inferiorly and outside the capsule. As the humerus is gradually externally rotated, the inferior capsule is released from the articular side with electrocautery in an anterior to posterior direction until 90 degrees of external rotation is achieved. The rotator interval is then opened by sharp release to the anterosuperior glenoid margin.

Other options for releasing the subscapularis tendon include a direct release from bone or osteotomizing the lesser tuberosity.[2] These options may be beneficial in cases with significant internal rotation contracture when the subscapularis tendon is significantly contracted and extra length is needed. Z-lengthening of the subscapularis has also been described in cases with severe contracture. However, in our experience, this approach can weaken the tendon, compromise the repair, and predispose to failure.[3,4]

After release of the subscapularis the inferior capsule should be released directly off the humeral neck using electrocautery, with the goal of achieving 90 degrees of external rotation. Gently moving the arm in extension and external rotation will dislocate the humeral head anteriorly. If a modular humeral head has been used, it should be removed. This will enhance exposure of the glenoid and facilitate circumferential releases. We will not address techniques related to humeral component revision here; these will be considered in other chapters. However, the version of the humeral component should be carefully assessed because malpositioning can contribute to instability. The use of a modular head will allow the option of upsizing or downsizing based on a careful assessment of soft tissue tension.

The proximal humerus should be retracted posteriorly using a levering type retractor. The retractor should be placed behind the posterior glenoid rim, with care taken to avoid excess levering force. Retraction of the proximal humerus posteriorly will be easier if a modular humeral head has been removed. Monoblock humeral components will make glenoid exposure more challenging. With the proximal humerus retracted posteriorly, the initial glenoid exposure is obtained. The soft tissue surrounding the rim of the glenoid should be excised. This will allow a complete evaluation of the glenoid component for possible loosening and malposition. As noted, if revision of the glenoid component is necessary, the techniques to be used will be discussed in other chapters. Depending on the relevant clinical factors, a more extensive glenoid exposure may be necessary. In shoulders that are excessively tight, mobilization of the soft tissues that surround the glenoid will facilitate postoperative range of motion. Therefore a careful, systematic 360-degree release around the glenoid should be performed to enhance soft tissue excursion and thereby improve the potential for satisfactory postoperative range of motion. We prefer to begin anteriorly. The interval between the capsule/subscapularis and the anterior glenoid neck should be released carefully using electrocautery (Fig. 13.1).

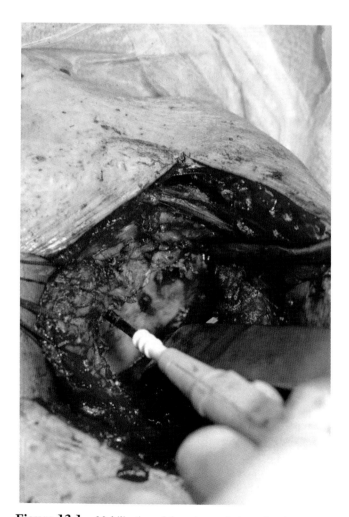

Figure 13.1. Mobilization of the subscapularis tendon is performed by releasing the capsular attachments at the anterior glenoid margin. This allows exposure of the anterior glenoid neck. The use of an elevator along the glenoid neck will further enhance subscapularis mobilization.

Once the initial release is performed at the glenoid edge, a blunt elevator should be used to elevate the soft tissue along the anterior glenoid neck. When this has been performed a levering retractor can be placed along the glenoid neck to further expose this area. Attention is then directed superiorly. If the biceps tendon remains, we prefer to perform a biceps tenodesis in the bicipital groove and excise the proximal portion by resecting it at the superior glenoid and just proximal to the tenodesis site. Electrocautery is used to release the superior capsular insertion to the glenoid. A small elevator is used to elevate this area and should not extend beyond 1 cm medial to the glenoid edge. This will minimize the risk of injury to the suprascapular neurovascular bundle. A small levering retractor is then placed superiorly. Attention is then turned to the inferior glenoid (Fig. 13.2). This is often an area of significant scarring. A Darrach elevator should be placed on the inferior capsule just beyond the inferior glenoid edge. This will place the inferior capsule under tension. The electrocautery is then used to carefully release the capsular attachments beginning at the anterior/inferior glenoid rim and

progressing inferiorly to the posterior/inferior glenoid rim (Fig. 13.2A). After the initial release at the rim, a blunt elevator is used to elevate the soft tissue from the inferior glenoid neck (Fig. 13.2B). This should allow improved excursion of the inferior soft tissues. The posterior glenoid can then be evaluated. Often, the placement of an angled posterior retractor performs an acceptable release. However, if additional posterior releases are necessary, the retractor should be removed and lateral traction placed on the proximal humerus using a bone hook. The capsular attachments posteriorly should be released with electrocautery and a curved elevator used to elevate the soft tissues from the posterior glenoid. After the capsular releases have been completed, the enhanced exposure of the glenoid will facilitate any further evaluation of the glenoid.

Of particular importance is the assessment of the excursion and mobility of the subscapularis tendon. Release of the anterior capsule along the anterior glenoid rim should facilitate subscapularis mobilization. At times the excursion of the subscapularis is limited by adhesions between the superior portion

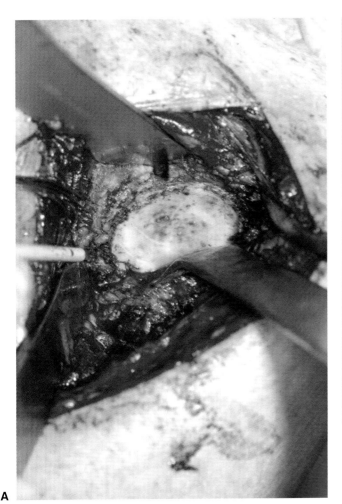 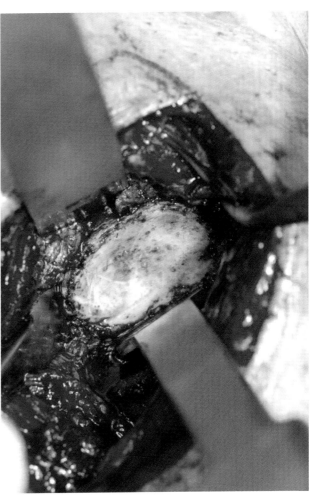

A   **B**

Figure 13.2. With the proximal humeral component retracted posteriorly, the circumferential glenoid exposure can be obtained. A levering retractor is inserted superiorly, and an anterior retractor is placed along the glenoid neck. Release of the inferior capsule from the interior glenoid should be performed carefully. **(A)** A Darrach elevator is used to place the inferior capsule under tension and the electrocautery is used for the initial release. **(B)** A blunt elevator is then used to release the capsule more medially along the inferior glenoid neck. These maneuvers provide a circumferential capsule release from the glenoid to enhance mobilization of the periglenoid soft tissues.

and the coracoid. The adhesions on the superficial aspect of the subscapularis tendon should be released with a combination of blunt finger dissection on the anterior surface and sharp dissection at the base of the coracoid. Opening the rotator interval to the base of the coracoid will facilitate the mobilization. We prefer to perform these releases with electrocautery. A small blunt elevator is then used to further release the superior edge of the subscapularis tendon from the coracoid, with care taken to avoid medial dissection.

After all soft tissue releases have been performed, soft tissue balancing should be assessed by evaluating glenohumeral motion, including forward elevation, internal/external rotation with the arm at the side, and at 90 degrees of abduction. If a modular humeral head is used, assessments can be made with different-sized humeral heads to determine the optimal combination of range of motion and stability. If an eccentric modular humeral head is used, the position of the head can be used to assist soft tissue balancing. Care should be taken to avoid excessive superior position of the humeral head in relation to the greater tuberosity. If a monoblock humeral component is in place, these options are not available and a decision will be necessary as to whether the soft tissue balancing is acceptable or additional releases should be performed. In some situations, a monoblock humeral component may require revision to achieve appropriate balancing.

At this point, closure is begun. The most important aspect of the closure is repair of the subscapularis. The technique used will be determined based on the type of subscapularis release performed. If a tenotomy was used, secure repair using nonabsorbable suture is essential. If the subscapularis is released directly from bone, a direct tendon-to-bone repair using sutures passed through bone tunnels should be performed (Fig. 13.3). If a lesser tuberosity osteotomy is performed, a bone-to-bone repair should be performed. The specific technique used is important in that it should provide a secure repair with minimal risk of disruption. We also prefer to perform a rotator interval repair. This is performed with the humerus in maximal external rotation after the subscapularis repair is performed. Nonabsorbable sutures are passed across the rotator interval to enhance the stability of the

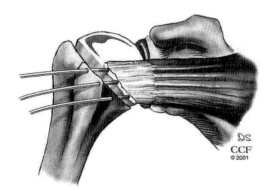

Figure 13.3. If the subscapularis tendon is released directly from its insertion to bone, it should be reattached with sutures passed through drill holes. This can be performed using a variety of techniques, including bone tunnels with simple or horizontal mattress sutures or use of suture anchors. (From Brems J. Complications of shoulder arthroplasty: infections, instability, and loosening, *Instr Course Lect* 2002;5:29–39.)

repair. We find that this also decreases the tension on the subscapularis repair. When the subscapularis reattachment is completed and rotator interval closure has been performed, the amount of external rotation should be assessed. This should be documented and incorporated into the postoperative rehabilitation program. The remainder of the repair is performed in standard fashion. The use of a drain should be determined based on the potential for postoperative hematoma formation. The patient is usually placed in a standard arm sling.

The postoperative rehabilitation program is an essential component of the overall treatment plan. We prefer to perform these procedures under regional anesthesia so that the patient can be started on an exercise regimen in the postanesthesia care unit. Our therapist begins an exercise regimen consisting of passive range of motion exercises for forward elevation, external rotation limited to the range determined intraoperatively, and internal rotation to the chest wall. The patient is instructed in passive stretching exercises that are continued during the first 4 weeks after the procedure. Use of the sling can be extended for a longer time if there is concern about the status and security of the subscapularis repair. When the sling is discontinued an active range-of-motion program is initiated, combined with continued stretching to increase the overall range. The stretching program is essential to maintain the gains in motion obtained intraoperatively. The patient should understand that dedication to the postoperative rehabilitation program is essential in to obtain an optimal result.

SOFT TISSUE FAILURE

Soft tissue failure, involving the capsule, rotator cuff, or both, manifesting itself in instability is one of the most common reasons for revision.[5–9] Patients may present with signs and symptoms of instability and/or rotator cuff dysfunction. Because stability following total shoulder arthroplasty is largely dependent on properly balanced soft tissues, significant overlap between rotator cuff tears and glenohumeral joint instability exists. Clinically significant isolated rotator cuff tears after shoulder arthroplasty are less commonly encountered[10]; therefore we will consider rotator cuff tears in the context of instability.

Instability can generally be attributed to soft tissue failure, inadequate soft tissue tensioning, or component malposition (Fig. 13.4); frequently more than one factor is involved.[11,12] Component malpositioning will be addressed in other chapters; this discussion will focus primarily on soft tissue failure. Globally lax and asymmetrically tight soft tissues can result in instability. For example, patients with circumferential soft tissue laxity, such as occurs when an undersized humeral head is used, are at risk for multidirectional instability. Paradoxically, patients with asymmetrically tight structures are at risk for rupture of the tight structures as they are stressed and subsequent instability in the same direction. In addition, patients with asymmetrically tight structures are also at risk for instability in the opposite direction as a result of the soft tissue imbalance. This is encountered more commonly in patients with tight anterior structures and lax posterior structures that result in posterior instability.

Acute dislocations can be diagnosed rather easily by history, physical examination, and radiographs. The diagnosis of more subtle instability can be difficult because patients may complain of only vague symptoms such as discomfort or even feeling that their shoulder is "not stable."[13] When patients present with acute instability, there is often an association with a specific traumatic event. Presentation early postoperatively should result in a high index of suspicion for soft tissue disruption. When anterior dislocation occurs, subscapularis description would be considered likely. If acute posterior dislocation occurs

as a result of an injury, rotator cuff disruption should be considered. Patients with rotator cuff rupture will complain of weakness and loss of motion[4]; however, the literature has not confirmed the clear association between postarthroplasty rotator cuff tears and activity altering pain.[14,30] Certainly a high level of suspicion is appropriate in patients who have risk factors for soft tissue failure. Patients with underlying neuromuscular disorders (Parkinson's disease[16]) or a history of recurrent instability before primary arthroplasty are at increased risk for subsequent instability. Risk factors for subscapularis tendon disruption and

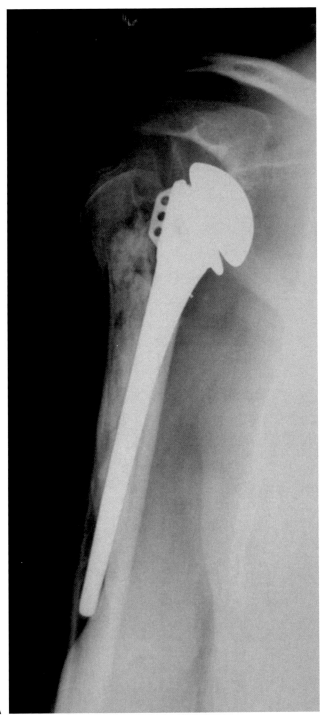

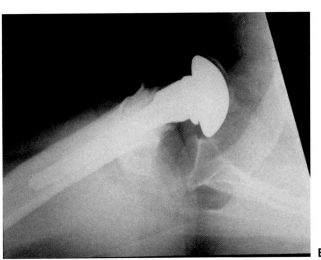

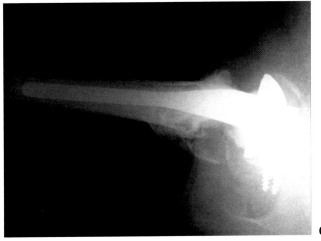

Figure 13.4. A 36-year-old woman underwent proximal humeral replacement for treatment of a comminuted fracture as a result of a high-speed motor vehicle collision. Anteroposterior (**A**) and lateral (**B**) radiographs obtained 4 months postoperatively show the component to be dislocated anteriorly, a large retained head fragment posteriorly, and absence of a lesser tuberosity fragment anteriorly. Instability in this case results from deficiency of the anterior soft tissues, component malposition, and retained bone. The patient underwent component revision combined with Achilles tendon allograft to reconstruct the anterior soft tissues. Postoperative axillary (**C**), lateral

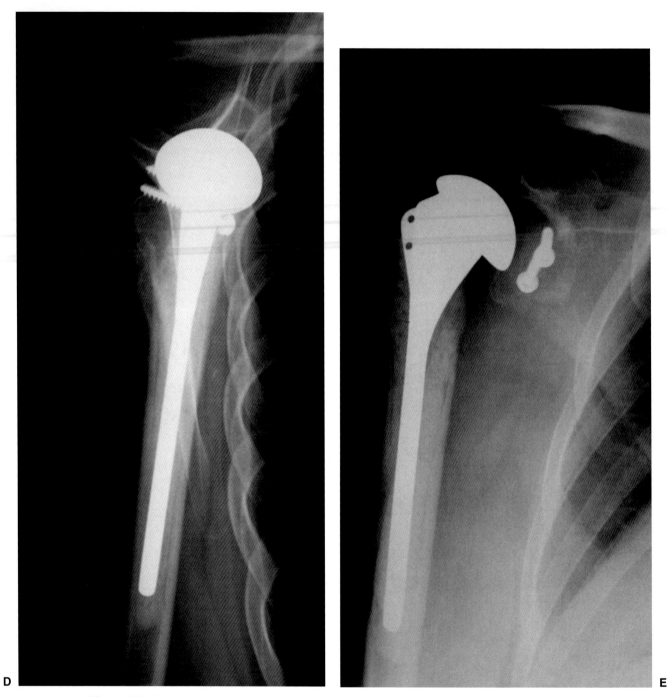

D   E

Figure 13.4. *(continued)* **(D),** and anteroposterior **(E)** radiographs show centralization of the humeral head on the glenoid. (From Zuckerman JD, Hurd JL. Revision total shoulder arthroplasty for instability. In: Zuckerman JD, ed. *Advanced Reconstruction: Shoulder.* Rosemont, Ill: American Academy of Orthopaedic Surgeons; 2007:639.)

subsequent instability include multiple previous operations; overstuffing of the joint; overly aggressive postoperative therapy, specifically involving external rotation during the early postoperative period; and tendon compromised by different lengthening techniques.[4,17] In addition, most patients with inflammatory arthritis have attritional changes of the rotator cuff that cause structural compromise, resulting in both dysfunction and a higher risk for disruptions—both of which would contribute to the development of instability.

In patients with an acute dislocation the physical findings may be quite obvious. Anterior dislocation will result in anterior prominence and an exaggerated appearance of the posterior acromion. Posterior dislocation can present with posterior prominence and an exaggerated prominence of the anterior acromion. In the acute setting, active and passive range of motion will be limited and painful. The neurological status, particularly with respect to axillary nerve deficits, should be carefully evaluated. A complete radiographic evaluation should be performed, including scapular anteroposterior, scapular lateral, and supine axillary views. This will confirm the position of the humeral head with respect to the glenoid and determine the presence of anterior or posterior dislocation.

The clinical signs are often more limited in patients with subtle instability. Failure to regain active motion and strength following shoulder arthroplasty may be indicative of rotator cuff failure. However, this finding can be nonspecific because there are many factors that contribute to a failure to regain active motion that are not associated with instability. In addition, most patients have some degree of postoperative pain and limitation of motion that should gradually improve over time. Failure to improve and progress in the overall recovery can be an indication that a problem exists. Sudden weakness and a decrease in active motion after a period of postoperative improvement may be more suggestive of a rotator cuff disruption. Patients with a subscapularis disruption may display increased passive external rotation accompanied by positive lift-off and/or abdominal compression tests. Recent literature suggests that the abdominal compression test is unreliable in the postoperative period.[14] Armstrong et al[14] demonstrated a sensitivity of only 25% and specificity of 73% for the diagnosis of subscapularis disruption. The diagnosis of subscapularis disruption can be difficult to make, and careful assessment of clinical findings is necessary, along with maintaining a high index of suspicion when progress does not occur.

Radiographic evaluation in patients with subtle or gradual progression of instability may be limited. Radiographs should include scapular anteroposterior views with the humerus internally rotated, scapular anteroposterior views with the humerus externally rotated, and scapular lateral and supine axillary views. These radiographs may show superior subluxation of the humeral head on the anteroposterior view consistent with rotator cuff disruption. The axillary view may show anterior translation of the humeral head in relation to the glenoid, consistent with a subscapularis disruption. Of course, when posterior subluxation is evident, the possibility of rotator cuff disruption and/or posterior soft tissue laxity should be considered. Using modified fast spin-echo sequencing, magnetic resonance imaging (MRI) after shoulder arthroplasty has been shown to have a 91% sensitivity and 88% specificity with regard to full-thickness rotator cuff tears.[18] Unfortunately, standard MRI will not adequately visualize soft tissues around the shoulder after an arthroplasty because of the metal artifact. A specialized MRI sequence, as described, will need to be developed with the radiologist to obtain useful information. Ultrasound evaluation has also shown some promise for the diagnosis of rotator cuff tears in postoperative patients following rotator cuff repair.[14,19] However, it is not clear whether ultrasound can play a role in the evaluation of rotator cuff tears following arthroplasty. In institutions without specialized MRI capabilities or experience with ultrasound, computed tomography (CT) arthrography is an option. However, its sensitivity may be less than ideal because of postoperative scarring.[20]

Successful revision of an unstable total shoulder arthroplasty depends on identifying the underlying causes of instability and appropriately addressing each factor. The timing of instability may be helpful in determining the cause as well as determining treatment. As noted, early instability (<6 weeks) is most often caused by static factors such as errors in soft tissue tensioning, component positioning at the time of surgery

and/or, disruption of the subscapularis repair. Late instability (>6 weeks after surgery) is most commonly caused by dynamic factors such as gradual rotator cuff compromise.[21,22]

An important clue to the cause of instability is its direction. Rupture of the subscapularis tendon is the most common cause of anterior instability. Wirth and Rockwood[15,23] found that either subscapularis rupture or incompetency of the coracoacromial ligament was required for anterior instability. The most common causes of posterior instability are component malposition, that is, excessive humeral component retroversion and/or glenoid component retroversion, and excessive posterior soft tissue laxity—usually in the context of preoperative posterior subluxation—will frequently be contributing factors. Inferior subluxation is most often caused by failure to restore humeral height and inadequate soft tissue tension. Superior instability, or, in its extreme, anterosuperior escape, occurs in the context of significant rotator cuff dysfunction and an incompetent coracoacromial arch.

ANTERIOR INSTABILITY

Anterior instability resulting from subscapularis disruption can be a challenging problem to treat. In all cases, the musculotendinous unit retracts medially, deep to the conjoined tendon. Depending on the acute or chronic nature of the disruption, mobilization may be relatively straightforward or impossible. In acute disruptions that are addressed promptly, the edge of the subscapularis tendon can usually be identified deep to the conjoined tendon muscle along the anterior glenoid margin. When identifying the plane between a conjoined tendon and the subscapularis, care must be taken not to cause further damage to the tendon. It is also essential to be aware of the location of the coracoid. Dissection should be lateral to the coracoid to minimize the risk of neurovascular injury. When the edge of the subscapularis tendon is identified, traction sutures should be inserted. Then the gradual process of mobilization begins by releasing adhesions along the glenoid neck as well as between the subscapularis and the conjoined tendon. Adhesions at the base of the coracoid should also be released with extension into the rotator interval area. The release along the anterior glenoid neck should be done directly off bone to avoid injury to the subscapularis itself. With adequate mobilization, the subscapularis tendon can be primarily repaired. The technique of repair should ideally be different from the repair initially used. A direct tendon-to-bone repair is strongly preferred, using either sutures passed through bone tunnels or suture anchors. Repair of the rotator interval will help decrease tension on the suture line and should be performed with the arm in external rotation. Of course, before repair the position of the humeral component should be evaluated to make certain that excessive anteversion is not present. In addition, the presence of overstuffing of the glenohumeral joint, by an oversized humeral head or by placing the implant too high, will also place increased tension on the subscapularis repair and predispose to failure. If these factors are present, revision will be necessary to avoid recurrent subscapularis failure.

In cases of chronic subscapularis ruptures in which mobilization of the subscapularis is not possible, a reconstructive procedure will be necessary. Chronic ruptures can represent as an acute disruption that was unrecognized or an attritional failure. In these situations the retraction of the musculotendinous unit is significant and makes it impossible to identify and mobilize the subscapularis tendon. Even if the tendon edge could be identified, the quality is often insufficient to allow mobilization and repair. Therefore reconstruction using allograft should be performed. An Achilles tendon allograft is useful to reconstruct the anterior soft tissues (Fig. 13.4).[24] In this technique the insertion of the Achilles tendon onto the calcaneus is secured to the glenoid neck using lag screws. The tendon is then secured to the proximal humerus using either suture anchors or sutures passed through bone tunnels. The graft is then sutured back to itself medially and, if sufficient length is available, brought back laterally to further secure the repair. In areas where the graft crosses itself, sutures are used to secure the graft in position. If a portion of the subscapularis remains either medially or laterally, or if capsule can be identified medially or inferiorly, the host tissue is secured to the graft to enhance the fixation and encourage vascular ingrowth. The rotator interval also should be repaired to the superior aspect of the graft.

Another option when mobilization and repair of the subscapularis is not possible is pectoralis major or pectoralis minor transfer.[12,25] This technique has the potential benefit of restoring active muscular power compared to the static reconstruction with Achilles tendon allograft. In this approach, the conjoined tendon, the tendon of the pectoralis major, and the anterior surface of the proximal humerus, are exposed using the deltopectoral approach (Fig. 13.5). Fibrous tissue that has filled the defect around the anterior aspect of the glenohumeral joint should be excised so that a clean bed is available. The superior half to two thirds of the pectoralis major tendon is detached from its insertion. The amount of tendon to be transferred will be determined, in part, by the size of the defect. After detaching the section of the tendon from its insertion into the humerus, the muscle fibers are split approximately 10 cm in line with its fibers. This effectively allows mobilization of the clavicular portion of the pectoralis major. Traction sutures are inserted into the tendon edge to enhance mobilization.

The next step is to develop the interval between the conjoined tendon and the pectoralis minor. This is developed by blunt dissection. The musculotaneous nerve should be identified either by palpation or, preferably, by visualization to minimize the risk of injury. The interval between the nerve and the overlying conjoined tendon should be developed. The interval between the pectoralis minor tendon and the conjoined tendon will be the path for the transferred pectoralis major. The traction sutures are first passed through the interval and then used to pass the pectoralis major tendon under the conjoined tendon but over the musculotaneous nerve. If additional length is needed, additional mobilization of the pectoralis major will be necessary. The tendon should be advanced to its insertion point at the lesser tuberosity. A bony trough is prepared just lateral to the bicipital groove for reattachment of the pectoralis major tendon. Bone tunnels are prepared lateral to the bony trough, with care taken to make certain that an adequate bone bridge is present. No. 2 or 5 nonabsorbable sutures are used for the tendon-to-bone repair. We prefer horizontal mattress sutures passed through overlapping bone tunnels. When the transfer is completed the position of the musculotaneous nerve should be assessed to make certain that excessive tension is not present. If there appears to be excessive tension, it may be necessary to thin the pectoralis major muscle belly to remove any potential for compression.[26] Any remaining inferior capsule should be used to reinforce the inferior aspect of the transfer. In addition, a rotator interval repair should be performed, if possible, to further enhance the security of the transfer and anterior stabilization. When the repair is completed, stability and range of motion should be assessed. The amount of external rotation should be documented because this will guide the postoperative rehabilitation program. After standard closure the upper extremity is placed in a sling.

We prefer to progress slowly in the postoperative rehabilitation program. The sling is used for at least 6 weeks to allow sufficient healing of the transfer. During this time, active range of

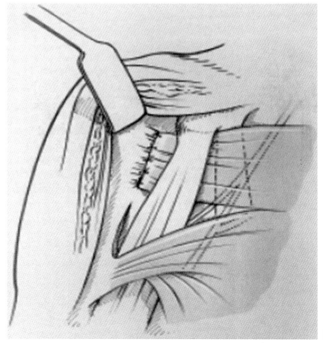

A

B

Figure 13.5. A subcoracoid transfer of the pectoralis major tendon can be used to restore the anterior soft tissues. The subcoracoid transfer provides a more anatomic path for the transferred tendon. Transfer is shown intraoperatively (**A**) and schematically (**B**). CP, coracoid process; CT, conjoined tendon; H, humerus; P, pectoralis.

motion of the elbow, wrist, and hand is allowed. Passive range of motion in the shoulder is allowed through a limited range. We allow forward elevation to 90 degrees with the humerus in internal rotation. External rotation with the arm at the side can be performed within the limits of external rotation documented at the time of surgery. We specifically avoid the combination of abduction and external rotation, as well as forward elevation and external rotation. The goal is to reduce the stress on the transfer. When the sling is removed, active range of motion is initiated. In addition, stretching above 90 degrees of forward elevation can be performed. We prefer to wait an additional 2 weeks or more before allowing stretching beyond the limits of external rotation. Patient compliance with the postoperative rehabilitation regimen is essential to maximize the possibility of a successful outcome. Isometric strengthening can be performed when the sling is discontinued. Resistance strengthening is started only when active forward elevation to 90 degrees has been achieved.

POSTERIOR INSTABILITY

The patient with osteoarthritis and posterior glenoid wear will develop posterior subluxation of the humeral head. This, in turn, results in posterior capsular laxity and anterior soft tissue contractures.[17,27] It has been reported that up to 60% of shoulders with posterior instability following glenohumeral arthroplasty have associated posterior capsular laxity.[28] If the anterior soft tissue contracture and posterior capsular laxity are not addressed at the time of arthroplasty, posterior instability is likely to occur. In patients with posterior instability, the underlying causes should be carefully assessed (Fig. 13.6). Component malposition, specifically excessive retroversion of the humeral component and retroversion of the glenoid component, is an important predisposing factor that may require component revision. These issues will be considered in other chapters. However, in patients who present with posterior instability and the absence of component malposition, the most likely ideology is excessive posterior capsular laxity that was not addressed at the time of the initial surgery. As with anterior instability, an acute traumatic event can result in posterior instability. This is very uncommon, and, if it is encountered, the possibility of significant rotator cuff disruption should be considered. In patients with gradual progression of posterior instability, surgery will most probably be required to address tight anterior structures and excessive posterior capsular laxity. Patients with limited external rotation preoperatively will require mobilization of the anterior soft tissues to achieve appropriate balancing. Following the initial exposure as described previously, the subscapularis insertion should be carefully evaluated. Mobilization and functional lengthening of the subscapularis can be accomplished with various methods. Release of the subscapularis tendon directly off bone and reinsertion in a more medial location will achieve functional lengthening. However, complete subscapularis mobilization should be performed as described to obtain as much length as possible. This includes extramuscular mobilization under the conjoined tendon muscles and release of the capsular attachments to the anterior glenoid neck. Elevation of the subscapularis tendon off the anterior glenoid neck will further enhance mobilization and lengthening. A Z-lengthening of the subscapularis tendon has

also been described, but our experience has been less successful and, most importantly, the soft tissue repair is less secure. Therefore we prefer other methods of mobilization to achieve subscapularis length.

When a modular humeral head is present, downsizing can be considered to effectively lengthen the anterior soft tissues. However, this has to be considered carefully in the context of posterior instability because of its effect on overall laxity. Modular eccentric humeral heads should be rotated posteriorly to effectively tighten the posterior structures. This may enhance the overall stability that can be achieved with the soft tissue repairs. Of course, with monoblock components these options are not possible.

The most common finding in the context of posterior instability is posterior capsular laxity. Therefore it is essential to address this finding at the time of surgery. Reducing the posterior capsular laxity/redundancy can be achieved through a posterior capsular plication. This is usually performed from inside the glenohumeral joint. When a modular humeral head is present, exposure is not problematic. When a monoblock humeral component is in place, exposure may be problematic and may necessitate a posterior approach with exposure of the capsule for imbrication. However, even with a monoblock component in place, lateral traction should be performed in an effort to obtain adequate exposure.

With the proximal humerus retracted laterally, there are different techniques that can be used to perform a capsular placation. The use of a purse-string suture has been described using a heavy, nonabsorbable suture.[29,30] The suture is passed through the medial capsular tissue, progressing superiorly, then progressing laterally, and then inferiorly with multiple passes. The distance between the most medial suture and most lateral suture should be at least 1.5 to 2 cm and should be gauged based on the amount of imbrication necessary. In addition, the superior and inferior dimensions of the purse string should encompass at least two thirds of the height of the glenoid. This suture can then be tied, with lateral traction released and the humerus in external rotation to facilitate closure. Another technique is placement of a series of three sutures lateral to the posterior glenoid margin in a vertical mattress fashion. Three sutures are placed in similar fashion laterally approximately 1.5 to 2.0 cm from the medial row. These sutures are then tied to each other, beginning with the superior sutures, followed by the middle sutures and the inferior sutures. This achieves a medial-to-lateral capsular plication. Passing of the sutures using either technique can be difficult using a standard needle and needle holder. We have found the use of an arthroscopic suture lasso to be helpful for passing these sutures.

After the capsular plication has been completed, the modular humeral head should be replaced and the instability assessed. There should be less than 50% posterior translation of the humeral head on the glenoid with stress testing. Additional fine tuning of the soft tissue tension can be accomplished using a larger humeral head or by rotating an eccentric humeral head into a more posterior position. Of course, care has to be taken to avoid making the shoulder excessively tight.

It has been noted that with a monoblock component in place exposure of the posterior capsule can be difficult. We have had success in passing sutures in this situation; however, in some cases a posterior approach has been necessary. In these cases it is important to properly position and prepare the patient to allow

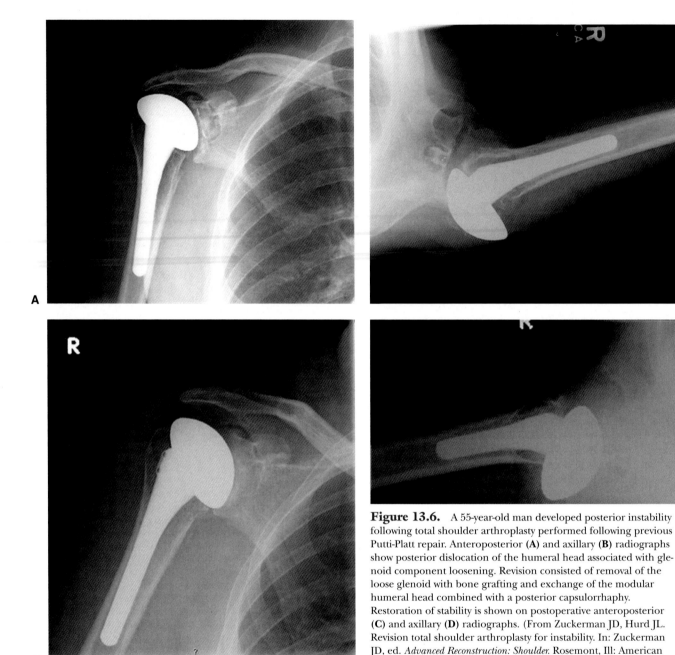

Figure 13.6. A 55-year-old man developed posterior instability following total shoulder arthroplasty performed following previous Putti-Platt repair. Anteroposterior (**A**) and axillary (**B**) radiographs show posterior dislocation of the humeral head associated with glenoid component loosening. Revision consisted of removal of the loose glenoid with bone grafting and exchange of the modular humeral head combined with a posterior capsulorrhaphy. Restoration of stability is shown on postoperative anteroposterior (**C**) and axillary (**D**) radiographs. (From Zuckerman JD, Hurd JL. Revision total shoulder arthroplasty for instability. In: Zuckerman JD, ed. *Advanced Reconstruction: Shoulder.* Rosemont, Ill: American Academy of Orthopaedic Surgeons; 2007:640.)

a posterior approach if necessary. Using a posterior axillary incision a standard approach and exposure are used. After splitting the deltoid, the infraspinatus and teres minor are isolated. We prefer to elevate the muscles off the capsule and then perform a capsular plication. Dividing the capsule with repair of the lateral flaps medially and the medial flap laterally is one approach. The adequacy of the plication can then be evaluated anteriorly by assessing posterior displacement.

The postoperative management of patients who have undergone revision for posterior instability, particularly with posterior capsular plication, has to be carefully designed. We prefer the use of a gunslinger-type orthosis with the humerus in 15 degrees of abduction, neutral flexion-extension, and neutral rotation. The duration of immobilization will vary from 3 to 6 weeks

based on the adequacy of the repair and the intraoperative assessment. Although this does result in some stiffness, we are willing to accept some stiffness in an effort to provide stability. Our experience has been that patients will regain range of motion with a structured and supervised rehabilitation program. When patients are in the orthosis, we allow limited range of motion out of the orthosis as long as neutral or external rotation is maintained. Patients can perform passive forward elevation to 90 degrees as long as neutral rotation is maintained. Range in motion of the elbow, wrist, and hand is also allowed.

Postoperatively, we obtain standing scapular anteroposterior and lateral views in the gunslinger orthosis to document that the humeral head is well reduced on the glenoid. We obtain similar radiographs during the immobilization and after the removal of the orthosis to confirm the reduction. Active range of motion movement can be initiated when the orthosis is discontinued. We generally try to avoid the position of elevation, adduction, and internal rotation for the first 8 to 10 weeks after the surgery. Of course, this can be modified based on the stability achieved and the security of the repair.

INFERIOR INSTABILITY

Inferior instability is quite uncommon and most often is caused by failure to restore humeral height. With current techniques in arthroplasty this is uncommonly encountered. Frequently, in the early postoperative period, some degree of inferior subluxation may be encountered. This is generally secondary to deltoid atony and will resolve with an isometric exercise regimen. However, the possibility of axillary nerve injury should be evaluated. If the inferior subluxation does not resolve, electrodiagnostic studies should be performed to make certain that neurological deficit is not present. In the vast majority of cases of deltoid atony, the inferior subluxation will resolve with appropriate rehabilitation.[22,31] If inferior subluxation does not resolve and the neurological examination is intact, revision should be considered and will consist of humeral component revision. When revision is performed,

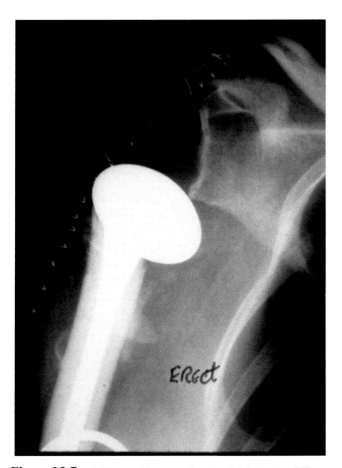

Figure 13.7. A 66-year-old woman developed inferior instability after humeral head replacement. Inadequate restoration of humeral height resulted in significant soft tissue laxity. Postoperative deltoid atony also contributed to the inferior instability.

there is also a benefit of adding an inferior capsular shift to tighten the inferior structures.

SUPERIOR INSTABILITY

Superior instability or, in its most severe form, anterosuperior escape, occurs in the context of significant rotator cuff defects and an incompetent coracoacromial arch. This form of instability is extremely difficult to treat with soft tissue repairs. It generally involves disruption of the supraspinatus and the infraspinatus combined with a subscapularis defect. Because of the massive nature of the rotator cuff tear and its chronicity, primary repair is not an option. Hemiarthroplasty with attempts to restore the soft tissue envelope by primary reconstruction have resulted in disappointing outcomes. However, more recently, revision to a reverse shoulder arthroplasty has been used as an effective treatment alternative. Reverse total shoulder arthroplasty effectively medializes the center of rotation and lengthens the deltoid. The constrained design creates a stable fulcrum that allows the deltoid to compensate for the loss of rotator cuff function, thereby allowing arm elevation to take place.[20,32]

Successful outcome after glenohumeral arthroplasty relies on the soft tissues, probably more so than any other joint replacement procedure in orthopaedic surgery. The spectrum of soft tissue problems ranges from significant stiffness to global instability. The etiology of these problems is generally multifactorial, and they will require careful assessment to determine the important contributing factors. Revision surgery directed at correcting soft tissue problems will require careful planning and meticulous technique to achieve successful outcomes. Soft tissue repairs will often be performed in combination with component revision to achieve improved outcomes.

REFERENCES

1. Hasan SS, Leith JM, Campbell B, et al. Characteristics of unsatisfactory shoulder arthroplasties. *J Shoulder Elbow Surg* 2002;11:431–441.
2. Gerber C, Pennington SD, Yian EH, et al. Lesser tuberosity osteotomy for total shoulder arthroplasty: surgical technique. *J Bone Joint Surg Am* 2006;88(suppl 1, Pt 2):170–177.
3. Ibarra C, Craig EV. Soft-tissue balancing in total shoulder arthroplasty. *Orthop Clin North Am* 1998;29:415–422.
4. Miller BS, Joseph TA, Noonan TJ, et al. Rupture of the subscapularis tendon after shoulder arthroplasty: diagnosis, treatment, and outcome. *J Shoulder Elbow Surg* 2005;14:492–496.
5. Bohsali KI, Wirth MA, Rockwood CA Jr. Complications of total shoulder arthroplasty. *J Bone Joint Surg Am* 2006;88:2279–2292.
6. Cofield RH, Chang W, Sperling JW. Complications of shoulder arthroplasty. In: Iannotti JP, Williams GR Jr, eds. *Disorders of the Shoulder: Diagnosis and Management*. Philadelphia: Lippincott Williams & Wilkins; 1999:571–593.
7. Cofield RH, Edgerton BC. Total shoulder arthroplasty: complications and revision surgery. *Instr Course Lect* 1990;39:449–462.
8. Gerber A, Ghalambor N, Warner JJ. Instability of shoulder arthroplasty: balancing mobility and stability. *Orthop Clin North Am* 2001;32:661–670.
9. Warren RF, Coleman SH, Dines JS. Instability after arthroplasty: the shoulder. *J Arthroplasty* 2002;17(4 suppl 1):28–31.
10. Chin PY, Sperling JW, Cofield RH, et al. Complications of total shoulder arthroplasty: are they fewer or different? *J Shoulder Elbow Surg* 2006;15:19–22.
11. Jahnke AH Jr, Hawkins RJ. Instability after shoulder arthroplasty: causative factors and treatment options. *Semin Arthroplasty* 1995;6:289–286.
12. Sanchez-Sotelo J, Sperling JW, Rowland CM, et al. Instability after shoulder arthroplasty: results of surgical treatment. *J Bone Joint Surg Am* 2003;85:622–631.
13. Neer CS 2nd, Watson KC, Stanton FJ. Recent experience in total shoulder replacement. *J Bone Joint Surg Am* 1982;64:319–337.
14. Armstrong A, Lashgari C, Teefey S, et al. Ultrasound evaluation and clinical correlation of subscapularis repair after total shoulder arthroplasty. *J Shoulder Elbow Surg* 2006;15:541–558.

15. Wirth MA, Rockwood CA Jr. Complications of total shoulder-replacement arthroplasty. *J Bone Joint Surg Am* 1996;78:603–616.

16. Koch LD, Cofield RH, Ahlskog JE. Total shoulder arthroplasty in patients with Parkinson's disease. *J Shoulder Elbow Surg* 1997;6:24–28.

17. Brems JJ. Complications of shoulder arthroplasty: infections, instability, and loosening. *Instr Course Lect* 2002;51:29–39.

18. Sperling JW, Potter HG, Craig EV, et al. Magnetic resonance imaging of painful shoulder arthroplasty. *J Shoulder Elbow Surg* 2002;11:315–321.

19. Prickett WD, Teefey SA, Galatz LM, et al. Accuracy of ultrasound imaging of the rotator cuff in shoulders that are painful postoperatively. *J Bone Joint Surg Am* 2003;85: 1084–1089.

20. Kwon YW, Sajadi KR. Revision total shoulder arthroplasty. In: Zuckerman JD, ed. *Advanced Reconstruction: Shoulder.* Rosemont, Ill: American Academy of Orthopaedic Surgeons; 2007:623–633.

21. Craig EV: Complication in shoulder arthroplasty. *Semin Arthroplasty* 1990;1:160–171.

22. Hennigan SP, Iannotti JP. Instability after prosthetic arthroplasty of the shoulder. *Orthop Clin North Am* 2001;32:649–659.

23. Wirth MA, Rockwood CA Jr. Glenohumeral instability following shoulder arthroplasty. *Orthop Trans* 1995;19:459.

24. Moeckel BH, Altchek DW, Warren RF, et al. Instability of the shoulder after arthroplasty. *J Bone Joint Surg Am* 1993;75:492–497.

25. Resch H, Povacz P, Ritter E, et al. Transfer of the pectoralis major muscle for the treatment of irreparable rupture of the subscapularis tendon. *J Bone Joint Surg Am* 2000;82:372–382.

26. Norris TR, Lipson SR. Management of the unstable prosthetic shoulder arthroplasty. *Instr Course Lect* 1998;47:141–148.

27. Miller SL, Hazrati Y, Klepps S, et al. Loss of subscapularis function after total shoulder replacement: a seldom-recognized problem. *J Shoulder Elbow Surg* 2003;12:29–34.

28. Neer CS II. Replacement arthroplasty for glenohumeral osteoarthritis. *J Bone Joint Surg Am* 1974:56:1–13.

29. Hill JM, Norris TR. Long-term results of total shoulder arthroplasty following bone-grafting of the glenoid. *J Bone Joint Surg Am* 2001;83:877–883.

30. Namba RS, Thornhill TS. Posterior capsulorrhaphy in total shoulder arthroplasty. *Clin Orthop* 1995;313:135–139.

31. Gill TJ, Warren RF, Rockwood CA Jr, et al. Complications of shoulder surgery. *Instr Course Lect* 1999;48:359–374.

32. Zuckerman JD, Hurd JL. Revision total shoulder arthroplasty for instability. In Zuckerman JD, ed. *Advanced Reconstruction: Shoulder.* Rosemont, Ill: American Academy of Orthopaedic Surgeons; 2007:635–643.

Shawn W. O'Driscoll

Arthroscopic Applications in Revision Shoulder Arthroplasty

INTRODUCTION

Arthroscopy has potential diagnostic and therapeutic applications in revision shoulder arthroplasty. The concept of visualizing a joint after replacement is not new; it has been used in the knee for several indications.[1–8]

Bonutti et al[9] used arthroscopy to evaluate glenoid component loosening in nine patients and found it to be a valuable technique to assess glenoid stability. They confirmed their arthroscopic findings with a subsequent open procedure, at which time they addressed the glenoid component instability.

Hersch and Dines[10] reported diagnostic arthroscopy in 10 patients, with 12 failed total shoulder arthroplasties. Arthroscopic treatment included acromioplasty, debridement of the biceps tendon, capsular release, and removal of loose bodies, including cement fragments. They found arthroscopy to be useful not just diagnostically but also therapeutically.

ARTHROSCOPIC REMOVAL OF PAINFUL LOOSE GLENOID COMPONENT

Although total shoulder arthroplasty enjoys a successful clinical track record for pain relief and improvement of function, there are significant concerns regarding the prevalence of glenoid lucent lines and therefore the possibility of glenoid component loosening long term.[11,12] Treatment options for symptomatic glenoid loosening include revision of the component or conversion to hemiarthroplasty by removal of the loose glenoid component with or without bone grafting the glenoid.[11,13] The philosophy of managing component loosening by glenoid removal is based on reports of humeral hemiarthroplasty without a glenoid component, which has been reasonably successful in the treatment of glenohumeral arthritis.[3,14–21] I have found that it is possible to remove a symptomatic loose glenoid component and underlying cement arthroscopically with complete pain relief in 3 of 5 patients and partial relief in 2 at 4 years follow-up.[22]

SURGICAL TECHNIQUE

Standard posterior and anterior portals are used initially, and accessory anterior and/or posterior portals are made as needed.

A 7-mm cannula is placed in the high anterior portal and a standard 30-degree, 4-mm arthroscope is used. Orientation can be difficult because of distorted reflections off the polished metal humeral head. The first step is to perform a local synovectomy and debridement around the anterior, superior, and posterior margins of the glenoid component. Confirm glenoid component looseness with a probe. Next, a curved osteotome (4–6 mm) through the anterior portal is used to make three sets of cuts (Fig. 14.1) so that the prosthesis can be removed in four pieces. The first cut (1a) transects the glenoid prosthesis diagonally from anterosuperior to posteroinferior (Fig. 14.2). The second cut (1b) divides the remaining intact polyethylene between the cut portion of the face plate and the underlying keel (Fig. 14.2b). The superior third of the glenoid face plate can be withdrawn through the anterior portal by grasping it at the tip and taking advantage of the "aerodynamic" shape created by the diagonal cut (Figs. 14.2 and 14.3). A second set of similar cuts (2a and b) detaches the inferior third of the glenoid face plate from the middle portion and from the keel (Fig. 14.3). The osteotome is then passed beneath the remaining middle part of the face plate (cut 3), separating it from the keel (Fig. 14.4). The keel is removed by backing it out with a twisting motion, apex first. Strong graspers are recommended because the soft tissues around the portal need to stretch to permit component extraction. A Ferris-Smith grasper, normally used to extract an intervertebral disc or intramedullary cement, is useful. The cement is then removed in pieces, breaking it up with a curved osteotome as necessary. A curette is used to clean the glenoid cavity. A total synovectomy is performed if there is significant synovitis present. Finally, a capsulotomy can be performed to improve motion if necessary.

Techniques that have not been found useful include grinding the component with a burr or cutting it into small pieces with bone-biting instruments. In one case the unwise decision was made to fully amputate the keel, but that rendered the remainder of the glenoid component unstable and difficult to cut.

Postoperatively, patients are given a sling for comfort for the first few days, but are encouraged to start moving the limb right away and pursue activities as tolerated. The procedure is generally performed on an outpatient basis, unless there is concern about the preoperative general medical status.

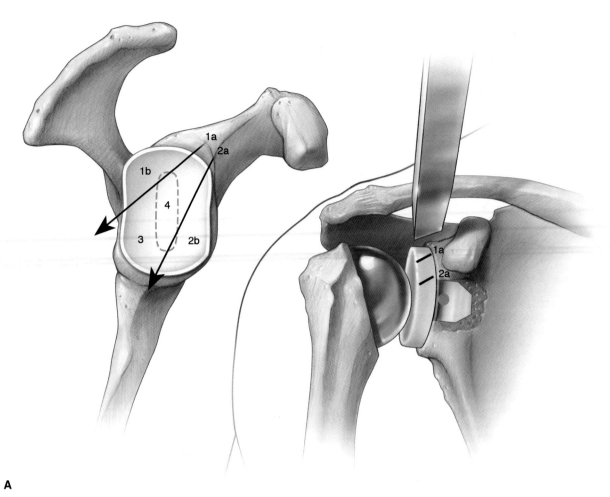

A

B

Figure 14.1.   The glenoid is cut into four pieces with three sets of cuts, designed to create aerodynami-
cally shaped pieces and to take advantage of the keel to hold the component in place until the final cut has
been made. Each of the cuts is made using a 4- to 6-mm osteotome through the anterior portal. (Figs. 14.1
through 14.4 are adapted from O'Driscoll SW, Petrie RS, Torchia ME. Arthroscopic removal of the glenoid
component for failed total shoulder arthroplasty. A report of five cases. *J Bone Joint Surg* 2005;87:858–863.)

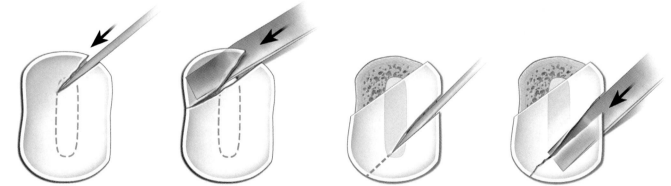

Figure 14.2.   Cut *1a* separates the superior to posterior third of
the glenoid face plate from the remainder of the face plate, leaving a
small attachment to the underlying keel. Cut *1b* separates the component fragment from the keel to permit removal.

Figure 14.3.   Cuts *2a* and *2b*, similar to cuts *1a* and *1b* above, separate the anterior to inferior third of the face plate from the middle
portion and from the keel.

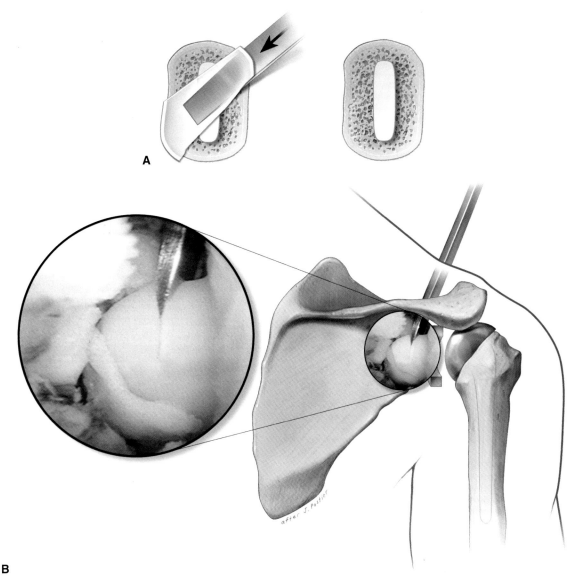

Figure 14.4. The third and fourth segments of the glenoid component (middle portion of face plate and keel, respectively) are separated by cut *3* using the osteotome. The technique with the osteotome coming from the anterior portal in this combined segmatic/arthroscopic view.

RECOMMENDATIONS

Arthroscopic removal of a loose glenoid component and its cement represents an appealing alternative to open revision surgery for failed total shoulder arthroplasty caused by symptomatic glenoid loosening. The concept is practicable; the questions that remain to be answered are: is it predictable, is it successful, and what are the indications, contraindications, and complications? A larger series with longer follow-up will be needed to answer these questions.

In addition, there are some limitations and potential pitfalls to this technique. Only all-polyethylene components and associated PMMA can be removed; removal of metal components is unrealistic. It is difficult to bone graft glenoid defects, should this be deemed necessary.

Damage to the surface of the prosthetic humeral head can occur as a result of scuffing by the instruments, and this could theoretically lead to component wear.[23]

The issue of total arthroplasty component damage from the arthroscopic instruments has received scant attention in the literature. I observed that the humeral components scuffed following this procedure. I suspect that it is highly unlikely that the procedure could be performed without contacting and marking the humeral component. The issue of how this relates to the longevity of the implant is unknown at this time. This maybe an important consideration if, in the future, a revision glenoid component is implanted. This would result in a scuffed/roughened humeral component articulating on a polyethylene component, which could potentially lead to increased polyethylene wear and early failure to the prosthesis. Therefore

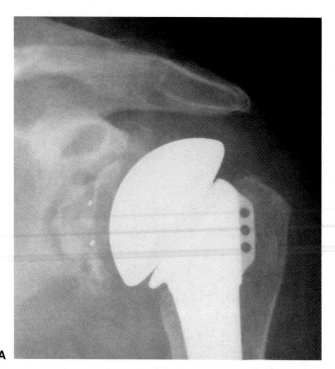

A

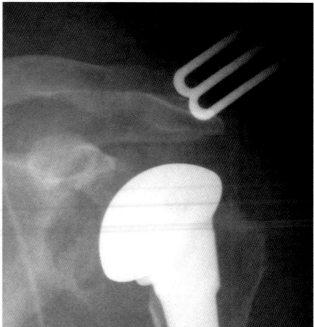

B

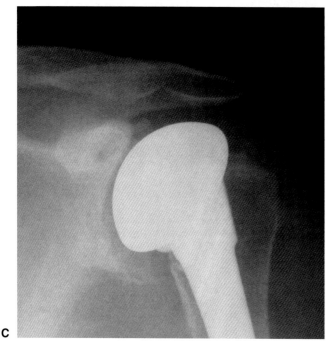

C

Figure 14.5. (A) A preoperative radiograph showing a wide, complete radiolucent line around a loose cemented glenoid component. (B) Postoperative radiograph taken 1 day after arthroscopic removal of the glenoid component and its cement. (C) Radiograph taken 58 months after arthroscopic glenoid component removal, showing concentric remodeling of the remaining glenoid. This patient had complete relief of pain.

I do not recommend this technique if implantation of a revision glenoid component is a likely possibility. At the current time, there are no plans to reimplant a glenoid component in my patients.

There are alternatives that were not employed in these patients, including bone grafting the glenoid cavity, that could be considered in future clinical applications. If reimplantation of a glenoid component is anticipated in the future, arthroscopic removal of a loose glenoid component (and cement) combined with bone grafting of the defect might theoretically be used as an interim procedure to restore glenoid bone stock.

Synovectomy, potentially an important part of the procedure, was performed in each patient in this series and may have contributed to pain relief. In follow-up there has not been any conclusive evidence of progressive bone loss resulting from erosion of the glenoid (Fig. 14.5).

SUMMARY

Arthroscopic removal of a loose glenoid component along with its cement can be considered for patients who have a painful loose polyethylene glenoid component due to rotator cuff deficiency or in the absence of any treatable cause for failure of the total shoulder arthroplasty. It should be considered in elderly or frail patients for whom the need to minimize further surgery is even more important. Relative contraindications would be the presence of a metal-backed glenoid component and severe bone loss that compromises the bony rim of the glenoid such that containment of the humeral component in the glenoid is not possible after removal of the glenoid component.

REFERENCES

1. Allardyce TJ, Scuderi GR, Insall JN. Arthroscopic treatment of popliteus tendon dysfunction following total knee arthroplasty. *J Arthroplasty* 1997;12:353–355.

2. Bocell JR, Thorpe CD, Tullos HS. Arthroscopic treatment of symptomatic total knee arthroplasty. *Clin Orthop* 1991;271:125–134.

3. Boyd AD Jr, Thomas WH, Scott RD, et al. Total shoulder arthroplasty versus hemiarthroplasty: indications for glenoid resurfacing. *J Arthroplasty* 1990;5:329–336.

4. Flood JN, Kolarik DB. Arthroscopic irrigation and debridement of infected total knee arthroplasty: report of two cases. *Arthroscopy* 1988;4:182–186.

5. Johnson DR, Friedman RJ, Mcginty JB, et al. The role of arthroscopy in the problem total knee replacement. *Arthroscopy* 1990;6:30–32.

6. Markel DC, Luessenhop CP, Windsor RE, et al. Arthroscopic treatment of peripatellar fibrosis after total knee arthroplasty. *J Arthroplasty* 1996;11:293–297.

7. Nordt W, Giangarra CE, Levy IM, et al. Arthroscopic removal of entrapped debris following dislocation of a total hip arthroplasty. *Arthroscopy* 1987;3:196–198

8. Wasilewski SA, Frankl U. Arthroscopy of the painful dysfunctional total knee replacement. *Arthroscopy* 1989;5:294–297.

9. Bonutti PM, Hawkins RJ, Saddemi S. Arthroscopic assessment of glenoid component loosening after total shoulder arthroplasty. *Arthroscopy* 1993;9:272–276.

10. Hersch JC, Dines DM. Arthroscopy for failed shoulder arthroplasty. *Arthroscopy* 2000; 16:606–612.

11. Wirth MA, Rockwood CA Jr. Complications of shoulder arthroplasty. *Clin Orthop* 1994; 307:47–69.

12. Torchia ME, Cofield RH, Settergren CR. Total shoulder arthroplasty with the Neer prosthesis: long-term results. *J Shoulder Elbow Surg* 1997;6:495–505.

13. Petersen SA, Hawkins RJ. Revision of failed total shoulder arthroplasty. *Orthop Clin North Am* 1998;29:519–533.

14. Groh GI, Badwey TM, Rockwood CA. Treatment of cysts of the acromioclavicular joint with shoulder hemiarthroplasty. *J Bone Joint Surg* 1993;5:90–94.

15. Bell SN, Geschwend N. Clinical experience with total arthroplasty and hemiarthroplasty of the shoulder using the Neer prosthesis. *Int Orthop* 1986;10:217–222.

16. Jonsson E, Brattstrom M, Lidgren L. Evaluation of the rheumatoid shoulder function after hemiarthroplasty and arthrodesis. *Scand J Rheumatol* 1988;17:17–26.

17. Kay SP, Amstutz HC. Shoulder hemiarthroplasty at UCLA. *Clin Orthop* 1988;22:842–848.

18. Marmor L. Hemiarthroplasty for the rheumatoid shoulder joint. *Clin Orthop Relat Res* 1977;122:201–203.

19. Williams GR, Rockwood CA. Hemiarthroplasty in rotator cuff–deficient shoulders. *J Shoulder Elbow Surg* 1996;5:362–367.

20. Field LD, Dines DM, Zabinski SJ, et al. Hemiarthroplasty of the shoulder for rotator cuff arthropathy. *J Shoulder Elbow Surg* 1997;6:18–23.

21. Levine WN, Djurasovic M, Glasson J-M et al. Hemiarthroplasty for glenohumeral osteoarthritis: results correlated to degree of glenoid wear. *J Shoulder Elbow Surg* 1997;6:449–454.

22. O'Driscoll SW, Petrie RS, Torchia ME. Arthroscopic removal of the glenoid component for failed total shoulder arthroplasty. A report of five cases. *J Bone Joint Surg* 2005; 87-A(4):858–863.

23. Raab GE, Jobe CM, Williams PA et al. Damage to cobalt-chromium surfaces during arthroscopy of total knee replacements. *J Bone Joint Surg Am* 2001;83:46–52.

15

Mark A. Frankle

Revision of Reverse Shoulder Arthroplasty

INTRODUCTION

With the advances in medical care the average life expectancy continues to increase worldwide.[1] Rotator cuff pathology affects a significant segment of the population, and its prevalence most likely will increase as the general population ages. Treatment of rotator cuff disease has evolved over the years, and reverse shoulder arthroplasty has become an effective treatment for the management of the rotator cuff deficient shoulder.[2-6] As orthopaedic surgeons become comfortable performing reverse shoulder arthroplasty the number of these procedures that are performed each year has steadily increased since the release of these implants in the United States.[7] The long-term survivorship of these implants continues to be studied, and similar to other joint arthroplasties, these implants can be expected to have failures associated with them. Given that, we anticipate the need for revision reverse shoulder arthroplasty will become more prevalent as these devices fail and more information is gathered regarding their performance. To date we have performed 54 revision reverse arthroplasties and more than 700 reverse shoulder arthroplasties. Our experience has provided a wealth of information on management of the pathological processes present in the revision setting. This chapter discusses the various modes of failure, indications for revision surgery, and appropriate management of the problems that occur after reverse shoulder arthroplasty.

FAILURE OF REVERSE SHOULDER ARTHROPLASTY

In discussing mechanical failure of reverse shoulder arthroplasty, we feel it is easiest to divide the causes into glenoid-side and humeral-side failures. On the glenoid side of the implant the three predominant modes of failure have been described as scapular notching,[8] mechanical failure of the baseplate,[2] and glenosphere dissociation.[3] On the humeral side of the implant, failure has been related to recurrent dislocation, humeral loosening, polyethylene failure, and periprosthetic fracture.

GLENOID-SIDE MODES OF FAILURE

Scapular notching has been a radiographic finding in multiple series.[3,5,9] This notching is a documented feature with certain reverse shoulder prosthesis designs and is thought to be due to impingement of the humeral cup against the inferior scapular neck (Fig. 15.1). The clinical relevance of scapular notching has been disputed, although it has been associated with a poorer clinical outcome, polyethylene wear, chronic inflammation of the joint capsule, and local osteolysis.[9] It has been postulated that progressive abrasion of the humeral cup against the scapular neck may lead to osteolysis and cause significant bone loss around the inferior screw of the baseplate and ultimately compromise glenoid fixation. Sirveaux et al[3] reported on a multicenter study evaluating 77 patients (88 shoulders) treated with the Delta III prosthesis for cuff tear arthropathy; 63% demonstrated some evidence of scapular notching at last follow-up examination.[3] Progressive loosening was noted in five glenoid components, two of which had been revised at the time of publication. As more long-term follow-up studies are performed the overall effects of scapular notching may become clearer and may potentially be a cause for reverse shoulder arthroplasty failure.

Mechanical failure of the baseplate (Fig. 15.2) is another type of glenoid-side failure that has been reported.[2,3] The stresses on the baseplate in reverse shoulder arthroplasty are related to both the type of fixation used for the baseplate and the center of rotation of the glenosphere that is implanted. In a study by Harman et al[10] the fixation and offset of the glenosphere component were evaluated with respect to the forces and micromotion at the baseplate-bone interface. The authors found that using a glenosphere with a lateral center of rotation 27 mm from the glenoid resulted in a 69% increase in the moment at the baseplate-bone interface compared with the traditional Grammont design, which has a glenosphere with 16 mm of offset.

Also of note in the study was the effect that screw fixation had on micromotion at the interface (Fig. 15.3). The authors showed that 3.5-mm nonlocked screws were sufficient in limiting micromotion at the baseplate-bone interface to less than 150 microns (generally the accepted threshold for bony in-growth) in the

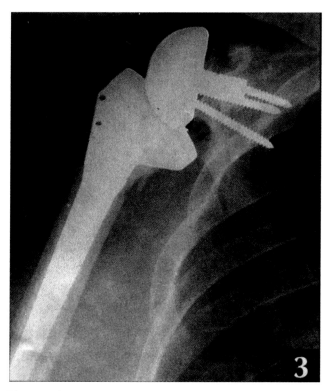

Figure 15.1. A true anteroposterior radiograph demonstrating scapular notching in a reverse shoulder arthroplasty.

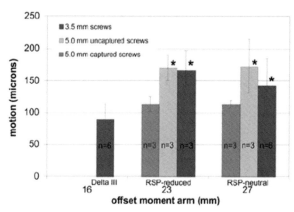

Figure 15.3. Graph showing the effects of lateral offset and screw type on the micromotion at the baseplate-bone interface.

Grammont-type design; however, they were unsuccessful at limiting the micromotion beneath this threshold in the glenosphere with more lateral offset. The authors were able to show that with the use of 5.0-mm peripheral locking screws this micromotion was decreased below the 150-micron threshold in the glenospheres with more lateral offset. This may explain why in some early series using lateral-offset glenospheres with 3.5-mm

nonlocked peripheral screw fixation the failure rate approached 12%.[2] Later series investigating the use of lateral center of rotation glenospheres with 5.0-mm peripheral locking screws have not shown problems with mechanical failure, further illustrating the value of improved fixation. Mechanical failure of the baseplate has also been reported in studies using the more medial center of rotation in the Grammont design. This has been linked to the previously mentioned scapular notching, in which the erosion of the scapular neck compromised the fixation of the baseplate and led to failure.[3]

Glenosphere dissociation (Fig. 15.4) is a rare potential mode of glenoid-side failure.[11] This mode of failure varies depending on the way the glenosphere is secured to the baseplate. In the early Grammont design, the glenosphere screwed onto the baseplate and in some series simply unscrewed and dissociated from the baseplate. More modern designs use a Morse taper similar to that used in other orthopaedic implants. Our group has had three patients require revision surgery as a result of glenosphere dissociation from the baseplate because

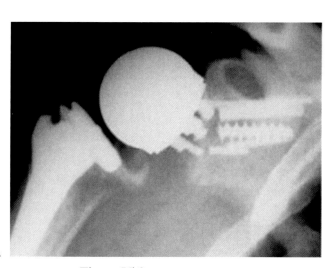

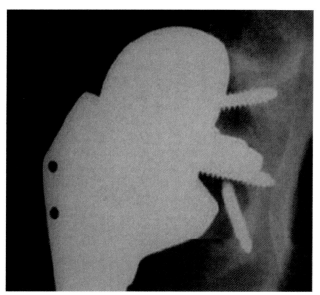

A

B

Figure 15.2. True anteroposterior radiograph of a mechanical baseplate failure of a glenosphere with a center of rotation lateral to the glenoid (**A**) and a glenosphere with center of rotation located at the glenoid (**B**).

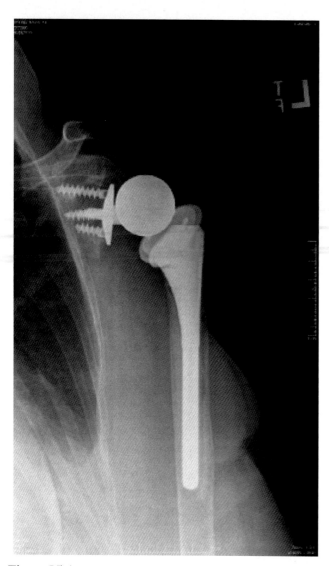

Figure 15.4. Radiograph demonstrating glenosphere dissociation.

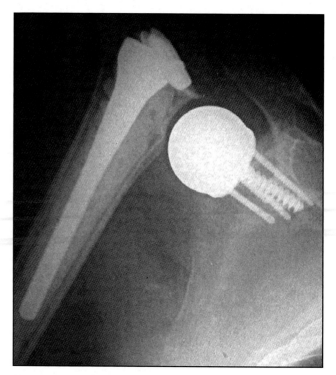

Figure 15.5. Radiograph showing a dislocated reverse shoulder replacement.

the Morse taper was disengaged. Multiple factors are felt to contribute to possible dissociation of Morse tapers. Improper taper impaction, contamination of the taper socket with fluid or solid material, improper taper design or manufacturing, distraction forces at the shoulder joint, and material failure via corrosion have been shown to negatively affect Morse tapers.[12] In our experience, both trauma and technical error in not properly seating the glenosphere have been causes of dissociation. We have subsequently taken steps to limit this technical error, and they are discussed later in the chapter.

HUMERAL-SIDED MODES OF FAILURE

Dislocation of reverse shoulder (Fig. 15.5) replacements is one of the most common complications of this arthroplasty[7] and, if recurrent in nature and unable to be treated by closed means, often necessitates revision surgery. Stability of the reverse articulation is dependant on multiple factors. Improper version of the glenosphere or humeral component is a common factor that can lead to instability. Different authors recommend different degrees of version in which they place their components, but

the ultimate key to stability is to ensure that there is no gross mismatch in the version between components that could result in recurrent instability. The soft tissue tension in the shoulder is another factor that plays a role in instability. It is felt that extreme laxity in the soft tissue envelope after reduction can lead to instability. Attempting to assess this soft tissue tension after reduction can be difficult and may require experience for a clear appreciation of this factor.

Finally, the level of bone loss on the glenoid or humeral side of the articulation is often overlooked as a cause of instability. In cases in which severe glenoid erosion has occurred the joint line can become medialized in relation to its normal location. Surgeons should be wary of this because medialization of the joint line caused by severe erosion may produce relative laxity in the soft tissues surrounding the shoulder joint, resulting in an unstable reverse articulation. This is especially common if in the primary procedure a glenosphere with a medial center of rotation was placed in this medialized position (Fig. 15.6).

A different mechanism of instability can result in patients having substantial proximal humeral bone loss. Many of these patients had a previous hemiarthroplasty that was converted to a reverse shoulder arthroplasty. In some instances, secondary to either resorption of the tuberosities resulting from a previous fracture or as a result of loss of some proximal humerus at the time of previous implant extraction, the patient may be lacking a significant amount of proximal humerus. This leads to the change in the vector of the deltoid that occurs when a substantial amount of the proximal humeral bone is missing (Fig. 15.7). With loss of the proximal humerus, the deltoid loses its natural contour and, in this position, as it contracts, actually provides a slight laterally directed distractive force. This is in contrast to the normal joint compressive force of the deltoid and is believed to

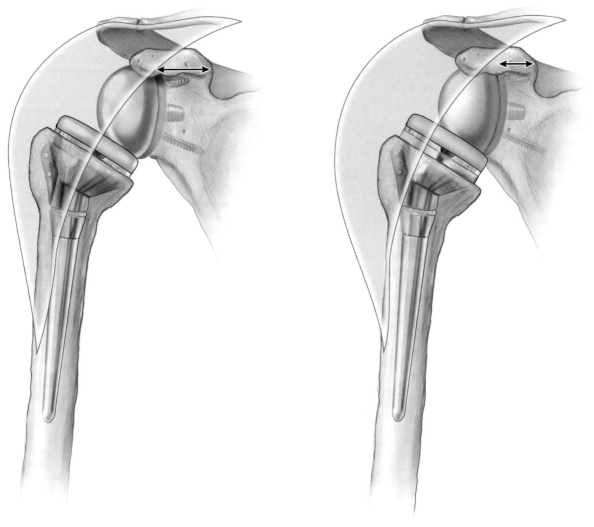

A   **B**

Figure 15.6. **(A)** The vector of the deltoid in a shoulder with no significant glenoid erosion. **(B)** Note that with significant medial erosion the deltoid now produces a distractive force.

be a potential cause of instability. Another humeral-side mode of failure that may lead to revision surgery is loosening of the humeral component. Reverse shoulder arthroplasty is by design a constrained implant, and, given that, forces from the articulation are transmitted to both the humerus and scapula. The most common scenario in which we have seen early humeral loosening is in patients who have had a hemiarthoplasty that was converted to a reverse shoulder arthroplasty in the setting of significant proximal humeral bone loss that was not reconstituted (Fig. 15.8). In these cases, lack of metaphyseal support for the implant allows the forces of the constrained articulation to be transmitted to the stem with the diaphysis. On multiple occasions we have seen this result in early humeral loosening that occurred without evidence of a concomitant pathological process such as an infection to help explain the loosening.

Humeral socket failure after primary reverse shoulder arthroplasty is another mode of failure we have treated with revision surgery. In some patients, trauma led to fracture or dissociation of the polyethylene (Fig. 15.9). However, some polyethylene failures may be directly related to impingement of the polyethylene on the scapular neck. Abrasion of the polyethylene can lead to wear particles and possibly osteolysis in the surrounding bone.

In earlier reverse shoulder arthroplasty, humeral component designs required substantial humeral bone stock to support the proximal humeral component. In the earlier design of the Encore Reverse Prosthesis System (Encore, Austin, Texas), the polyethylene socket had little metal support; thus in circumstances with proximal humeral bone loss, disassociation could occur at the polyethylene-metal junction. Similarly, in the earlier Grammont design the proximal humeral stem screwed into the distal segment so that when there was a proximal humeral deficiency, humeral stem unscrewing could occur.

Periprosthetic fracture is another potential cause for revision (Fig. 15.10). The majority of patients who undergo reverse shoulder arthroplasty are elderly, and the procedure is more commonly performed on women than men. Given that, many of these patients will have some degree of osteoporosis. The difference in the modulus of elasticity between the metal humeral stem and the osteoporotic bone can predispose patients to periprosthetic fracture if they suffer a fall or other trauma. The type of fracture, location, and condition of the implant often determine whether revision surgery is indicated.

As in all arthroplasty, periprosthetic infection can lead to pain and radiographic loosening, requiring revision surgery.

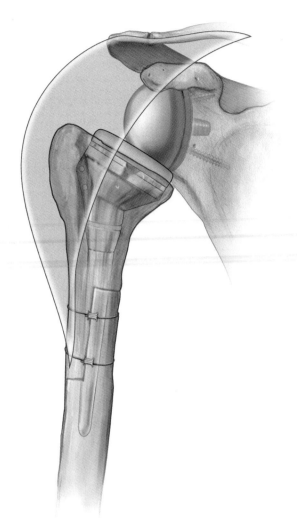

Figure 15.7. Proximal humeral allografting re-establishes the normal deltoid contour, thereby producing a joint compressive force. By replacing the missing proximal humeral bone stock, the deltoid is displaced farther away from the center of rotation.

The infection rate after reverse shoulder arthroplasty has been reported to be between 3% and 7%[3,4] for primary reverse shoulder arthroplasty. The number is higher than in conventional total shoulder arthroplasty. Many authors attribute this to the increased dead space present around the articulation, which often allows for hematoma formation.[11] If infection is diagnosed, the need for revision surgery is clearly indicated, as in most other arthroplasties.

INDICATIONS FOR REVISION REVERSE ARTHROPLASTY

As in all revision surgery, a patient's willingness to undergo surgery must be dependent on the severity of the symptoms the patient is experiencing, a thorough understanding of the symptoms as they relate to the mechanical problem, and the ability to expectantly improve the mechanical problem as to alleviate the symptoms. The indication for revision surgery in patients with scapular notching has not been previously described. In

our experience, patients develop progressive pain associated with radiographic findings consistent with notching. Patients with symptomatic scapular notching may have difficulty fully adducting their operative arm and may experience pain on attempted full adduction as a result of the medial aspect of the humeral component impinging on the inferior scapular neck. This has been termed an "adduction deficit."[13] We have been reluctant to offer surgery unless the pain has been unremitting for at least for 1 year and other causes of pain, such as infection, have been ruled out. Indications for revision arthroplasty in patients with mechanical failure of the glenoid include patient willingness to undergo revision surgery and adequate bone stock for reimplantation of a new glenoid component. Similarly, in patients with glenoid component disassociation, securing a new glenosphere on the existing baseplate should proceed only with adequate understanding of the mechanism for the separation of the glenosphere from the baseplate; this will vary for each prosthetic system.

Indications for humeral-side failure are similar to those for glenoid-side failure. Instability surgery is most challenging because the causes can be multifactorial; thus a high degree of confidence in identifying the factors may be impossible to define. This may diminish confidence in one's ability to predictably alleviate this condition; thus the severity of patient symptoms should be carefully defined.

Indications for revision surgery in the face of infection is dependent on whether the infection is acute or chronic. In patients who develop an acute infection in the early postoperative period or an acute infection arising from hematogenous seeding, early recognition with surgical debridement with retention of components can be considered. In chronic infections a more conservative staged procedure with prosthetic removal is considered.

The decision to revise a failed reverse prosthesis to another reverse prosthesis or to perform other revision surgeries such as conversion to a hemiarthroplasty has been mostly dependent on our ability to technically understand the failure mechanism, overcome technical problems of bone stock, and take into account soft tissue considerations.

PREOPERATIVE PLANNING AND SURGICAL TREATMENT

In planning for revision surgery, certain preoperative steps are taken in preparation for the procedure. Obtaining a detailed history and performing a physical examination are the first steps in evaluating these patients. Careful attention is paid to clinical signs or symptoms that may indicate that an infection could account for failure of the previous arthroplasty. If there is clinical suspicion, we routinely order a complete blood count, erythrocyte sedimentation rate, and C-reactive protein level for baseline laboratory data that may indicate possible infection. During the physical examination we focus on the patient's prior incisions, range of motion (ROM), and provocative maneuvers or activities that may reproduce the pain. Patients with mechanical failure of the baseplate and those with glenosphere dissociation frequently present with limited but variable ROM that is often painful. Patients with instability may be able to perform certain maneuvers and reproduce subluxation of their implant. Those with a dislocation often present with pain and a significantly limited

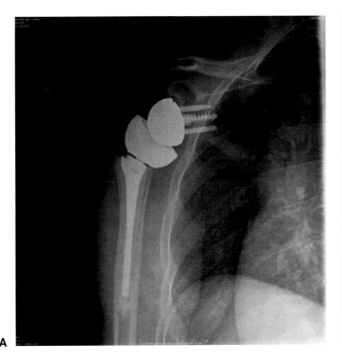

A

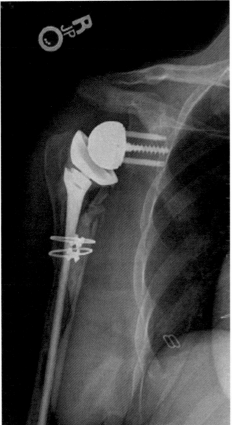

C

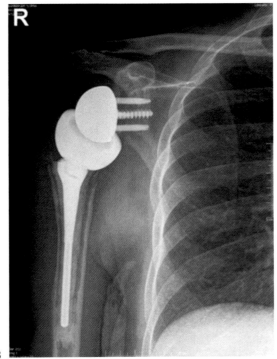

B

Figure 15.8. (A) A reverse shoulder arthroplasty that was performed after a failed hemiarthroplasty. Note the bone loss and lack of metaphyseal support for the implant because of this loss of bone. (B) This patient had early humeral loosening secondary to the lack of proximal bone as all the forces of the articulation are transferred to the diaphyseal portion of the implant. (C) This patient was treated with revision to a long-stemmed component with proximal humeral allografting.

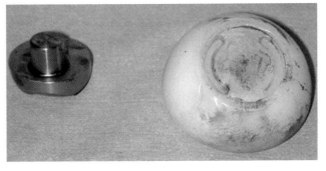

Figure 15.9. A retrieved implant showing the failure of the polyethylene component of the reverse shoulder arthroplasty.

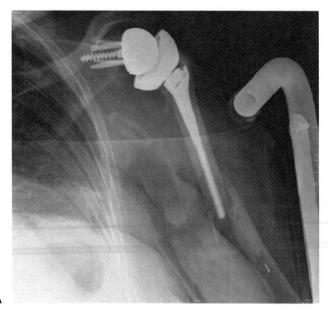

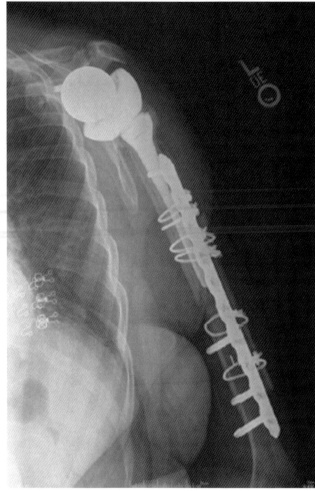

Figure 15.10. (A) This patient sustained a periprosthetic fracture after a fall. (B) The patient's fracture was treated with cables, a locking plate, and a strut allograft.

ROM. Patients with humeral loosening of their implant may present with a dull arm pain that is made worse with ROM movements. Finally, those with periprosthetic fracture typically have some history of trauma and their ROM is limited by pain.

Preoperative imaging should include a full series of shoulder radiographs (true anteroposterior, internal and external rotation, outlet, and axillary views). Radiographs are examined closely for evidence of scapular notching, bone loss, implant or screw breakage, radiolucencies around any of the components, and evidence of instability. In cases in which large amounts of humeral bone loss is observed, bilateral humeral scanograms to assess the overall loss of humeral length may also be helpful. If possible, an attempt should be made to obtain prior postoperative radiographs for comparison to try to determine the progression to failure of the implant. A preoperative CT scan is obtained on all patients as well. This often allows for a closer determination of the remaining bony architecture of the scapula, which aids in defining available bone stock for placement of the glenoid baseplate. Based on the patient's history and physical examination, and the imaging studies obtained, the surgeon should gain an understanding of the previous implant that was placed and what potentially led to failure of the implant, to develop a surgical plan for revising the implant. Each of the modes of failure described often has special circumstances that must be taken into consideration in performing revision surgery; these will be discussed in the following section.

PATIENT POSITIONING AND SURGICAL APPROACH

For surgery the patient is positioned in the upright beach chair position and is administered a general anesthetic in addition to a scalene block. The skin incision may make use of previous skin incisions if they are close to the deltopectoral interval. If the previous incision is not in close proximity to the deltopectoral groove, a separate skin incision must be made. This incision is centered directly over the deltopectoral groove and is often longer than the incision used for primary surgery. Making the incision slightly longer allows for identification of undisturbed tissue planes and can assist in defining normal anatomic planes.

Meticulous dissection must be done in a layered approach and often takes additional time because of thick scar formation. Large subcutaneous flaps are created to correctly identify the deltoid and the pectoralis major. Once the correct location of the deltopectoral interval is found it can then be divided. First, the deltoid needs to be identified and adequately mobilized. We try to begin proximally, as described previously, and find the triangular fat interval between the proximal deltoid and pectoralis major. If this plane has become obscured because of scar tissue, we start distally, separating the distal deltoid from the humeral shaft, and then working proximally. Hohman retractors placed under the proximal deltoid and under the acromion may help to develop the subdeltoid and subacromial spaces, which must be freed. Often the pectoralis major may be scarred down to the conjoined tendon. Additional time is taken to identify the pectoralis major and separate it from the underlying conjoined tendon. Separating these two structures is necessary to find the lateral edge of the conjoined tendon. Once this is found the subcoracoid space can then be identified and freed from the underlying subscapularis, which can be scarred to the conjoined tendon. The axillary nerve can then be palpated and a tug test performed.

If the subscapularis tendon is intact, it is released subperiosteally from the proximal humerus. The humeral capsule is released circumferentially from the humeral neck. At this point the reverse articulation of the glenophere with the humeral socket should be clearly exposed. We typically then use slight lateral traction, and a black-handled retractor is placed between the articulation. Once this is accomplished, gentle external rotation can allow disarticulation and delivers the humeral component anteriorly. At this point the surgeon can make the planned necessary revisions. We will discuss the surgical technique of each of the failure mechanisms in detail.

SURGICAL TECHNIQUES FOR GLENOID-SIDE FAILURES

For patients with both scapular notching and mechanical failure of the baseplate there is similar pathology that must be addressed in the revision setting. In revising each of these failures the surgeon will most likely be faced with glenoid bone loss. In the setting in which scapular notching has led to osteolysis and loss of bone on the inferior glenoid and scapular neck, the surgeon should have two primary goals at the time of revision. The first should be to limit further impingement of the humeral component on the scapula, and the second should be to place a new glenosphere that will achieve stable fixation into the remaining available bone stock.

To treat patients with symptomatic notching an understanding of what factors can be used to treat or avoid this problem is necessary. Gutierrez et al[13] performed a biomechanical study evaluating different implant positions and combinations to find ways to limit scapular impingement of the humeral socket on the inferior aspect of the glenoid, which results in the previously mentioned adduction deficit. The authors performed this biomechanical study using varying combinations of humeral neck-shaft angle, baseplate position on the glenosphere, center of rotation offset of the glenosphere, and inferior tilt of the glenosphere to develop a hierarchy of the factors that may limit scapular impingement of the humeral socket. After testing all possible combinations and performing a regression analysis the authors determined that, in order of importance, using a humeral neck-shaft angle with a more varus angle of inclination (135 degrees) was the best way to limit scapular notching (Table 15.1). Placing the baseplate in the inferior third of the glenoid, choosing a glenosphere with a more lateral center of rotation, and inferiorly tilting the glenosphere followed this.

Knowledge of this hierarchy of factors to limit scapular notching gives the surgeon choices at the time of revision. Certain humeral components offer a more varus inclination of the humeral socket. If the humeral socket has been significantly damaged by scapular impingement, the surgeon may want to consider extracting the humeral component and placing a stem and socket that has a more varus angle of inclination. Given the morbidity associated with stem removal, and if the humeral component is salvageable, the surgeon may choose to revise the glenoid side of the device (Fig. 15.11). In planning for revision of the glenoid, we hope to optimize this hierarchy of factors on the glenoid side of the articulation to limit future scapular impingement. We attempt to place a baseplate in the inferior third of the glenoid; use a more lateral center of rotation than is present in the Grammont design, which is the implant most associated with notching[3,4,8]; and attempt to inferiorly tilt the implant. Inferiorly tilting the implant can be difficult and is not always achieved given the level of bone loss that often accompanies these revision cases; however, these are methods we keep in mind during the procedure.

TABLE 15.1	Humeral Neck-Shaft Angle to Limit Scapular Notching		
Study Factor	Condition	Number with No Adduction Deficit	Percentage (%)
Humeral angle (degrees)	130	49	61
	150	17	21
	170	0	0
Location	Inferior	41	51
	Neutral	13	16
	Superior	12	15
Tilt	Inferior	30	37
	Neutral	23	28
	Superior	13	16
COR Offset (mm)	10	32	40
	5	22	27
	0	12	15
Diameter (mm)	42	28	35
	36	21	26
	30	17	21

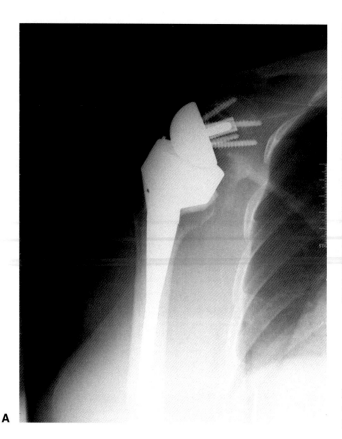

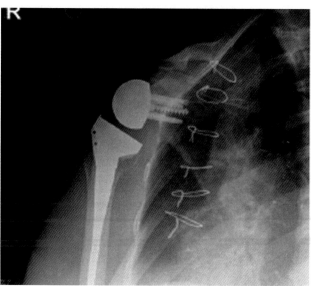

Figure 15.11. (A) This patient developed symptomatic scapular notching. (B) The patient was treated with a revision to a glenosphere with lateral offset to minimize scapular impingement.

In approaching the glenoid the different implant designs vary in how the glenosphere must be removed from the baseplate. Some method must be employed by the surgeon to remove the glenosphere from the baseplate. The implant we currently use allows a T-handled device that threads into the apex of the glenosphere to facilitate easy disimpaction of the Morse taper and glenosphere removal. This is not available on all designs, and removing the glenosphere can be a struggle depending on the previous implant used. Once the glenosphere is removed, adequate glenoid exposure is the next step. Glenoid exposure is accomplished by retracting the proximal humerus posteriorly using a posterior glenoid retractor and performing an aggressive 360-degree subperiosteal periglenoid capsular release. A Hohman retractor is then placed anteriorly on the glenoid neck, and a second Hohman retractor is placed at the superior aspect of the glenoid. With protection of the axillary nerve, the inferior capsule is then resected. After glenoid exposure the baseplate is extracted as well, and all hardware and broken screws that can block placement of a new baseplate should be removed. In most instances, several of the broken screws are left in place when removal is not required. At this point the surgeon must do a careful visual assessment of the available glenoid bone stock and take note of the areas of glenoid deficiency.

In patients who demonstrate minimal glenoid bone loss the ideal position of the central screw will follow the path of the centering line described by Matsen,[7] in which the central screw exits anteriorly on the scapular body. This typically will provide at least 25 mm of bone for the screw to achieve purchase. However, in cases of severe glenoid bone loss this position of the center screw

will provide for an inadequate amount of bone to secure the screw (<25 mm). Therefore a different orientation of the screw should be achieved to increase the amount of bone captured by this screw. In our work examining cadaveric shoulders, as well as our operative experience, we have found that a dense column of bone is present in the area where the scapular spine meets the scapular body (Fig. 15.12). When evaluating the CT scan in the

Acromion

Glenoid

Coracoid

Figure 15.12. At the junction of the scapular spine and scapular body there is a dense column of bone.

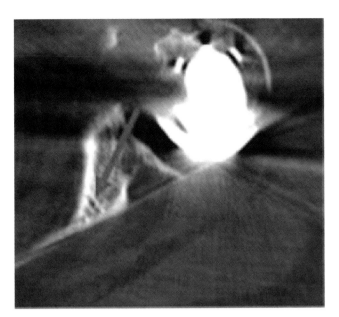

Figure 15.13. Preoperative computed tomography scan with area indicating the dense region of bone to be captured with the central screw.

preoperative setting, we try and identify the anticipated trajectory of the center screw (Fig. 15.13). Additionally, in these circumstances of significant glenoid bone loss, restoration of glenoid bone stock with bone grafting techniques has been helpful.

It can be challenging reconstructing the glenoid side and achieving stable fixation when there is minimal bone stock present. In addition to loss of the peripheral bone, a varying degree of the central cavitation of the glenoid may be present secondary to the previous implant's fixation. The following method has been used to deal with glenoid bone loss. In cases of severe glenoid bone loss (Fig. 15.14), it is critical to obtain adequate purchase with the central screw of the baseplate. As noted previously, a dense column of bone is present in the area where the scapular spine meets the scapular body. To access this column of dense bone, we orient the drill slightly more posteriorly than we would for a primary reverse shoulder prosthesis with no glenoid bone loss, while at the same time attempting to incorporate 10 to 15 degrees of inferior tilt (Fig. 15.15). This posterior trajectory allows penetration of this thick bony area at the base of the scapular spine. In tapping this area after drilling, we have been able to achieve an impressive amount of purchase despite the level of bone loss (Fig. 15.16). The superior and inferior screws are in line with the central screw of the baseplate; therefore, if the central screw is properly positioned, the superior and inferior screws typically will have excellent purchase as well. Once this central position is felt to be adequate, we place a structural bone graft around the 6.5-mm tap and secure with Kirschner wires. The glenoid is then reamed to allow the grafted region to match the rest of the glenoid (Fig. 15.17). In global defects, which can be encountered after failed reverse shoulder arthroplasty, the entire glenoid has been eroded and the only remaining bone is the junction of the coracoid base with the scapular body. Despite this level of bone loss in several cases, this technique of central screw fixation down the column of bone between the scapular spine has been successful.

The baseplate is then placed via the central screw, and the superior, inferior, anterior, and posterior screws are placed to

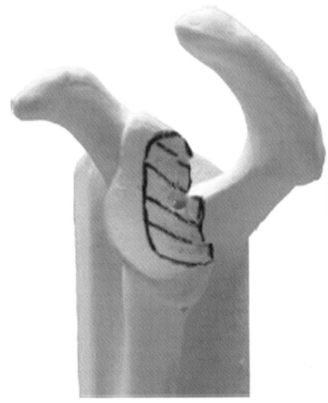

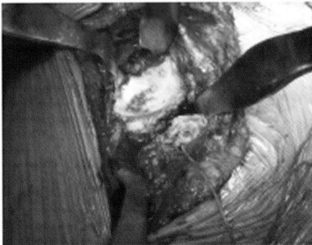

Figure 15.14. Sawbones model and intraoperative image showing severe posterior glenoid erosion.

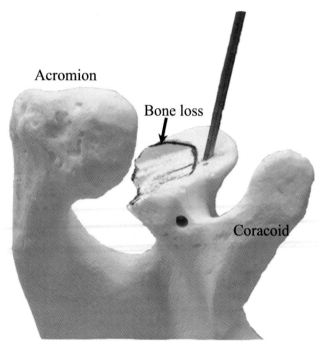

Figure 15.15.   This posterior trajectory is used to attempt to engage the dense column of bone at the junction of the scapular spine and scapular body.

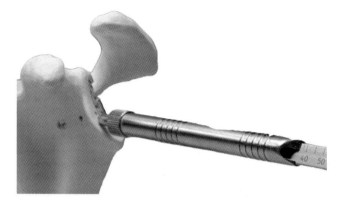

Figure 15.16.   Depth gauge showing the orientation used during drilling.

secure the baseplate (Fig. 15.18). We currently use 5.0-mm peripheral locking screws for fixation of the baseplate. In the previously referenced study by Harman et al,[10] 5.0-mm peripheral locking screws provided excellent fixation and limited the micromotion at the baseplate bone interface to less than 150 microns, which is generally the accepted threshold to allow for bony ingrowth. If the baseplate were inserted with 10 to 15 degrees of inferior tilt, we believe that too would augment fixation. In a study by Gutierrez et al[13] a glenosphere placed in 15 degrees of inferior tilt produced a compressive load at the baseplate-bone interface and decreased the shear stress at the superior and inferior

aspects of the baseplate compared to a glenosphere placed in neutral or 15 degrees of superior tilt. Since incorporating the 5.0-mm peripheral locking screws, along with an inferiorly tilted glenosphere, we have yet to have a mechanical failure of the baseplate in 405 cases to date. Therefore, in revision cases such as a previously failed baseplate with accompanying bone loss, we find this fixation extremely advantageous.

As noted previously, we prefer to use a glenosphere with a lateral center of rotation to move the humeral component away from the scapula to provide a greater impingement-free arc of motion. The implant we use offers modularity with respect to the amount of lateral offset available (10, 6, 4, and 0 mm). Clearly, the more lateral offset that is selected, the greater the moment arm and resultant forces at the baseplate-bone interface will be. Given that, in these revision cases that often require glenoid bone grafting, a slightly more medial center of rotation (0.4 mm) is typically selected. This type of glenosphere offers an extended hooded coverage that may be used to dial into any remaining defect, thereby protecting the graft and providing additional support of the graft and a decreased amount of force across the baseplate-glenoid interface (Fig. 15.19). We have found this strategy successful regardless of the location of bone

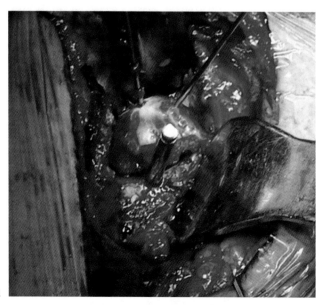

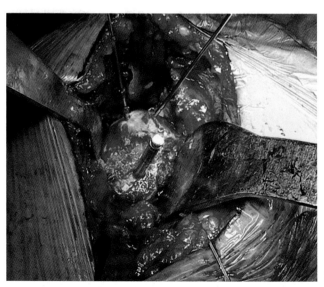

Figure 15.17.   **(A,B)** The graft is reamed to match the native glenoid.

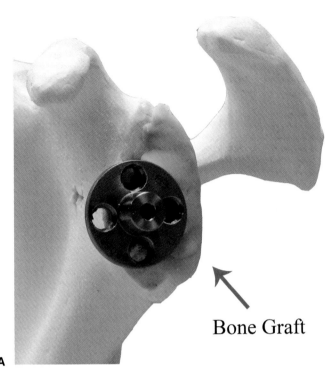

A

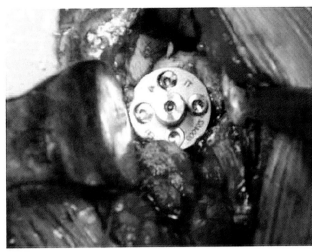

B

Figure 15.18.   **(A,B)** Sawbones model and intraoperative image of a grafted glenoid defect.

Bone Graft

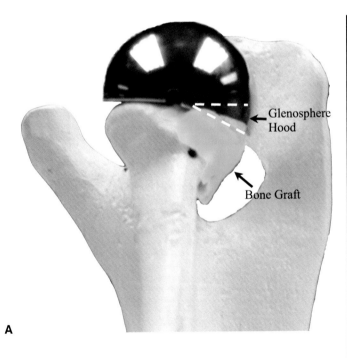

A

Glenosphere Hood

Bone Graft

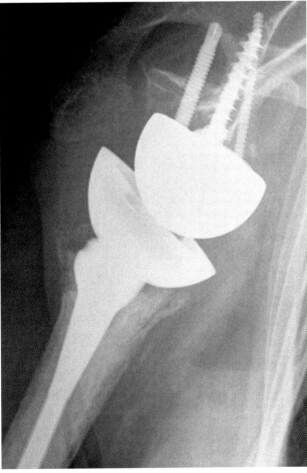

B

Figure 15.19.   **(A)** Sawbones model with the glenosphere with extended hood coverage to protect and further compress the graft. **(B)** Postoperative radiograph of a case in which the glenoid was grafted because of severe glenoid bone loss.

loss, be it posterior, superior, or anterior; this is the method we use in revision in patients with glenoid-side failure resulting from scapular notching or mechanical failure of the implant.

The last type of glenoid-side failure that warrants discussion is glenosphere dissociation. As stated earlier, technical error can lead to this complication. To this end we now employ several techniques to ensure proper taper impaction and stability at the time of surgery. To avoid the need for revision surgery, we make every effort to keep the taper dry at the time of glenosphere placement. After impaction of the glenosphere the connection is checked via a distraction force that is applied with a T-handled instrument that is threaded into the glenosphere. If the connection is stable, the glenosphere will remain stable. We also use a retaining screw to augment taper connection in all cases. The surgical tactics are similar to the approach for other causes of glenoid failure but require special attention in ensuring all bone and soft tissue are cleaned around the baseplate and some sort of intraoperative verification that the locking mechanism for the prosthetic system used is clearly understood.

SURGICAL TECHNIQUES FOR HUMERAL-SIDE FAILURES

In attempting to surgically treat recurrent dislocation we believe it is valuable to have a have a device that offers modularity with respect to glenosphere size and offset, as well as options on the humeral side with varying thickness in the socket and levels of constraint.

We use a deltopectoral approach, as previously described in this chapter, to provide exposure. Once the implants are exposed the joint can often be reduced and the shoulder placed through ROM movements to assess stability. We pay careful attention to the position of arm adduction, internal rotation, and extension because we think this is the position of greatest potential instability. In evaluating the articulation, one factor that may become apparent is that the version of one or both of the components may be responsible for the recurrent instability. In certain instances the glenosphere may have been placed in an anteverted position, leading to anterior instability. Similarly, malrotation of the humeral component can be a factor as well and can often be observed by carefully inspecting the orientation of the component throughout the ROM at the revision setting. Ideally, in cases of mismatched version, one would prefer to retain the glenosphere and baseplate because removal and reorientation would provide significant potential morbidity if it were well fixed and in-grown into the glenoid. Altering the humeral version to match the glenoid may be a more reasonable option to reestablish stability of the articulation.

In many cases it is not simply version mismatch that accounts for instability. The soft tissue tension of the shoulder plays a substantial role in the stability of the reverse articulation. In assessing the stability of the articulation the surgeon may discover that laxity in the soft tissues accounts for an inability to hold the articulation reduced through ROM. In these instances the surgeon must have options to increase the soft tissue tension in the shoulder. Depending on the implant used previously, the options as to how to adjust the soft tissue tension varies. If a glenosphere with a more medial center of rotation had previously been implanted, at the time of revision one could place a glenosphere with a more lateral center of rotation to increase the soft tissue tension. Using a larger diameter glenosphere may

also impart added stability by increasing the volume within the shoulder and thereby increasing the overall soft tension as well. On the humeral side, most implant systems offer varying thickness polyethylene sockets with different amounts of constraint (neutral-semiconstrained, +4 mm, +4 mm semiconstrained, +8 mm, +8 mm semiconstrained) to assist in increasing the soft tissue tension and stability of the reduction. The surgeon should test these various humeral combinations in an effort to find a stable reduction. In selecting an implant with more constraint the surgeon may sacrifice some ROM of the articulation and at the same time increase the forces across the implant as a result of this increased constraint.

In certain instances when a glenosphere with a medial center of rotation was used, scapular impingement may potentially lead to the humeral component levering out of the articulation, leading to dislocation. In these instances, revising the glenosphere to a more lateral center of rotation is often necessary. By moving the center of rotation laterally the humeral component will then have a greater impingement-free arc of motion and thus more stability of the articulation.

The role of bone loss in instability is an often overlooked factor. Both glenoid-side and humeral-side bone loss may play a role in recurrent dislocation. In cases in which severe glenoid erosion has occurred the joint line can become medialized in relation to its normal location. In these instances, the surgeon may attempt to place a glenosphere with a slightly more medial center of rotation (6, 4, or 0 mm) to decrease the forces at the baseplate-bone interface given the amount of bone loss. The surgeon should be wary of this in that the medialization of the joint line from this severe erosion may produce a relative laxity in the soft tissues surrounding the shoulder joint, resulting in an unstable reverse articulation (Fig. 15.20). In these cases we have occasionally chosen to use a glenosphere with the most lateral amount of center of rotation offset (10 mm) in an effort to compensate for this medialization and attempt to restore some soft tissue tension.

As noted previously in this chapter, a different mechanism of instability can result in patients having substantial proximal humeral bone loss and is related to the vector of the pull of the deltoid in these cases. We feel that placing a reverse shoulder arthroplasty in these cases without restoring the proximal humeral bone can lead to potential problems, one of them being instability. One of the benefits of restoring the proximal humerus via allografting, as we have described in the literature,[6] is that it allows the deltoid to maintain its normal contour and vector and thereby provide a compressive force at the articulation (Fig. 15.21).

In performing proximal humeral allografting the previously mentioned deltopectoral approach is used. On the back table a fresh-frozen humeral allograft is prepared to match the proximal humerus. To do this, we cut the humeral head of the proximal humeral allograft at the level of the anatomic neck and remove all the cancellous allograft bone from the intramedullary canal. We then determine the appropriate height of the allograft by determining the amount of diaphyseal bone remaining and estimating the amount of proximal humerus that must be replaced to restore the bone stock and allow for a stable reduction (Fig. 15.22). An oscillating saw is then used to create a step-cut of the metaphyseal bone where 5 cm of bone remains laterally, creating a lateral plate, and 1 to 2 cm of bone remains medially (Fig. 15.23). All soft tissue is removed, with the exception of the subscapularis tendon,

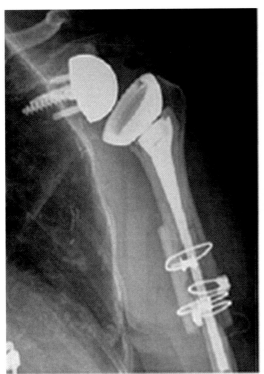

A

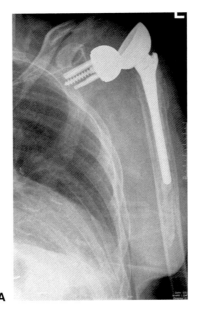

A

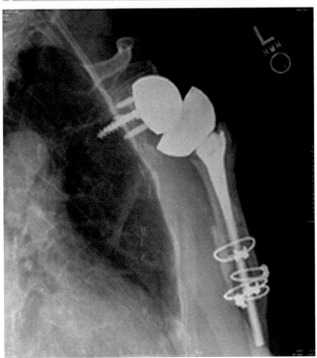

B

Figure 15.20. (**A,B**) This patient had severe glenoid erosion resulting in soft tissue laxity and subsequent dislocation, treated with revision to a glenosphere with the maximum lateral offset to restore soft tissue tension.

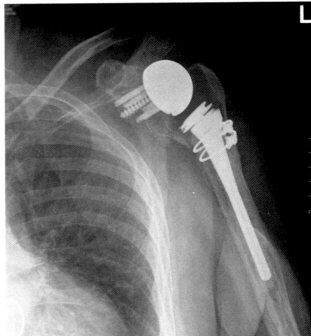

B

Figure 15.21. (**A**) This patient originally had a hemiarthroplasty with cuff deficiency treated with a reverse prosthesis, but the proximal humeral bone loss was not restored when the original reverse shoulder arthroplasty was implanted. Insufficient deltoid tension was present postoperatively and the shoulder was unstable. (**B**) Subsequently the surgery was revised with proximal humeral allograft and a larger glenosphere. Adequate deltoid tension was restored and the shoulder instability resolved.

which can later be used for repair of the patient's subscapularis. The proximal humeral allograft is then cabled to the native humerus, and a humeral guide is used to ensure that the humeral stem and allograft are oriented correctly (Fig. 15.24). The humeral component is cemented into this construct and the cables tightened (Fig. 15.25). It is in these revi-

sion cases particularly that we test and consider the various humeral implants (neutral, neutral-semiconstrained, +4 mm, +4 semiconstrained, +8 mm, +8 semiconstrained), depending on the soft tissue balancing and degree of instability.

As noted previously, another humeral-side mode of failure that may lead to revision surgery is loosening of the humeral component. In these cases, that lack of metaphyseal support of the implant allows all of the forces of the constrained

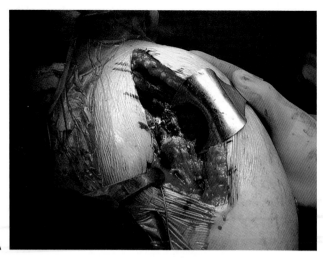

A

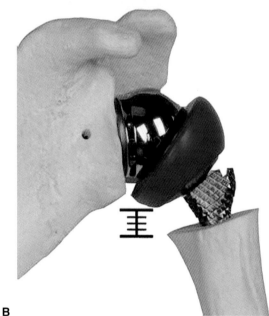

B

Figure 15.22. **(A)** Intraoperative image of severe proximal humeral bone loss. **(B)** The amount of bone stock that needs to be restored is measured with the trial implant in place. **(C)** Intraoperative image demonstrating amount of proximal humeral bone that needs to be compensated for with allografting.

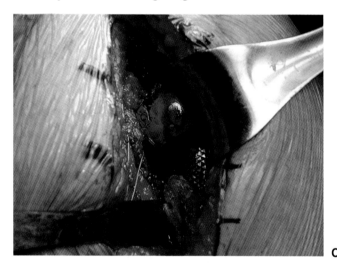

C

articulation to be transmitted to the stem with the diaphysis. In these cases we revise the humeral component and place a proximal humeral allograft to reconstitute the proximal humerus (Fig. 15.26). The allografted metaphyseal portion of the proximal humerus is then in a position to share the load of the forces transmitted to the humeral side of the articulation.

Humeral socket failure after primary reverse shoulder arthroplasty is another mode of failure we have treated with revision surgery. Treatment of the complication depends on the mode of failure. In some patients, if trauma has led to fracture or dissociation of the polyethylene, simply exchanging the polyethylene may be sufficient. However, some polyethylene failures may be directly related to impingement of the polyethylene on the scapular neck. In these patients, further consideration must be given to possibly revising the glenosphere to a more lateral center of rotation to give the humeral component a greater impingement-free arc of motion.

Periprosthetic fracture management most typically depends on the status of the implant. If, along with the fracture, the prosthesis remains stable, it may be possible to treat the patient nonoperatively or with an open reduction and internal fixation using plates, cables, or strut grafting, depending on the level of the fracture. However, if the humeral component is loose, revision of the implant is necessary. In these cases, we often use an extended deltopectoral approach that reaches into the anterolateral approach to the humerus. We use intraoperative fluoroscopy, and given the level of the fracture, we are prepared for the possible use of long-stemmed implants if necessary.

TREATMENT OF INFECTION AFTER REVERSE SHOULDER ARTHROPLASTY

Treatment of infection after reverse shoulder arthroplasty can be approached in a fashion similar to that in other infected

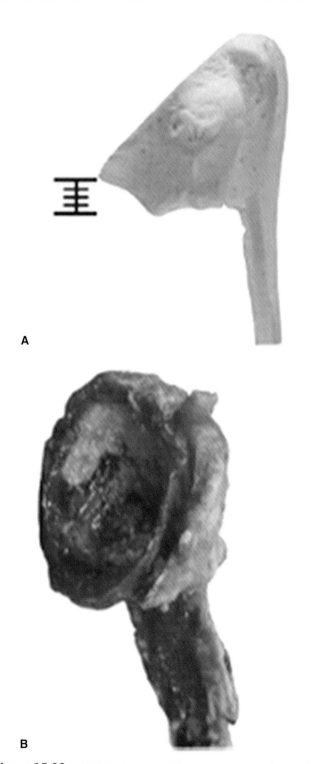

A

B

Figure 15.23. **(A,B)** Sawbones model and intraoperative image of a proximal humeral allograft.

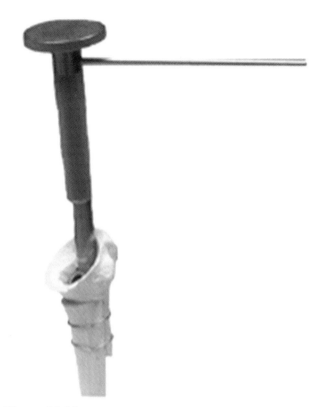

Figure 15.24. Sawbones model demonstrating how the proximal humeral allograft is cabled to the native humerus and a version guide is used to ensure the correct orientation as the humeral stem is placed into the allograft construct.

performed a single-stage conversion of an infected reverse arthroplasty to perform only one surgical insult in the patient. To date we have not had a recurrence of infection in either of these groups of patients, be it two stage or one stage.

POSTOPERATIVE PROTOCOL AND REHABILITATION

Postoperatively we place all patients in a shoulder immobilizer. The patient begins pendulum exercises on postoperative day 1, along with active elbow, wrist, and hand ROM exercises. The patient wears the immobilizer for the first 6 weeks, performing the pendulum exercises on a daily basis, but does no other active or active-assisted ROM exercises of the operative shoulder. At postoperative week 6 the immobilizer is discontinued and the patient is progressed to passive ROM exercises of the operative extremity, working on forward elevation. The patient can begin using the arm for dressing, bathing, and feeding, but is still limited to lifting no weight greater than 2 lb with the operative extremity. At 3 months the patient is cleared to light strengthening and able to participate fully in hobbies such as golf. With respect to the use of the arm, we encourage patients to return to most of their preferred recreational activities. Activities of concern are contact sports because of the risk of fracture or dislocation and bowling because the weight of the ball produces a distractive force that could cause dislocation. If the patient wants to bowl, we discourage using balls heavier than 9 or 10 lb. We follow patients at 6 weeks, 3 months,

arthroplasties. The primary goal is elimination of the infection, and the secondary goal is future reconstruction of the shoulder. We think that in patients who are medically stable and without a significant number of comorbidities, the treatment of choice is a two-stage exchange of the implant using an antibiotic-impregnated spacer and 6 weeks of intravenous antibiotics, followed by conversion to a new reverse shoulder arthroplasty. In some patients with significant medical comorbidities, we have

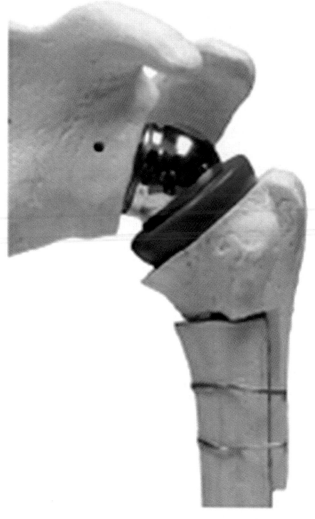

A

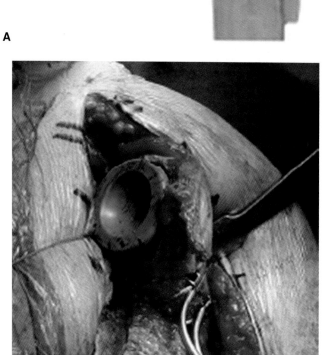

B

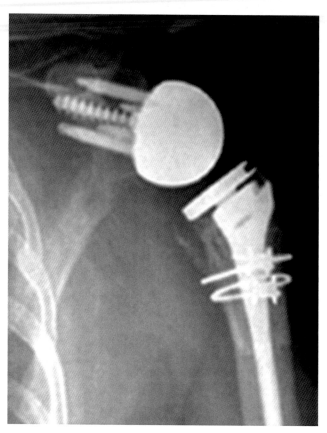

C

Figure 15.25.   (A) Sawbones, (B) intraoperative, and (C) post-operative images showing the final allograft-prosthetic construct.

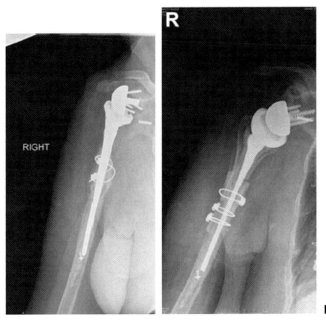

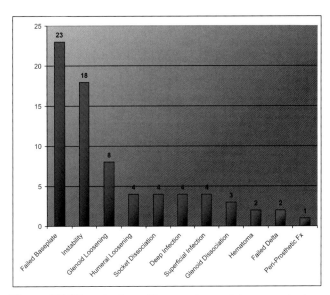

Figure 15.26. (A) Radiograph of a reverse shoulder prosthesis in which the proximal humerus has severe bone loss. This implant went on to loosen. (B) This was treated with revision and proximal humeral allografting.

Figure 15.27. This figure illustrates the conditions necessitating revision surgery. Some patients had a combination of problems that led to revision. For example, patients with infection could also have prosthetic loosening.

6 months, 9 months, and 1 year points and then yearly after that. We videotape all patients beginning at 3 months postoperatively performing a ROM protocol doing the best attempt at active forward elevation, abduction, external rotation, and internal rotation at each office visit. This is kept and catalogued for comparison to the preoperative ROM and for research purposes.

OUR EXPERIENCE WITH REVISION REVERSE ARTHROPLASTY

To date, we have preformed 56 revisions of reverse shoulder arthroplasty in 25 men (25 shoulders) and 30 women (31 shoulders) with average age of 71. The two most common indications for the revision surgery in our series included mechanical failure of the baseplate (23 patients) and instability (18 patients) (Fig. 15.27). Patients undergoing revision surgery were followed for an average of 44 months, during which time their outcome scores and patient satisfaction ratings were collected. While treating these patients, the mean American Shoulder and Elbow Surgeons (ASES) scores improved from 31 to 52 and simple shoulder test (SST) scores improved from 1.5 to 3.6. Preoperatively, Visual Analogue Scale (VAS) pain scores were 7 and improved to 3.8 postoperatively, and the VAS function scores were 2.8 preoperatively and improved to 4.3 postoperatively. Forward flexion improved from 58 to 85, abduction improved from 45 to 81, and external rotation improved from 14.8 to 19.6. In terms of patient satisfaction, 15 patients rated their outcome as excellent, 16 good, 11 satisfied, and 9 unsatisfied (5 patients did not have satisfaction ratings available).

COMPLICATIONS AFTER REVISION REVERSE ARTHROPLASTY

Revision of reverse shoulder arthroplasty has proven to be a procedure fraught with many potential complications. In the 56 revisions of reverse shoulder arthroplasty we performed, 36 complications occurred in 20 of the patients (37%) (Fig. 15.28). The most common complications were chronic instability (6) and humeral socket dissociation (5). Revision surgery using reverse shoulder arthroplasty to treat other failed arthroplasty has been reported to be as high as 50%.[4] The number of complications associated with revising reverse arthroplasty clearly speaks to the difficult nature of these procedures.

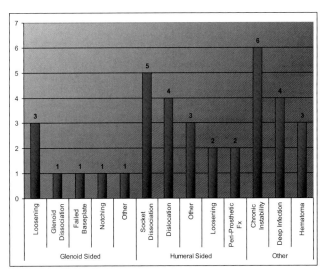

Figure 15.28. The frequency of complications seen in our series by glenoid-side, humeral-side, and others.

FUTURE DIRECTIONS AND CONCLUSION

Reverse shoulder arthroplasty remains a relatively new treatment in the armamentarium of shoulder surgeons. Good long-term studies are needed to better understand the longevity and ultimate modes of failure of these devices. With continued study, we hope that improved surgical technique and advancements in implant design and instrumentation will continue to help the learning curve progress as surgeons attempt to treat the difficult problem of a failed reverse shoulder arthroplasty.

REFERENCES

1. Lee RD, Carter L. Modeling and forecasting the time series of U.S. mortality, *J Am Stat Assoc* 1992;87:659–671.
2. Frankle M, Siegal S, Pupello D, et al. The reverse shoulder prosthesis for glenohumeral arthritis associated with severe rotator cuff deficiency: a minimum 2-year follow-up study of 60 patients. *J Bone Joint Surg Am* 2005;87:1697–1705.
3. Sirveaux F, Favard L, Oudet D, et al. Grammont-inverted total shoulder arthroplasty in the treatment of glenohumeral osteoarthritis with massive rupture of the cuff: results of a multicentre study of 80 shoulders. *J Bone Joint Surg Br* 2004;86:388–395.
4. Werner C, Steinmann P, Gilbart M, et al. Treatment of painful pseudoparesis due to irreparable rotator cuff dysfunction with the Delta III reverse-ball-and-socket total shoulder prosthesis. *J Bone Joint Surg Am* 2005;87:1476–1486.
5. Valenti PH, Boutens D, Nerot C. Delta III reversed prosthesis for arthritis with massive rotator cuff tear: long-term results (>5 years). In: Walch G, Boileau P, Molé D, eds. *2000 Shoulder Prosthesis: 2- to 10-Year Follow-up.* Montpellier, France: Sauramps Medical; 2001:253–259.
6. Levy JC, Virani N, Pupello D, et al. Use of the reverse shoulder prosthesis for the treatment of failed hemiarthroplasty in patients with glenohumeral arthritis and rotator cuff deficiency. *J Bone Joint Surg Br* 2007;89:189–195.
7. Matsen FA III, Boileau P, Walch G, et al. The reverse total shoulder arthroplasty. *J Bone Joint Surg Am* 2007;89:660–667.
8. Simovitch RW, Zumstein MA, Lohri E. Predictors of scapular notching in patients managed with the Delta III reverse total shoulder replacement. *J Bone Joint Surg Am* 2007;89:588–600.
9. Nyffeler RW, Werner CM, Simmen BR, et al. Analysis of a retrieved Delta III total shoulder prosthesis. *J Bone Joint Surg Br* 2004; 86:1187–1191.
10. Harman M, Frankle M, Vasey M, et al. Initial glenoid component fixation in "reverse" total shoulder arthroplasty: a biomechanical evaluation. *J Shoulder Elbow Surg* 2005;14:S162–S167.
11. Guery J, Favard L, Sirveaux F, et al. Reverse total shoulder arthroplasty: survivorship analysis of 80 replacements followed for 5 to 10 years. *J Bone Joint Surg Am* 2006;88:1742–1747.
12. Blevins FT, Deng X, Torzilli PA, et al. Dissociation of modular humeral head components: a biomechanical and implant retrieval study. *J Shoulder Elbow Surg* 1997;6:113–124.
13. Gutierrez S, Greiwe R, Frankle M, et al. Biomechanical comparison of component position and hardware failure in the reverse shoulder prosthesis. *J Shoulder Elbow Surg* 2007;3S:9–S12.

Jay Smith
Jonathan T. Finnoff

Postoperative Rehabilitation

"When a surgeon realizes that technical expertise is responsible for only a small part of the success picture, and that a well-designed and executed rehabilitation program is mandatory, a successful outcome can be realized."—John Brems, MD[1]

INTRODUCTION

Patients undergoing revision or complex primary total shoulder arthroplasty are by definition a challenging patient population for shoulder surgeons to successfully manage. Bone loss, rotator cuff insufficiency, scarring, and nerve injury not only dictate the range of usable components but may also necessitate modification of component placement, bone grafting, soft tissue release or repair, or concomitant tendon transfer.[2,3] Furthermore, candidates for revision or complex primary total shoulder arthroplasty are typically older patients with multiple comorbidities. Successful management of these patients requires a skillful surgeon working in conjunction with the patient, the patient's family and caregivers, and a qualified rehabilitation team.[4]

Regardless of the complexities of any individual case, the primary goal of the surgical and rehabilitation process is to restore optimal, pain-free function within the anatomic and physiological constraints of the patient and his or her shoulder. Although individualization of the rehabilitation program is a necessity, each program should be based on fundamental principles reflective of the current, admittedly limited, scientific knowledge and accumulated, collective clinical experience.[1,4–6] Multiple total shoulder arthroplasty rehabilitation programs have been detailed in the literature.[1,4–8] The primary purpose of this chapter is to familiarize surgeons with the contemporary principles of rehabilitation as they apply to revision and complex primary total shoulder arthroplasty. These principles form the foundation on which surgeons can work with their rehabilitation team to create rational and modifiable rehabilitation programs for individual patients (Table 16.1).

ESTABLISH EFFECTIVE COMMUNICATION

Effective communication among the surgeon, patient, patient's family and caregivers, and rehabilitation team members is essential for a successful outcome.[1,4,7,9] Preoperatively, the surgeon should meet with the patient and the patient's family to outline the surgical procedure and establish realistic goals based on the complexities of the individual case. For many revision and complex primary total shoulder arthroplasties, pain relief is the primary goal, whereas range of motion (ROM), strength, and functional improvements may be secondary.[3,8] It is essential that the expectations are outlined and agreed on before the surgery. This includes not only the ultimate expected outcomes but also the anticipated duration of time to achieve these outcomes.[1,4]

The patient should also meet with the physical therapist during the preoperative period.[1,4,7] The surgeon should communicate to the therapist the case-specific challenges that may be encountered during postoperative rehabilitation and anticipated modifications to the program. The therapist ensures that the patient and his or her family and other supporters understand their central role in the rehabilitation process, reinforces the expected outcomes as determined by the surgeon, and outlines the general aspects of the rehabilitation program. The therapist also educates the patient regarding pain and stiffness in the postoperative period, and methods that may be used to improve patient comfort. This discussion serves to reduce patient anxiety and fear. Finally, as time permits, preoperative exercise instruction may be provided. Areas of particular focus include functional lower limb strength and balance training, posture exercises, scapulothoracic ROM exercises, and isometric strengthening exercises. These exercises may be started immediately to improve the patient's balance and potentially prevent a devastating fall in the postoperative period, as well as initiate the process of optimizing the function of the scapulothoracic articulation, which is a key component for shoulder function after arthroplasty.[10,11]

ENSURE ADEQUATE PAIN CONTROL

The importance of maintaining adequate pain control in the postoperative period cannot be overemphasized. Pain relief is the primary goal of shoulder arthroplasty surgery. Failure to control pain in the postoperative period can easily be misconstrued by the patient as a failure of the operation itself and thereby sabotage the rehabilitation process. First, the patient must have the motivation to participate in the rehabilitation process. Second, pain reflexively inhibits shoulder girdle muscle control and may result in potentially damaging muscle activation and co-contraction during rehabilitative exercises.[12–14]

TABLE 16.1	Principles of Rehabilitation Following Revision and Complex Primary Total Shoulder Arthroplasty

Establish effective communication
   Surgeon, patient, family, rehabilitation team
   Preoperative and postoperative
Obtain adequate pain control
   Preemptive analgesia for exercise sessions
   Medications
   Modalities
Initiate early, atraumatic motion
   Individualized parameters
   Position of stability (e.g., plane of the scapula)
   Include the scapulothoracic articulation
Optimize upper limb function
   Realistic goals established preoperatively, modified as necessary
   Appropriate strengthening
   Address kinetic chain to support shoulder
Modify program based on case specifics
   Patient factors
   Surgical factors

It is essential to discuss pain control during the preoperative visit, as noted earlier. Some pain should be expected and the management methods outlined. This educational process should be continued postoperatively. The patient should be reassured that some degree of pain and stiffness is normal, that measures will be taken to control it, and that it will improve over time. The surgeon and rehabilitation team should also emphasize the importance of early mobilization in reducing pain and facilitating the rehabilitation process.[15]

The surgeon should work closely with the anesthesiologists to ensure adequate analgesia, accounting for patient-specific comorbidities. The increased use of interscalene blocks has facilitated the early rehabilitation process because patients are able to visualize the intraoperative and early postoperative motion and realize that there are no mechanical blocks to motion.[1,4] Analgesic medications should be administered 30 minutes before therapy so that their optimal effects may coincide with the exercise session. Similarly, after the acute inflammatory phase subsides, a hot pack applied 30 minutes before therapy will facilitate muscle relaxation and increased blood flow to the area in preparation for the session.[1,4,16] Following exercise, application of an ice pack or cooling device will reduce the pain and inflammation incurred by the session itself.[16,17] The appropriate use of analgesics, heat, and cryotherapy can significantly facilitate the rehabilitation process, particularly when applied correctly.[16,17] As necessary, these interventions may be supplemented by other pain-relieving modalities, such as electrical stimulation (e.g., transcutaneous electrical nerve stimulation [TENS]) and biofeedback, unless otherwise contraindicated.[16]

INITIATE EARLY ATRAUMATIC MOTION

Adequate ROM is a prerequisite for optimal functional outcome. The ROM goals for any patient should be established in the preoperative period and modified postoperatively as appropriate. For some patients, pain relief may be the primary surgical goal

and the role of ROM exercises may simply be to prevent stiffness, minimize muscle atrophy, and facilitate pain control through proprioceptive mechanisms.[15,18] Other patients may be expected to regain arm elevation above 90 degrees and therefore require a more structured ROM rehabilitation program to provide a foundation for subsequently implemented resistive and functional exercises. In all cases, early ROM exercise is also necessary to promote collagen synthesis and alignment and minimize contracture and scar formation.[19,20] These benefits should be weighed against the potential for overly aggressive ROM exercises to result in pain and potentially injure the healing soft tissues.

Advances in surgical techniques, including deltoid preservation, improved component design and placement, and restoration of myofascial sleeve tension, have facilitated early ROM exercises in patients who have undergone shoulder arthroplasty.[1,4,7] Despite these advances, there is no single ROM program that can be used for all patients. Each patient's program must be modified based on case-specific factors. Whereas previous articles and chapters have outlined an array of specific exercises to facilitate motion in the postoperative period, this section will focus on important concepts in designing and modifying ROM exercise progressions for patients after revision or complex primary total shoulder arthroplasty.[1,4,6,7]

IMMOBILIZATION

Many surgeons will immobilize postperatively patients who have undergone shoulder arthroplasty. In the absence of guiding scientific evidence, the type and duration of immobilization is based primarily on surgeon preference, collective clinical experience, and the complexities of the specific case. Immobilization has ranged from a simple sling worn for a week in uncomplicated arthroplasty to 6 weeks in 30 to 40 degrees of abduction and 30 to 40 degrees of rotation for reverse total shoulder arthroplasty supplemented by latissimus dorsi and teres major tendon transfer.[2,5] In general, the type and duration of immobilization is influenced by component design and placement, intraoperative stable ROM, extent and quality of soft tissue repair, and presence or absence of concomitant tendon transfers.

During this early period of immobilization, the patient may perform wrist, hand, and elbow ROM exercises. In addition, lower limb strengthening, balance, and posture exercises may be implemented. Lower limb strengthening will facilitate improved balance during immobilization and potentially reduce fall risk. Posture exercises such as deep breathing and scapular retraction promote thoracic extension and scapulothoracic control.[21-23] In addition, deep breathing may promote muscle relaxation and facilitate pain control.

It is also possible for patients to initiate scapulothoracic ROM exercises during periods of immobilization, as addressed later in this section.

ESTABLISHING THE RANGE OF MOTION PROGRAM

As the period of immobilization and protection is completed, the patient enters the period of remobilization. Several concepts are relevant during this phase and will be reviewed.

In general, patients tolerate multiple short-duration sessions per day better than one or two prolonged sessions.[1,4,8] In practice, three to five 5- to 10-minute sessions per day should be implemented. This high-frequency, short-duration exercise regimen provides several advantages. First, its simplicity improves compliance. Second, short-duration sessions minimize the risk for incurring fatigue or tissue injury during any particular session. Shoulder muscle fatigue has been documented to result in force-couple imbalance, scapulothoracic dyskinesis, and reduced proprioception.[24–26] Third, from a motor-learning standpoint, frequent short-duration sessions are advantageous to facilitate restoration of neuromuscular control. Fourth, the more frequent exercise sessions minimize the risk of stiffness from prolonged immobility between sessions. The primary disadvantage of the program pertains to the scheduling challenges of the therapist and/or nursing staff to supervise the exercises. However, it is possible to have the patient's caregivers supervise some sessions as part of the educational process in anticipation of hospital dismissal. The frequency of sessions can be modulated based on patient response.

The allowable arcs of motion should be defined by the surgeon, specifically discussed with the physical therapist, and conveyed to the patient, nursing staff, and caregivers. Exceeding motion limitations and the resultant tissue injury is probably the most feared aspect of the postoperative rehabilitation program for the majority of surgeons and rehabilitation team members. Once the allowable arcs of motion are defined, the therapist can initiate a logical progression of passive, active-assisted, and active ROM/resistive exercises. Passive ROM movement is used initially to prevent stiffness, enhance circulation to the healing tissues, and inhibit pain via proprioceptive feedback.[6,15] When performed by a skilled therapist, electromyographic activity of the rotator cuff musculature is minimal, which is an important consideration in cases of arthroplasty with concomitant rotator cuff repair.[27] Typical exercises performed during this phase include pendulum exercises, as well as elevation and external rotation performed by the physical therapist, within the allowable arcs of motion.[27,28] Therapists may also initiate scapulothoracic motion exercises, as described later. Although pendulum exercises are done in a standing position, the other exercises are typically performed in a supine position to promote patient relaxation and mitigate against gravitational loads that may trigger a damaging muscle contraction. The passive ROM program may continue for days to weeks following any initial period of postoperative immobilization.

The progression from passive ROM to active-assisted ROM (AAROM) depends primarily on the surgeon's perceived need to protect a concomitant rotator cuff repair or tendon transfer. AAROM includes some assistance provided by an external force, such as a wand, cane, or pulley device. AAROM initiates the rehabilitation phase during which the patient's own musculature submaximally contracts. This controlled muscle activation, in turn, facilitates restoration of neuromuscular control (or the retraining process in cases of tendon transfer) and stimulates collagen reformation and soft tissue remodeling.[19,20] The transition to AAROM is a precarious point in the rehabilitation process because there is a paucity of science to assist the therapist in controlling the amount of muscle contraction and subsequent stress to the shoulder. Based on the available literature and clinical experience, some guidelines can be provided that will be of assistance to surgeons. First, electromyographic

activity in the rotator cuff during AAROM exercises is generally less during motions performed while supine compared to those performed while seated or standing, likely because of increased gravitational loads during upright exercises.[27,28] Second, in some cases, therapist-assisted AAROM has been shown to produce more rotator cuff electromyographic activity compared to the same motions completed by a patient using a wand or cane.[27,28] This phenomenon remains unexplained, but may in part be related to the patient subconsciously attempting to resist the therapist's motions. Third, data suggest that some closed kinetic chain exercises may be beneficial during this phase of arthroplasty rehabilitation. Table slides, table walk-aways, and wall slides are performed with the patient's hand and upper limb partially supported (Fig. 16.1). Although not specifically studied in the postarthroplasty population, these exercises have been demonstrated to elicit low levels of electromyographic activity in the rotator cuff and scapular stabilizer muscles.[12,29,30]

Commonly used AAROM exercises are well outlined elsewhere and include supine-assisted elevation, external rotation, and internal rotation; supine-assisted elevation-abduction; standing-assisted internal rotation; and pulley-assisted elevation.[1,4,6–8,27,28] Execution is crucial to optimize benefits and minimize adverse effects. Restoration of elevation is paramount to success and is the primary goal of specific surgeries such as the reverse total shoulder arthroplasty.[2,3] Patients typically progress from supine-assisted elevation to upright pulley-assisted exercises. It should be noted that to optimize pulley-assisted exercise efficacy, the pulley should be placed at least 12 inches above the patient's head and behind the patient.[1,4,6] This typically requires the pulley to be attached to a door or doorframe with the patient facing away from the door or doorframe (Fig. 16.2). Failure to do this will significantly compromise the ROM gains and promote a slouching posture in the patient, adversely affecting scapulothoracic and therefore glenohumeral mechanics.[1,4,6,23,30] Table walk-aways can also be implemented during the pulley-assisted exercise phase. As the patient progresses with these exercises, table slides and wall slides can be added as a prelude to the strengthening phase.[12,29]

External rotation is the second most important motion to restore because significant functional limitations are incurred if the patients cannot achieve 30 to 45 degrees of external rotation.[7] During the AAROM phase, two points are worthy of mention with respect to external rotation. First, external rotation goals are often limited in revision or complex primary total shoulder arthroplasty because of component or soft tissue restrictions (e.g., reverse total shoulder arthroplasty).[2,3] In cases in which some restoration of external rotation is feasible, the allowable arc of motion is typically limited to 20 degrees or less to prevent functionally limiting stiffness while allowing subscapularis healing. Second, when external rotation exercises are performed, it is beneficial to maintain elbow flexion at 90 degrees. This elbow position will facilitate application of a more pure external rotation force to the shoulder. Otherwise, patients will substitute shoulder abduction for external rotation and not achieve expected motion gains. Common exercises to restore external rotation include supine cane- or wand-assisted external rotation, supine therapist-assisted external rotation, standing doorframe external rotation, and standing cane-, wand-, or therapist-assisted external rotation. Details of these exercises have been published previously.[1,4,6–8] Regardless of which exercise(s) is/are chosen, surgeons should be aware that active scapular retraction should be incorporated into the external rotation motion to facilitate scapulothoracic rehabilitation and improve functional upper limb external rotation.[12,22]

THE PLANE OF THE SCAPULA

During ROM exercises, whether passive, active-assisted, or resistive-strengthening, the surgeon and members of the rehabilitation team should recognize the importance of the plane of the scapula. The plane of the scapula is 30 to 45 degrees horizontally adducted from the coronal plane.[31] All motions should be initiated in the plane of the scapula for the following reasons. First, the plane of the scapula is inherently the most stable position for the glenohumeral joint.[32–35] Second, the scapular plane provides the largest impingement-free ROM in the shoulder.[32–34] Third, the scapula exhibits the largest degree of upward rotation in the plane of the scapula.[36] Fourth, assuming a balanced soft tissue envelope about the shoulder, the plane of the scapula provides minimal tension on the surrounding rotator cuff musculature.[1,4,37] Fifth, motion and strength gained in the scapular plane translate into the sagittal and coronal planes.[1,4,38]

In practice, elevation and external rotation motions are initiated in the plane of the scapula. During therapist-assisted motions, the therapist places the patient's limb in the scapular plane. During supine wand- or cane-assisted exercises, rolled towels are placed under the elbow to achieve the plane of

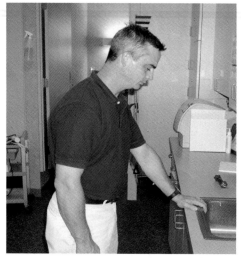
A1

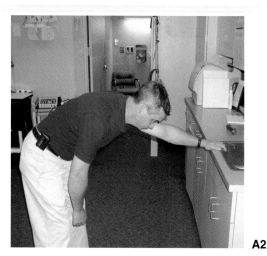
A2

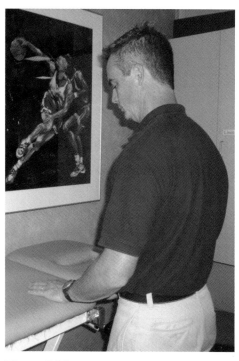
B1

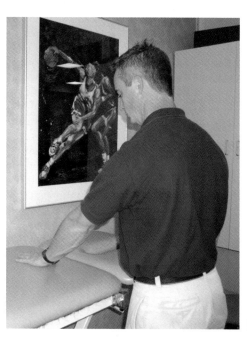
B2

Figure 16.1. **(A)** Table walk-away. The hand stays on the table top and the patient walks away from table, thus achieving arm elevation with relatively little shoulder girdle muscle activation. **(B)** Table slide. The subject slides hand in multiple directions on a table top to achieve active assisted range of motion in a closed kinetic chain environment. The movement direction as well as table height can be adjusted.

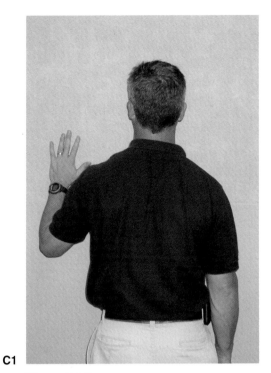
C1

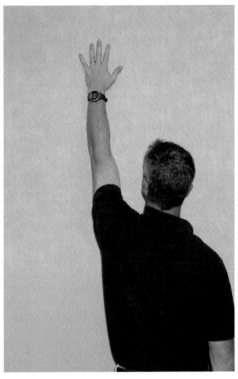
C2

Figure 16.1. *(continued)* **(C)** Wall slides. The patient's hand partially supported on a wall in an elevated position. The patient can perform a variety of upper limb motions with the partial support of the wall. The direction and amplitude of motions can be manipulated.

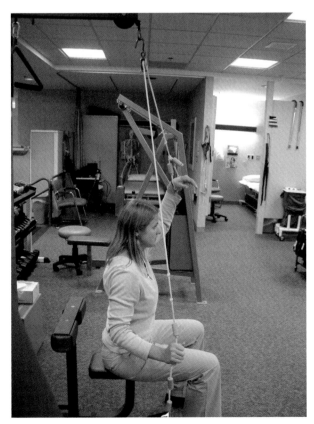

Figure 16.2. The pulley is properly positioned over or slightly behind the patient to ensure optimal elevation during this active assisted ROM exercise.

the scapula (Fig. 16.3). As the patient moves to upright pulley- and wall-assisted motion exercises, he or she is counseled and monitored to maintain the scapular plane. Finally, resisted motion/strengthening exercises are initiated in the scapular plane. As the patient's strength and neuromuscular control improve, the arc of acceptable horizontal adduction-abduction relative to the scapular plane can be widened based on need.

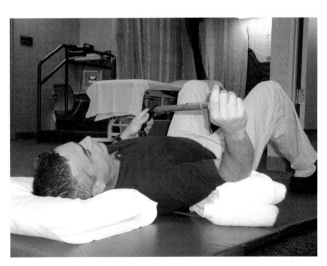

Figure 16.3. Appropriate positioning for active-assisted ROM into external rotation. Note the elbow is flexed to 90 degrees, a towel positions the upper limb in the plane of the scapula, and the force imparted by the cane is perpendicular to the arm to produce relatively pure external rotation.

Although not conclusive, preliminary evidence suggests that patients with reverse total shoulder arthroplasties may progress out of the scapular plane faster than patients with total shoulder arthroplasty or hemiarthroplasty. As a final note in this regard, it is recognized that the plane of the scapula, that is, the plane of maximal glenohumeral congruity, may be altered surgically and would need to be considered during the rehabilitation process as determined intraoperatively by the surgeon and communicated to the rehabilitation team.

THE SCAPULOTHORACIC ARTICULATION

The importance of the scapulothoracic articulation in the rehabilitation of patients with total shoulder arthroplasty has received little direct attention in the literature. The importance of the scapula for optimal shoulder function and its role in shoulder dysfunction have been emphasized and clarified in recent years.[12,22,23,30,39–41] Motion at the scapulothoracic articulation significantly contributes to total upper limb motion and is a determinant of overall function.[30,31] Consequently, abnormal scapular positioning (typically protraction) and scapulothoracic dyskinesis can result in a reduction of available upper limb motion, as well as contribute to increased soft tissue strain about the shoulder, instability, and pain.[23,36]

With specific reference to the shoulder arthroplasty population, kinematic studies have clearly documented an increased contribution of the scapulothoracic articulation to upper limb elevation during functional motions.[11,42,43] Consequently, focusing rehabilitative efforts on maximizing scapulothoracic motion and optimizing scapulothoracic control via strengthening and proprioceptive exercises provides the opportunity to optimize motion and therefore functional outcomes for patients undergoing revision and complex primary total shoulder arthroplasty. Reassuringly, with the exception of concomitant tendon transfers or nerve injury, most of these patients have normal or near normal anatomy of the scapulothoracic articulation and intact scapular stabilizer muscles (e.g., rhomboids, trapezii, serratus anterior).

Specific exercises and functional progressions for scapulothoracic rehabilitation are detailed elsewhere.[29,30,44] Conceptually, scapulothoracic rehabilitation may start postoperatively during immobilization. The therapist or caregiver can perform passive ROM movement of the scapulothoracic articulation, focusing on the important motions of scapular retraction and upward rotation.[30,44] Early scapular stabilizer muscle activation may also be performed during immobilization and progressed thereafter. While the patient is in an immobilizer, the therapist may have the patient perform manually resisted isometric scapulothoracic exercises in elevation, retraction, protraction, and depression. By using manual resistance, the therapist can easily control scapulothoracic and glenohumeral position and the respective forces crossing these articulations. When performing any active or resisted scapulothoracic exercises, the patient is instructed not to press his or her hand into the abdomen, which will activate the subscapularis muscle.[45] During immobilization, the patient may also perform intentional movements with the nonimmobilized upper limb, including straight forward, cross-body, and downward reaches (Fig. 16.4). Although not studied specifically in arthroplasty patients, the stabilization demands imparted by these motions have been demonstrated to elicit scapular stabilizer muscle activity in the immobilized shoulder girdle, while

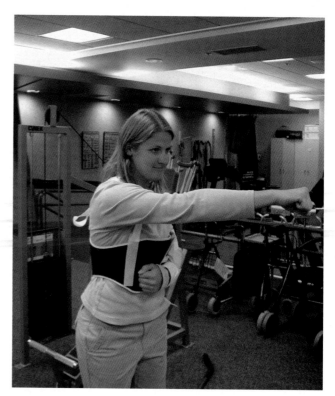

Figure 16.4.   Subject demonstrating a cross body reach with the unaffected arm, which produces electromyographic activity in the immobilized shoulder girdle musculature (see text for discussion).

concomitantly producing minimal rotator cuff activation.[46] As allowed by pain and soft tissue healing, the scapulothoracic rehabilitation program can be advanced to include exercises such as active-assisted and -resisted isotonic contractions, active scapulothoracic ROM exercises, scapular clocks, wall slides, and table slides.[29,30,44] Particularly for patients with rotator cuff deficiency after arthroplasty, scapulothoracic rehabilitation represents an essential and potentially outcome-limiting aspect of the rehabilitation process.

OPTIMIZE UPPER LIMB FUNCTION

As previously stated, it is essential to determine the goal of the arthroplasty in the preoperative period and modify it postoperatively as necessary. Pain reduction is paramount, followed by restoration of ROM based on the limitations of the patient's anatomy and physiology. As the ROM program progresses from active- to active-assisted ROM, re-establishment of neuromuscular control about the shoulder girdle is initiated. The primary goal of this aspect of postarthroplasty rehabilitation is to establish and maintain a level of neuromuscular control about the shoulder girdle to achieve the surgeon's and patient's functional goals without sacrificing stability or comfort. This requires not only strength but a balance of strength and coordinated muscle activity about the shoulder—thus the more general term neuromuscular control (NMC) is used. To develop strength and NMC a muscle needs to be challenged by an external force, whether it be gravity, a therapist's hand, or some resistive device such as a free weight or elastic tubing. In the simplest sense, active ROM exercise in a gravitational environment is the most fundamental method to reestablish NMC, provided that the motions are performed correctly. In fact, for many patients with revision and complex primary shoulder arthroplasty, the end point for the rehabilitation program is the point at which the patients are performing elevation and external rotation (if possible) actively against gravity. Whether this end point is desirable or sufficient, compared to more advanced strengthening, is decided and agreed on by the surgeon, patient, caregivers, and rehabilitation team.

Specific exercises and functional progressions for strengthening after arthroplasty are detailed elsewhere.[1,4,6,8] However, surgeons managing patients who undergo arthroplasty should be aware of several important concepts to consider when designing and supervising strengthening programs for these patients.

The surgeon, patient, family, and rehabilitation team should decide and agree on the end point for strengthening during rehabilitation. For some patients with limited goals, the strengthening phase may consist merely of active movements performed in a gravitational environment, without the use of manual resistance, free weights, or elastic bands. Other patients with greater functional goals would benefit from the application of progressive external loading to optimize NMC. Regardless, both groups of patients would benefit from a scapulothoracic rehabilitation program as highlighted earlier.

Isometric contractions are generally safe to use early in the rehabilitation period and may be directed at the scapulothoracic and glenohumeral articulations. Patients may maintain and increase strength by performing several brief isometric contractions each day.[47–49] These contractions can be performed by the patient or with manual resistance by the therapist. The intensity of the contractions can be easily controlled, the primary caveat being that isometric strength gains are angle specific (i.e., strength gains occur at the angle of the exercise, with 15 degrees in either direction).[50] Therefore isometric contractions at multiple angles should be performed when indicated. Isometric exercises can also be combined with active ROM exercises, such that the therapist or caregiver assists the patient in performing isometric contractions at the end ROM. In such cases the external force may be imparted from multiple directions while the patient holds the position, a technique known as rhythmic stabilization; it has been proposed to promote stability.[50,51]

As isometric exercises progress and ROM improves, active assisted and resisted motions are implemented. During these motions, muscles are contracting while simultaneously either shortening (concentric contraction) or lengthening (eccentric contraction). Although not purely isotonic, these types of movements are often referred to as isotonic. Active-assisted ROM in a gravitational field is the most fundamental of the isotonic exercises. The key during this phase is to determine which motions to train and what level of resistance is necessary, gradually increasing the resistance toward the goal. Resisted movements in a reduced gravitational field can be achieved in several ways: (a) using the assistance of a therapist, pulley, cane, or wand; (b) positioning the body and the shoulder differently with respect to gravitational pull (e.g., active shoulder elevation in a supine versus upright position); or (c) changing the normal moment arm of the upper limb (e.g., elevation with the elbow bent versus straight). Ultimately, the minimum goal is to achieve the end-point ROM in elevation and external rotation

(if possible), in an upright position against gravity. Thereafter, where appropriate, patients may be instructed in a variety of elevation and external rotation exercises against additional external loads imparted by free weights or elastic tubing. Patients using elastic resistance should be instructed on appropriate positioning and monitored for increased pain during the strengthening phase; the nonphysiological resistance provided by these bands can commonly result in overstressing or understressing the target musculature.

Similar to the discussion with respect to ROM, all strengthening exercises should be performed initially within the scapular plane and advanced as the clinical situation allows. Additionally, many patients progress faster by performing less intense strengthening sessions twice per day as opposed to one intense session daily.[1,4,6] Finally, patients should be taught to self-monitor for fatigue and not exercise beyond the point of fatigue because of the adverse effects of fatigue on shoulder function.[24–26]

PROGRAM MODIFICATION BASED ON CASE-SPECIFIC FACTORS

The primary purpose of this chapter was to outline important rehabilitation concepts that should be considered when designing programs for patients following revision or complex total shoulder arthroplasty. These concepts provide the framework to effectively manage patients with a wide variety of complexities following their surgeries. As a final point, surgeons should recognize the common need to modify rehabilitation programs and protocols based on case-specific factors. The skillful surgeon understands normal shoulder mechanics and the pathomechanics incurred postoperatively. Atypical components, bone or soft tissue grafts, soft tissue reconstructions, tendon transfers, tissue quality, repair quality, and nonstandard component positioning must all be considered when determining the need for and duration of immobilization, when to initiate ROM exercises, which motion arcs to protect and for how long, whether strengthening is appropriate, and ultimately the expected outcome of the surgery in terms of pain relief, motion, and function. The surgeon must consider these issues, formulate an expected outcome, and effectively communicate this information to the patient, family, and rehabilitation team members. Postoperatively, by implementing and monitoring a logical, progressive rehabilitation program, the surgeon, family, and rehabilitation team can provide the patient with the best opportunity to realize his or her best outcome.

REFERENCES

1. Brems J. Rehabilitation following total shoulder arthroplasty. *Clin Orthop* 1994;307:70–85.
2. Boileau P, Trojani C, Chuinard C. Latissimus dorsi and teres major transfer with reverse total shoulder arthroplasty for a combined loss of elevation and external rotation. *Tech Shoulder Elbow Surg* 2007;8:13–22.
3. Matsen F, Boileau P, Walch G, et al. The reverse total shoulder arthroplasty. *J Bone Joint Surg Am* 2007;89:660–667.
4. Brems J. Rehabilitation after total shoulder arthroplasty: current concepts. *Semin Arthroplasty* 2007;18:55–65.
5. Boardman N, Cofield R, Bengston K, et al. Rehabilitation after total shoulder arthroplasty. *J Arthroplasty* 2001;16:483–486.
6. Brown D, Friedman R. Postoperative rehabilitation following total shoulder arthroplasty. *Orthop Clin North Am* 1998;29:535–547.

7. Wilcox R, Arsalanian L, Millet P. Rehabilitation following total shoulder arthroplasty. *J Orthop Sports Phys Ther* 2005;35:821–836.

8. McCluskey GI, Uhl T. Total shoulder replacement. In: Donatelli R, ed. *Physical Therapy of the Shoulder*. New York: Churchill Livingstone; 1997:459–476.

9. Maybach A, Schlegel T. Shoulder rehabilitation for the arthritic glenohumeral joint: preoperative and postoperative considerations. *Semin Arthroplasty* 1995;6:297–304.

10. Mahfouz M, Nicholson G, Komistek R, et al. In vivo determination of the dynamics of normal, rotator cuff deficient, total, and reverse replacement shoulders. *J Bone Joint Surg Am* 2005;87S107–S113.

11. Veeger H, Magermans D, Nagels J, et al. A kinematical analysis of the shoulder after arthroplasty during a hair-combing task. *Clin Biomech* 2006;21:S39–S44.

12. Kibler W. Shoulder rehabilitation: principles and practice. *Med Sci Sports Exerc* 1998;30:S40–S50.

13. Warner J, Micheli L, Arslanian L, et al. Patterns of flexibility, laxity, and strength in normal shoulders and shoulders with instability. *Am J Sports Med* 1990;18:366–375.

14. Brox J, Roe C, Saugen E, et al. Isometric abduction muscle activation in patients with rotator cuff tendinosis of the shoulder. *Arch Phys Med Rehabil* 1997;78:1260–1267.

15. Melzak R, Wall P. Pain mechanisms: a new theory. *Science* 1965;150:971–979.

16. Weber D, Brown A. Physical agent modalities. In: Braddom R, ed. *Physical Medicine and Rehabilitation*. Philadelphia: WB Saunders; 1996:449–463.

17. Singh H, Osbahr D, Holovacs T, et al. The efficacy of continuous cryotherapy on the postoperative shoulder: a prospective randomized investigation. *J Shoulder Elbow Surg* 2001;10:522–525.

18. Muller E. Influence of training and of inactivity on muscle strength. *Arch Phys Med Rehabil* 1970;51:449–462.

19. Aren A, Madden J. Effects of stress on healing wounds. *J Surg Res* 1976;20:93–97.

20. Halar E, Bell K. Immobility. In: DeLisa J, Gans B, eds. *Rehabilitation Medicine: Principles and Practice*. Philadelphia: Lippincott-Raven; 1998:1015–1034.

21. Kibler W, Livingston B, Bruce R. Current concepts in shoulder rehabilitation. *Adv Operative Orthop* 1995;3:249–300.

22. Kibler W. The role of the scapula in athletic shoulder function. *Am J Sports Med* 1998;26:325–337.

23. Kebaetse M, McClure P, Pratt N. Thoracic position effect on shoulder range of motion, strength, and three-dimensional scapular kinematics. *Arch Phys Med Rehabil* 1999;80:945–950.

24. Voight M, Hardin J, Blackburn T, et al. The effects of muscle fatigue on and the relationship of arm dominance to shoulder proprioception. *J Orthop Sports Phys Ther* 1996;23:348–352.

25. Ellenbecker T, Roetert E. Testing isokinetic muscular fatigue of shoulder internal and external rotation in elite junior athletes. *J Orthop Sports Phys Ther* 1999;29:275–281.

26. McQuade K, Dawson J, Smidt G. Scapulothoracic muscle fatigue associated with alterations in scapulohumeral rhythm kinematics during maximum resistive shoulder elevation. *J Ortho Sports Phys Ther* 1998;28:74–80.

27. Dockery M, Wright T, LaStayo P. Electromyography of the shoulder: an analysis of passive modes of exercise. *Orthopedics* 1998;21:1181–1184.

28. McCann P, Wootten M, Kadaba M, et al. A kinematic and electromyographic study of shoulder rehabilitation exercises. *Clin Orthop Rel Res* 1993;288:179–188.

29. Uhl T, Carver T, Mattacola C, et al. Shoulder musculature activation during upper extremity weight-bearing exercise. *J Ortho Sports Phys Ther* 2003;33:109–117.

30. Kibler W, McMullen J. Scapular dyskinesis and its relation to shoulder pain. *J Am Acad Orthop Surg* 2003;11:142–151.

31. Inman V, Saunders M, Abbot L. Observations on the function of the shoulder joint. *J Bone Joint Surg* 1944;27:1–30.

32. Saha A. Mechanism of shoulder movements and a plea for recognition of the zero position of the glenohumeral joint. *Clin Orthop* 1983;173:3–10.

33. Saha A. Mechanics of elevation of the glenohumeral joint: its application in rehabilitation of flail shoulder in brachial plexus injuries and poliomyelitis and in replacement of the upper humerus by prosthesis. *Acta Orthop Scand* 1973;44:668–678.

34. Lippett S, Matsen F. Mechanisms of glenohumeral joint stability. *Clin Orthop* 1993;291:20–28.

35. Johnston T. Movements of the shoulder joint: a please for the use of the "plane of the scapula" as the plane of reference for movements occurring at the humeroscapular joint. *Br J Surg* 1937;25:252–260.

36. Borsa P, Timmons M, Sauers E. Scapular-positioning patterns during humeral elevation in unimpaired shoulders. *J Athl Train* 2003;38:12–17.

37. Jobe C. Superior glenoid impingement. *Orthop Clin North Am* 1997;28:137–143.

38. Greenfield B, Donatelli R, Wooden M, et al. Isokinetic evaluation of shoulder rotational strength between the plane of the scapula and the frontal plane. *Am J Sports Med* 1990;18:124–128.

39. Kibler W, Sciascia A, Dome D. Evaluation of apparent and absolute supraspinatus strength in patients with shoulder injury using the scapular retraction test. *Am J Sports Med* 2006;34:1643–1647.

40. Smith J, Kotajarvi B, Padgett D, et al. Effect of scapular protraction and retraction on isometric shoulder elevation strength. *Arch of Phys Med Rehabil* 2002;83:367–370.

41. Smith J, Dietrich C, Kotajarvi B, et al. The effect of scapular protraction on isometric shoulder rotation strength in normal subjects. *J Shoulder Elbow Surg* 2006;15:339–343.

42. Boileau P, Walch G, Liotard J. Radiocinematographic study of active elevation of the prosthetic shoulder. *Rev Chir Orthop* 1992;78:355–364.

43. Friedman R. Biomechanics of total shoulder arthroplasty: a preoperative and postoperative analysis. *Semin Arthroplasty* 1995;6:222–232.

44. Burkhart S, Morgan C, Kibler W. The disabled throwing shoulder: spectrum of pathology. Part III: The SICK scapula, scapular dyskinesis, the kinetic chain, and rehabilitation. *Arthroscopy* 2003;19:641–646.

45. Smith J, Dahm D, Kaufman K, et al. Electromyographic activity in the immobilized shoulder girdle during scapulothoracic exercises. *Arch Phys Med Rehabil* 2006;87:923–927.

46. Smith J, Padgett D, Dahm D, et al. Electromyographic activity in the immobilized shoulder girdle musculature during contralateral upper limb movements. *J Shoulder Elbow Surg* 2004;13:583–588.

47. Lieberson W. Brief isometric exercises in therapeutic exercise. In: Basmajian J, ed. *Therapeutic Exercise*. Baltimore: Williams & Wilkins; 1984.

48. Carolan B, Cafarelli E. Adaptations in coactivation after isometric resistance training. *J Appl Physiol* 1992;73:911–917.

49. Garfinkel S, Cafarelli E. Relative changes in maximal force, EMG, and muscle cross-sectional area after isometric training. *Med Sci Sports Exer* 1992;24:1220–1227.

50. Davies G. A compendium of isokinetics in clinical usage. 2nd ed. LaCrosse, Wi: S&S Publishers; 1985.

51. Wilk K, Meister K, Andrews J. Current concepts in the rehabilitation of the overhead throwing athlete. *Am J Sports Med* 2002;30:136–151.

Robert H. Cofield
Mark E. Morrey
John W. Sperling

Reconstructive Techniques Used at the Mayo Clinic in Revision Shoulder Arthroplasty

INTRODUCTION

Understanding our experience with reconstruction in revision shoulder arthroplasty required examination of the actual cases. We reviewed the revision shoulder arthroplasty experience of one surgeon (RHC) from 1980 through 2005 to better understand the problems encountered and the chosen solutions. Early in the review process it became clear it would aid understanding of the material to divide these cases into four categories: failures of hemiarthroplasty initially performed at the Mayo Clinic, failures of total shoulder arthroplasty initially performed at the Mayo Clinic, failures of hemiarthroplasty referred to us for evaluation and treatment, and, finally, failures of total shoulder arthroplasty that were referred.

MAYO CLINIC HUMERAL HEAD REPLACEMENTS

Of the humeral replacements we performed between 1980 and 2005, 38 shoulders required revision procedures. The reason for revision was usually isolated and very straightforward (Table 17.1). In 34 shoulders, painful glenoid arthritis had developed and a glenoid component was placed. In two there was a periprosthetic humeral shaft fracture and the humeral component was replaced with a long-stemmed device and cerclage cables. In one there was humeral component loosening and a new stem was placed, fixed in position with bone cement. Finally, in one shoulder there was posterior glenohumeral instability addressed with posterior shoulder capsule tightening. Among these cases there were only a few secondary reasons for revision surgery. In one of the cases with painful glenoid arthritis there was also humeral component loosening that was addressed with placement of a long-stemmed, uncemented component. In four shoulders there was also rotator cuff tearing. In two the rotator cuff could be readily repaired, and in two the component was revised to a reverse type total shoulder arthroplasty. Figure 17.1 illustrates a shoulder with painful glenoid arthritis and the conversion to total shoulder arthroplasty. Figure 17.2 illustrates a shoulder with a hemiarthroplasty and painful glenoid arthritis, combined with a large extent of rotator cuff tearing that was converted to a reverse-type implant system.

In this group of shoulders, because of the simplicity of the revision surgery, it was straightforward to analyze the adjunctive procedures that were necessary to accomplish the surgery. In 24 shoulders it was necessary to remove the monoblock humeral component to achieve glenoid exposure. In 10 with a modular system the humeral head could be removed, leaving the stem in place. The head was then replaced with another head of a similar or slightly adjusted size. In 23 shoulders, subscapularis lengthening was necessary—freeing the musculotendinous unit from scar, freeing the anterior shoulder capsule from the subscapularis, and often incising the subscapularis and anterior shoulder capsule from the bone of the humerus, moving it medially approximately 1 cm. In only one shoulder was Z-lengthening possible and required. Inferior capsule lengthening was required for 21 shoulders; in all instances this release was done from the humeral neck. Posterior shoulder capsule lengthening was necessary in four shoulders. This was accomplished by division of the posterior shoulder capsule from the posterior glenoid rim. The superior shoulder capsule was released from the superior aspect of the glenoid rim in two shoulders. Adjunctive glenoid bone grafting was needed in only three shoulders. In one shoulder, subacromial impingement was recognized and an acromioplasty performed.

In summarizing this group, one can easily recognize that the problems were focused and the solutions were quite direct. There seems to be no doubt, at least in our patient population, that if a humeral head replacement is to fail, it is almost always because of the development of painful glenoid arthritis.

TABLE 17.1	Revisions of Humeral Head Replacements Performed at the Mayo Clinic (n = 38)	
Reasons for Revision	*Number of Shoulders*	*Treatment*
PRIMARY REASONS		
Painful glenoid arthritis	34	Glenoid placed
Periprosthetic humeral fracture	2	Long-stem + cerclage
Humeral loosening	1	New stem (cemented)
Posterior instability	1	Posterior capsule repair
Secondary reasons		
Humeral loosening	1	Long stem
Rotator cuff tear	4	Repair 2
		Reverse arthroplasty 2
ADJUNCTIVE PROCEDURES		
Remove monoblock stem for exposure	24	
Remove or replace humeral head	10	
Subscapularis lengthening	23	
Inferior capsule lengthening	21	
Posterior capsule lengthening	4	
Superior capsule lengthening	2	
Glenoid bone graft	3	
Acromioplasty	1	

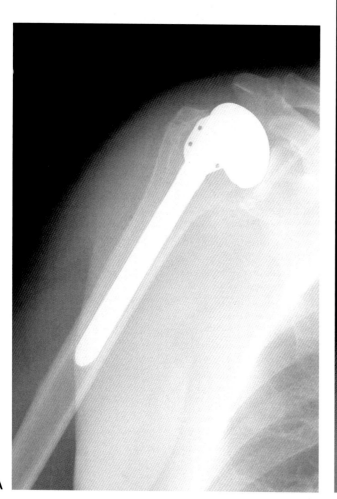

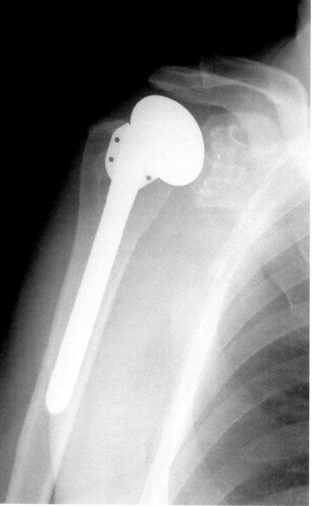

A   B

Figure 17.1.   A typical failed humeral head replacement. There is a single reason for failure—the accrual of pain related to glenoid arthritis. The solution was also simple. The modular humeral head was removed, the glenoid component was placed, and a modular humeral head was repositioned. Pre- **(A)** and postoperative **(B)** radiographs.

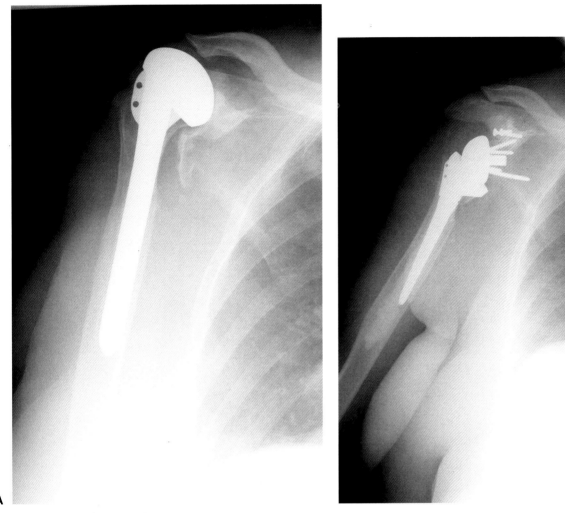

Figure 17.2.   A humeral head replacement that failed related to two problems—glenoid arthrosis associated with pain and progressive rotator cuff insufficiency with anterosuperior humeral head translation. For revision the humeral component was removed. Bone from the proximal humerus was used to graft the deficient superior aspect of the glenoid, and a reverse type shoulder arthroplasty was placed. Pre- **(A)** and postoperative **(B)** radiographs.

MAYO CLINIC TOTAL SHOULDER ARTHROPLASTIES

During this same period, there were 39 primary total shoulder arthroplasties performed at the Mayo Clinic that subsequently required revision shoulder arthroplasty. This excludes those cases with metal-backed glenoid components, focusing only on the commonly placed all-polyethylene type of glenoid. There were two major reasons for revision surgery, glenoid component loosening and instability, and again the needs during revision were quite focused (Table 17.2). There was glenoid loosening in 21 shoulders, with an associated glenoid component fracture in one shoulder, in addition to the osteolysis that occurred. The glenoid component was simply removed in four shoulders. It was removed, and the hollow glenoid cavity was grafted with particulate allograft bone in ten. There was enough bone remaining to replace the glenoid with a cemented all-polyethylene component in seven. There were several associated problems in this group of shoulders with glenoid component issues. There was also humeral loosening in 11, no doubt largely related to

the osteolytic response associated with polyethylene wear and cement debris. This was addressed with cementing the new humeral component in eight—using a long-stemmed component in three, using an in-growth component in two, and press-fitting a new humeral component in one. Additionally, in eight shoulders the humeral component was changed for exposure. A monoblock component was removed in five, and a modular humeral head was changed in three. There was associated rotator cuff tearing in four shoulders that could be completely repaired in three. There was posterior instability in one, addressed with change of the humeral head size and posterior capsule tightening.

The second major complication in this patient group was instability. There was posterior instability in seven and anterosuperior instability in six. To address the posterior instability there was posterior capsule tightening in all seven, anterior capsule and subscapularis lengthening was necessary in six, and the humeral head size was changed in six. In those six with anterosuperior instability there was disruption of the rotator interval, with stretching of the anterior aspect of the supraspinatus and the

TABLE 17.2	Revisions of Total Shoulder Arthroplasties Performed at the Mayo Clinic (n = 39)	
Main Reasons for Revision	*Number of Shoulders*	*Treatment*
Glenoid loosening	20	Remove component and bone graft 10,
Glenoid component fracture	1	replace component 7, remove component 4
Associated problems		
Humeral loosening	11	Cemented component 8, long stem 3
Humerus changed for exposure	8	Monoblock 5, head 3
Rotator cuff tear	4	Repair 3
Posterior instability	1	Capsule tightening + head change
Instability		
Posterior	7	Posterior capsule repair 7, anterior release 6, change humeral head 6
Anterior-superior	6	Repair 6, change humeral head 6
Infection	2	Excision arthroplasty + bone cement spacer
Periprosthetic humeral fracture with loosening	1	Long-stem cemented component with bone graft
Humeral component loosening	1	Standard-length component fixed with cement
Rotator cuff tear	1	Repair

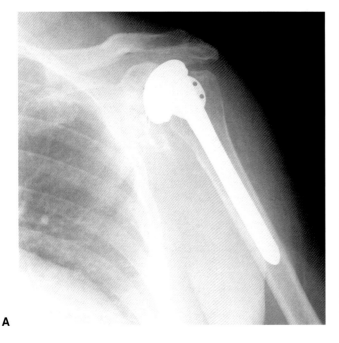

A

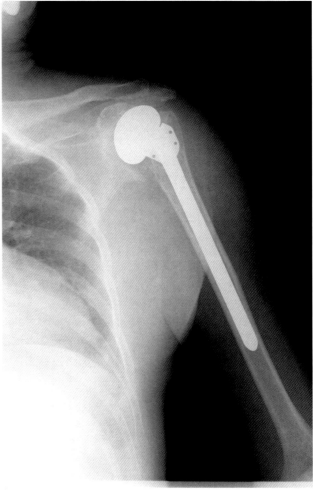

B

Figure 17.3. Glenoid-component loosening with shifting of the glenoid component position centrally and inferiorly and shifting of the monoblock humeral head centrally and superiorly. The rotator cuff was slightly stretched and thin but intact. The monoblock humeral component was removed. The glenoid component with underlying cement and histiocytic debris was removed. Allograft bone was packed into the glenoid cavity. An intermediate-length bone ingrowth humeral stem was positioned. The humeral head was adjusted in size to accommodate for the space needed to fill the shoulder joint to create stability yet allow nearly full motion as determined at the time of surgery. Pre- (**A**) and postoperative (**B**) radiographs.

superior aspect of the subscapularis, in other words, a partial detachment of the upper portion of the subscapularis. In these six cases the humeral head size was changed and the anterosuperior structures were tightened, with firm rotator interval closure.

Of these 39 revisions, two were done for infection using a two-stage treatment protocol—removing the components, debriding the shoulder, placing an antibiotic-impregnated bone cement spacer, and eight or more weeks later performing a reinsertion hemiarthroplasty. There was isolated humeral component loosening in one, addressed with fixing a new humeral component in place with cement. There was a large rotator cuff tear in one, addressed by repairing the rotator cuff, reinforcing it with a latissimus dorsi transfer, and changing the humeral component to a slightly smaller size. Finally, there was one periprosthetic humeral fracture with loosening addressed by placing a long-stemmed humeral component fixed in position with cement and cerclage cables and adding autogenous iliac crest bone graft material. Figures 17.3 through 17.6 illustrate the typical preoperative and postoperative radiographic appearances of those with glenoid or glenoid and humeral loosening and fixed or recurrent shoulder instability.

REFERRED HUMERAL HEAD REPLACEMENTS

Between 1980 and 2005, 84 shoulders having had humeral head replacement elsewhere (with ongoing discomfort and functional limitations) were revised by us. Similar to our own humeral head replacements that failed, 64 had revision surgery for painful glenoid arthritis (Table 17.3). It was possible to place a glenoid component in 61. In three it was determined at surgery that there was an inadequate amount of bone to support a glenoid component and the glenoid was reshaped.

Unlike in our cases, several other problems were identified. The humeral component was malpositioned in 22. Malpositioning was of all types—too high, too low, too anterior, too posterior, too anteverted, or too retroverted. In 18 of these 22 shoulders with humeral component malpositioning there was also painful glenoid arthritis. Of the 22 shoulders, it was possible to correct the malpositioning with a change of the humeral head only in one. In the other 21 shoulders the stem had to be removed. The stem was replaced in a

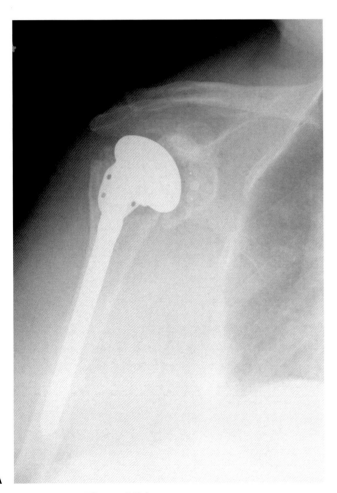

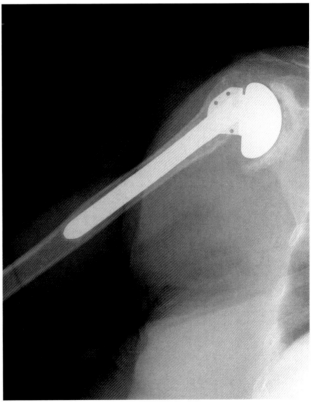

A   **B**

Figure 17.4.   Glenoid- and humeral-component loosening, with shifting of the glenoid component medially and the humeral component distally and into valgus. Both components were removed, along with underlying glenoid cement and histiocytic debris. A larger bone in-growth humeral stem was positioned. Allograft bone chips were used to fill the glenoid cavity, and the humeral head was adjusted to create stability and allow movement. Pre- **(A)** and postoperative **(B)** radiographs.

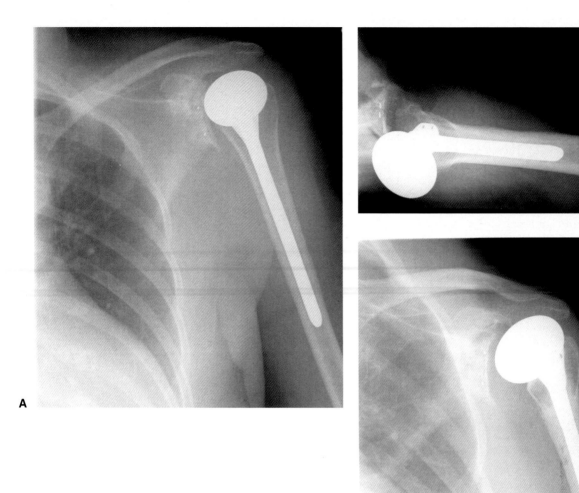

Figure 17.5. Fixed posterior shoulder dislocation 6 weeks after the initial surgical procedure. The humeral component was placed in anatomic position. In this patient that represented 50 to 60 degrees of retroversion. At revision surgery the glenoid was found to be secure and in good position. The humeral component was removed, a new component was cemented in 20 degrees of retroversion. This effectively tightened the posterior shoulder capsule and eliminated the posterior instability. Pre- **(A,B)** and postoperative **(C)** radiographs.

cemented fashion in 12, in a press-fit manner in three, or by use of a bone in-growth component in two. Long stems were used in four; these were cemented in two and press-fitted in two.

In addition, 17 of the humeral components were loose. This included 11 with press-fitting and six with cement fixation. These were managed by placing a new cemented component in eight, a press-fit component in one, and an in-growth compo-

nent in one. In addition, long-stemmed components were placed in seven, cement was used in five, and press-fitting in two. Only one of these 17 shoulders with component loosening was recognized to have an infection. This was a late, chronic infection with coagulase-negative staphylococcus grown on two of three cultures. Three histological specimens were obtained at surgery; one was benign, one was questionable for acute inflammation, and one definitely had acute inflammation. A primary

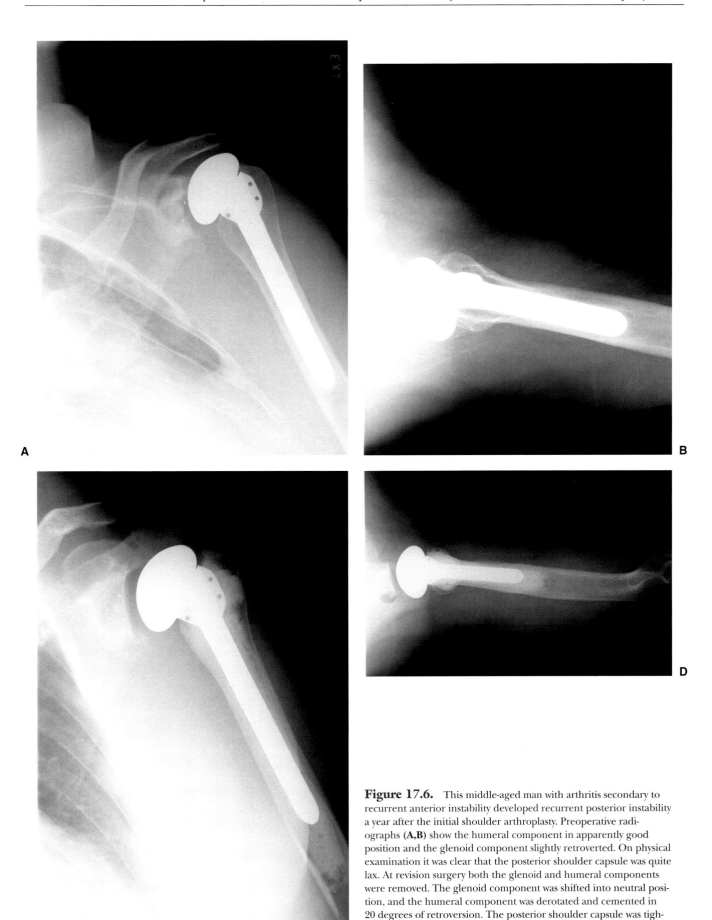

A

B

C

D

Figure 17.6. This middle-aged man with arthritis secondary to recurrent anterior instability developed recurrent posterior instability a year after the initial shoulder arthroplasty. Preoperative radiographs (**A,B**) show the humeral component in apparently good position and the glenoid component slightly retroverted. On physical examination it was clear that the posterior shoulder capsule was quite lax. At revision surgery both the glenoid and humeral components were removed. The glenoid component was shifted into neutral position, and the humeral component was derotated and cemented in 20 degrees of retroversion. The posterior shoulder capsule was tightened, and the shoulder was maintained in a brace in neutral arm rotation for 6 weeks. (**C,D**) Postoperative component positioning.

TABLE 17.3	Revisions of Referred Humeral Head Components (n = 84)	
Main Reasons for Revision	*Number of Shoulders*	*Treatment*
Glenoid arthritis	64	Glenoid placed 61
		Bone reshaped 3
Rotator cuff tear	27	Repair 26
Humeral component malposition	22 (glenoid arthritis in 18)	Standard length stem 17
		Cement 12
		Long stem 4
		Cement 2
		Head changed 1
Humeral component loosening	17	Standard length stem 10
		Cement 8
		Long stem 7
		Cement 5
Instability	14	Humerus changed 11
		Glenoid placed 9
		Rotator cuff repair 7
		Capsule tightening 2
Periprosthetic humeral fracture	5	Standard length stem 1
		Cement 1
		Long stem 4
		Cement 3
		Bone graft 5
Infection	1	Primary exchange
		Antibiotics in bone cement

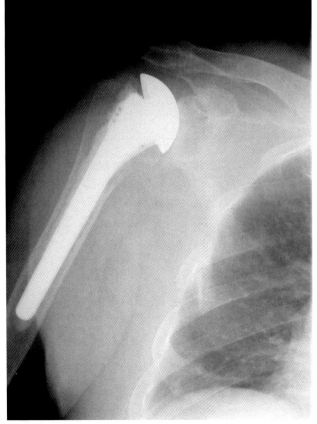

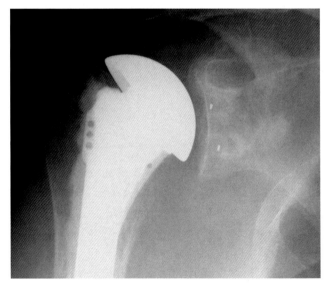

Figure 17.7.   After a humeral head replacement done elsewhere, pain developed over time related to a glenoid arthritis. In this patient the humeral component was well positioned and it was modular. This allowed removal of the modular head, placement of a glenoid component, and repositioning of the humeral head component. A rather straightforward revision case in a humeral head replacement failure referred from elsewhere. Pre- **(A)** and postoperative **(B)** radiographs.

exchange was performed, inserting the new humeral component with antibiotic-impregnated cement.

There were also five periprosthetic humeral shaft fractures. In three of these shoulders the implant was loose. These were addressed by a standard-length cemented component in one, a long-stemmed cemented component in three, and a long-stemmed press-fit component in one. Cerclage cables were used, and bone graft was added to all fractures.

In addition, there were a large number of soft tissue problems. There was rotator cuff tearing in 27, involving the supraspinatus and infraspinatus in 16; the subscapularis, supraspinatus, and infraspinatus in seven; the subscapularis and supraspinatus in two; and the supraspinatus in two. The rotator cuff tearing was able to be repaired in all but one case.

Instability also occurred in 14 shoulders. It was anterosuperior in seven, anterior in four, and posterior in three. To address the instability the humeral component was changed in 11, a glenoid component was placed in nine, the rotator cuff was repaired in seven, and the capsule in the direction of the instability was tightened in two.

Again, for failure of a humeral head component the primary factor involved was glenoid arthritis, but in these referred cases there were several other associated problems, as one can see from the earlier discussion, including humeral component malposition, humeral component loosening, periprosthetic humeral shaft fractures, rotator cuff tearing, instability, and one case with infection. Figures 17.7 through 17.15 illustrate some of the problems encountered and the methods of surgical treatment.

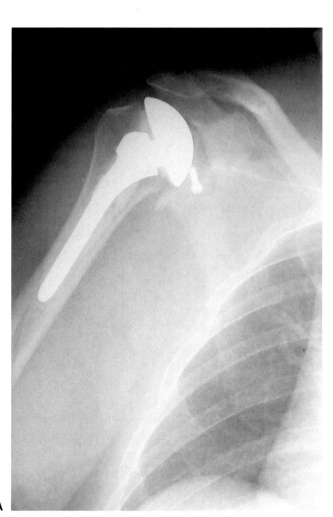
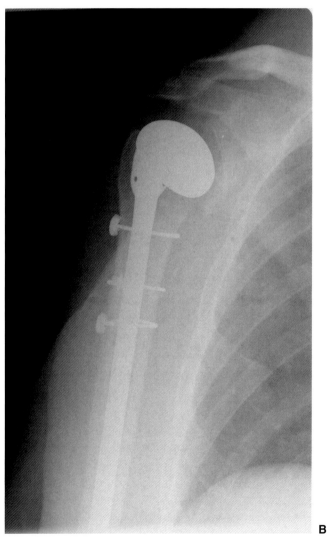

A   **B**

Figure 17.8.   A shoulder with previous instability surgery, the development of arthritis, and placement of a cemented nonmodular humeral head prosthesis. Glenoid arthritis and pain developed. This required removing the well-cemented humeral stem. The entrance to the humeral canal was blocked by the humeral head portion of the component. A longitudinal split was created on the anterolateral aspect of the proximal humerus. By slowly spreading this split and the bone and cement with osteotomes, the component could be loosened and driven free. This then allowed further cleaning of the cement from the humeral canal and exposure for placing the glenoid component. An intermediate-length bone in-growth stem was placed. The split in the humerus was controlled with cerclage cables. Pre- **(A)** and postoperative **(B)** radiographs.

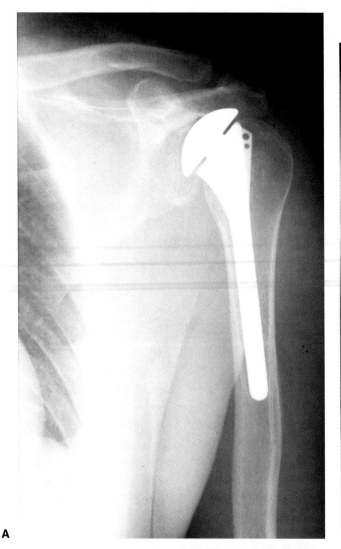

A

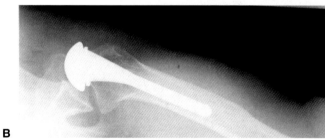

B

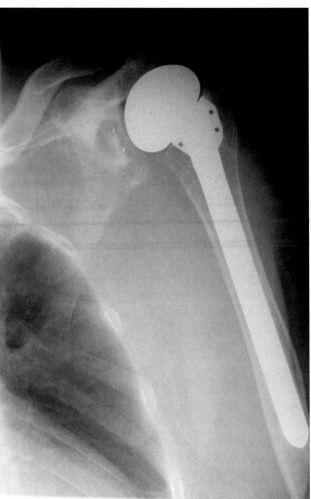

C

Figure 17.9. A painful and poorly functioning humeral head replacement referred from elsewhere. There is wear of the anterosuperior aspect of the glenoid. The humeral component is placed in varus, effectively overtightening the glenohumeral joint and anterior in the humeral metaphysis, creating a moderate degree of anterior instability and eccentric glenoid wear. The malpositioning of the humeral component could not be corrected by changing humeral head size or eccentricity. The humeral component required removal. A glenoid component was placed, related to the eccentric glenoid wear. An intermediate-length bone in-growth humeral component was seated with appropriate axial alignment and positioning in the metaphyseal region of the humerus. The humeral head size was then adjusted to maintain stability yet allow a nearly full range of motion after subscapularis repair, at the time of revision surgery. Pre- **(A,B)** and postoperative **(C)** radiographs.

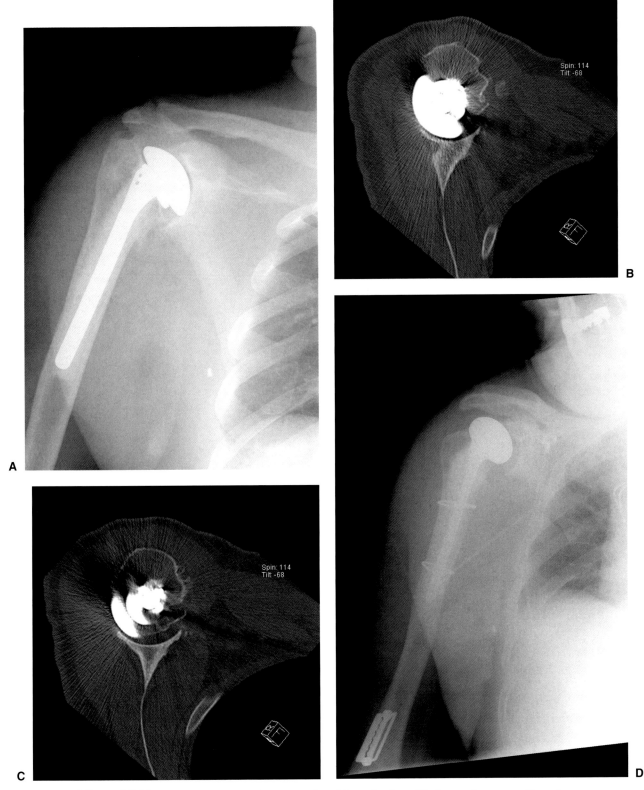

Figure 17.10. A humeral head replacement referred from elsewhere. The humeral component is positioned in varus and too inferior related to the top of the humeral tuberosity. There is also glenoid cartilage and central bone erosion. The humeral component was removed using the longitudinal split through bone and cement, driving the humeral component free. Cement was then removed from the interior of the humerus. **(A)** Preoperative radiograph. **(B,C)** Preoperative computed tomography (CT) imaging. **(B)** represents a CT cut just below the level of the coracoid process, and **(C)** represents a cut at the junction of the lower and middle third of the glenoid. Both cuts implied there was ample glenoid bone remaining to allow placement of the glenoid component and also strongly suggested that the humeral component was seated in too much retroversion. The glenoid component was successfully placed, and a new humeral stem was cemented in better position. The split was controlled with cerclage cables, and the modular humeral head was adjusted to create stability yet allow excellent movement. **(D)** Postoperative radiograph.

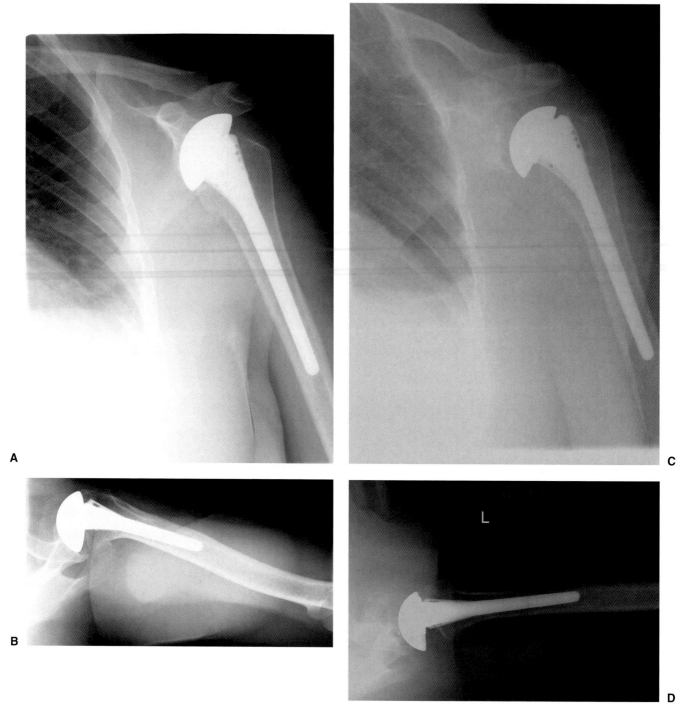

Figure 17.11.   Perhaps to emphasize the point further, this series represents yet another humeral component problem, in part the result of the patient's native anatomy. The humeral component on this occasion being placed somewhat too superiorly and in 10 to 15 degrees of retroversion. This is associated with anterior glenohumeral subluxation and anterior glenoid wear. The humeral head component was removed. A glenoid component was placed, and a new eccentric humeral head component was repositioned and seated. **(A,B)** Preoperative radiographs. **(C,D)** The glenoid is in place and the more central position of the humeral component has a slightly increased humeral offset posteriorly.

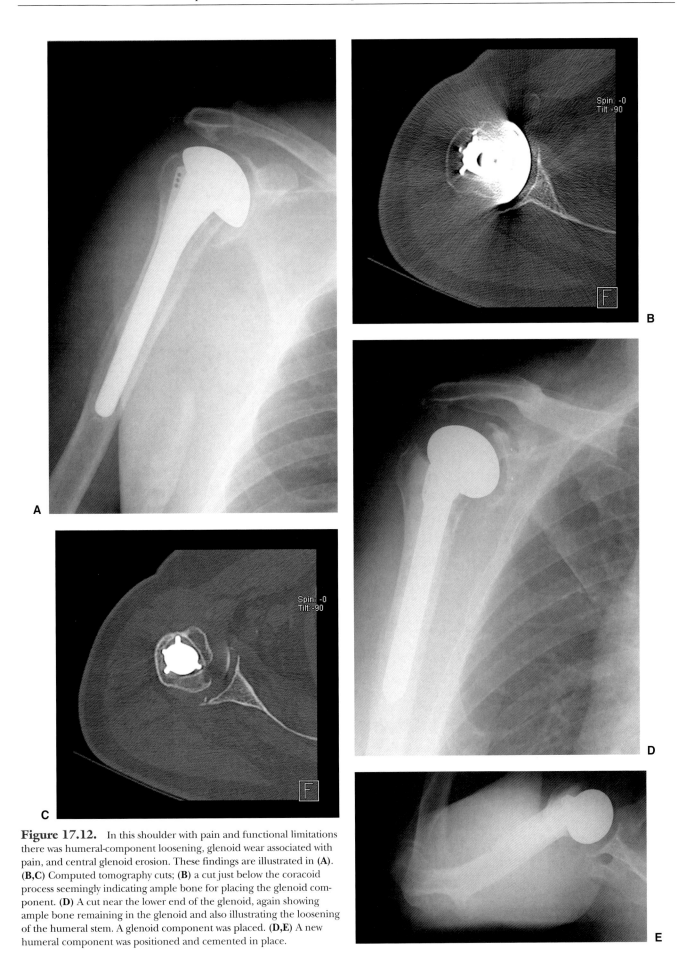

Figure 17.12.   In this shoulder with pain and functional limitations there was humeral-component loosening, glenoid wear associated with pain, and central glenoid erosion. These findings are illustrated in (**A**). (**B,C**) Computed tomography cuts; (**B**) a cut just below the coracoid process seemingly indicating ample bone for placing the glenoid component. (**D**) A cut near the lower end of the glenoid, again showing ample bone remaining in the glenoid and also illustrating the loosening of the humeral stem. A glenoid component was placed. (**D,E**) A new humeral component was positioned and cemented in place.

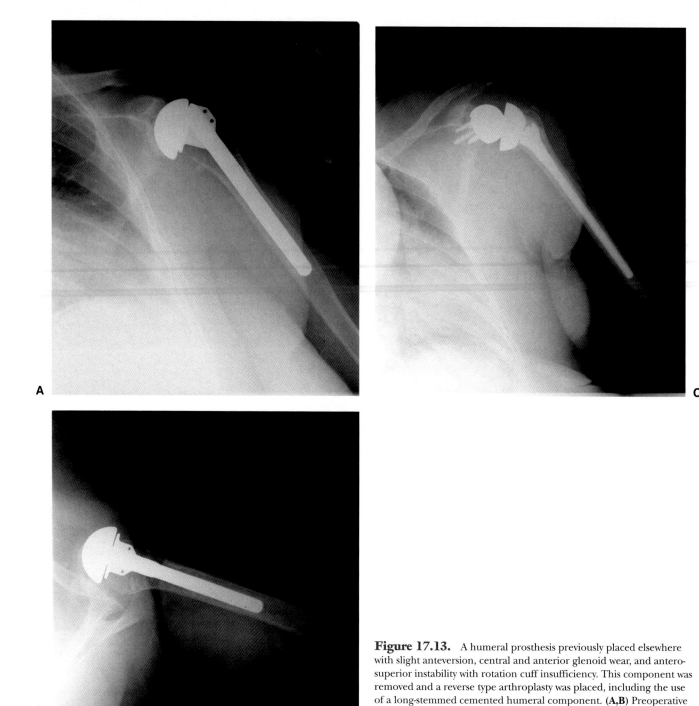

Figure 17.13. A humeral prosthesis previously placed elsewhere with slight anteversion, central and anterior glenoid wear, and antero-superior instability with rotation cuff insufficiency. This component was removed and a reverse type arthroplasty was placed, including the use of a long-stemmed cemented humeral component. (**A,B**) Preoperative radiographs. (**C**) Component postoperative positioning.

REFERRED TOTAL SHOULDER ARTHROPLASTIES

During the period from 1980 to 2005, 96 failed total shoulder arthroplasties were directed to us and underwent revision arthroplasty (Tables 17.4 and 17.5). In 88 shoulders there were difficulties with the glenoid; this included glenoid loosening in 66, substantial glenoid wear often with involvement of underlying metal in 14, glenoid material fracture in six, and

substantial malposition in two. Eighty-three of these required treatment directed toward the glenoid. The glenoid was removed in 55, the surface was recontoured only in 16, and the surface was recontoured and the cavity filled with allograft bone in 39. In 28 a glenoid component was reinserted. The complete glenoid was replaced in 23, and new plastic was applied to a metal-backed component in five.

As we discovered with the hemiarthroplasty failures that were referred to us for revision surgery, often there was not an

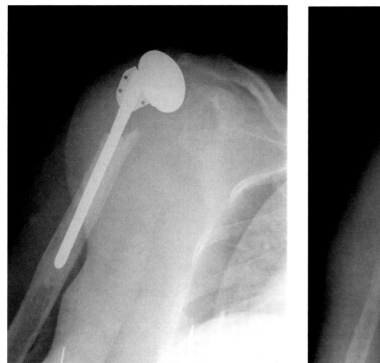
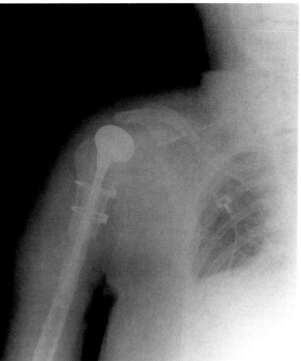

A

B

Figure 17.14. This middle-aged woman had a complex proximal humeral fracture. The upper end of the humerus was resected, and the rotator cuff was repaired to the remaining humeral shaft. Not unexpectedly, instability ensued. A proximal humeral bulk allograft with retained rotator cuff was positioned about the prosthesis, and secured with cerclage cables, and the allograft rotator cuff and native rotator cuff that remained nicely in position were strongly sutured one to the other to effect greater component stability. Pre- (**A**) and postoperative (**B**) radiographs.

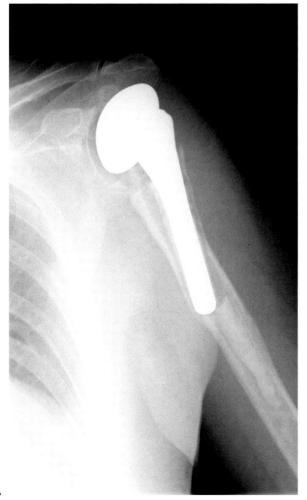
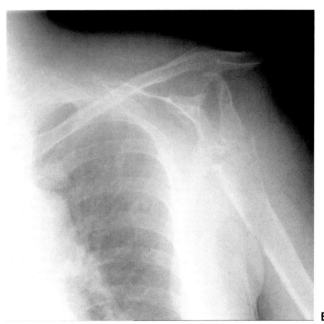

B

Figure 17.15. A middle-aged man with a complex proximal humeral fracture who had a humeral head prosthesis placed. He had substantial pain and quite poor function. Further evaluation demonstrated an active infection. The component and cement were removed. There was such extensive destruction of the glenoid, the shoulder capsule, and rotator cuff that the shoulder was left as a resection arthroplasty. (**A**) Preoperative radiograph. (**B**) After resection.

A

179

TABLE 17.4	Revisions of Referred Total Shoulder Arthroplasties (n = 96)
Reasons for Revision	*Number of Shoulders*
Glenoid component issues	88
Glenoid loosening	66
Wear	14
Fracture	6
Malposition	2
Instability	44
Posterior	23
Anterior-superior	9
Anterior	9
Superior	3
Humeral component issues	41
Malposition	26
Loosening	14
Too small	1
Rotator cuff tear	26
Supraspinatus, infraspinatus	10
Subscapularis, supraspinatus	6
Supraspinatus	4
Subscapularis	3
Infraspinatus	3
Late infection	2
Periprosthetic humeral fracture	1

TABLE 17.5	Treatment of Referred Total Shoulder Arthroplasties (n = 96)
Procedure	*Number of Shoulders*
Glenoid component issues	
Remove component and bone graft	39
Remove and reinsert new component	28
Remove and recontour bone	16
Humeral component issues	
Place new standard length component	25
Cement	17
Place long-stem component	18
Cement	14
Change humeral head	41
Change humeral head or stem	3
for exposure only	
Bone graft humerus	14
Rotator cuff repair	24
Shoulder capsule tightening	11
Posterior	9
Anterosuperior	2
Infection	
Primary exchange	1
Resection and spacer	1

isolated problem but a combination of problems that existed in many of the shoulders. For example, in addition to the glenoid issues outlined above, 44 shoulders also presented with glenohumeral instability. This was posterior in 23, anterior in nine, anterosuperior in nine, superior in three.

In 26, there was rotator cuff tearing. This involved the supraspinatus and infraspinatus in ten, the subscapularis and supraspinatus in six, the supraspinatus only in four, the subscapularis only in three, and the infraspinatus in three. These tears could be re-repaired in 24 cases.

The humeral component was found to be loose in 14 shoulders. The humeral component was malpositioned and required positional correction with stem removal in 26. The humeral head was dramatically undersized in one, and tension across the joint was addressed by enlarging the humeral head.

There was only one periprosthetic fracture. This was addressed by converting the short stem to a long-stemmed, cemented humeral component and adding a bone graft to the fracture site.

There were two late infections. One underwent resection related not only to the infection but also to severe soft tissue deficiencies. In one the infection was of quite low grade; the shoulder underwent a primary exchange to new components supported by antibiotic-impregnated bone cement. Figures 17.16 through 17.25 illustrate several of the issues encountered and their methods of correction.

LESSONS LEARNED

Patients with unsuccessful shoulder arthroplasties typically present with a combination of pain and functional limitations, often stiffness, but occasionally instability or weakness. We have

observed, as outlined previously, with assessment of our own failed cases, that there is usually an isolated issue such as glenoid arthritis in hemiarthroplasty or glenoid wear with osteolysis and loosening in total shoulder arthroplasty. These isolated problems offer opportunities for a rather direct approach and hopefully a high frequency of success. For many arthroplasties that presented to us from elsewhere, there were a combination of factors associated with a failure. Thus we have learned to be very cautious in evaluation, being patient in listening to the history and reviewing outside records, being careful about physical examination, obtaining accurately positioned high-quality radiographs[1] and obtaining adjunctive images if necessary. We are also very mindful of the possibility of there being an occult low-grade infection,[2] because many of these shoulders have very little in the way of infection identifiable preoperatively but have positive intraoperative cultures.

Additional images might include bone scanning to identify focal increased uptake around the glenoid component or a generalized increased activity around the shoulder, indicative of an inflammatory process. Indium-labeled white cell scans are sometimes a useful adjunct to understanding the overall picture but do not often appear to be diagnostic in and of themselves. With a suspicion of infection, aspiration is useful, both for cell count with differential and obtaining a specimen for aerobic and anaerobic culture. Arthrography can be useful to outline the shoulder and assess the level of synovitis; assess whether or not the dye tracks around the components, implying component loosening; or, of course, determine whether there is rotator cuff tearing or not. Computed tomography (CT) evaluation can be helpful in further understanding the glenoid, whether or not the component is loose, identifying how much glenoid bone remains; adjunctively, CT can define the rotator cuff muscles fairly well to identify whether substan-

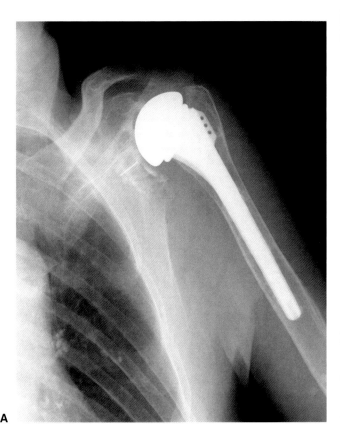

A

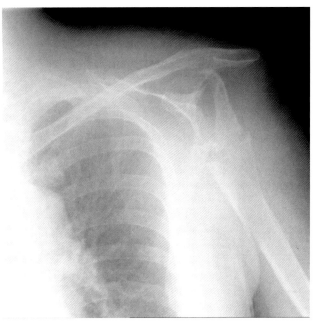

B

Figure 17.16. Glenoid-component loosening with medial shifting of the glenoid component and extensive cavitation of the glenoid cavity. The humeral component is well positioned and secure. Revision was performed, including removal of the glenoid component, cement, and histiocytic membrane. Allograft bone was placed in the glenoid cavity, and humeral head size was adjusted to affect stability and ample motion. Pre- (**A**) and postoperative (**B**) radiographs.

tive atrophy is present. Magnetic resonance imaging could also outline the muscles quite nicely, but the metal artifact in the joint greatly obscures the rotator cuff tendons and subtleties about the implants and the bone immediately surrounding the implants. Ultrasonography can further define the subscapularis and supraspinatus tendons.

When there is pain in the shoulder but all other aspects of the evaluation are normal, we have been very reluctant to undertake revision surgery. In this setting there probably is a problem that is just not yet identifiable. In these cases, we follow the patients over time to assess whether the pain continues or diminishes and also to further the search for structural changes becoming evident that were not definable at the earlier evaluation.

AT SURGERY

For revision and primary cases we have typically used interscalene block anesthesia supplemented by a light general anesthetic. A beach chair position is used, with ample exposure of the shoulder anteriorly, superiorly, and posteriorly, and draping the arm free. We use a Mayo stand, movable in position and height, to assist in arm support throughout the case.

The previous skin incision is carefully considered. Often the old skin incision is excised to create a fresh incision line on closure. Sometimes the incisions are so far medial, lateral, or transverse that they cannot be incorporated into an incision for an anterior approach, but this is uncommon. Usually, after being excised, the old incision is either used alone or incorpo-

rated into a new incision that might be somewhat more extensile. For approximately 90% of revision cases, a deltopectoral exposure is used. The deltoid is identified proximally at its attachment on the clavicle, and the line along the medial border of the anterior deltoid is developed separating the deltoid from the cephalic vein and the pectoralis major, which are allowed to remain medial. The incision line is extended distally, often freeing the anterior-most aspect of the deltoid insertion on the humerus to make sure the deltoid is flexible and can be brought aside without undue stress on it. We then develop the interval between the deltoid and the underlying structures from medial to lateral and from distal to proximal, identifying planes in those areas and following them proximally and laterally. The area beneath the coracoacromial ligament is incised and the plane on top of the rotator cuff defined, separating it from the overlying acromion process. This plane is then extended laterally and posteriorly to meet the plane that has been developed beneath the deltoid muscle. Often the most difficult part of the exposure is the area immediately beneath the lateral border of the acromion; by changing humeral positions in several ways, one can connect the superior and lateral areas of dissection to completely mobilize the subacromial-subdeltoid space, protecting the axillary nerve and its extensions as it courses around the posterior aspect of the humerus, across the subdeltoid space, and on to the undersurface of the deltoid muscle. The area beneath the conjoined tendon group is then developed. This is usually most easily accomplished by starting superiorly, just distal to the coracoid process where the conjoined group is pulled away from the underlying subscapularis by virtue of the support of the coracoid process. If this proves

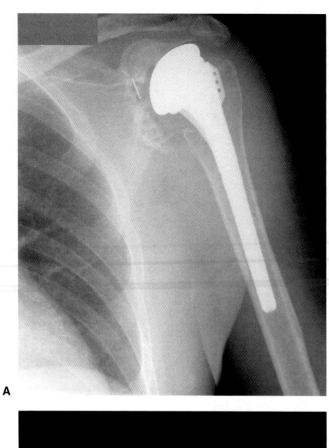

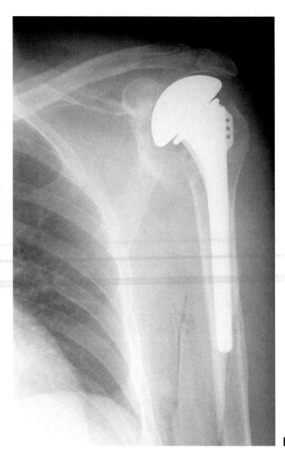

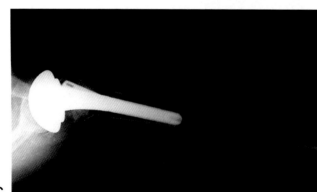

Figure 17.17. Glenoid-component loosening and extensive central glenoid erosion. The modular humeral component was well fixed in a reasonable position. The loosened glenoid component, cement, and histiocytic membrane were removed. The glenoid cavity was bone grafted with allograft bone chips, and the humeral head size was adjusted. **(A)** Preoperative radiograph. **(B,C)** Postoperative radiographs, with **(C)** nicely illustrating the even concavity reformed after remodeling of the allograft bone.

too difficult, one can then approach the conjoined group distal to the subscapularis and work proximally and then work from lateral to medial to carefully elevate the coracobrachialis and short head of the biceps brachii off the underlying subscapularis while at the same time protecting the neurovascular structures, particularly the axillary and musculocutaneous nerves. One must note that the extension of the brachial plexus is nearby and must be carefully protected. Finally, knowledge of the location of the branches of the nerves to the subscapularis muscle must be considered during this dissection.[3,4]

For approximately 10% of revision procedures we prefer an anteromedial approach to the shoulder.[5] This includes developing the deltopectoral interval, but when attempting to free the deltoid from the underlying tissues the exposure is converted to the anteromedial approach because it is recog-

nized that dissection is so difficult that one is worried about damaging the branches of the axillary nerve on the undersurface of the anterior deltoid, the anterior deltoid is so thin from previous injury and surgery that one is quite worried about stretching and tearing it, the distortion of anatomy is so extreme that greater general exposure is needed, or the bone is so osteopenic from generalized disease as in rheumatoid arthritis or arthroplasty-induced osteolysis one wishes to place less stress on these structures throughout the case. We have not found using the anteromedial approach with release of the anterior deltoid from the clavicle and anterior acromion to be a negative. In our cases we have never had detachment of the deltoid reattachment postoperatively, because in the postoperative period the underlying repair is protected and this in turn protects the anterior deltoid repair.

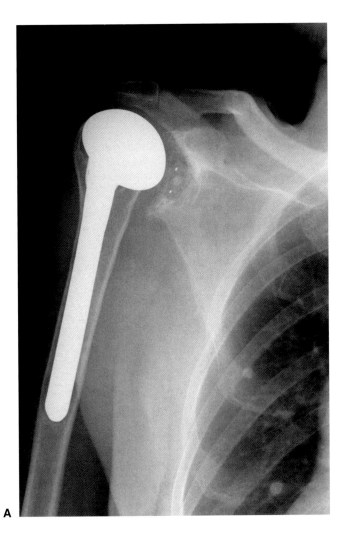

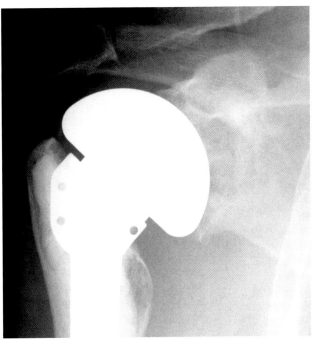

Figure 17.18. Both glenoid- and humeral-component loosening with some osteolysis at the lower end of the humeral stem. Both the glenoid and humeral components were removed, along with underlying glenoid bone cement and all histiocytic debris. The glenoid was packed with allograft bone chips. A new humeral component was cemented in place. Pre (**A**) and postoperative (**B**) radiographs.

After freeing the subdeltoid, subacromial, and subconjoined group layer thoroughly, the rotator cuff is assessed and the shoulder is again taken through a range of motion (ROM). Occasionally freeing this layer allows much more glenohumeral motion than one would anticipate, but that is the exception rather than the rule in failed arthroplasty cases. At this point when performing the arthrotomy we incise low in the interval area just above the upper border of the subscapularis muscle tendon unit. We free the contractures that are present around the base of the coracoid. If there is 30 degrees or more of passive external rotation with the arm at the side or if there is very little lesser tuberosity remaining (the lesser tuberosity has been filled with an implant or bone cement), we will incise the subscapularis and anterior shoulder capsule 5 mm medial to the capsule insertion to the bone of the humerus. This will then allow us to do a direct capsule and tendon repair at the end of the case. If there is less than 30 degrees of external rotation available and there is ample lesser tuberosity to sew back to at the end of the case, we will release the subscapularis from bone, release the anterior capsule from bone, and then continue the release distally through the upper portion of the pectoralis major and upper portions of the latissimus dorsi and teres major. This creates a rather long anterior arthrotomy. It also then allows us to slowly externally rotate the humerus and free the inferior capsule safely from the humeral neck.[6] As we

rotate the humerus externally, more inferior capsule comes into view; typically this is released past the 6 o'clock position to the 4 o'clock position in a right shoulder and the 8 o'clock position in a left shoulder. Care is taken to stay completely on the bone to avoid iatrogenic damage to the axillary nerve.

After all of these releases the humeral head can typically be subluxated forward with very little force. The humeral component is assessed for its position anterior to posterior, medial to lateral, and superior to inferior and for rotational alignment. Most implants currently are modular, and the modular humeral head can be removed. The humeral component is then forcefully stressed in rotation and the axial direction assessing for tightness or looseness, often using the holder for the humeral component designed for that particular implant system. Unfortunately, as can be seen from the earlier discussion of cases, all too often the humeral stem has been malpositioned and consideration must be given to its removal, if position cannot be successfully corrected with alteration of head position using the eccentric head options that are available for some systems.

The joint is now distracted laterally. Specimens are taken for frozen section histology, and multiple cultures are obtained, usually 3 to 5 in number. The synovium is inspected for its characteristics, and the glenoid is assessed or the glenoid prosthesis is evaluated for wear, position, and looseness or tightness.

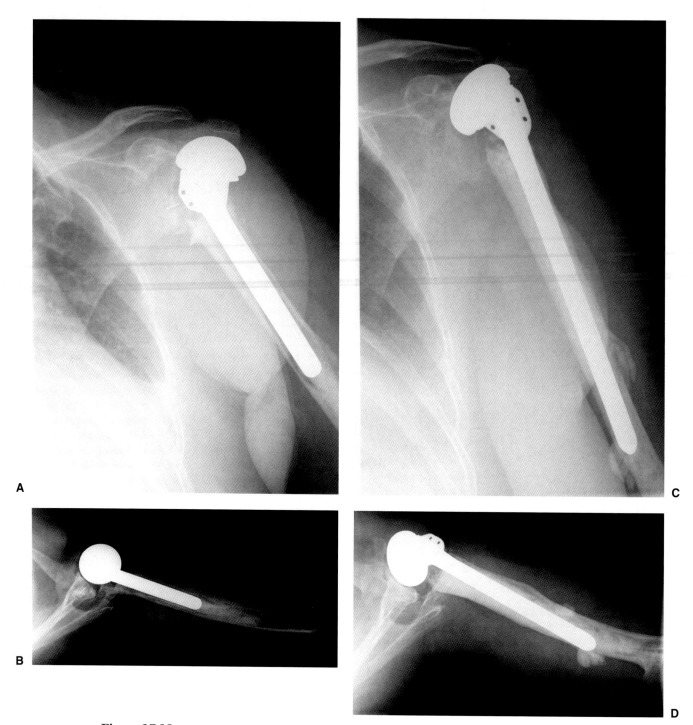

Figure 17.19.   Loosening of both the glenoid and humeral components. Previous resection of the upper portion of the humerus and tuberosities had been performed secondary to complex fracturing. Anterolateral rotation of the loosened humeral component and anterior shoulder instability. Both of the loosened components were removed. The hollow glenoid cavity was packed with allograft bone chips. A new humeral component was secured in appropriate position. The anterior shoulder capsule structures were firmly repaired. This created a reconstruction similar to a primary procedure one might undertake for rotator cuff tear arthropathy in the face of insufficient glenoid bone to support a reverse component. Pre- **(A,B)** and postoperative radiographs **(C,D)**.

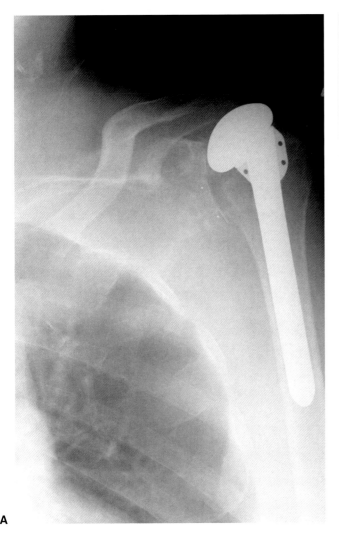

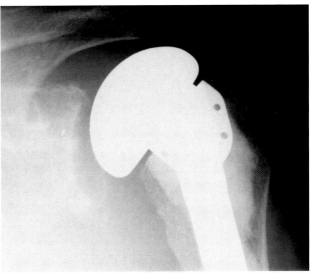

Figure 17.20. A painful malfunctioning total shoulder arthroplasty. The glenoid component was positioned too low. The humeral component was positioned too high. At revision surgery both components were removed. The glenoid component was positioned 1 cm more superior than it had been, and the humeral component was positioned 1 cm lower than it previously had been positioned. Pre- (**A**) and postoperative (**B**) radiographs.

If the humeral stem does not need to be removed, the humerus is retracted posteriorly. To obtain more flexibility for the anterior structures, the anterosuperior shoulder capsule is incised at the glenoid rim and this incision is continued laterally along the superior band of the inferior glenohumeral ligament to free the subscapularis and anterosuperior shoulder capsule from contracture. Hypertrophic scar within the joint is excised. If the posterior capsule is too tight, incision is made along the posterior aspect of the glenoid rim, and an elevator is carefully inserted in this area to enhance the freedom of movement of the posterior muscles and tendons, without tethering by the capsule insertion on the posterior aspect of the glenoid. The humeral head is then more fully subluxated in the posterior direction, and the glenoid or glenoid implant is thoroughly assessed. If there is substantial glenoid component wear, malposition, or loosening, the component is removed. This is readily done by use of the small microsagittal router, an instrument that cuts through polyethylene like a hot knife through butter. The surface of the glenoid component is cut around the pegs and removed. The margins of the polyethylene pegs are then cut and the pegs extracted. If a keel has been used earlier, the margin of the keel is cut and removed. Loose underlying cement, if present, is then removed and the

bone is cleaned. If two thirds of the glenoid subchondral plate and bone within the glenoid vault remain intact, a new glenoid component can be inserted. When only half of these bony elements remain, fixation quality is more marginal, and certainly when two thirds of the glenoid face and internal aspect of the glenoid vault bone are absent, one is very concerned about the ability to place a secure glenoid component. In our practice it seems that approximately two thirds of the time there is enough glenoid bone loss that placing a new glenoid component does not seem wise. The glenoid surface is then reshaped to a gentle concavity. Allograft of bone is impacted into the deficient areas.[7]

If the humeral stem needs to be removed, there are several options for doing this. The most simple and direct is to cut around the top part of the implant, or implant and cement, removing cement whenever possible. This again is most readily accomplished by a pencil-like router that can extend for approximately 5 cm down the humeral canal. Also, if the humeral stem rests medially and firmly against the medial cortex of the proximal humerus, a small V-shaped section can be removed from the medial cortex to facilitate detaching the implant or implant and cement from the upper humerus.[8] It is quite helpful when doing this to have the specific humeral

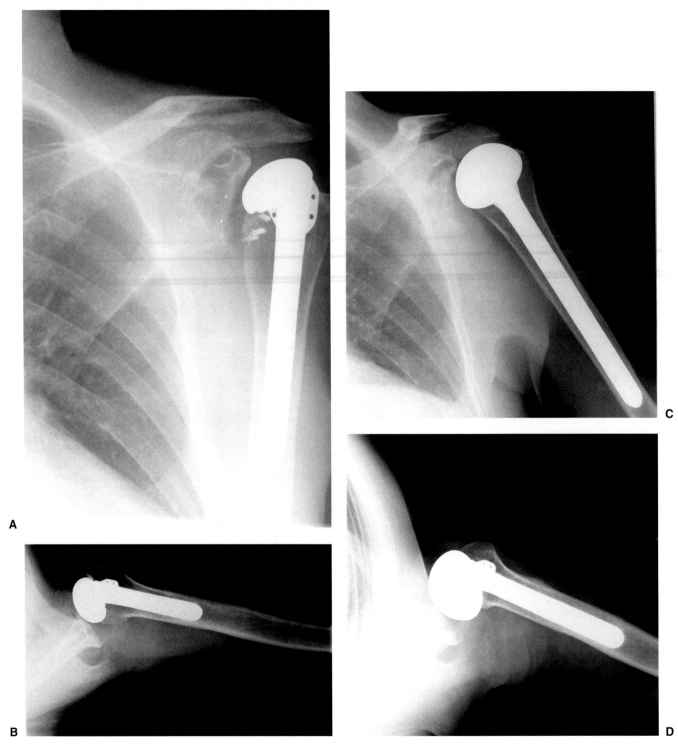

Figure 17.21.   Total shoulder arthroplasty with anterior shoulder instability. In addition to the soft tissue deficiency the humeral head seemed slightly undersized for a person of this stature and the humeral component was positioned in 20 degrees of retroversion. At revision surgery the humeral component was repositioned in 35 degrees of retroversion. The humeral head size was increased to match the size of the person. The surrounding capsule and rotator cuff musculature and the soft tissues were meticulously repaired. After surgery the arm was supported in internal rotation for 1 month. **(A,B)** Preoperative radiographs. **(C,D)** Postoperative radiographs illustrating a residual anterior instability. This illustrates not only the reconstructive techniques used but how difficult it is to consistently eliminate instability once it has developed.

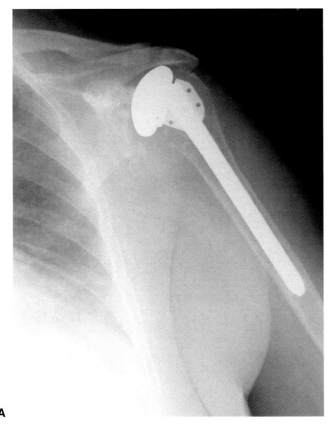

A

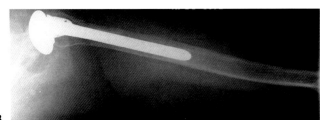

B

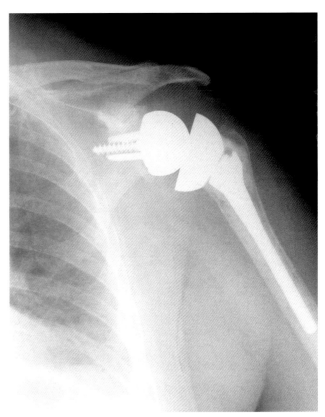

C

Figure 17.22. A total shoulder arthroplasty with glenoid-component loosening and dislodgement from the glenoid fossa coupled with anterior-superior shoulder instability as a result of rotator cuff tearing. **(A,B)** Glenoid-component position in the posterior subdeltoid pouch. **(C)** Reverse shoulder arthroplasty following removal of both components and grafting of the glenoid using bone from the proximal humerus.

holder/extractor available for the system that was placed. After freeing around the upper third of the humeral component, one can often hold the humerus downward and try to disimpact the humeral stem upward.

If the humeral stem will not come free after doing this, the problem becomes much more difficult. If the humeral stem is cemented in place, it seems most useful to further free the anterior aspect of the deltoid insertion from the humerus and develop a longitudinal split in the humerus through bone and cement down to the humeral implant for the full length of the implant. One can then use osteotomes and quite carefully spread the split, separating the metallic implant from the cement and bone. Unless the humeral implant is too textured, one can with caution then drive the implant out of the humerus, remove any loose cement, re-prepare the internal surface of the remaining cement, and use cement within cement fixation for a new humeral component. We prefer to fix the humerus after doing this maneuver with two to three cerclage cables that are available in fracture management systems. If it does not seem that a longitudinal split will be ample, because a more fully textured stem is right up against the

humeral cortex, or there is a very thin layer of cement present, an anterior humeral window approximately 1 cm wide and extending the full length of the humeral component is a useful osteotomy method to reach the internal aspect of the humeral canal and free the malpositioned humeral component from the humerus. When reconstructing this we prefer to use a longer stem to go past the window and cement the stem in the distal aspect of the humerus. Sometimes cement is used proximally, but often the area surrounding the proximal aspect of the humeral stem is filled with allograft bone graft material and the window is repositioned and secured in place with heavy cerclage sutures.

Instability is a very special issue in failed shoulder arthroplasty. This is not uncommon and is often seen in association with malpositioned components or with rotator cuff tearing. Thankfully, posterior instability can usually be corrected by appropriate component position and adjusting humeral head size. If this will not be adequate, one can tighten the posterior shoulder capsule either internally with longitudinal and transverse suturing from within the joint or externally by developing a trap door–like flap of the infraspinatus and underlying shoulder

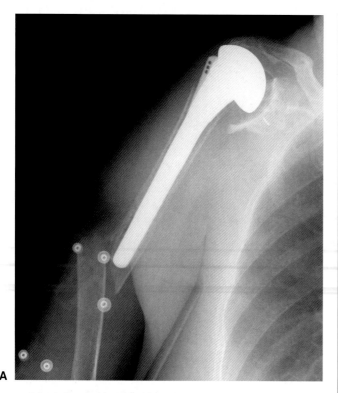

A

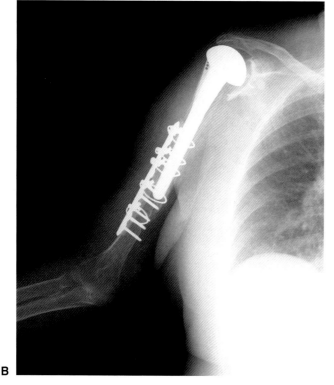

B

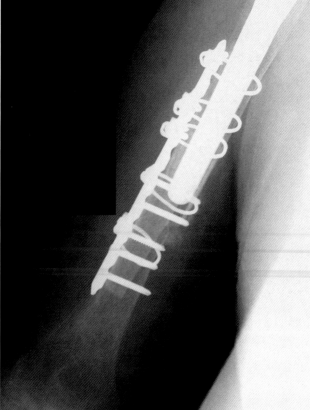

C

Figure 17.23. A periprosthetic humeral shaft fracture through osteopenic bone. The humeral component is secure in its position, and the shoulder arthroplasty was functioning well despite rotator cuff tearing before the fall. The fracture was fixed with a lateral plate, screws, pins, and cables. Because of anticipation of a rather weak healing response, a strut allograft was placed anteriorly in addition to placing particulate autogenous bone graft material. **(A)** The fracture, **(B)** early following fracture fixation, and **(C)** later, when consolidation has occurred. The patient was managed postoperatively with a sling and shoulder immobilizer for 3 months until there was ample evidence of bone consolidation.

capsule and advancing it laterally on the humerus, suturing these structures more tightly. The side opposite the instability must be made quite flexible so that in the postoperative period, when, for example, attempting external rotation, the humeral head is not forced posteriorly, recreating the posterior instability. In the patients we have encountered we have found that anterior instability is often associated with component malposition (usually neutral or anteversion of the humeral component) plus

stretching of the anterior shoulder structures. Repositioning the components helps a great deal toward regaining anterior stability. The subscapularis can often be resutured firmly to the humerus, and occasionally this needs to be reinforced with a portion of the pectoralis major. Anterosuperior instability is very difficult to control. This is associated with rotator cuff tearing of the upper subscapularis and anterior aspect of the supraspinatus. Rotator cuff repair is possible in this setting and may be preferable to other treatment alternatives, but the chances of success are low.[9,10] For many patients in this setting, if they are older, conversion to a reverse type prosthesis will probably prove to be the better choice.

Late periprosthetic humeral shaft fractures come in a variety of locations and shapes, extent of displacement, and condition of the humeral stem and surrounding proximal bone. Certainly if the humeral stem is loose and there is a great deal of osteolysis, one must in this circumstance strongly consider performing revision total shoulder arthroplasty and at the same time fixing the fracture with a variety of tools, usually including a lateral plate, cables, and screws with pins inserted throughout the plate wherever practically possible during cable application. If the bone is somewhat weakened, a cortical allograft strut can be added. If the fracture is acute, we have not developed the habit of using adjunctive bone graft; however, if there is any chronicity to the fracture, the combination of autogenous iliac crest bone graft and allograft seems to be very reasonable.[11] On the other hand, if the humeral component is secure, but the periprosthetic fracture is not well aligned or too unstable to allow conservative treatment with a sling and brace, one can consider internal fixation of the fracture itself with a plate with or without an allograft strut and with a combination of screws and cables. These fractures seem to take a very long time to heal, and quite ample internal fixation seems to be the best choice rather than marginal fixation methods.[12–14]

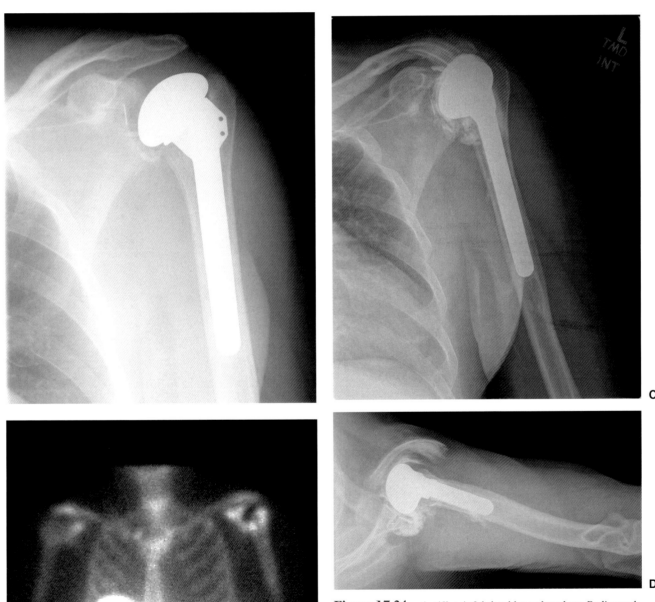

Figure 17.24. A stiff, painful shoulder arthroplasty. Radiograph illustrates loosening of the glenoid component and settling of the humeral component distalward within the humerus (**A**). Technetium bone scan (**B**) illustrating considerable activity about the glenohumeral joint and lesser but increased activity within the humeral shaft. The shoulder was aspirated and an arthrogram performed. Bacteria grew from the aspirate (**C,D**).

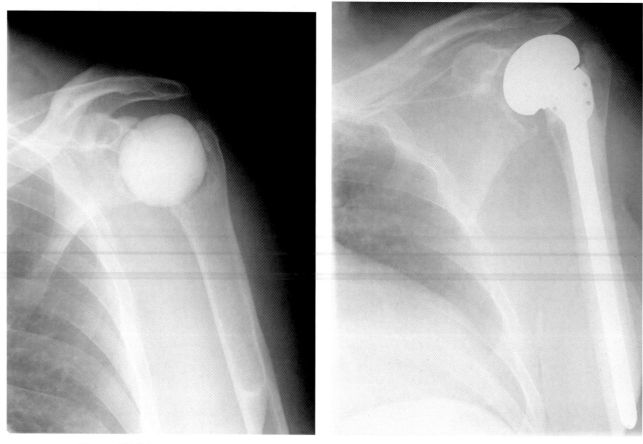

E   F

Figure 17.24. *(continued)* Arthrographic pictures show considerable synovitis within the joint and dye tracking around the glenoid component, confirming loosening. A two-stage revision was performed. The components were removed. The shoulder was thoroughly debrided, and an antibiotic spacer was positioned within the glenohumeral joint (**E**). Eight weeks later this was removed and a new humeral head prosthesis was placed, fixed in position with antibiotic-impregnated bone cement (**F**).

Thinking continues to evolve in the care of infected shoulder arthroplasties.[15] It seems that during these times the most common type of infection problem encountered is a positive culture at the time of revision surgery for glenoid component loosening in the absence of any other preoperative or interoperative factors indicative of infection. Related to this, and recognizing this is a reality, we at the time of revision surgery do a thorough joint debridement, a thorough joint cleansing with pulsatile lavage, and careful inspection of the implant bone interface and use antibiotics in bone cement that is used for reinsertion of components. We also consider mixing antibiotics with particulate allograft bone when that is used as a part of the reconstructive procedure.

If there is a known chronic infection in an older patient and the infection is of rather low grade in terms of its aggressiveness, we may well consider a primary exchange removing the components and cement, thorough debridement, thorough irrigation, and reinserting new parts fixed in place with antibiotic-impregnated bone cement. Currently, though, if the cultures are positive at the time of this revision surgery our infectious disease consultants think these patients must be kept on antibiotics for a long time, so this method seems from a practical point of view very difficult for middle-aged people. Typically, if chronic infection is identified, we at this point prefer a two-stage revision procedure removing all components

and cement, thorough debridement, thorough lavage, and placing an antibiotic-impregnated bone cement spacer. Intravenous antibiotics are then continued for 6 weeks. Several weeks later the second stage procedure is undertaken, removing the antibiotic-impregnated spacer and placing a new component or components. If the cultures are positive, antibiotics are usually continued for a long period. If the cultures are negative at that time, further antibiotic care is not provided.

Rarely, there will be such extensive tissue destruction by infection that it does not seem practically possible to replace components. This occurs when the capsule and rotator cuff or the rotator cuff attachments to the humerus have been destroyed by the infectious process and when the glenoid has been so terribly eroded that it would not support any kind of new component; in this setting, resection arthroplasty is performed. Usually this cures the infection and provides comfortable use with the arm near the side, but at least a third of patients have more pain than they would want to have and the overall function of the shoulder is poor.

Following any revision procedure it is important to use ample arm support in the form of a shoulder immobilizer, sling, or brace to protect the vulnerable soft tissues. We typically direct the support be used for 6 weeks. The passive rehabilitation program[16] will be commenced on the first postoperative day if healing of a torn rotator cuff or repair for instability

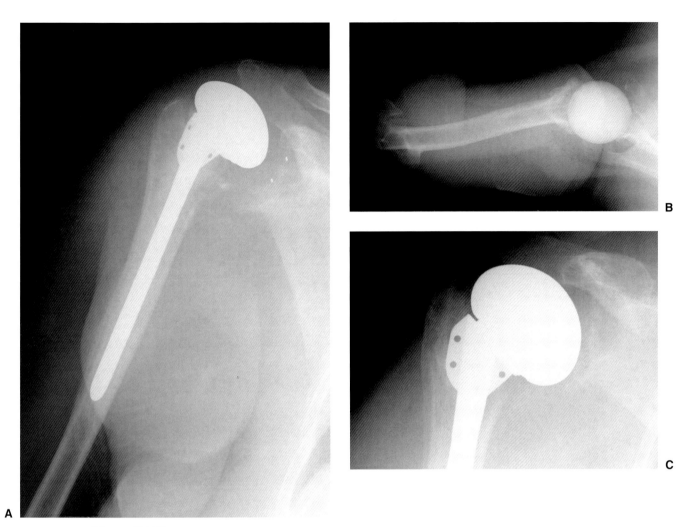

Figure 17.25. This shoulder presented with substantial pain, stiffness, and slight redness on the anterior aspect of the shoulder. **(A)** Illustrating resorption of the proximal humerus, particularly in the calcar region. On aspiration there were multiple white cells and bacteria grew. At revision surgery, because of polishing of the distal three quarters of the humeral component, the humeral component could be removed from above by cutting around the upper end of the component and then driving it free from the bone cement. The bone cement was then removed, as was a loosened glenoid component. The glenohumeral space was filled with bone cement impregnated with multiple units of antibiotics **(B)**. Eight weeks later this spacer was removed and a new humeral head component was placed. Enough humeral bone remained to allow positioning with an in-growth humeral component **(C)**.

has not been undertaken as a part of the procedure. If these two things have been important components of the procedure, we will often defer rehabilitation to allow these repaired structures to heal, knowing that it is very difficult to obtain healing of these structures with the maintenance of shoulder stability in revision shoulder arthroplasty.

REFERENCES

1. Kelleher IM, Cofield RH, Becker DA, et al. Fluoroscopically positioned radiographs of total shoulder arthroplasty. *J Shoulder Elbow Surg* 1992;1:306–311.
2. Topolski MS, Chin PYK, Sperling JW, et al. Revision shoulder arthroplasty with positive intraoperative cultures: the value of preoperative studies and intraoperative histology. *J Shoulder Elbow Surg* 2006;15:402–406.
3. Lynch NM, Cofield RH, Silbert PL, et al. Neurologic complications after total shoulder arthroplasty. *J Shoulder Elbow Surg* 1996;5:53–61.
4. Boardman ND 3rd, Cofield RH. Neurologic complications of shoulder surgery. *Clin Orthop* 1999;368:44–53.
5. Gill GRJ, Cofield RH, Rowland C. The anteromedial approach for shoulder arthroplasty: the importance of the anterior deltoid. *J Shoulder Elbow Surg* 2994;13:532–537.
6. Cofield RH. Integral surgical maneuvers in prosthetic shoulder arthroplasty. *Semin Arthroplasty* 1990;1:112–123.
7. Antuña SA, Sperling JW, Cofield RH, et al. Glenoid revision surgery after total shoulder arthroplasty. *J Shoulder Elbow Surg* 2001;10:217–224.
8. Sperling JW, Cofield RH. Humeral windows in revision shoulder arthroplasty. *J Shoulder Elbow Surg* 2005;14:258–263.
9. Sanchez-Sotelo J, Sperling JW, Rowlan CM, et al. Instability after shoulder arthroplasty: results of surgical treatment. *J Bone Joint Surg Am* 2003;85:622–631.
10. Hattrup SJ, Cofield RH, Cha SS. Rotator cuff repair after shoulder replacement. *J Shoulder Elbow Surg* 2006;15:78–83.
11. Krakauer JD, Cofield RH. Periprosthetic fractures in total shoulder replacement. *Oper Tech Orthop* 1994;4:243–252.
12. Wright TW, Cofield RH. Humeral fractures after shoulder arthroplasty. *J Bone Joint Surg Am* 1995;77:1340–1346.
13. Kumar S, Sperling JW, Haidukewych GH, et al. Periprosthetic humeral fractures after shoulder arthroplasty. *J Bone Joint Surg Am* 2004;86:680–689.
14. Cofield RH, Sperling JW, Morrey BF, et al. Periprosthetic fractures of the elbow and shoulder. In: Bucholz RW, Heckman JD, Court-Brown CM, eds. *Rockwood and Green's Fractures in Adults.* 6th edition. Philadelphia: Lippincott Williams & Wilkins; 2006:681–703.
15. Sperling JW, Kozak TK, Hanssen AD, et al. Infection after shoulder arthroplasty. *Clin Orthop* 2001;382:206–216.
16. Boardman ND III, Cofield RH, Bengtson KA, et al. Rehabilitation after total shoulder arthroplasty. *J Arthroplasty* 2001;16:483–486.

Specific Types of Reconstruction

Thomas W. Wright

Periprosthetic Humeral Fractures

INTRODUCTION

Fractures of the humerus associated with shoulder arthroplasty have a reported incidence of 0.5% to 3%.[1,2] These fractures occur both intraoperatively and postoperatively. They can range in complexity from stable, nondisplaced fractures to comminuted, highly unstable ones. Predisposing patient factors include advancing age, osteoporosis, rheumatoid arthritis, female gender,[2] prior proximal humerus fracture, and revision shoulder arthroplasty. Predisposing surgical factors include difficult or less extensive exposure by the surgeon.

Intraoperative fractures occur much more frequently than postoperative fractures and generally involve bone about the prosthesis. Patients undergoing revision shoulder arthroplasty are at especially high risk for this complication. Periprosthetic humeral fractures that occur intraoperatively are stable or unstable. The stable variety occurs when broaching and final impacting of the prosthesis results in a minimally displaced metaphyseal fracture. These fractures are usually benign and require minimal treatment. On occasion, a surgeon might want to place a proximal cerclage wire to augment these fractures, but in most cases no internal fixation is necessary. The unstable variety of intraoperative periprosthetic fractures are usually secondary to reaming of the humeral diaphysis (the humerus is not a femur) and less complete surgical exposure. The fracture occurs with rotation as the shoulder is being dislocated or reduced or with attempts at glenoid exposure. These fractures are long oblique or spiral and extend past the tip of the implant, rendering the implant unstable. This type of fracture must be recognized and treated at the time of surgery. Unfortunately, these fractures may be increasing in frequency with the advancing popularity of uncemented humeral prosthetic designs, in an effort by the surgeon to obtain a true press fit.[1]

Humeral fractures occurring around a shoulder prosthesis after surgery generally are the result of a low-energy fall[2] and are more often located distal to the prosthesis, as opposed to intraoperative fractures. The humerus is particularly at risk if there is associated poor-quality bone or the diaphysis has been aggressively reamed. Rheumatoid patients with an ipsilateral shoulder and elbow arthroplasty are at particular risk for fractures developing between the two rigid implants.[3,4] Reverse shoulder arthroplasty, which is becoming a relatively common procedure in the United States, may also lead to an increased risk of humeral periprosthetic fractures because of their constrained nature when a patient falls.

There are several classification systems for periprosthetic humeral fractures. One system describes the fractures based on anatomic location. In type A there is fracture about the tip of the stem extending proximally, in type B fracture about the stem tip extending distally, and in type C fractures distal to the prosthesis[5] (Fig. 18.1[6]). Worland et al[7] proposed a classification based on location of fracture and stability. In type A there are fractures about the tuberosities, in type B1 spiral fracture about the stem (stem stable), in type B2 short oblique/transverse fracture about the stem (stem stable), in type B3 fracture about the prosthesis with stem unstable, and in type C fractures distal to the tip of the stem. Regardless of the system used, the predominant issue is to determine whether the prosthesis is stable.[7]

EVALUATION

Postoperative periprosthetic fractures should be evaluated with good-quality radiographs, including a true anteroposterior view of the glenohumeral joint (30 degrees external oblique), axillary, anteroposterior, and lateral views of the humerus. It is important to know the radiographic and clinical status of the shoulder arthroplasty before surgery. If the implant was performing poorly before fracture, a further workup might include a computed tomography scan to evaluate the glenoid and look for evidence of rotator cuff atrophy, as well as an infection workup with erythrocyte sedimentation rate and C-reactive protein values. For example, a patient who had a poorly functioning total shoulder arthroplasty with a loose glenoid before fracture would be treated very differently from a patient with a good prefracture functional status of the shoulder arthroplasty.

Patient factors are also of significant importance, because revision shoulder surgery with a humeral fracture is major surgery, associated with substantial blood loss. The patient's medical status needs to be optimized, and very frail patients may best be treated nonoperatively or in a manner that will result in the least amount of blood loss.

TREATMENT OPTIONS

There is no one method for treatment of periprosthetic humerus fractures. Issues of paramount importance in determining treatment are the fracture destabilizing the implant, in-

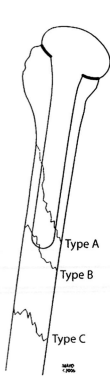

Figure 18.1. Classification system for periprosthetic fractures as proposed by Wright and Cofield.[5] (By permission of Mayo Foundation Education and Research. All rights reserved.)

stability of the fracture itself, patient health, status of the arthroplasty before fracture, and surgeon experience. By far the most important issue is to determine if the implant is stable. If the fracture has not destabilized the implant, nonoperative treatment is a reasonable option; however, a higher rate of nonunion compared to an isolated humeral shaft fracture should be anticipated. A trial with a sling and humeral fracture brace is a reasonable option when the implant is stable. If the patient is not making progress toward union by 3 months, operative intervention should be strongly considered.[8]

Patients with a periprosthetic fracture that destabilizes the implant or that cannot be managed effectively by a fracture brace orthosis should be encouraged to undergo surgical treatment. If the implant is unstable, or stable but the fracture is displaced markedly, open reduction with internal fixation (ORIF) with a 4.5-mm narrow locking plate is an excellent option. The fracture can be fixed with a combination of unicortical locking screws and bicortical screws. The 4- and 5-mm unicortical locking screws are as short as 8 mm if they are taken from the periprosthetic fracture locking plate system. The 8-mm locking screws will generally be short enough to engage the plate before hitting the prosthesis. If need be, cerclage cables can be used as an augmentation for the fixation (use extreme caution near the radial nerve) (Fig. 18.2). The fracture site should be bone grafted, or an osteoinductive graft of the surgeon's choice should be used.

In the situation in which the implant is unstable or the pre-fracture functional status of the implant was poor, the prosthesis should be revised. Options are a long-stemmed implant, which might be part of a revision total shoulder arthroplasty; hemiarthroplasty; or a reverse arthroplasty. The implant should

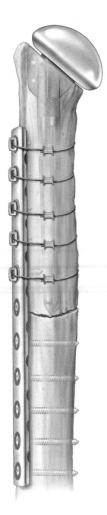

Figure 18.2. Schematic diagram showing open reduction with internal fixation with 4.5-mm locking plate with short locking proximal and distal screws providing compression with bicortical fixation. This construct can be augmented with cerclage wires if necessary. If the cortex is very thin, further augmentation can be made with the use of an allograft onlay graft placed adjacent to the plate and held in place with cables. This fixation works well with a functional implant that was stable before the fracture (cemented or press fit). It precludes the need for revision of the entire implant and tends to be a less traumatic approach to periprosthetic humeral fractures that occur postoperatively.

pass the fracture site by at least three cortical diameters. Cement should be kept out of the fracture site. A short locking plate can add needed rotational stability. Grafting as with the ORIF procedure should be performed. Cortical strut allografts can be added as an onlay graft to restore bone stock (Fig. 18.3). The struts are held in place with cerclage wires.

SURGICAL TECHNIQUE

Preoperative planning is mandatory when undertaking surgery for a periprosthetic humerus fracture. The surgeon should anticipate the status of the humeral stem and have a plan that will focus predominantly on ORIF of the humerus versus a plan for revision of the entire implant. Equipment needs include a

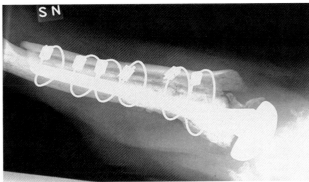

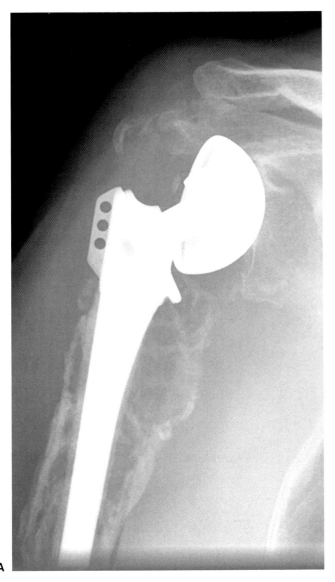

Figure 18.3. Periprosthetic fracture secondary to removal of a bipolar arthroplasty associated with severe osteolysis. **(A)** Preoperative radiograph. The implant was revised to a long-stemmed hemiarthroplasty, bypassing the fracture by three diameters. Because of the very poor bone quality the fixation was further augmented by an allograft onlay graft held in place with cables. **(B)** Postoperative radiograph. This patient sustained a permanent radial nerve injury in the course of the revision, possibly caused by either the cables or bone cement.

4.5-mm locking plate, cable cerclage system, allograft strut graft, several units of packed red blood cells, and an osteoinductive graft. If revision arthroplasty is planned, a long-stemmed shoulder arthroplasty or reverse arthroplasty component should be at hand. If the current humeral stem is cemented, equipment for cement removal needs to be present.

With a well-cemented stem in a patient with a good functioning arthroplasty before fracture, strong preference should be given to the ORIF method of treatment over the long-stemmed revision because of the amount of damage that can occur to the humerus in the process of removing a well-fixed stem. This same consideration should be given to some of the older in-growth stems that can be difficult to remove.

SURGICAL TECHNIQUE FOR OPEN REDUCTION WITH INTERNAL FIXATION

The humeral fracture is approached through a long deltopectoral incision that is extended into an anteriolateral incision. Steinmann and Cheung[6] have done an excellent job of

describing the various approaches to the humerus for the treatment of periprosthetic humeral fractures. The fracture site is exposed using a minimal periosteal stripping technique. (Remember, the endosteal blood flow has already been disrupted by an intramedullary implant.) A long, narrow, 4.5-mm locking plate is used and generally requires no or little contouring. The plate needs to be longer proximal to the fracture site than one used with a typical humeral diaphyseal fracture because of the challenge of proximal fixation in and through and about a stem and cement. To fit this long plate it will be necessary to elevate the anterior third of the deltoid insertion footprint. The fracture is reduced and the plate placed. The plate can be positioned slightly to one side or the other to facilitate passing screws about the stem. Usually one or two screws can be angled around the stem to obtain good bicortical purchase. If cement is present, plan to have multiple drill bits because they will dull rapidly. Once provisional proximal fixation is obtained, the fracture site is compressed through the plate, with a bicortical screw placed distally. Distal to the fracture, bicortical screws usually can be used easily and can be locked or nonlocked depending on the quality of the bone. Proximal fixation can then be completed with unicortical locking screws. In some cases the implant will be contacted before insertion of even the shortest locking screw. If this occurs in multiple holes, proximal fixation will need to be augmented with cerclage cables. However, with the advent of 4- and 5-mm locking screws from the periprosthetic locking plate system, screws as short as 8 mm can be obtained and are generally sufficient to engage the bone before contacting the prosthesis. If cable fixation is necessary, it is best to place them around the humerus, avoiding the area of the spiral groove. The purpose of the plate being longer proximally than distally, is to allow a minimum of four to six locked holes, with six ideal, proximal to the fracture site. With six locked unicortical screws proximal to the fracture site, the need for cables can be minimized or eliminated. Although cables are very useful, they do increase the risk of radial nerve injury. The osteoinductive graft of choice should then be placed about the fracture site.

SURGICAL TECHNIQUE FOR REVISION LONG-STEMMED ARTHROPLASTY

A discussion concerning the glenoid is beyond the scope of this chapter. Nevertheless, its status and that of the subscapularis and the rest of the rotator cuff should be taken into account when choosing the type of long-stemmed implant to be used in the revision. If the rotator cuff or subscapularis is deficient and the patient is elderly, the surgeon may opt to revise the implant with a long-stemmed reverse prosthesis. If none of these conditions are present, then a long-stemmed standard prosthesis will work well.

A standard deltopectoral approach is used. If access to the fracture site is needed, and it generally is, this approach can be extended into an anterolateral approach. The implant is removed after tenotomizing the subscapularis or osteotomizing the lesser tuberosity. All soft tissue along the proximal humeral neck medially is released, protecting the axillary nerve and preserving the rotator cuff. If the implant is modular, the head is removed. Frozen sections are obtained routinely at our institution in all cases of revision implant surgery. If the frozen sections are negative, revision surgery proceeds as planned. Some shoulder arthroplasty systems will have a distracting device for attaching to the humeral component and removing it. If there is not one present, exposure of the anteromedial humerus under the collar of the stem and placement of a bone tamp with the use of a mallet will usually work. If the stem is well cemented, removal of proximal cement will be necessary, followed by using the bone tamp technique for removal. If this still does not work in a cemented stem, access to the stem through the fracture site will be necessary. Unfortunately, this approach requires significant periosteal stripping and devascularization of bone. A bone tamp can then be used after removing distal cement to remove the stem from distal to proximal. If the stem comes out at this time, and most of the cement does not, it may be necessary to remove only the terminal plug, not all of the cement. It may be possible to revise with a smaller diameter long-stemmed prosthesis and cement it into the old cement mantle. This procedure will not work if the initial implant had a small diameter. When ce-

menting into the old cement mantle is not an option, it is best to place a controlled vascularized window the length of the entire proximal humerus. This window is created by exposing a very small area of the anterior humerus, no more than 5 mm wide. Multiple drill holes are placed linearly and at an angle to the surface, about 3 mm apart, starting at the fracture site and extending to the proximal end of the humerus. Using a drill guide and beginning about 5 mm more medially, another set of holes is made parallel to the first, but placed directly through the soft tissue and approximately 5 mm apart. A thin osteotome is used to connect the first row of periosteal stripped holes. Once these holes have been connected, multiple wide curved osteotomes are placed into the osteotomy and the vascularized window is pried open slowly. If done correctly, a hinge will be left on one side and the window will be in one piece with soft tissue connecting to it (Fig. 18.4). The bone cement can then be removed with relative ease.

A long-stemmed humeral prosthesis is then put in place. It should pass the fracture site distally by at least three humeral diameters. Cement should be placed distally but kept out of the fracture site. If a window is used, the proximal humerus can be cemented through it, keeping cement out of the fracture and osteotomy sites. This is usually done by finger packing when the cement is doughy. If there is no cortical window, a minimal proximal cement technique is used. The key is to obtain stability with cement but keep it out of the fractures site and off the radial nerve. After placing the implant, if there are concerns about rotational control about the fracture site, a short locking 3.5-mm plate can be used. Generally, two screws on each side of the fracture site are adequate, with intramedullary stability conferred by the long-stemmed implant (Fig. 18.5). Optionally, a long cortical onlay allograft strut can be held in place with cerclage wires. Some surgeons prefer cerclage, primarily to augment fixation. The surgeon must be very careful to keep these wires subperiosteal if passing them near the radial groove. With the advent of unicortical locking plates, the risk of neurological injury is less because frequently cerclage wire fixation is unnecessary.

SURGICAL TECHNIQUE FOR TREATMENT OF INTRAOPERATIVE FRACTURES

Intraoperative fractures occur in two varieties. One is a minor split of the proximal humerus resulting from final implantation of the stem. The second is a highly unstable long oblique or spiral fracture, usually acquired while dislocating or reducing the humerus or in the course of glenoid preparation. The stable variety generally can be ignored or, if displaced more than a couple of millimeters, may be treated by a simple cerclage wire around the proximal humerus (Fig. 18.6). The unstable variety needs to be treated. Assuming the stem has not been cemented when this fracture occurs, removal of the prosthesis and replacing it with a long-stemmed prosthesis is the most prudent course of action. If there is still concern about rotational stability after placing the long stem, it can be cemented (keeping cement out of the fracture site, which is often difficult) or a short locking plate can be added to provide the needed rotational control. The surgeon must not leave the operating room without obtaining a stable construct.

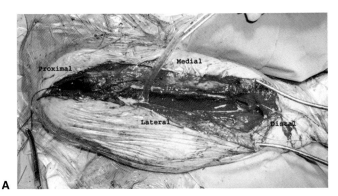

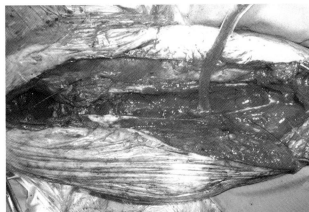

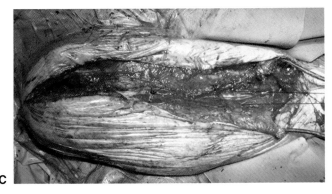

Figure 18.4. **(A)** Intraoperative image of the vascularized humeral window, allowing excellent exposure of the entire humeral canal. **(B)** Intraoperative image of the window with monofilament suture placed through drill holes that will allow for closure of the window. **(C)** Intraoperative image showing the window closed.

RESULTS

Based on a biomechanical study by Choo et al[9] and considering the high incidence of poor bone quality in this patient population, it is surprising that periprosthetic humeral fractures are not more common. They reported that strain in the reamed diaphysis increased 30% as it was reamed and broached and the implant was placed. Of even more significance is that their results revealed a decrease in torsional strength of 33%.

There is a paucity of large studies demonstrating the correct treatment method for periprosthetic humeral fractures. All of the studies in the literature were retrospective and treated the variety of fractures with a myriad of different treatment techniques. All of them agree that fracture stability and implant stability are of paramount importance.[10,11] Of the four largest studies, none had more than 21 patients—Wright and Cofield,[5] 9 patients; Campbell et al,[12] 21 patients; Worland et al,[7] 6 patients; and Kumar et al,[8] 16 patients. The results of these studies are nicely summarized in a chapter written by Steinmann and Cheung.[6] Care must be used when interpreting these articles because most were written before the advent of unicortical locking plates[5,7,12] and most of the treatment group in the study by Kumar et al[8] likely had surgery before the locking plates used now were widely available. The trend then was to treat most patients with long-stemmed revision implants augmented with cerclage wires. By using unicortical locking plates, more of these fractures can be treated with ORIF without revising to a long-stemmed prosthesis.

A number of smaller studies using specialized implants have reported high union rates when treating periprosthetic humeral fractures, including Kent et al,[13] using a locking compression plate; Christoforakis et al,[14] using a Dall-Miles plate and cables; Lill et al,[15] using a Mennen clamp-on plate[16]; and Kligman and Roffman,[17] using a Mennen plate.

Kumar et al[8] recommend that type C fractures or fractures distal to the implant should have a 3-month trial of nonoperative treatment. After that time, if they cannot be managed appropriately with a fracture orthosis or are not progressing to union, they should be converted to operative management. Kim et al[18] reported on the successful management of two patients treated with functional bracing.

COMPLICATIONS

Periprosthetic humeral fractures are a complex complication of shoulder arthroplasty. They are challenging to treat, and additional complications are common and, unfortunately, often severe. Significant morbidity can result. Treatment of periprosthetic humeral fractures is major surgery that may result in prolonged operating time and substantial blood loss. More serious complications can occur in the host patient, who is often elderly and may be frail from the prolonged anesthesia and fluid shifts. The most challenging complication to manage is a periprosthetic fracture treated appropriately but that subsequently becomes infected. Treatment of this dreaded complication requires removal of the entire implant, all cement, all hardware, and any allograft used. These patients invariably end up with a poor result and are often left with a nonunited humerus and a resection arthroplasty. Other significant complications include persistent nonunion, radial nerve palsy, axillary nerve palsy, brachial plexus injury, and stiffness of the shoulder and or elbow. Radial nerve palsies are usually temporary, but permanent injuries can and do occur, especially if the nerve comes into contact with cement or a cerclage wire is put around or through the nerve.

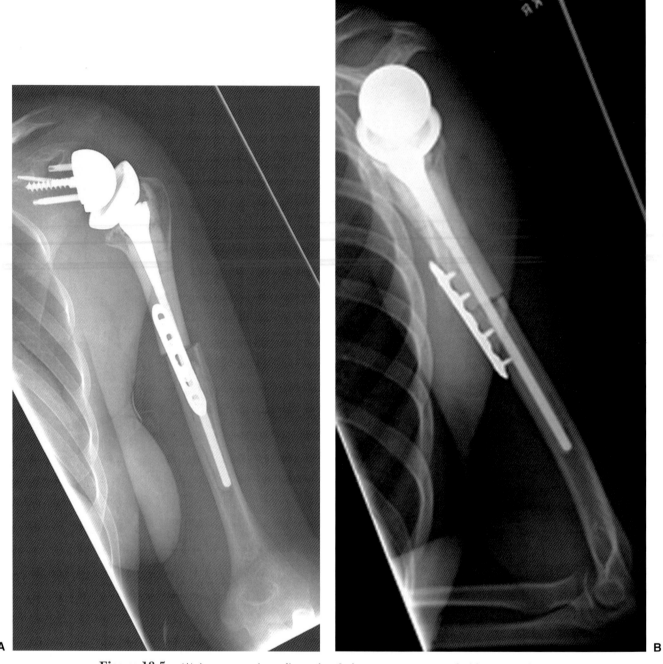

A   B

Figure 18.5.   **(A)** Anteroposterior radiography of a humerus reconstructed with a composite massive allograft long-stemmed reverse prosthesis. When intramedullary fixation is good the mode of failure will be rotational instability. Rotational stability can be significantly augmented by using a short locking plate; usually two short locking screws on each side of the fracture will suffice. This fixation is not to be confused with treatment of a periprosthetic fracture without revision to a long stem; in that case the plate is the primary mode of fixation and must be long. **(B)** Lateral radiograph of the same patient.

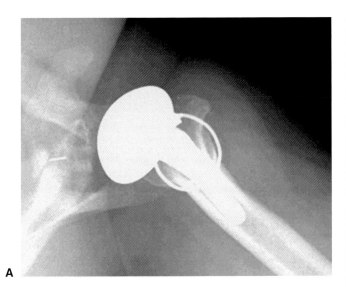

A

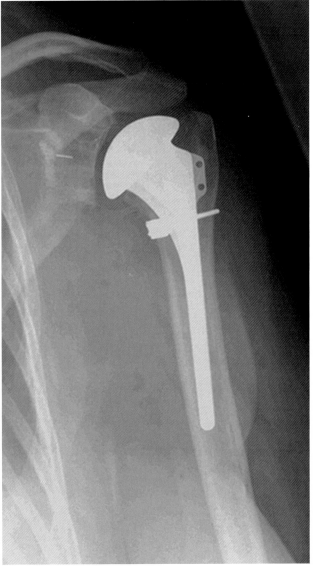

B

Figure 18.6. (**A**) Lateral radiograph of a proximal metaphyseal split fracture occurring during broaching, fixed with a single cerclage wire. (**B**) Anteroposterior radiograph of the same patient.

CONCLUSION

Periprosthetic humeral fractures are not common but are a significant complication of shoulder arthroplasty. Treatment is complex, and complications can be severe and result in significant patient morbidity. Poor-quality bone is the main predisposing factor. These fractures can occur intraoperatively or postoperatively, with the intraoperative variety being more common. Prevention is the best approach to minimize the intraoperative variety. To allow for nonforceful exposure of the glenoid, the soft tissue release should be performed meticulously and the humerus should not be overreamed. Treatment is based on the stability of the fracture and implant. Stable fractures and implants may be treated with no or minimal fixation (intraoperative simple cerclage alone). Unstable fractures and implants require revision to a long-stemmed prosthesis augmented with cerclage wires, cement, or locking plates or ORIF with unicortical locking plate alone. Bone grafting with an osteoinductive graft of choice will promote union because some of these fractures take a long time to unite. Fractures distal to the implant may be treated with functional bracing. If progress is not satisfactory, the fracture can be treated with compression or locking plates, as is standard for humeral shaft fractures.

Treatment as outlined will result in a high union rate of the humerus, but, unfortunately, ultimate function of the shoulder may be decreased because of immobilization time, the additional trauma of the periprosthetic fracture itself, and the surgical treatment. The best treatment by far for the intraoperative fracture is avoidance, which is possible in the majority of patients with strict adherence to the principles outlined. Revision shoulder arthroplasty is the exception, however, and is likely to continue to be a problem area.

REFERENCES

1. Williams GR, Ianotti JP. Management of periprosthetic fractures: the shoulder. *J Arthroplasty* 2002;17(4 suppl 1):14–15.
2. McDonough EB, Crosby LA. Periprosthetic fractures of the humerus. *Am J Orthop* 2005;34:586–591.
3. Gill DR, Cofield RH, Morrey BF. Ipsilateral total shoulder and elbow arthroplasties in patients who have rheumatoid arthritis. *J Bone Joint Surg Am* 1999;81:1128–1137.

4. Plausinis D, Greaves C, Regan WD, et al. Ipsilateral shoulder and elbow replacements: on the risk of periprosthetic fracture. *Clin Biomech (Bristol Avon)* 2005;20:1055–1063.
5. Wright TW, Cofield RH. Humeral fractures after shoulder arthroplasty. *J Bone Joint Surg Am* 1995;77:1340–1346.
6. Steinmann SP, Cheung E. Open reduction and internal fixation. In: Zuckeman JD, ed. *Advanced Reconstruction Shoulder.* Indianapolis: American Academy Orthopaedic Surgeons; 2007:351–357.
7. Worland RL, Kim DY, Arrendo J. Periprosthetic humeral fractures: management and classification. *J Shoulder Elbow Surg* 1999;8:590–594.
8. Kumar S, Sperling JW, Haidukewych GH, et al. Periprosthetic humeral fractures after shoulder arthroplasty. *J Bone Joint Surg Am* 2004;86:680–689.
9. Choo AM, Hawkins RH, Kwon BK, et al. The effect of shoulder arthroplasty on humeral strength: an in vitro biomechanical investigation. *Clin Biomech (Bristol Avon)* 2005;20:1064–1071.
10. Cameron B, Iannotti JP. Periprosthetic fractures of the humerus and scapula: management and prevention. *Orthop Clin North Am* 1999;30:305–318.
11. Chin PY, Sperling JW, Cofield RH, et al. Complications of total shoulder arthroplasty: are they fewer or different? *J Shoulder Elbow Surg* 2007;15:19–22.
12. Campbell JT, Moore RS, Iannotti JP, et al. Periprosthetic humeral fractures: mechanisms of fracture and treatment options. *J Shoulder Elbow Surg* 1998;7:406–413.
13. Kent ME, Sinopidis C, Brown DJ, et al. The locking compressions plate in periprosthetic humeral fractures: a review of two cases. *Injury* 2005;36:1241–1245.
14. Christoforakis JJ, Sadiq S, Evans MJ. Use of a Dall-Miles plat and cables for the fixation of a periprosthetic humeral fractures. *Acta Orthop Belg* 2003;69:562–565.
15. Lill H, Hepp P, Rose T, et al. Mennen clamp-on plate fixation of periprosthetic fractures of the humerus after shoulder arthroplasty: a report on three patients. *Acta Orthop Scand* 2004;75:772–774.
16. De Smet L, Debeer P, Degreef I. Fixation of a periprosthetic humeral fractures with CCG-cable system. *Acta Chir Belg* 2005;105:543–544.
17. Kligman M, Roffman M. Humeral fracture following shoulder arthroplasty. *Orthopedics* 1999;22:511–513.
18. Kim DH, Clavert P, Warner JJ. Displaced periprosthetic humeral fracture treated with functional bracing: a report of two cases. *J Shoulder Elbow Surg* 2005;14:221–223.

Matthew H. Griffith
David M. Dines

Instability after Shoulder Arthroplasty

INTRODUCTION

The number of shoulder arthroplasties performed in the United States continues to grow rapidly. It is estimated that more than 18,000 shoulder arthroplasties are performed each year. Recent studies with long-term follow-up after shoulder arthroplasty show very good outcomes, with 92% of the results rated as good or excellent and a 10-year survivorship of 93% to 96%.[1,2] Despite the excellent results reported, the systematic review by Bohsali et al[3] found an overall complication rate of 14.7%. With a continued increase in the number of shoulder arthroplasties performed each year, the shoulder surgeon must be prepared to deal with the paralleled increase in frequency of complications requiring revision.

Approximately 30% of complications after shoulder arthroplasty are attributed to instability, with only rotator cuff tears occurring more frequently.[4] The overall rate of instability after shoulder arthroplasty is 4.9%, with 80% of cases resulting from anterior and superior instability.[3] Instability has been found to cause significant pain and dysfunction after arthroplasty and is a frequent cause of reoperation.[5] Despite early reports of success using a nonoperative approach to the treatment of unstable shoulder arthroplasties,[6] more recent studies have shown these shoulders to commonly require operative treatment.[7,8]

ETIOLOGY AND CLASSIFICATION

Normal glenohumeral joint stability is maintained through its wide range of motion by the interaction of several static and dynamic stabilizing forces. Minimal stability is provided by the conforming bony articulation and the adhesive and cohesive properties of the articular cartilage and joint fluid.[9] These factors, along with the slight negative intra-articular pressure within the joint, help to center the humeral head on the glenoid surface in the normal shoulder. The remaining stabilizing forces contribute to the concavity-compression mechanism of stability.[9] This involves passive and active forces that compress the humeral head against the concavity of the glenoid and coracoacromial arch. The deltoid and rotator cuff provide the primary active forces compressing the humeral head against

the coracoacromial arch and glenoid, respectively. The ligaments of the shoulder joint (including the glenohumeral ligaments, coracohumeral ligament, and rotator interval capsule) provide compression passively in certain shoulder positions, where the rotator cuff tendons cannot produce an appropriate stabilizing force.[3]

In shoulder arthroplasty, minimal constraint is offered by the conformity of the components and a metal-on-polyethylene bearing surface does not possess the adhesive and cohesive properties found in the native joint. In addition, standard techniques for shoulder arthroplasty involve extensive capsular releases or resection without later repair. Therefore many of the static stabilizing forces found in the native joint are lost. Stability of the glenohumeral joint after arthroplasty is reliant primarily on proper component orientation and balanced rotator cuff function.

Another important factor contributing to joint stability is scapular kinematics. It is the role of the periscapular musculature to position the scapula in space so that it is in line with the joint reactive force resulting from the activity that is being performed. In a shoulder with normal kinematics, the scapula is positioned so that the glenoid center line is aligned with the axis of the joint reactive force.[9] Any malalignment between these two axes will result in a translational force vector. After shoulder arthroplasty, if scapular kinematics is not restored, this type of imbalance can lead to subluxation, dislocation, or edge loading of the glenoid component, with subsequent loosening. An anteverted or retroverted glenoid component produces a similar effect. Even with an appropriate scapular position in space, a glenoid that is not aligned perpendicular to the axis of the scapula will result in eccentric loading and shear forces.

Instability of the prosthetic shoulder is classified by the direction of displacement—superior, anterior, posterior, or inferior (Table 19.1). It can be further described by the cause (soft tissue dysfunction, component malalignment, or a combination) or the degree of instability (subluxation or dislocation), both having an impact on treatment and outcome. This section will review the classification system and the causes of each type of instability, as well as discuss the preventive measures at index arthroplasty that may be employed to optimize stability.

TABLE 19.1	Classification of Instability after Shoulder Arthroplasty
Direction	*Causes*
Superior	Rotator cuff insufficiency
	Humeral component too high
	Glenoid component superior inclination
Anterior	Subscapularis rupture
	Humeral component anteversion
	Glenoid component anteversion
	Anterior deltoid dysfunction
Posterior	Glenoid component retroversion
	Humeral component retroversion
	Tight subscapularis
	Loose posterior soft tissue structures
Inferior	Low implantation of the humeral component
	Insufficiency of SGHL and rotator interval
	Pseudosubluxation

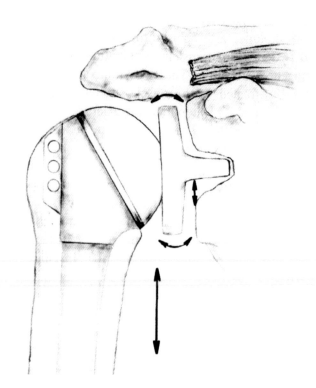

Figure 19.1. The rocking horse glenoid. Deficiency of the rotator cuff causes superior subluxation, micromotion and component loosening. (From Craig EV, ed. *Textbook of Orthopaedic Surgery*. Philadelphia: Williams & Wilkins; 1998, with permission.)

SUPERIOR INSTABILITY

Superior subluxation or migration is the most common type of instability after shoulder arthroplasty, representing 61% of cases.[3] It is usually due to rotator cuff insufficiency secondary to a massive tear, severe fatty infiltration, or significant thinning of the tendons, as seen in cases of inflammatory arthropathy or after multiple operations.[3,10–13] In addition, improper component selection can lead to rotator cuff failure. A large glenoid component can cause attritional wear of rotator cuff tendons with time. Increasing the lateral offset of the joint by varus stem position, a high offset humeral head, or a thick glenoid component places excess tension on the rotator cuff tendons. This may result in decreased motion, increased pain, and eventual tendon failure.[14]

Rotator cuff insufficiency leads to an imbalance in the concavity-compression mechanism. Without adequate centering of the humeral head by the rotator cuff, the shear force produced by the deltoid muscle subluxes the humeral head superiorly. Superior migration has been shown to result in worse functional outcomes and increased pain.[13] It has also been shown to be responsible for the "rocking-horse" glenoid,[15] as a result of increased stresses on the superior aspect of the glenoid component (Fig. 19.1). Eccentric loading of the glenoid leads to micromotion, failure of fixation, and early loosening. This mode of failure is the rationale behind recommendations against the implantation of a glenoid component in patients with massive irreparable rotator cuff tears.[16]

Another factor that can contribute to superior subluxation is increasing the humeral height by implanting the humeral component proud. When implanting the humeral component, a line tangent to the superior-most aspect of the humeral head should be 5 to 8 mm above the greater tuberosity.[14] Nyffeler et al[11] showed in a cadaveric study that implanting the humeral component 5 to 10 mm too high causes premature tightening the inferior ligaments in abduction and decreases the maximum abduction angle that can be achieved. In addition, they showed in this study that a proud humeral component raises the joint center of rotation above the force vectors of the infraspinatus and subscapularis muscles. This decreases

the moment arms of the infraspinatus and subscapularis 20% to 50% and 50% to 100%, respectively, and increases the moment arms of their antagonists.[11] Anatomic placement of the humeral head helps optimize the balance between the stabilizing forces of the shoulder, thus maximizing motion and preventing subluxation.

Finally, glenoid inclination can contribute to superior subluxation. Normal glenoid inclination in the coronal plane is vertical.[17] The glenoid should be implanted with no more than 10 degrees of superior or inferior inclination. A glenoid with superior inclination cannot effectively balance the compressive forces acting on the humeral head. This results in superior shear forces and subluxation (Fig. 19.2).

ANTERIOR INSTABILITY

The most common cause of anterior instability after shoulder arthroplasty is disruption of the subscapularis tendon. The subscapularis is critical for maintaining stability after shoulder arthroplasty. It is the primary anterior compressor and balances the posterior muscles, as well as acting as a static soft tissue restraint to subluxation.[9] Moeckel et al[7] reported on 7 cases of anterior instability, all of which had a subscapularis tear. Subscapularis tears have been attributed to multiple surgeries that violate the tendon, poor tissue quality, lengthening procedures for internal rotation contracture, previous anterior stabilization procedures, lateralization the of the joint center of rotation placing increasing tension on the repair (Fig. 19.3), and aggressive physical therapy or activity in the early postoperative period that exceed

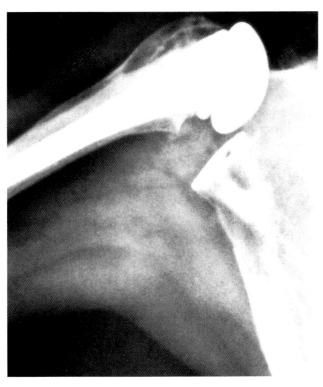

Figure 19.2. Radiograph of a superiorly inclined glenoid component causing superior instability. (From Warren RF, Craig EV, Altchek DW, eds, *The Unstable Shoulder*. Philadelphia: Lippincott-Raven; 1999, with permission.)

the limitations of the repair.[3,7,18–22] Miller et al[20] reported a rate of reoperation for subscapularis tear after shoulder arthroplasty of 5.8%. Improved results have been shown if subscapularis repair is done early, possibly because of progressive fatty infiltration of the muscle with time.[23]

Subscapularis function after shoulder arthroplasty was evaluated by Miller et al[24] in a retrospective study of 41 patients after total shoulder arthroplasty. The lift-off examination was abnormal in 67.5%, and the belly-press test was abnormal in 66.5%. They concluded that subscapularis dysfunction results in suboptimal outcome, and they now perform lesser tuberosity osteotomy rather than splitting the tendon. Other authors have reported lesser tuberosity osteotomy techniques and have shown excellent healing and improved subscapularis function after arthroplasty.[22,25,26] The literature has not yet demonstrated that a lesser tuberosity osteotomy decreases the rate of anterior dislocation after shoulder arthroplasty but it is intuitive that optimizing subscapularis healing is critical.

Anterior deltoid dysfunction can occur as a result of axillary nerve injury or thinning from multiple surgeries. Loss of the anterior deltoid leads to a muscle imbalance, with an anteriorly directed force resulting from the unopposed posterior and middle heads of the deltoid. This can lead to significant functional impairment with few treatment options.

Component malposition can also contribute to anterior instability.[3] Hasan et al[5] found a direct correlation between instability and component malposition. Humeral or glenoid component anteversion can cause anterior instability. Wirth and Rockwood[10] found all of their total shoulder arthroplasties

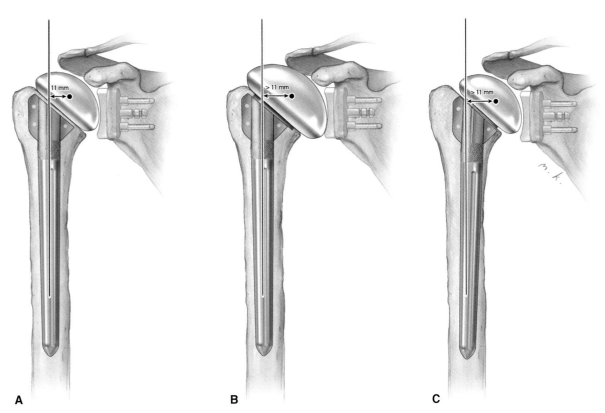

Figure 19.3. Normal offset is approximately 11 mm from the center of the medullary canal (**A**). Increased offset caused by a large head (**B**) or varus stem placement (**C**) places increased tension on the rotator cuff.

treated operatively for anterior instability to have an anteverted humeral component. Normal humeral head retroversion is 10 to 40 degrees to the epicondylar axis.[14] Care must be taken when performing the humeral osteotomy to recreate anatomic retroversion. Various cutting guides are available to help ensure that an optimal neck osteotomy is made. Another rough landmark is to place the fin of the humeral component 1 cm posterior to the bicipital groove.[27] Implanting the humeral component in an anteverted position can limit external rotation and lead to anterior instability.[14]

Normal glenoid version in the axial plane should be neutral ±10 degrees.[14] An anteverted glenoid component can result from improper technique or unrecognized anterior bone loss. Anteversion of the glenoid results in an anteriorly directed joint reactive force (Fig. 19.4). It is recommended that computed tomography (CT) be performed preoperatively to assess the glenoid version and bone stock.[17,28–31] If imaging studies reveal bone loss anteriorly, eccentric reaming should be performed to correct version and to prevent glenoid component anteversion.[32] Approximately 1 cm of bone can be removed with eccentric reaming and still leave enough bone to enable glenoid implantation. If more than this must be removed to correct the version, structural bone grafting may be required.[29,33–35]

Even with optimal glenoid version, stability may be compromised if a small glenoid component is implanted.[18] With a small component, less translation is required for dislocation. This can result in anterior or posterior instability. Care should be taken to obtain adequate exposure to allow placement of a proper-size component.

POSTERIOR INSTABILITY

In the systematic review by Bohsali et al,[3] 20% of instability cases were posterior. Causes include humeral or glenoid component retroversion and soft tissue imbalance, with most cases being multifactorial. In the study by Moeckel et al,[7] three cases

of posterior instability were identified, and contributing factors included retroversion of the glenoid, retroversion of the humeral component, and a tight subscapularis. In the series reported by Godeneche et al,[8] there were four cases of posterior instability, all with B2 glenoids preoperatively as classified by the system described by Walch et al.[36]

Posterior glenoid erosion is commonly seen in osteoarthritis and capsulorrhaphy arthritis. It is a relatively common mistake to place the glenoid component in retroversion because of inadequate correction of the deformity. Each degree of glenoid retroversion results in 0.5 mm of posterior humeral displacement. In addition, with greater than 20 degrees of glenoid retroversion, the subluxation rate is 85%.[37] Finite element analysis has revealed significant increases in stress on the cement mantle with retroversion greater than 10 degrees, increasing the risk of early loosening.[38] It can be very difficult to assess the version on preoperative axillary radiographs because of inaccuracies created by patient positioning. A preoperative CT scan is very helpful in evaluating the version and deformity.[17,28–31] The glenoid erosion, if severe, may lead to posterior subluxation of the humeral head and soft tissue contracture preoperatively. These shoulders are at increased risk for postoperative posterior instability, and it is essential to correct the glenoid version and to carefully balance the soft tissues.[29]

Abnormal glenoid version should be corrected in the primary arthroplasty to prevent early loosening or instability (Fig. 19.4). Options for correcting glenoid retroversion include reaming down the high side in smaller deformities and structurally bone grafting larger deformities.[17] Obtaining proper version may be assisted by using a K wire placed down the axis of the scapula and a special goniometer to guide reaming.[17] Other authors have described computer-assisted navigation to assist in optimizing glenoid alignment.[30] Habermeyer et al[37] reported that 83% of their patients with preoperative subluxation treated with correction of glenoid version and soft tissue balancing had humeral heads centered on the glenoid component at follow-up.[37]

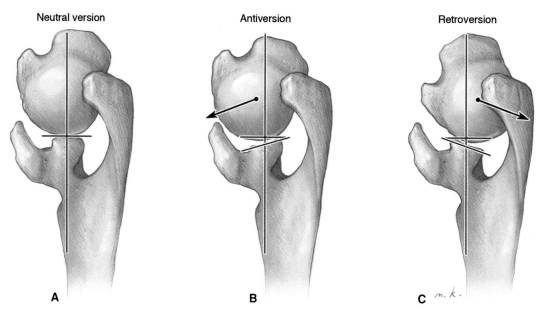

| Neutral version | Antiversion | Retroversion |

A   **B**   **C**

Figure 19.4. Normal glenoid version is neutral ±10 degrees (**A**). Excess anteversion (**B**) or retroversion (**C**) of the glenoid component can lead to instability.

Structural bone grafting is rarely required in primary cases.[33] In Neer's report on 463 total shoulder arthroplasties, 65 glenoids had significant bone loss necessitating grafting, with 20 being structural.[33] In this series, only two had such severe bone loss that glenoid implantation was impossible.[33] There were no patients with loosening or migration requiring reoperation at an average follow-up of 4.4 years.

Soft tissue balance is critical to avoid instability. Posterior instability can occur in patients with a tight subscapularis. In the report by Sperling et al[31] on patients who underwent shoulder arthroplasty for arthritis after previous anterior instability surgery, three required revision for posterior instability caused by tight anterior structures.[39] Wirth et al[10] outlined their guidelines for management of the subscapularis. In patients with greater than 40 degrees of external rotation preoperatively, no alteration in technique is required. If external rotation is limited to 15 to 20 degrees, they recommend that the subscapularis be taken down directly off its insertion on the lesser tuberosity and reattached to the neck medially. A partial release of the pectoralis major tendon may also be required to regain motion. In patients with less than 15 degrees of external rotation preoperatively, a coronal Z-lengthening may be performed. One centimeter of lengthening gains about 20 degrees of external rotation. As noted previously, lengthening procedures of the subscapularis have been shown to increase the risk for rupture and insufficiency postoperatively.

In patients with prior posterior dislocations or chronic subluxation of the humeral head, the posterior capsule can become lax and patulous. A general rule is that after the soft tissues are balanced, anterior or posterior translation of the humeral head should not exceed 30% to 50% of the glenoid diameter and should spontaneously recenter after the translational force is released.[7,40] If posterior translation exceeds 50% or if the head does not self-reduce, a posterior capsulorrhaphy should be performed.

INFERIOR INSTABILITY

Inferior instability most commonly is due to failure to restore appropriate humeral height after prosthetic treatment of a proximal humeral fracture. In three- and four-part proximal humerus fractures, comminution can disrupt bony landmarks, making it difficult to determine the proper anatomic height to recreate. A humeral component that is implanted with the center of rotation shifted inferiorly results in suboptimal tension in the deltoid and rotator cuff, with apparent inferior subluxation on the glenoid. This has been shown to result in worse outcomes, with a limited ability to abduct the arm.[3] In addition, with an inferiorly placed humeral component, the greater tuberosity is higher than the implant and can impinge on the coracoid.[18] Murachovsky et[41] al described a method to reference humeral head height off the pectoralis major tendon, which is usually intact after proximal humerus fracture. The superior-most aspect of the humeral head is 5.6 ± 5 mm from the proximal border of the pectoralis major tendon.[41]

Insufficiency of the superior glenohumeral ligament and rotator interval capsule may also contribute to inferior instability. Release or resection of these structures is common in shoulder arthroplasty, and it is unlikely that insufficiency of these structures alone will result in inferior subluxation if component positioning and muscle balance are optimal. However, it

has been demonstrated that closure of the rotator interval may decrease inferior translation.[42]

A temporary cause of inferior subluxation seen on postoperative radiographs in the recovery room is pseudosubluxation. It is caused by a combination of muscle laxity from the regional block, hematoma, and venting of the capsule with loss of the negative intra-articular pressure.[43] This condition is usually asymptomatic and self-limited. It can be minimized by supportive sling use in the postoperative period until muscle control is regained.

PATIENT EVALUATION

Evaluation of the unstable arthroplasty begins with a thorough history. Patients may present with a spectrum of symptoms ranging from pain to frank dislocation.[5] It is important to recognize that not all patients with dysfunction resulting from instability present complaining of subluxation or dislocation. Instability should be included in the differential for any patient complaining of pain and dysfunction after shoulder arthroplasty. Activities or positions that aggravate the symptoms can give insight into the diagnosis and direction of instability. Patients with anterior instability may complain of pain or apprehension when attempting to externally rotate the abducted shoulder, and patients with posterior instability may experience symptoms with shoulder flexion, adduction, and internal rotation.

The onset of symptoms should also be determined. Instability usually presents earlier than other modes of failure, with an average time of 2.1 years from the index procedure.[2] Patients with component malposition may have instability symptoms in the immediate postoperative period. Subscapularis rupture often presents early in the postoperative course as a discreet pop felt in external rotation or extension.[20] In more subtle cases, the patient may complain only of pain. Component oversizing or excess lateral offset may lead to attritional wear of the cuff and late instability.

The indication for the index arthroplasty may also give insight into the pathology involved. Patients with osteoarthritis often have posterior glenoid wear predisposing to a retroverted glenoid component. This can also be seen after anterior stabilizing surgery with tightening of the anterior soft tissues. These patients have been shown to have increased risk for posterior instability after shoulder arthroplasty.[39] An arthroplasty performed for a proximal humerus fracture may have humeral component malposition or problems with tuberosity healing, leading to cuff dysfunction.[44,45] Patients with rheumatoid arthritis frequently have poor soft tissues, and rotator cuff pathology is common.[12,13] Prior anterior surgeries that involved take-down or lengthening of the subscapularis place the patient at risk for subscapularis rupture. It is valuable to obtain previous operative reports to gather information regarding the surgical approach used, the soft tissue and bone quality, and whether any capsular or tendinous balancing procedures were performed.

A careful physical examination is critical to the diagnosis of instability after arthroplasty, helping to identify contributing factors and guiding treatment. Inspection of the incision and surrounding skin is important when ruling out infection, and one must also look for any muscular atrophy that may be present. Scapular motion should be observed from behind as the patient actively elevates the arm. Passive and active motion is evaluated and positions of apprehension are noted. Increased external rotation may be seen after a rupture of the subscapularis. A thorough motor and sensory examination should be performed. This should focus on the deltoid and rotator cuff as well as distal muscle groups. Axillary nerve palsy is a contraindication to shoulder arthroplasty, so its function must be carefully assessed.[46] The lift-off and belly-press tests should be performed to assess the subscapularis.[23,24] The sulcus test can reveal inferior laxity, and the load-and-shift and modified load-and-shift tests are valuable in assessing for increased anterior and posterior translation. Performing the sulcus test in 30 degrees of external rotation evaluates the integrity of the rotator interval structures. It is also important to examine the cervical spine, including range of motion (ROM), tenderness, reflexes, and specialty tests for cord and root compression (Lhermitte and Romberg tests).

Radiographic studies should include an anteroposterior image of the glenohumeral joint, a scapular Y view, and an axillary view. The anteroposterior radiograph shows implant position and relationship. Comparison to previous radiographs can help reveal progressive osteolysis, implant loosening, and superior migration of the humeral head resulting from rotator cuff failure. An acromial-humeral distance of less than 5 mm is considered to be diagnostic of an irreparable rotator cuff tear.[17] The scapular Y lateral can add information regarding implant position and joint reduction. The axillary view can show anterior or posterior subluxation of the joint and allows evaluation of glenoid version. Greater than 5 mm of anterior subluxation on the axillary radiograph is indicative of subscapularis insufficiency.[17] There can be significant variation in the measurement of glenoid version using the axillary view because of patient positioning and imaging technique.[35,47] Therefore most surgeons now recommend CT for the evaluation of glenoid version and assessing remaining bone stock. Internal and external rotation views of the humerus can be helpful in evaluating the tuberosities if malunion or nonunion is suspected. In cases of superior or inferior subluxation, a full-length humeral radiograph with a contralateral image for comparison allows accurate determination of humeral length.[27,48] Magnetic resonance imaging (MRI) may also be of value to assess the soft tissues. Newer protocols allow accurate imaging even with implants in place. Rotator cuff tears can be diagnosed using MRI with a sensitivity of 91% and a specificity of 80% after arthroplasty.[49]

TREATMENT

NONOPERATIVE TREATMENT

After thorough evaluation, with identification of the direction of instability and the contributing factors, treatment options can be considered. Several authors have reported modest success with nonoperative treatment.[2,6,15] Prompt closed reduction should be performed after any dislocation. With stable implants and an intact rotator cuff, it is reasonable to attempt a course of physical therapy to strengthen stabilizing muscles and optimize scapular kinematics. However, from the small series available in the literature, it appears that 25% to 100% of patients with instability after shoulder arthroplasty require operative treatment.[2,6–8,50,51] As discussed previously, instability after shoulder arthroplasty is often multifactorial in nature.

The following discussion will review the surgical treatment options for each potential contributing factor.

SUBSCAPULARIS RUPTURE

Subscapularis rupture is the most common cause of anterior instability. Miller et al[20] reported that 5.8% of patients in their series required reoperation for subscapularis rupture. Several factors come into play when considering repair options. In acute tears with healthy tissue, direct repair to bone may be performed. With poor tissue quality resulting from multiple surgeries, previous lengthening or inflammatory disease, augmentation is recommended.[52] Moeckel et al[7] described a technique using an Achilles tendon allograft to create an anterior static soft tissue restraint between the scapula and humerus. This type of reconstruction may restore stability but risks limiting motion. Thin subscapularis tissue can be augmented with a piece of Achilles allograft.[46] This maintains the subscapularis as the primary anterior dynamic stabilizer but is reliant on good muscle quality. Preoperative CT or MRI scans should be reviewed for fatty infiltration of the muscle. A muscle with fatty infiltration that is stage 3 or higher as classified by the system of Goutallier[53,54] will have poor function, and a tendon transfer should be considered.[48]

A good option for adding an anterior dynamic stabilizer to substitute for the subscapularis is a pectoralis major transfer. The tendon can be passed deep or superficial to the conjoined tendon and is then attached to the lesser tuberosity.[52,55–57] Some surgeons feel that a subcoracoid transfer (deep to the conjoined tendon) provides a better antagonistic force to balance the posterior rotator cuff and deltoid.[57] If tendon transfer is not possible because of previous surgeries or inadequate tissues, a salvage procedure such as a reverse total shoulder arthroplasty may be required to restore stability.

GLENOID MALALIGNMENT

Abnormal glenoid alignment in patients with instability must be corrected by revising the component. Loosening of the glenoid in the unstable shoulder is also an indication for component revision. A major issue when considering glenoid revision in these patients is bone quality. Bone loss can be classified as cavitary (cancellous bone loss), segmental (rim loss), or combined. Cavitary lesions may be grafted with particulate autograft or allograft. If the defect is large, glenoid fixation may not be possible and must be abandoned. In this case, the patient will be left with a hemiarthroplasty articulating on the grafted bone. Later component implantation can be performed after healing if pain is significant. When grafting a large cavity, the cancellous bone can be secured in place by sewing a soft tissue flap such as fascia lata or allograft over the cavity.[17]

Segmental bone loss requires structural grafting (Figs. 19.5 and 19.6). Attempts at using custom implants or built-up cement to fill the gaps have demonstrated poor results with early failure.[17,58] In Neer and Morrison's series of 20 patients requiring segmental bone grafting at the index arthroplasty,[33] there were no cases with glenoid loosening or reoperation for component migration at 4.4 years. Hill and Norris[59] reported less promising results in their series of 17 patients with long-term follow-up who underwent structural bone grafting and single-stage implantation of a glenoid component. All patients in their series had preoperative instability. Despite correction of

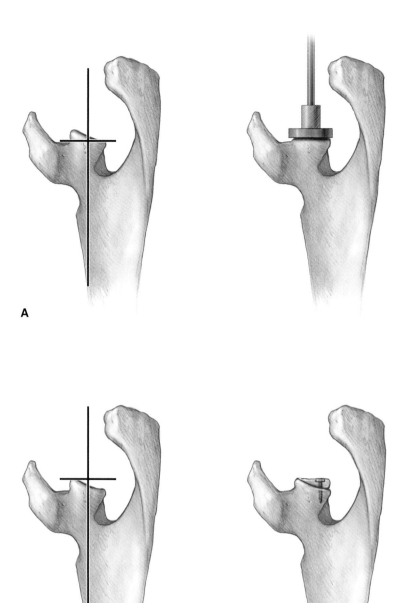

A

B

Figure 19.5. Small abnormalities in glenoid version with adequate remaining bone can be corrected with eccentric reaming (**A**). Segmental bone loss and large deviations from neutral version are treated with structural bone grafting to restore neutral glenoid version (**B**).

glenoid version and careful soft tissue balancing, eight of the 17 patients had some form of postoperative instability and five had failure of glenoid fixation. This study illustrates the difficulty in restoring stability in patients with significant preoperative instability and bone loss.

Some surgeons have recommended against structural bone grafting in one stage because of graft resorption.[46] It is hypothesized that in a two-stage technique the bone graft is unloaded, allowing more opportunity for healing. Antuña and Sperling[60] reviewed 48 shoulder arthroplasties that underwent revision of the glenoid component. Thirty shoulders that had adequate bone had a new implant placed, and the remaining cases underwent bone grafting without reimplantation. The group who had a glenoid implanted had significantly higher pain relief and satisfaction. They recommended placing a glenoid component if possible. If bone stock is insufficient, the defect can be grafted and glenoid implantation may be performed in a second stage if pain persists.

Previous studies have recommended placing the humeral component in anteversion as a treatment for glenoid retroversion.[7,10,33,61] However, recent data suggest that this technique does not improve stability. In a cadaveric study by Iannotti et al,[14,62] it was shown that rotating the humeral component within the humerus does not change the length-tension relationship of the soft tissues. The glenoid version remains abnormal, and the posteriorly directed shear force is unchanged. In addition, with anteversion of the humeral component, the offset is decreased slightly, which may actually make the shoulder less stable. They concluded that the best solution is to correct glenoid version and restore anatomic alignment of the components.

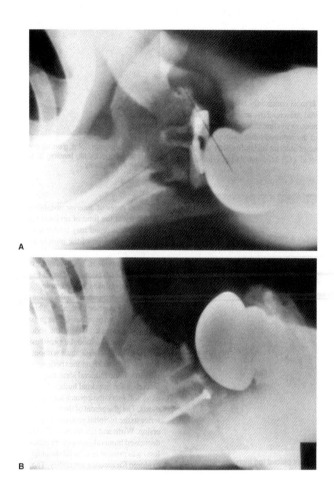

Figure 19.6. Axillary radiograph demonstrates posterior instability resulting from component retroversion (**A**). Glenoid component revision with structural bone grafting restores neutral glenoid version and centers the humeral head (**B**). (From Warren RF, Craig EV, Altchek DW, eds. *The Unstable Shoulder*. Philadelphia: Lippincott-Raven 1999, with permission.)

HUMERAL MALALIGNMENT

Humeral malalignment may also contribute to instability. Whether it is placed with abnormal version height or offset, the humeral component must be revised in the unstable shoulder if its position is not acceptable. The normal height of the humeral component is 5 to 8 mm above the greater tuberosity, normal retroversion is 10 to 40 degrees from the epicondylar axis, neck-shaft angle is 35 to 45 degrees from vertical, and offset of the humeral head center is about 11 mm from the center of the shaft.[14] At revision, the humeral component is removed, as well as the cement mantle if present. This can be difficult, and care should be taken to preserve as much bone as possible. Techniques of creating humeral windows have been described to enable cement removal.[63,64] After removal of the implant and cement, the humeral component can be revised with the goal of recreating anatomic positioning in all planes.

SOFT TISSUE IMBALANCE

Soft tissue imbalance can be a major contributing factor to instability and must be corrected at revision. In the revision setting, much of the capsule may be thin or absent, and usually

circumferential releases are performed to improve exposure. After component implantation, the position of the humeral head on the glenoid should be noted. Using the criteria described previously, soft tissue balance is assessed. If the humeral head can be translated on the glenoid anteriorly or posteriorly greater than 50% of its diameter, soft tissue balancing should be performed. If adequate tissue is present, a capsular plication can be performed and translation retested. If this is not possible or does not sufficiently balance the joint, shortening of the corresponding rotator cuff tendon can be considered. However, this may compromise the integrity of the tendon and should be performed judiciously. Another option for increasing soft tissue static restraint is augmentation with allograft tissue. The technique described by Moeckel et al[7] restored stability in their patients with anterior instability after shoulder arthroplasty but risks limiting motion. Conversely, if soft tissue contractures restrict translation to less than 25% of the glenoid diameter or cause the head to have fixed subluxation, releases should be performed. Extensive capsular and soft tissue releases can be performed and if this fails then lengthening procedures for the rotator cuff may be considered. Caution must be used when lengthening the cuff tendons because iatrogenic disruption of the rotator cuff can be an extremely disabling complication. If soft tissue restraints are insufficient to restore reasonable stability, use of a constrained implant (reverse total shoulder arthroplasty) must be considered.

Failure of the infraspinatus and teres minor tendons may contribute to posterior instability. Failure to counterbalance the anterior muscle forces results in a posteriorly directed joint reactive force. Repair of the tendons should be performed if possible. Healthy tendon tissue is required, and fatty infiltration on CT or MRI should be no higher than Goutallier stage 2. If these criteria are not met, it is possible to augment or substitute for the posterior rotator cuff tendon with a latissimus dorsi tendon transfer.[65–69] This may successfully balance the shoulder and improve function.

CORACOACROMIAL ARCH INSUFFICIENCY

The coracoacromial arch is made of the coracoid, acromion, and intervening coracoacromial ligament. Disruption of any part of the arch may result in an inability to counteract the compressive forces of the deltoid. This results in anterosuperior instability or escape when in combination with a large tear of the rotator cuff.[70] The coracoacromial ligament may be disrupted in an overly aggressive subacromial decompression or in open surgical approaches that involve release of the ligament.[71] The acromion or coracoid may be disrupted as a result of fracture malunion, nonunion, or prior surgeries. Anterosuperior escape has proved to be a very difficult condition to treat and is quite debilitating for the patient. Several techniques of reconstruction of the arch have been attempted using allograft tissue.[72,73] Results have generally been poor and the problem remains unsolved. Salvage with a reverse prosthesis may be the best treatment option.

SALVAGE

In refractory cases of instability after shoulder arthroplasty, standard revision techniques may be unable to provide satisfactory stability, function, and pain relief. In these cases, salvage with a reverse total shoulder replacement, resection arthroplasty, or arthrodesis may be the only treatment option.

The reverse total shoulder arthroplasty shifts the center of rotation of the joint inferiorly and medially. The prosthesis has increased constraint compared with conventional total shoulder arthroplasty and relies less on the capsule and rotator cuff to provide stability. The compressive force of the deltoid is the primary stabilizer. Indications for using a reverse total shoulder arthroplasty when revising an unstable shoulder arthroplasty include massive irreparable rotator cuff tear and coracoacromial arch insufficiency with anterosuperior escape. Contraindications include deltoid dysfunction, axillary nerve palsy, infection, and insufficient glenoid bone. However, Norris et al[74] recently reported a technique of reverse total shoulder arthroplasty as a treatment of cuff insufficiency with severe glenoid bone loss or erosion. This involves one-stage iliac crest bone grafting using a custom baseplate with a long central peg.

In a multicenter study of 457 reverse total shoulder arthroplasties, 24 were revisions of failed total shoulder arthroplasty.[75] Causes of failure included six resulting from anterior instability, six with glenoid loosening, and three with posterior instability. At an average follow-up of 38.3 months, there was a significant increase in Constant score from 23.3 to 51.2 and 81% were satisfied or very satisfied. However, there was a 50% complication rate, with 5 of the 10 adverse events being dislocations. The revision rate in this series was 20%, with two of the five patients with dislocation after reverse total shoulder arthroplasty requiring revision. They recommended repairing the anterior soft tissue structures and augmenting a deficient subscapularis with a pectoralis major transfer to minimize the risk of postoperative instability. They concluded that a reverse prosthesis is a good option for revision of the unstable total shoulder arthroplasty, especially when rotator cuff pathology is present.

Shoulder arthrodesis should be reserved as a salvage procedure for severe refractory cases. Indications include loss of deltoid and rotator cuff function, recurrent debilitating instability, failed revision total shoulder arthroplasty, and chronic infection.[76] Although satisfaction has been reported to be as high as 80%,[76] other studies have found outcomes to be less predictable. Hawkins and Neer[77] reported on 17 patients with an average follow-up of 40 months. Nine of the 17 patients rated their outcome as unsatisfactory, with chronic pain being a common problem. This echoed the results previously reported by Cofield et al,[78] who noted a 25% rate of significant postoperative pain. Component resection is another salvage option available when no other treatment is appropriate. Pain may be relieved but function is generally poor.

POSTOPERATIVE CARE

It is critical to allow soft tissues to heal after revision of the unstable shoulder arthroplasty. Several authors have stressed the importance of determining the limits of motion intraoperatively.[7,79] This should be noted in the operative report and is used to guide rehabilitation. It is advisable to communicate directly with the therapist to customize the protocol and to clearly establish the limitations of motion. If intraoperative stability is at all questionable, prolonged bracing or splinting in a safe position should be considered.[79]

RESULTS OF TREATMENT

Few studies have reported specifically on the treatment of instability after arthroplasty. Moeckel at al[7] reported on the treatment in ten cases of instability (seven anterior, three posterior) from their series of 236 total shoulder arthroplasties. All seven of the anteriorly unstable shoulders were stable at follow-up, although three required two operations to achieve stability. Of the three that were unstable posteriorly, two were stable at follow-up examination. The third failed two revisions and finally underwent component removal. This study demonstrates a 90% rate of stability after revision but had a reoperation rate of 50% to achieve these results.

In the multicenter study performed by Ahrens et al,[50,51] there were 80 cases of instability. Fifty-one of the shoulders had anterior instability and 29 had posterior instability. All of the patients failed nonoperative treatment. Of the patients with anterior instability, 87% had a tear of the subscapularis. They reported success in restoring stability in 40% of the anterior group and 53% of the posterior group.

Sanchez-Sotelo et al[80] reported their results after treating 33 unstable shoulder arthroplasties. Their series included 26 total shoulder arthroplasties and seven hemiarthroplasties, with 19 unstable anteriorly and 14 unstable posteriorly. Revision was performed in 32 of the 33 arthroplasties, and only nine were stable after the first operation (28%). Eleven of the shoulders that were unstable after revision underwent reoperation. At final follow-up, 14 of 32 shoulders were stable (44%), with 23 being unsatisfactory on the Neer grading system. Nineteen of the revision shoulder arthroplasties were performed using the anteromedial approach, with take-down and later reattachment of the anterior deltoid. It is unclear from the data available whether the approach had an effect on the outcome and previous reports have shown no increased risk of instability using this approach.[6,81]

An outcomes analysis study on revision shoulder arthroplasties from our institution reported on 78 revision total shoulder arthroplasties with an average follow-up of 76 months.[72] The five cases of instability that were due to soft tissue deficiency had significantly worse outcomes than those who had component malposition. The revisions performed for soft tissue problems included three with coracoacromial arch reconstruction and two with pectoralis major transfer. Two were fair and three had poor outcomes at follow-up.

These studies demonstrate the difficulty involved with treating the unstable shoulder arthroplasty. Patients should be counseled carefully that the risk for complication, recurrence, and reoperation is high. Failure to restore stability may be as high as 50%, with worse outcomes associated with soft tissue failures.

INSTABILITY AFTER REVERSE TOTAL SHOULDER REPLACEMENT

Instability is one of the most common complications after reverse total shoulder arthroplasty, with an incidence ranging from 0 to 8.6%.[82-88] Potential causes include component malalignment, subscapularis tightness or insufficiency, inferior cam effect, or overly aggressive rehabilitation.[88] In the multicenter study of reverse total shoulder arthroplasty performed in Europe,[88] there were 22 cases of instability (4.8%). There was a statistically significant increase in instability in the group who underwent arthroplasty via the deltopectoral approach versus the superolateral approach. The authors thought that extensive anteroinferior release that is unique to the deltopectoral approach is a risk for postoperative instability. An inferiorly placed humeral component placed below the tuberosities was also a potential cause for instability, with this finding noted in 15 of the 22 unstable shoulders. They found that the type of instability had an effect on outcome. Patients with early frank dislocation who underwent revision generally had better outcomes with fewer recurrences than patients who presented later or had static inferior subluxation. This study shows that when early instability is due to an inferiorly placed humeral component, revision with placement of a spacer to increase the deltoid tension appears to successfully restore stability. Salvage options for the persistently unstable reverse total shoulder arthroplasty include hemiarthroplasty, resection arthroplasty, and arthrodesis.

SUMMARY

Instability is the second most common complication following shoulder arthroplasty. A careful evaluation must be performed to determine what factors are contributing to the instability. If nonoperative treatment fails, revision arthroplasty can be performed, taking care to correct any component malalignment and properly balance the soft tissues. Expected results are modest at best, and preoperative patient counseling is important. Salvage procedures such as reverse total shoulder arthroplasty, implant removal, or arthrodesis may be the only options in the debilitating, refractory case of instability after shoulder arthroplasty.

REFERENCES

1. Adams JE, Sperling JW, Schleck CD, et al. Outcomes of shoulder arthroplasty in Olmsted County, Minnesota: a population-based study. *Clin Orthop Relat Res* 2007;455:176–182.
2. Deshmukh AV, Koris M, Zurakowski D, et al. Total shoulder arthroplasty: long-term survivorship, functional outcome, and quality of life. *J Shoulder Elbow Surg* 2005;14:471–479.
3. Bohsali KI, Wirth MA, Rockwood CA, Jr. Complications of total shoulder arthroplasty. *J Bone Joint Surg Am* 2006;88:2279–2292.
4. Chin PY, Sperling JW, Cofield RH, et al. Complications of total shoulder arthroplasty: are they fewer or different? *J Shoulder Elbow Surg* 2006;15:19–22.
5. Hasan SS, Leith JM, Campbell B, et al. Characteristics of unsatisfactory shoulder arthroplasties. *J Shoulder Elbow Surg* 2002;11:431–441.
6. Neer CS 2nd, Watson KC, Stanton FJ. Recent experience in total shoulder replacement. *J Bone Joint Surg Am* 1982;64:319–337.
7. Moeckel BH, Altchek DW, Warren RF, et al. Instability of the shoulder after arthroplasty. *J Bone Joint Surg Am* 1993;75:492–497.
8. Godeneche A, Boileau P, Favard L, et al. Prosthetic replacement in the treatment of osteoarthritis of the shoulder: early results of 268 cases. *J Shoulder Elbow Surg* 2002;11:11–18.
9. Matsen FA 3rd, Chebli CM, Lippitt SB. Principles for the evaluation and management of shoulder instability. *Instr Course Lect* 2007;56:23–34.
10. Wirth MA, Rockwood CA Jr. Complications of shoulder arthroplasty. *Clin Orthop Relat Res* 1994;307:47–69.
11. Nyffeler RW, Sheikh R, Jacob HA, et al. Influence of humeral prosthesis height on biomechanics of glenohumeral abduction: an in vitro study. *J Bone Joint Surg Am* 2004;86:575–580.
12. Stewart MP, Kelly IG. Total shoulder replacement in rheumatoid disease: 7- to 13-year follow-up of 37 joints. *J Bone Joint Surg Br* 1997;79:68–72.
13. Trail IA, Nuttall D. The results of shoulder arthroplasty in patients with rheumatoid arthritis. *J Bone Joint Surg Br* 2002;84:1121–1125.
14. Iannotti JP, Spencer EE, Winter U, et al. Prosthetic positioning in total shoulder arthroplasty. *J Shoulder Elbow Surg* 2005;14(1 suppl S):111S–121S.
15. Barrett WP, Franklin JL, Jackins SE, et al. Total shoulder arthroplasty. *J Bone Joint Surg Am* 1987;69:865–872.
16. Bishop JY, Flatow EL. Humeral head replacement versus total shoulder arthroplasty: clinical outcomes—a review. *J Shoulder Elbow Surg* 2005;14(1 suppl S):141S–146S.
17. Gerber A, Warner JJ. Management of glenoid bone loss in shoulder arthroplasty. *Tech Shoulder Elbow Surg* 2001;2:255–266.
18. Brems JJ. Complications of shoulder arthroplasty: infections, instability, and loosening. *Instr Course Lect* 2002;51:29–39.
19. Greis PE, Dean M, Hawkins RJ. Subscapularis tendon disruption after Bankart reconstruction for anterior instability. *J Shoulder Elbow Surg* 1996;5:219–222.
20. Miller BS, Joseph TA, Noonan TJ, et al. Rupture of the subscapularis tendon after shoulder arthroplasty: diagnosis, treatment, and outcome. *J Shoulder Elbow Surg* 2005;14: 492–496.
21. Wirth MA, Rockwood CA Jr. Complications of total shoulder-replacement arthroplasty. *J Bone Joint Surg Am* 1996;78:603–616.
22. Ponce BA, Ahluwalia RS, Mazzocca AD, et al. Biomechanical and clinical evaluation of a novel lesser tuberosity repair technique in total shoulder arthroplasty. *J Bone Joint Surg Am* 2005;87(suppl 1 2):1–8.
23. Gerber C, Krushell RJ. Isolated rupture of the tendon of the subscapularis muscle: clinical features in 16 cases. *J Bone Joint Surg Br* 1991;73:389–394.
24. Miller SL, Hazrati Y, Klepps S, et al. Loss of subscapularis function after total shoulder replacement: a seldom-recognized problem. *J Shoulder Elbow Surg* 2003;12:29–34.
25. Gerber C, Yian EH, Pfirrmann CA, et al. Subscapularis muscle function and structure after total shoulder replacement with lesser tuberosity osteotomy and repair. *J Bone Joint Surg Am* 2005;87:1739–1745.
26. Gerber C, Pennington SD, Yian EH, et al. Lesser tuberosity osteotomy for total shoulder arthroplasty: surgical technique. *J Bone Joint Surg Am* 2006;88(suppl 1 Pt 2):170–177.
27. Kenter K, Dines DM. Instability after prosthetic arthroplasty. In: Warren RF, Craig EV, Altchek DW, eds. *The Unstable Shoulder.* Philadelphia: Lippincott-Raven Publishers; 1999: 479–489.
28. Wirth MA, Tapscott RS, Southworth C, et al. Treatment of glenohumeral arthritis with a hemiarthroplasty: surgical technique. *J Bone Joint Surg Am* 2007;89(Pt 1 suppl 2):10–25.
29. Klepps S, Hazrati Y, Flatow E, et al. Management of glenoid bone deficiency during shoulder replacement. *Tech Shoulder Elbow Surg* 2003;4:4–17.
30. Stanley RJ, Edwards TB, Sarin VK, et al. Computer-aided navigation for correction of glenoid deformity in total shoulder arthroplasty. *Tech Shoulder Elbow Surg* 2007;8:23–28.
31. Kwon YW, Powell KA, Yum JK, et al. Use of three-dimensional computed tomography for the analysis of the glenoid anatomy. *J Shoulder Elbow Surg* 2005;14:85–90.
32. Warren RF, Coleman SH, Dines JS. Instability after arthroplasty: the shoulder. *J Arthroplasty* 2002;17(4 suppl 1):28–31.
33. Neer CS 2nd, Morrison DS. Glenoid bone-grafting in total shoulder arthroplasty. *J Bone Joint Surg Am* 1988;70:1154–1162.
34. Steinmann SP, Cofield RH. Bone grafting for glenoid deficiency in total shoulder replacement. *J Shoulder Elbow Surg* 2000;9:361–367.
35. Friedman RJ, Hawthorne KB, Genez BM. The use of computerized tomography in the measurement of glenoid version. *J Bone Joint Surg Am* 1992;74:1032–1037.
36. Walch G, Badet R, Boulahia A, et al. Morphologic study of the glenoid in primary glenohumeral osteoarthritis. *J Arthroplasty* 1999;14:756–760.
37. Habermeyer P, Magosch P, Lichtenberg S. Recentering the humeral head for glenoid deficiency in total shoulder arthroplasty. *Clin Orthop Relat Res* 2007;457:124–132.
38. Farron A, Terrier A, Buchler P. Risks of loosening of a prosthetic glenoid implanted in retroversion. *J Shoulder Elbow Surg* 2006;15:521–526.
39. Sperling JW, Antuna SA, Sanchez-Sotelo J, et al. Shoulder arthroplasty for arthritis after instability surgery. *J Bone Joint Surg Am* 2002;84:1775–1781.
40. O'Brien SJ, Schwartz RE, Warren RF, et al. Capsular restraints to anterior/posterior motion of the shoulder. *Orthop Trans* 1988;12:143.
41. Murachovsky J, Ikemoto RY, Nascimento LG, et al. Pectoralis major tendon reference (PMT): a new method for accurate restoration of humeral length with hemiarthroplasty for fracture. *J Shoulder Elbow Surg* 2006;15:675–678.
42. Harryman DT III, Sidles JA, Harris SL, et al. The role of the rotator interval capsule in passive motion and stability of the shoulder. *J Bone Joint Surg Am* 1992;74:53–66.
43. Warner JJ, Deng XH, Warren RF, et al. Superiorinferior translation in the intact and vented glenohumeral joint. *J Shoulder Elbow Surg* 1993;2:99–105.
44. Boileau P, Krishnan SG, Tinsi L, et al. Tuberosity malposition and migration: reasons for poor outcomes after hemiarthroplasty for displaced fractures of the proximal humerus. *J Shoulder Elbow Surg* 2002;11:401–412.
45. Boileau P, Trojani C, Walch G, et al. Shoulder arthroplasty for the treatment of the sequelae of fractures of the proximal humerus. *J Shoulder Elbow Surg* 2001;10:299–308.
46. Ankem HK, Blaine TA. Revision shoulder arthroplasty. *Tech Shoulder Elbow Surg* 2005;6: 189–198.
47. Nyffeler RW, Jost B, Pfirrmann CW, et al. Measurement of glenoid version: conventional radiographs versus computed tomography scans. *J Shoulder Elbow Surg* 2003;12:493–496.
48. Boileau P, Sinnerton RJ, Chuinard C, et al. Arthroplasty of the shoulder. *J Bone Joint Surg Br* 2006;88:562–575.
49. Sperling JW, Potter HG, Craig EV, et al. Magnetic resonance imaging of painful shoulder arthroplasty. *J Shoulder Elbow Surg* 2002;11:315–321.
50. Ahrens P, Boileau P, Walch G. Anterior instability after unconstrained shoulder In: Walch G, Boileau P, Molé D, eds. *2000 Shoulder Prosthesis: 2- to 10-Year Follow-up.* Montpellier, France: Sauramps Medical; 2001:359–376.
51. Ahrens P, Boileau P, Walch G. Posterior instability after unconstrained shoulder arthroplasty. In: Walch G, Boileau P, Molé D, eds. *2000 Shoulder Prosthesis: 2- to 10-Year Follow-up.* Montpellier, France: Sauramps Medical; 2001:377–393.
52. Young DC, Rockwood CA Jr. Complications of a failed Bristow procedure and their management. *J Bone Joint Surg Am* 1991;73:969–981.
53. Goutallier D, Postel JM, Bernageau J, et al. Fatty infiltration of disrupted rotator cuff muscles. *Rev Rhum Engl Ed* 1995;62:415–422.
54. Goutallier D, Postel JM, Bernageau J, et al. Fatty muscle degeneration in cuff ruptures. Pre- and postoperative evaluation by CT scan. *Clin Orthop Relat Res* 1994;304:78–83.

55. Wirth MA, Rockwood CA Jr. Operative treatment of irreparable rupture of the subscapularis. *J Bone Joint Surg Am* 1997;79:722–731.

56. Resch H, Povacz P, Ritter E, et al. Transfer of the pectoralis major muscle for the treatment of irreparable rupture of the subscapularis tendon. *J Bone Joint Surg Am* 2000;82:372–382.

57. Galatz LM, Connor PM, Calfee RP, et al. Pectoralis major transfer for anterior-superior subluxation in massive rotator cuff insufficiency. *J Shoulder Elbow Surg* 2003;12:1–5.

58. Rodowsky MW, Weinstein DM, Pollock RG, et al. On the rate of component failure. *J Shoulder Elbow Surg* 1995;4:S13–S14.

59. Hill JM, Norris TR. Long-term results of total shoulder arthroplasty following bone-grafting of the glenoid. *J Bone Joint Surg Am* 2001;83:877–883.

60. Antuña SA, Sperling JW, Cofield RH, et al. Glenoid revision surgery after total shoulder arthroplasty. *J Shoulder Elbow Surg* 2001;10:217–224.

61. Cofield RH, Edgerton BC. Total shoulder arthroplasty: complications and revision surgery. *Instr Course Lect* 1990;39:449–462.

62. Spencer EE Jr, Valdevit A, Kambic H, et al. The effect of humeral component anteversion on shoulder stability with glenoid component retroversion. *J Bone Joint Surg Am* 2005;87:808–814.

63. Dodson CC, Nho SJ, Cordasco FA, et al. Anterior humeral window for revision shoulder arthroplasty. *Tech Shoulder Elbow Surg* 2006;7:111–115.

64. Sperling JW, Cofield RH. Humeral windows in revision shoulder arthroplasty. *J Shoulder Elbow Surg* 2005;14:258–263.

65. Codsi MJ, Hennigan S, Herzog R, et al. Latissimus dorsi tendon transfer for irreparable posterosuperior rotator cuff tears: surgical technique. *J Bone Joint Surg Am* 2007;89(Pt 1 suppl 2):1–9.

66. Gerber C, Vinh TS, Hertel R, et al. Latissimus dorsi transfer for the treatment of massive tears of the rotator cuff: a preliminary report. *Clin Orthop Relat Res* 1988;232:51–61.

67. Gerber C, Maquieira G, Espinosa N. Latissimus dorsi transfer for the treatment of irreparable rotator cuff tears. *J Bone Joint Surg Am* 2006;88:113–120.

68. Habermeyer P, Magosch P, Rudolph T, et al. Transfer of the tendon of latissimus dorsi for the treatment of massive tears of the rotator cuff: a new single-incision technique. *J Bone Joint Surg Br* 2006;88:208–212.

69. Pearle AD, Kelly BT, Voos JE, et al. Surgical technique and anatomic study of latissimus dorsi and teres major transfers. *J Bone Joint Surg Am* 2006;88:1524–1531.

70. Fagelman M, Sartori M, Freedman KB, et al. Biomechanics of coracoacromial arch modification. *J Shoulder Elbow Surg* 2007;16:101–106.

71. Wiley AM. Superior humeral dislocation: a complication following decompression and debridement for rotator cuff tears. *Clin Orthop Relat Res* 1991;263:135–141.

72. Dines JS, Fealy S, Strauss EJ, et al. Outcomes analysis of revision total shoulder replacement. *J Bone Joint Surg Am* 2006;88:1494–1500.

73. Krishnan SG, Burkhead WZ, Nowinski RJ. Humeral hemiarthroplasty with biologic resurfacing of the glenoid and acromion for rotator cuff tear arthropathy. *Tech Shoulder Elbow Surg* 2004;5:51–59.

74. Norris TR, Kelly JD. Management of glenoid bone defects in revision shoulder arthroplasty: a new application of the reverse total shoulder prosthesis. *Tech Shoulder Elbow Surg* 2007;8:37–46.

75. Wall B, Walch G, Jouve F, et al. The reverse shoulder prosthesis for revision of failed total shoulder arthroplasty. In: Walch G, Boileau P, Molé D, et al, eds. *Reverse Shoulder Arthroplasty*. Montepellier, France: Sauramps Medical; 2006:231–242.

76. Clare DJ, Wirth MA, Groh GI, et al. Shoulder arthrodesis. *J Bone Joint Surg Am* 2001;83:593–600.

77. Hawkins RJ, Neer CS 2nd. A functional analysis of shoulder fusions. *Clin Orthop Relat Res* 1987;223:65–76.

78. Cofield RH, Briggs BT. Glenohumeral arthrodesis: operative and long-term functional results. *J Bone Joint Surg Am* 1979;61:668–677.

79. Sperling JW, Pring M, Antuña SA, et al. Shoulder arthroplasty for locked posterior dislocation of the shoulder. *J Shoulder Elbow Surg* 2004;13:522–527.

80. Sanchez-Sotelo J, Sperling JW, Rowland CM, et al. Instability after shoulder arthroplasty: results of surgical treatment. *J Bone Joint Surg Am* 2003;85:622–631.

81. Gill DR, Cofield RH, Rowland C. The anteromedial approach for shoulder arthroplasty: the importance of the anterior deltoid. *J Shoulder Elbow Surg* 2004;13:532–537.

82. Werner CM, Steinmann PA, Gilbart M, et al. Treatment of painful pseudoparesis due to irreparable rotator cuff dysfunction with the Delta III reverse-ball-and-socket total shoulder prosthesis. *J Bone Joint Surg Am* 2005;87:1476–1486.

83. Frankle M, Levy JC, Pupello D, et al. The reverse shoulder prosthesis for glenohumeral arthritis associated with severe rotator cuff deficiency: a minimum 2-year follow-up study of 60 patients surgical technique. *J Bone Joint Surg Am* 2006;88(suppl 1 Pt 2):178–190.

84. Frankle M, Siegal S, Pupello D, et al. The reverse shoulder prosthesis for glenohumeral arthritis associated with severe rotator cuff deficiency: a minimum 2-year follow-up study of 60 patients. *J Bone Joint Surg Am* 2005;87:1697–1705.

85. Guery J, Favard L, Sirveaux F, et al. Reverse total shoulder arthroplasty: survivorship analysis of 80 replacements followed for 5 to 10 years. *J Bone Joint Surg Am* 2006;88:1742–1747.

86. Sirveaux F, Favard L, Oudet D, et al. Grammont inverted total shoulder arthroplasty in the treatment of glenohumeral osteoarthritis with massive rupture of the cuff: results of a multicentre study of 80 shoulders. *J Bone Joint Surg Br* 2004;86:388–395.

87. Seebauer L, Walter W, Keyl W. Reverse total shoulder arthroplasty for the treatment of defect arthropathy. *Oper Orthop Traumatol* 2005;17:1–24.

88. Nove-Josserand L, Walch G, Wall B. Instability of the reverse prosthesis. In: Walch G, Boileau P, Molé D, et al. *Reverse Shoulder Arthroplasty*. Montpellier, France: Sauramps Medical; 2006:247–260.

Surgical Management of the Infected Shoulder Arthroplasty

INTRODUCTION

Shoulder infection is in any situation a devastating event and will not only impair the function of the joint but also have a considerable impact on the future outcome of any revision surgery.[1–4]

The increased interest in the shoulder joint and its associated pathologies and their respective treatments has also increased the rate of infections as a sequence to the various therapies. The incidence for infection has been quoted as between 0% and 2.9%, with an increase in more constrained implants up to 15.4%.[5] In a multicenter study with 2,343 shoulder prostheses, the rate of infection was found to be 1.86% in primary arthroplasty and 4% in revision arthroplasty.[6] The outcome of arthroplasty surgery under these conditions becomes seriously impaired, with a loss in the respective function scores.[7,8]

Susceptibility to infection is determined by the state of the host defense, the route that the infection takes for contamination, and the local conditions found at the involved site. Most infections will be focused locally, although a true shoulder sepsis is relatively uncommon, usually found in patients affected by systemic diseases such as rheumatoid arthritis, inadequate immune competence, or a consuming disease.[9,10] Patients with diabetes are known to develop a higher rate of frozen shoulders and to have an increased incidence of infection.[11] A pseudogout may also mimic an infection.[12]

If a total joint arthroplasty is present in situ, it might act as a foreign body, enabling an infection to embed itself. Pathogens may enter the joint either directly at the time of surgery or by a secondary intervention such as an intra-articular or extra-articular injection.[13,14] A contagious spread through the underlying bone is rather rare, but a spontaneous hematogenous seeding through the supporting local blood supply of the joint is possible.[15]

The most common agents causing an infection are those as in any other joint infection, such as coagulase-negative staphylococci (30% to 40%), *Staphylococcus aureus* (12% to 23%), any of the streptococci family (9% to 10 %), gram-negative bacilli and enterococci each in 3% to 7%, and a mixed flora responsible in approximately 10% to 12%.[16,17] Recently propionibacterium has been identified as a main pathogen involving shoulder joint infections[18–20] and has been shown to be sometimes difficult to detect. The incidence of shoulder infection for this bacterium has been cited as being 16 times that in any other joints.[21]

HISTORY

Shoulder surgeries have been reported since the late 1800s, and the most commonly cited intervention for an arthroplasty is that by Dr. Jules-Émile Péan in 1893, when he attempted to reconstruct a tuberculous shoulder joint in a 30-year-old man.[22] Little or nothing is known about the outcome or a possibly needed revision and removal of the hand-made implant. This shows that it is easy to become famous with a heroic act, but only a few will follow the possible complications.

INFECTION PATHWAYS

Although it was thought at the beginning of understanding microbial infections that tuberculosis was the most common cause for osteomyelitis and infection of joints,[23] it became evident with better microbial testing and knowledge that other agents were more frequently responsible for joint infections.[17,21,24,25]

The anatomic pathway of a shoulder infection is usually a local inoculation of the joint at the time of an intervention such as a shoulder joint puncture for an injection, a penetrating injury by a weapon, or possibly even at the time of surgery. Open injuries rarely affect the shoulder joint and are usually associated only with very high-impact accidents.

Trueta et al[26] demonstrated the intramedullary vascular supply and its competence in the growing child. They showed that the epiphyseal vessels are patent until the age of approximately 1 year only. After that point the growth plate forms a complete barrier, so all vascular communication must follow the metaphyseal supply to reach the joint through the synovial layers in an extra-articular way.[27] Therefore we find osteomyelitis through the metaphyseal area, but almost never in the epiphyseal region. Only once the old growth plate has been penetrated by osteomyelitis can the infection involve the humeral head.[28,29]

Whereas the joint is closed in through the joint capsule, various bursae are located in the periarticular space.[30] Therefore the anatomic bridge-ways into the joint cavity are either the long head of biceps tendon sheath or a small physiological foramen, which might be present in the interval area and may open the joint to secondary contamination through the subacromial spaces. Obviously, a rotator cuff tear will also allow for free communication between the subacromial and intra-articular spaces, particularly with injections into the subacromial/subdeltoid bursa, rendering the joint more susceptible to secondary infection.[31]

A hematogenous pathway may allow bacterial penetration through the synovial vessels and in this way trigger the cascade of a local infection and later joint destruction. A resurfacing prosthesis (cap prosthesis), for instance, might induce local bony necrosis, and it is known that devitalized bone can provide the base for any bacterial colonization.[32]

EARLY VERSUS LATE INFECTION

Infections are usually classified into early and late, and this concept will also allow for a choice of therapeutic approaches to the patient. Early is classified as an event that will occur within the first 4 weeks after an intervention, and late is anything after this period. An infection that occurs within the first year might still be associated with the index surgery or intervention; infection developing after 1 year is considered to have followed the hematogenous pathway.[16]

The route of infection can be classified into either direct or primary intra-articular through an inoculation, be it through trauma or an intervention such as needle penetration at the time of an injection or aspiration or through surgery.[13,33] It also may occur secondarily through a continuous spread along the hematogenous pathway or through an infiltrating osseous spread through osteomyelitis. Tuberculosis, pseudomonas, *S. aureus,* and salmonella have all been reported to cause local osseous infiltrations. The pure hematogenous pathway is more common in children.[21,34] The most common cause for infection, however, is through internal or external osteosynthesis devices that have become contaminated, such as an external fixateur, internal fixation plates and screws, or a total joint arthroplasty.[35,36] More rare ports of entry can be an ipsilateral forearm fistula, such as in patients undergoing renal transplant and dialysis. Acupuncture for therapeutic or diagnostic purposes also may be associated with proximal infections.

BACTERIAL ADHERENCE

In implant-related infection, particularly with *Staphylococcus* species, such as *S. aureus* and *S. epidermidis,* the bacteria will develop a glycocalix that adheres to the surface of metal and bone[37,38] and may even change their morphology through minimal variant colony formation, thereby trying to escape direct antibiotic attack.[39–41] This is particularly the case in surface cartilage because it may still be present in a hemiarthroplasty and is susceptible to colonization, thereby fostering intra-articular spread and destruction of the joint surfaces. The same holds true for any foreign body, such as an implant, where a glycocalix

will form on the surface, thus protecting the bacterial coating from any direct attack except for mechanical abrasion.[25,42] The bigger the foreign body surface, the higher is the likelihood of an infection just because of the space provided for settling of the bacteria.

The most common causal organism for shoulder infection is still *S. aureus,* but as mentioned earlier, infection by *Propionibacterium* species seems to be on the increase.[20]

This might be associated with contamination at the time of intervention and the proximity of the axillary fold.

Frank osteomyelitis is rare and mainly present in immunocompromised patients or in children, account for 80% to 90% of all of cases. The causative agent here is usually *S. aureus* or to a lesser degree in sickle cell disease *Salmonella* or *Proteus* species.[43]

The opportunity for local infection is enhanced in rheumatoid arthritis, immunosuppressed patients who have undergone transplantation, the newborn, and pregnant women.[29,33,44] A static lymphedema, such as may be present after a breast operation and possibly radiation[45] or a urogenital tract infection, may also give a base to an infection. The mechanism is bacterial aggregation on the surfaces, forming a biofilm that can migrate and form colonies in a more distant spot. *S. aureus* is the major pathogen in biometal bone and tissue infections and the pathogen most commonly isolated in osteomyelitis.[46] Infections with propionibacterium are particularly difficult to detect because cultivation and isolation of the bacteria might take a longer time and clinical signs and symptoms might be less obvious than would be expected in a general joint infection. Therefore a high index of suspicion should be entertained for propionibacterium in the case of infection; at the time of surgery considerable tissue destruction by propionibacterium may be found.[47]

CLINICAL SIGNS

Clinical findings, symptoms, and signs of any infection are well known—reddening, pain, tumor, and warmth. The patient can present with signs of infection such as fever and skin effluence, which are most prominent with streptococci infection and erysipelas.

After the clinical examination, laboratory evaluation will be done, including the erythrocyte sedimentation rate, C-reactive protein value, and differential white blood count. Synovial fluid analysis can be done, and in septic arthritis will most likely show a high leukocyte count, a low glucose level, and more than 75% polymorphonuclear cells. Intraoperative frozen section has been used for verification of the presence of an infection. Banit et al[48] pointed out that this technique can be only an additive measure in detecting infection (>75% polymorphonuclear leukocytes per high power field is suggestive of an infection). Topolski et al[19] demonstrated that this is not always a reliable finding and a high index of suspicion for infection has to be retained despite negative findings in the synovial fluid analysis.

Joint aspiration and culture is still the gold standard for any type of infection to identify the causing agent. Although protein levels might well be elevated, polymorphonuclear leukocyte counts usually show a left shift in an acute infection. A Gram stain can be performed and is positive approximately

50% of the time, but false negative findings might occur as well. Therefore this can be only an additive measure but not necessarily used exclusively for determination of presence of a joint infection.

Aspiration and assertion of a joint culture is still the mainstay for any type of diagnosis and therefore has to be done correctly. The use of local anesthetics, particular of the ester type, might inhibit cell growth and therefore give a false negative result. Aspiration is done in a sterile environment under sterile conditions to avoid contamination of the probe. If the aspiration is negative, reaspiration may very well yield a positive result.[49] Any antibiotic therapy that the patient might have been started on erroneously will have to be stopped for at least 2 weeks in order not to compromise the results negatively.

RADIOGRAPHIC ANALYSIS

Standard radiographs will be taken to demonstrate any local erosions or secondary changes in an advanced infection. An effusion might be present, lateralizing the humeral component on the image.[50]

Frank loosening of the joint implant might indicate an advanced infection, giving rise to secondary mechanical irritation resulting from the loose implant in situ. Computed tomography (CT) will help in demonstrating the amount of loosening and bony destruction. Magnetic resonance imaging (MRI) will also show the soft tissue involvement at the same time.[51] Both CT and MRI will show metal image artifacts, which can be corrected through an imaging calculating program.

Specific scans such as a technetium diphosphate scan or an indium-labeled leukocyte scan will also help in revealing activity at the local area.[52] They will not help in proving infection, and false negative results can occur during the very acute phase of an infection or in patients who are immunocompromised and without an appropriate inflammatory response. This might also be true for the very elderly.

A CT scan can be useful in identifying osteomyelitis and associated bone disease. Positron emission tomography (PET) measures activated local glucose levels and can be used to demonstrate the extent of an infection, particularly around a total joint arthroplasty. This seems to be useful to identify the nidus and at the same time will more accurately help the physician in assessing the extent of the infection into the surrounding soft tissues.

Ultrasound is an inexpensive and noninvasive tool to assess a joint for fluid content and in high resolution also can demonstrate erosion around the bone.

THERAPY

Therapy will depend on the extent and timing of detection of an infection. Surgical therapy is the mainstay of therapy in these infections. Adequate debridement of any necrotic tissue allows systemic antibiotics provided during and after surgery to reach the joint.[53] Topical antibiotics will give a high antibiotic concentration locally without compromising renal function.[54] Antibiotic-impregnated beads may be indicated in certain cases of infection or in rare cases with osteomyelitis. Usually it will be

the surgical removal of any destroyed or necrotic tissue that will increase the chance of a surgical success.

ARTHROSCOPIC LAVAGE AND OPEN DEBRIDEMENT

An early infection might be treated through arthroscopic lavage of the involved joint, but one must determine whether the cartilage and tissues are involved so that all of the recesses can be reached by the lavage fluid. An adequate history must prove that the infection is present only within the previous 10 to 14 days to allow for success for this therapy. Irrigation systems with a disinfectant solution such as 0.01% Lavasept may help in the very early phase of infected joints (<14 days) and can be maintained for approximately 48 hours.[55] Secondary so-called highways or fluid street formation should be avoided with suction irrigation systems. Retrograde colonization of the tubing might occur after 48 hours. A disinfectant should not be used in cases in which a hemiarthroplasty only is present, to avoid injury to the remaining glenoid cartilage.

The results with arthroscopic irrigation are rather disappointing. Most authors agree that limited interventions are successful only if the infection was found early.[9,11,36,55,57]

A French multicenter study reports on 49 implants treated in this way, and inadequate antibiotics were cited as one of the problems of reinfection.[6] Jerosch and Schneppenheim[16] reported on their results, in which only one implant could be saved with an arthroscopic synovectomy. A chance for success with an intervention is given within the first 8 days after an infection.[9] If there is only minimal soft tissue involvement, surgical lavage combined with a disinfectant (Lavasept) might be able to save the implant.

Repeated needle aspirations of the infected joint in association with a concomitant intravenous antibiotic therapy have been attempted for joint salvage. If the bone is involved, repeated aspirations do not appear to yield any success and a surgical intervention with a possible resection arthroplasty will be more successful.[52]

If there is any doubt regarding success, we always opt for open debridement, allowing mechanical cleansing of all joint surfaces and at the same time, if possible, replacement of any polyethylene components, if they are of a modular type. The exchange of all polyethylene inlays, if they are modular, should be done to avoid increased adherence of bacteria to the surfaces. Sperling et al[11] reported on 26 shoulder infections, of which six were treated by open debridement, but only 50% of those were successful.

LOW-GRADE INFECTION

If the patient presents with a latent infection, or a so-called low-grade infection, one first must identify the underlying causative agent if possible. This will be done by aspiration and, if needed, reaspiration of the joint in an antibiotic-free interval. Often these patients will have been treated for their symptoms; sometimes even an allergy to the metal implant might be suggested as a cause for the symptoms.[58] Careful observation of tissues or joint fluid with the collaboration of an expert microbiologist may reveal a propionibacterium or corynebacterium infection in some cases.[9]

Late detection is usually associated with a delayed diagnosis, and often a more relevant type of infecting organism can become apparent. A possible persistent drainage through a fistula and later secondary osteomyelitis and bone destruction may develop.

ONE-STAGE EXCHANGE

Essential to the decision to perform a one-time exchange is the identification of the underlying causative agent. The combination of surgical debridement and topical antibiotics locally with systemic antibiotic therapy is the underlying key to success.[49] The advantages of a one-stage surgery are obvious, as follows:

- Less destruction/dissection of soft tissues and bone
- Immediate reconstruction
- Avoidance of secondary adhesions between the implantations as needed in a two-stage procedure
- Less anxiety for the patient
- Less hospitalization cost

The main problem will in any case be the soft tissues because the remaining rotator cuff will be affected, thereby rendering the necrotic tissues unsuitable for reconstruction.[59,60] They can sometimes be saved in the very early phase of an infection, if the rotator cuff is still preserved, but still all suture materials must be removed because as they will act as foreign bodies.

Soft tissue reconstruction at a later second stage, such as muscle transfer or muscle pedicle insertion, may be an option to keep in mind at the time of surgery.[61] But care must be taken to avoid compromising the joint surface with the extent of debridement, which might render the joint more susceptible to reinfection if not done completely.

Removal of the components can be challenging, particularly if the glenoid bone stock is of a more "cookie" type quality (hard and brittle) and could leave an empty cavity after implant removal.

On the humeral side, one has to determine whether the components can be removed properly without further bone loss or destruction. This can be very challenging in the case of a well-fixed uncemented arthroplasty stem in situ, in which case we extend the incision along the humeral shaft and do a longitudinal split, allowing the surfaces to be separated from the implant by long-bladed chisels. Gentle tapping from below will loosen the stem. A prophylactic cerclage may be used to prevent uncontrolled splitting distally, and a drill hole at the end of the split may prevent the stress riser extending any farther down the shaft.

If the implant has been cemented, all cement must be removed, which again can be challenging if the cement has extruded well below the implant into the canal.

Once the implants have been removed, proper mechanical washing with a lavage system should be used, taking care to not pulse-lavage the soft tissues, which might render them more susceptible to further necrosis. All mucosal layers must be removed from the joint surfaces, and the anterior and posterior walls along the glenoid neck have to be probed as well. If a glenoid had been fixed with screws, the screw holes have to be drilled out to remove all debris within the old threads.

In a one-stage exchange the instruments are changed before the insertion of the new implant to avoid secondary contamination as far as possible. Systemic antibiotic therapy is started once the tissue probes have been secured from the site of the infection, be it stem or glenoid.

Ince et al[62] reported on 16 patients who were followed for more than 2 years without occurrence of reinfection. Sperling et al[11] reported on a group of the Mayo Clinic, in which two patients were treated in this way, with one of them surviving.

TWO-STAGE REVISION

Two-stage revision is done for patients in whom the underlying causative agent could not be identified. The essentials are the same as in one-stage exchange surgery. One needs to identify if possible all of the causative agents, to effectively direct topical antibiotic therapy. The debridement must be just as carefully performed and as extensive as in a one-stage exchange operation.[63] A temporary spacer can be fashioned with a Steinman pin as an enforcement core, and the appropriate mix of antibiotics can be employed locally. The temporary spacer can be formed from a bulb syringe in order to fill the joint fully, and one should take care to not lose any more bone stock by implanting the spacer in a too-fixed fashion, making later removal difficult.[64]

The patients' laboratory values as well as the clinical signs are monitored for approximately 4 to 6 weeks before secondary reimplantation is considered. Monitoring of the clinical signs and laboratory values, particularly C-reactive protein, will help in choosing the best point for the secondary exchange surgery in these patients. An antibiotic-free interval of approximately 14 days will demonstrate whether any increase in the infection-related parameters takes place. The choice of antibiotics must be directed toward the underlying causative agents.[65–67] Reaspiration might well yield false negative results because the local spacer is bactericidal and may cause a false negative result. Careful debridement and thorough irrigation with the disinfectant Lavasept during reimplantation seems necessary. Before implantation the bone and tissues should be rinsed well with Ringer's or saline solution to remove any remnants of the disinfectant from the joint surfaces. It is then decided whether a secondary implant is feasible and what type (reverse[68,39] versus a cuff tear arthropathy type of humeral arthroplasty[70–72]) is appropriate. Hemiarthroplasty has to be considered (if the glenoid will not allow safe seating of an implant. An autologous bone graft impacted safely in the glenoid cavity may be of help later to restore some bone stock. The scarring might make dissection more difficult in the two-stage procedure, and particular care must be given to neural structures such as the axillary and musculocutaneous nerves.

In a hemiarthroplasty, reconstruction of the ventral wall might have to be considered for stability, such as in a muscle transfer (pectoralis transfer), at the same time. Because of the necrotic process, some soft tissue destruction or fibrosis is usually found in an infected joint. Therefore various types of flaps have been suggested, such as a pectoralis transfer or use of the latissimus dorsi[73] for reconstruction of the upper and ventral rotator cuff.

Most of these options will help in retaining a large ball head hemiarthroplasty but will not necessarily allow for better function. The reports so far are few.[74,75]

After surgery the same type of antibiotics are administered as before, but once the probes have been re-evaluated, an adjustment according to the pattern of resistance found might be needed.[17]

Jerosch and Schneppenheim[16] reported on their results with good success in ten patients who stayed infection-free. Eight of those were exchanged; two remained by patient wish, with the spacer prosthesis in situ, declining any further surgery.

Seitz and Damacen[76] reported on a two-stage procedure in eight patients with no recurrent infection. Functional results were poor, although with approximately 50% function compared to the other nonaffected patients. Sperling et al[11] reported on two patients having undergone a one-stage revision, with one replacement being still in situ without a major problem after 10 years and one having failed after 9 months.

A low-grade infection might tempt the surgeon to be not as aggressive as in a frank purulent infection, but again only diligent removal of all affected tissues will give a chance for success.

ANTIMICROBIAL THERAPY

The therapy chosen depends on the underlying bacteria found and their respective resistances. In the presence of a foreign body a contamination as low as 100 colony-forming units is sufficient to induce an infection in contrast to 10,000 units without foreign material.[17] This underlines the need for removal of any material that might act as a nidus for bacterial embedding. The effect is thought to be due to the reduced clearing capacity by phagocytosis of the leukocytes in the presence of foreign materials.

The choice of antibiotics will in most cases be a first- or second-generation cephalosporin, such as cefazolin, for preoperative prevention. In the case of an allergy to beta-lactam agents, vancomycin may be chosen. Glycopeptide prophylaxis has been considered as well, particularly as a result of the rise of methicillin-resistant infections by S. aureus or S. epidermidis (MRSA and MRSE). But trials have shown that beta-lactam–derived drugs can still be effective in coping with these infections, reducing in this way the risk for vancomycin resistance to develop. Ideally the antimicrobial agent should be bactericidal against biofilm-producing microorganisms. Rifampin can do this in combination with ofloxacin or ciprofloxacin and has been shown to be susceptible to development of resistance. Quinolones have shown improved efficacy in combination with rifampin, just as linezolid has demonstrated. Gentamycin-loaded cement has been used for a long time. In combination with clindamycin it has been manufactured in a premixed combination as a commercially available product, Copal. This, sometimes in combination with other antimicrobial agents such as vancomycin, has improved the success of the cemented revision substantially. An excellent summary of the agents of choice for various microorganisms is given by Zimmerli et al.[77]

REHABILITATION

Rehabilitation after one-stage or two-stage procedures is dependent on the type of implant used. If the ventral wall has been reconstructed, external rotation is limited to 0 degrees, with an abduction of approximately 30 degrees for the first 4 to 5 weeks. Depending on the remaining muscle function present, as can be assessed on the MRI before surgery for degeneration and fatty content,[78] this can then be increased gradually.

Active-assisted exercises under the supervision of a physiotherapist can later be initiated, and one can expect some improvement for the next 6 to 12 months.

In the case of an inverse prosthesis having been implanted, gentle abduction and elevation maneuvers are being started on the third postoperative day, moving into active-assisted motion after the first 10 days under the supervision of a physiotherapist. Usually the sling is being worn for approximately 4 to 6 weeks, particularly at night. Once patients have gained control over the implant, they will proceed with outpatient exercises to the pain limit. In inverse prosthesis, forced internal or external rotation exercises should be avoided because of the nature of the implant mechanics.[79]

RESECTION ARTHROPLASTY

Resection arthroplasty gives relatively good pain relief, as reported in the literature. The function, however, is poor, and traction pain has been reported as well.[80,81] The arm can sometimes be trained with maneuvers to reach the mouth, but because of loss of internal rotation, personal hygiene is severely impaired, as is, obviously, the strength of the arm.

Rispoli et al[82] reported on 34 patients, of whom 18 could be followed. Ten patients had significant improvement of pain; active elevation, although limited, was 70 degrees. Of those who underwent surgery because of infection, six experienced reinfection, ten were rated as fair to poor, and in eight of 11 shoulders followed for a longer period, a poor clinical grading was given. Four of the patients had reinfection despite a resection arthroplasty.

Resection arthroplasty should always be considered, particularly if a chronic fistula or a chronic infection has developed. This might be the only way to avoid recurrent infection.

SHOULDER ARTHRODESIS

Arthrodesis was for many years the only way to settle an infection and to attempt through a fusion some function without pain and drainage. External fixation will be used in only a few cases. The limited function that has to be expected will induce many patients and surgeons to attempt an arthroplasty revision before fusion. The use of a permanent draining fistula is poorly accepted, and suppressive therapy in terminal ill patients is also rarely acceptable. Arm ablation has been reported for acute infection and sepsis, representing the worst case scenario for any surgeon.[83,84]

SHOULDER ARTHROPLASTY FOR POSTINFECTIOUS ARTHRITIS

Shoulder arthroplasty for treatment of postinfectious arthritis has also been reported. Mileti et al[59] reviewed 12 shoulder joints with a mean follow-up of 9.7 years who underwent revision arthroplasty after having had a postinfectious arthritis. None of the patients became reinfected, with one having a positive culture at the time of repeat surgery treated with a 2-week course of antibiotics postoperatively. The functional outcome, however, was rather limited, and only six patients rated the overall results as significantly better than the preoperative state.

SUMMARY

Infection of an arthroplasty is still a major concern with an uncertain outcome. Infection after total shoulder arthroplasty is rare, although still a serious problem. The incidence is being cited as between 0% and 15%. This can depend on host susceptibility, such as with the presence of rheumatoid arthritis or diabetes mellitus, or the type of implant used.

Local injections are one of the causes leading to secondary infections, particularly if an arthroplasty had been performed in the past. With an unsatisfactory result, this might lead to the administration of local injections given repeatedly for pain relief. A deep infection necessitating the removal of the implant and leaving the patient with a resection arthroplasty may later develop as a result of contamination.

Early infections might be treated with arthroscopic lavage or, even better, open debridement, thereby retaining the joint, if the infection is detected and the intervention is done within the first 10 days. Systemic antibiotics directed toward the causative agent will help in securing the surgical success.

Once an infection has become manifest, the most important part is detecting the underlying causative agent to properly direct antibiotic therapy. If this is possible and particularly if the pathogen can be identified without major resistance to antimicrobial therapy, a one-stage exchange can give good results as far as infection eradication and function are concerned. The problem remains the degree of soft tissue destruction, be it through the infection or the necessary debridement.

If an implant can be placed, the choice is either a large-head prosthesis, such as a cuff tear arthropathy head, or an inverse type of prosthesis. The reverse type of prosthesis seems to give good functional results at this time. These results depend on whether one can still find good anchorage for a safe fixation of the glenoid component. It is essential that the muscle functional state, particularly that of deltoid muscle, be tested before the intervention to ensure proper function later.

Systemic antibiotics are started once the probes have been safely acquired during surgery. The systemic antibiotic therapy can be adjusted once the microbiologist has reported the results for the probes or any possible resistance to antibiotics.

The length of antibiotic therapy is empirical and depends on the clinical response of the patient. A treatment interval of 4 to 6 weeks has in some centers become a standard. The most important concept is identification of the underlying bacteria, as has been stated now many times, to direct the antibiotic therapy properly, be it topical or systemic, to the target. Adequate serum concentrations of the antibiotic have to be documented and side effects of the antibiotics monitored. The bacterial resistance test (mean inhibition concentration) is used to determine the adequacy of the therapy, being defined as a dilution of the patient's serum that will kill more than 99% of the infection organisms in vitro.

Close follow-up of the laboratory values, such as C-reactive protein, is mandatory to determine whether treatment is successful or resistance is evolving. A careful history must be obtained for any allergies before a systemic or topical medication is chosen.

Although systemic antibiotics are usually advantageous, oral antibiotics can be used if appropriate and have the economic advantage over intravenous therapy for patients requiring longer term treatment. In osteomyelitis treatment the therapy will be continued for approximately 2 to 3 months. Careful monitoring of these patients after discharge is mandatory. If a recalcitrant infection is suspected, all antibiotics have to be stopped for approximately 2 weeks before reaspiration is attempted.

In our institution the success of a one-stage procedure depends on careful patient selection and successful identification of the underlying causative bacteria. A surgical debridement with resection of all necrotic tissue is the mainstay for a successful revision in any case. Proper selection and administration of antibiotics topically will allow for a high local antibiotic load directed against underlying bacteria.[85,86] Because there is only one surgery, soft tissue handling will be less destructive, and rehabilitation seems to be easier without a prosthetic-less interval.

In the event that a negative culture is present and even a repeat aspiration cannot provide identification of the bacteria present, a two-stage revision becomes indicated. Signs of infection should be evaluated in the absence of the identification of an organism. Any antibiotic therapy must be stopped for at least 2 weeks to allow an appropriate aspiration without local anesthetics interference with the results. If the sedimentation rate remains elevated for more than 13 mm/hour or the C-reactive protein shows levels higher than 10 mg/L, there is a high likelihood for an ongoing infection. If a section taken at the time of surgery reveals more than five polymorphonuclear leukocytes to be present per high power field, an infection has to be suspected as well. Propionibacterium infection is a particular problem, as has been reported by Sperling et al[11,20] and seems to be on the rise. It is thought that contamination at the time of surgery through the proximity of the axillary fold might be one of the underlying reasons for these bacteria to be present. Detection is difficult, and microbiologists require a long period of observation and culture to isolate this species. Low-grade infection or aseptic loosening, as reported in the past, might well represent an infection with bacteria of this genus.

If in doubt, infection must be assumed to be present, despite a negative aspiration result or negative bone scans of any type. Identification of the underlying agent is the mainstay of the diagnostic process, and therapy is directed accordingly. The one-stage exchange seems to give good results, particularly because the invention of the inverse prosthesis allows for better function when the involved rotator cuff has been compromised. One-time exchange is appropriate only if antibiotic therapy can be directed toward the underlying cause, be it topical or systemic.[63] In the more common type of infection, extended systemic therapy has not been proved to be of any extra benefit versus a 2-week period of intravenous therapy after careful surgical debridement has been performed.

A multidisciplinary collaboration is needed, including an experienced microbiology department to give the needed support.[25,87]

Although the results given in the literature show a reasonable success for infection eradication, they all have in common relatively poor function and therefore limited success for subjective evaluation.[2,53,59,71,75,88,89] This is in many cases due to the implants used in the earlier studies that had to rely on a

TABLE 20.1	Demographics

Patient	Gender	Age (Years)	Follow-Up (Months)	Premorbidities	Previous Surgeries	Bacteria	Antibiotic Therapy (Topical)	Antibiotic Therapy (Systemic)	Flexion Preoperatively	Flexion Postoperatively
1	M	78	72	Impingement, rotator cuff lesion	Hemiarthroplasty 1990, two times revision, shoulder prosthesis exchange and glenoid–implantation 1994, glenoid exchange 2001	Staphylococcus capitis, Propionibacterium acnes	Copal (clindamycin + gentamycin)	Penicillin 3 × 1 Mega, Zinacef 3 × 1.5 g	20	60
2	M	78	65				Copal		30	
3	M	78	61	Impingement, rotator cuff lesion	Hemiarthroplasty 1990	Staphylococcus species	Copal + vancomycin		30	150
4	M	39	59			P. acnes	Copal		30	30
5	M	78	56	Shoulder arthritis, rotator cuff massive tear	Primary implantation Delta prosthesis April 23, 2003	P. acnes	Copal + vancomycin	Gentamycin 1 × 240, Zienam 4 × 500	30	60
6	F	71	72	Humeral head fracture	Primary implantation by fracture February 2002, septic exchange to Delta prosthesis December 2002	S. epidermidis	Gentamycin, ofloxacin, vancomycin	Levofloxacin 2 × 500, rifampicin 1 × 600	20	60
7	M	57	41	Humeral head fracture	Osteosynthesis 2002, hemiarthroplasty 2002, arthrolysis 2003	S. epidermidis	Vancomycin, gentamycin	Vancomycin 4 × 500, rifampicin 1 × 600, Targocid 1 × 400	20	30
8	M	46	41	Rheumatoid arthritis	Primary implantation Delta prosthesis 2002, periprosthetic infection left knee, arthrodesis with nail, S. epidermidis with shoulder involvement	S. epidermidis	Copal + vancomycin	Rifampicin 1 × 600, vancomycin 4 × 500, (später zus. linezolid 2 × 600)	0	120
9	M	45	40	Humeral head fracture		P. acnes	Copal	Imipenem 4 × 500	50	
10	M	57	35	Humeral head fracture	Hemiarthroplasty 1999, revision 2002, exchange to a Delta prosthesis 2004, postoperative dislocation	P. acnes	Copal	Penicillin G 4 × 5 Mega	150	180
11	M	63	30	Humeral fracture, elbow fracture	Elbow prosthesis (TOELL) 1975, TOELL exchange 1994 and 1997, Implantation Delta prosthesis 1998, exchange to a total humeral prosthesis with inverse shoulder, 2003 revision due to stem fracture 2005	P. acnes	Copal	Imipenem 4 × 500	0	
12	F	62	28	Humeral head necrosis radiation/ chemo breast -ca	Delta prosthesis 2002	S. epidermidis	Copal + vancomycin	Levofloxacin 2 × 500, rifampicin 2 × 300	50	90
13	F	70	23	Humeral head fracture	Hemiarthroplasty 2004, head exchange 2004	S. epidermidis	Copal	Staphylex 3 × 2 g	25	90
14	M	62	20	Shoulder arthritis	Schulterkappenprothesesis 1997, exchange to a Delta prosthesis 2003, soft tissue debridement and antibiotic therapy by fistulae and abcess 2005	P. acnes	Copal	Penicillin 4 × 5 Mega	150	150
15	M	57	13	Humeral head fracture	Osteosynthesis May 2004, revision by fistulae September 2004, revision and spacer implantation October 2004, spacer exchange November 2004, shoulder prosthesis January 2005, inlay exchange August 2006, new fistulae December 2006	S. epidermidis (two strains), S. faecalis, Finegoldia magna, Propionibacterium species, Proteus species		Rifampicin 2 ×450, Tavanic	20	
16	M	80	7	Shoulder arthritis	Primary implantation Delta prosthesis 2006	P. acnes	Copal	Penicillin 4 × 5 Mega	150	150
16	<>	63.8	41.43			<>			48.43	97.5

Adduction Postoperatively	Adduction Postoperatively	Patient's Satisfaction	Constant-Score Preoperatively	Constant-Score Postop	Remarks	Revision After (Months)	Revision Indication	Revision Operation	Radiography Findings	Lost to Follow-Up
0	60	Fair	5	20	Two Stage procedure: glenoid explantation + stem exchange to a Delta Prosthesis 2/02, in 11/02 glenoid reimplantation				Radiograph not available	—
10			0			6	Cranial migration	Glenoid and head exchange	Radiograph not available	No answer
0	120	Good	5	54					Radiograph not available	—
10	30	Good	41	26		50	Dislocation	Stem exchange	Cement augmentation, no loosening, no impingement	—
20	0	Bad	20	19		—	—	—	No loosening, no impingement	—
30	60	Bad	18	52		—	—	—	No loosening, no impingement	—
20	30	Fair	2	0		—	—	—	No loosening, no impingement	—
0	60	Good	5	45	Glenoid explantation	—	—	—	No loosening, no impingement	—
30			32		Glenoid explantation	—	—	—	No loosening, no impingement	Moved away
80	180	Very good	68	100		—	—	—	Radiograph not available	—
0			10			—	—	—	Radiograph not available	No answer
30	90	Good	36	70		—	—	—	Radiograph not available	—
5	60	Fair	21	31		—	—	—	No loosening, no impingement	—
80	150	Good	47	90		—	—	—	No loosening, no impingement	—
20			31			2	Recurrence S. epidermidis	Explantation, Resection arthroplasty.	Normal	No answer
140	120	Very good	73	90		—	—	—	No loosening, no impingement	—
29.68	**80**		**25.9**	**49.8**						

functional soft tissue envelope, particularly in a reconstructed rotator cuff, for proper range of motion. The advent of the inverse or Grammont prosthesis made it possible to use the deltoid muscle for function.[42,69,74,90–93] This allows for better results at this time, but still one needs a line of retreat from this implant because the glenoid bone will have to take all of the loading after reimplantation. In an infection situation this might not be possible, so a hemiarthroplasty, acting as a spacer rather than a valid prosthesis, is the last resort to turn to as a prosthesis.

OUR RESULTS

Between February 2002 and June 2007, 15 patients with 16 joints underwent one-stage revision. The average follow-up was 36.8 months; in nine cases surgery was on the right side and in seven cases on the left side. The average age was 63.8 years, ranging from 39 to 80 years.

Eight patients were available for personal radiographic and clinical follow-up. One patient was lost to follow-up because of relocation and not available for review.

At the time of surgery, *P. acnes* was the causative pathogen in seven cases, *S. epidermidis* in six, and *S. capitis*, *S. aureus*, *Enterococcus fecalis*, proteus, and *Finegoldia magna* in one case each. One patient underwent reoperation 2 months after the revision, going on to resection arthroplasty.

The preoperative Constant score[94] was 29.3; the postoperative Constant score 46.1. When asked whether they would undergo a second operation, six of the patients said yes and two said no.

The topical antibiotic used in 12 cases was Copal, a clindamycin and gentamycin combination. Vancomycin was added in four cases and flucloxacillin in one case. The patient undergoing re-revision had multiple bacteria present and had undergone two shoulder revisions before the most recent attempt for exchange. At this stage he is working as a physician and has remained infection-free with a resection arthroplasty for 12 months. The underlying pathology that led to the primary arthroplasty was fracture in seven cases, radiation therapy for same-side breast cancer in one case, primary omarthrosis in two cases, and mass rupture of the rotator cuff with cuff arthropathy in four cases. All patients having had fractures had undergone two or three previous surgeries before the prosthetic implantation, which then became infected secondarily. The demographics are provided in Table 20.1.

REFERENCES

1. Brems JJ. Complications of shoulder arthroplasty: infections, instability, and loosening. *Instr Course Lect* 2002;51:29–39.
2. Dines JS, Fealy S, Strauss EJ, et al. Outcomes analysis of revision total shoulder replacement. *J Bone Joint Surg Am* 2006;88:1494–1500.
3. Franta AK, Lenters TR, Mounce D, et al. The complex characteristics of 282 unsatisfactory shoulder arthroplasties. *J Shoulder Elbow Surg* 2007;16:555–562.
4. Magosch P, Habermeyer P, Lichtenberg S. Infectious arthropathy: destiny or indication for endoprosthetic joint replacement. *Z Orthop Ihre Grenzgeb* 2002;140:575–578.
5. Pahle J, Kvarnes L. Shoulder replacement arthroplasty. *Ann Chir Gynaecol* 1995;74:85–89.
6. Sirveaux F. Favard L, Oudet D, et al. Grammont-inverted total shoulder arthroplasty in the treatment of glenohumeral osteoarthritis with massive rupture of the cuff: results of a multicenter study of 80 shoulders. *J Bone Joint Surg Br* 2004;86:388–395.
7. Steindler A. *Orthopedic Operations: Indications, Techniques, and End Results*. Springfield, Ill: CC Thomas; 1940:304.
8. Wirth MA, Rockwood CA Jr. Complications of total shoulder replacement arthroplasty. *J Bone Joint Surg Am* 1996;78:603–616.
9. Rolf O, Stehle, J, Gohlke F. Treatment of septic arthritis of the shoulder and periprosthetic shoulder infections: special problems in rheumatoid arthritis *Orthopaede* 2007; 36:700–707.
10. Vainio K. Surgery of rheumatoid arthritis. *Surg Annu* 1974;6:309–335.
11. Sperling JW, Kozak TK, Hanssen AD, et al. Infection after shoulder arthroplasty. *Clin Orthop Relat Res* 2001;382:206–216.
12. Hughes GM, Biundo JJ Jr, Scheib JS, et al. Pseudogout and pseudosepsis of the shoulder. *Orthopedics* 1990;13:1169–1172.
13. Gowans JDC, Granieri PA. Septic arthritis: its relation to intra-articular injections of hydrocortisone acetate. *N Engl J Med* 1959;261:502–504.
14. Metha P, Schnall SB, Zalavras CG. Septic arthritis of the shoulder, elbow, and wrist. *Clin Orthop* 2006;451:42–45.
15. Kaandrop CJ, Van Schaardenburg D, Krijnen P, et al. Risk factors for septic arthritis in patients with joint disease: a prospective study. *Arthritis Rheum* 1995;38:1819–1825.
16. Jerosch J, Schneppenheim M. Management of infected shoulder replacement. *Arch Orthop Trauma Surg* 2003;123:209–214.
17. Zimmerli W, Ochsner PE. Management of infection associated with prosthetic joints. *Infection* 2002;33:99–108.
18. Berthelot P, Carricajo A, Aubert G, et al. Outbreak of postoperative shoulder arthritis due to *Propionibacterium acnes* infection in nondebilitated patients. *Infect Control Hosp Epidemiol* 2006;27:987–990.
19. Topolski MS, Chin PY, Sperling JW, et al. Revision shoulder arthroplasty with positive intraoperative cultures: the value of preoperative studies and intraoperative histology. *J Shoulder Elbow Surg* 2006;15:402–406.
20. Zeller V, Ghorbani A, Strady C, et al. Propionibacterium acnes: an agent of prosthetic joint infection and colonization. *J Infect* 2007;55:119–124.
21. Bernard L, Hoffmeyer P, Assal M, et al. Trend in the treatment of orthopaedic infections. *J Antimicrobial Ther* 2004;53:127–129.
22. Lugli T. Artificial shoulder joint by Péan (1893): the facts of an exceptional intervention and the prosthetic method. *Clin Orthop Relat Res* 1978;133:215–218.
23. Lizarralde Palacios E, Baraia-Etxaburu J, Gutiérrez-Macías A, et al. Infection of shoulder joint prosthesis by Mycobacterium tuberculosis. *Microbiol Clin* 2002;20:188.
24. Buchholz HW, Gartmann HD. Infektionsprophylaxe und operative Behandlung der schleichenden tiefen Infektion bei der totalen Endoprothese. *Chirurg* 1978;43:446–452.
25. Frommelt L. Periprosthetic infection. In: Learmonth ID, ed. *Bacteria and the Interface Between Prosthesis and Bone Interfaces in Total Hip Arthroplasty*. London: Springer-Verlag; 2000:153–161.
26. Trueta J. The normal vascular anatomy of the human femoral head during growth. *J Bone Joint Surg Br* 1957;39:358–394.
27. Bos CF, Mol, LJ, Obermann WR, et al. Late sequelae of neonatal septic arthritis of the shoulder. *J Bone Joint Surg Br* 1998;80:645–650.
28. Kelly PJ, Conventry MB, Martin WJ. Bacterial arthritis of the shoulder. *Mayo Clin Proc* 1965;40:695–699.
29. Smith AM, Sperling JW, Cofield RH. Outcomes are poor after treatment of sepsis in the rheumatoid shoulder. *Clin Orthop* 2005;439:68–73.
30. Codman EA. *The Shoulder: Rupture of the Supraspinatus Tendon and Other Lesions in or about the Subacromial Bursa*. 2nd ed. Malabar, Fla: Robert E. Kreiger; 1984.
31. Athwal GS, Sperling JW, Rispoli DM, et al. Deep infection after rotator cuff tears. *J Shoulder Elbow Surg* 2007;16:306–311.
32. Baier RE, Meyer AE, Natiella JR, et al: Surface properties determine bioadhesive outcomes: methods and results. *J Biomed Mater Res* 1984;18:337–355.
33. Karten I. Septic arthritis complicating rheumatoid arthritis. *Ann Intern Med* 1969;70:1147–1151.
34. Schmidt D, Mubarak S, Gelberman R. Septic shoulders in children. *J Pediatr Orthop* 1981;1:67–72.
35. Mileti J, Sperling JW, Cofield RH. Reimplantation of a shoulder arthroplasty after a previous infected arthroplasty. *J Shoulder Elbow Surg* 2004;13:528–531.
36. Rand JA, Morrey BF, Bryan RS. Management of the infected total joint arthroplasty. *Orthop Clin North Am* 1984;15:491–504.
37. Costerton JW, Geesey GG, Cheng K-J. How bacteria stick. *Sci Am* 1978;238:86–95.
38. Costerton JW, Stewart PS, Greenberg EP. Bacterial biofilms: a common cause of persistent infections. *Science* 1999;284:1318–1322.
39. Gristina AG. Biomaterial-centered infection: microbial adhesion versus tissue integration. *Science* 1987;237:1558–1595.
40. Gristina AG, Costerton JW. Bacteria-laden biofilms: a hazard to orthopedic prostheses. *Infect Surg* 1984;3:655–662.
41. Trampuz A, Osmon DR, Hanssen AD, et al. Molecular and antibiofilm approaches to prosthetic joint infection. *Clin Orthop* 2003;414:69–88.
42. Gristina AG, Costerton JW. Bacterial adherence to biomaterials and tissue: the significance of its role in clinical sepsis. *J Bone Joint Surg Am* 1985;67:264–273.
43. Epps, CH Jr, Bryant DD III, et al. Osteomyelitis in patients who have sickle cell disease: diagnosis and management. *J Bone Joint Surg Am* 1991;73:1281–1294.
44. Souter WA. The surgical treatment of the rheumatoid shoulder. *Ann Acad Med Singapore* 1983;12:243–255.
45. Chaudhuri K, Lonergan D, Portek I, et al. Septic arthritis of the shoulder after mastectomy and radiotherapy for breast carcinoma. *J Bone Joint Surg Br* 1993;75:318–321.
46. American Medical Association, Division of Drugs and Toxicology: *Antimicrobial Therapy for Common Infectious Diseases: Drug Elevations Annual 1995*. Chicago: American Medical Association; 1995:1277–1282.
47. Katzer A, Sickelmann F, Seemann K, et al. Two-year results after exchange shoulder arthroplasty using inverse implants. *Orthopedics* 2004;27:1165–1167.

48. Banit DM, Kaufer H, Hartford JM. Intraoperative frozen section analysis in revision total joint arthroplasty. *Clin Orthop Relat Res* 2002;401:230–238.
49. Steinbrink K, Frommelt L. Behandlung der periprothetischen Infektion der Hüfte durch einzeitige Austauschoperationen. *Orthopäde* 1995;24:335–343.
50. Hamada K, Fukuda H, Mikasa M, et al. Roentgenographic findings in massive rotator cuff tears: a long-term observation. *Clin Orthop Relat Res* 1990;254:92–96.
51. Hopkins KL, Li KC, Bergman G. Gadolinium-DTPA-enhanced magnetic resonance imaging of musculoskeletal infectious processes. *Skeletal Radiol* 1995;24:325–330.
52. Merkel KD, Brown ML, DeWanjee MK, et al. Comparison of indium-labeled leukocyte imaging with sequential technetium-gallium scanning in the diagnosis of low-grade musculoskeletal sepsis. *J Bone Joint Surg Am* 1985;67:465–476.
53. Gristina AG, Romano RL, Kammire GC, et al. Total shoulder replacement. *Orthop Clin North Am* 1987;18:445–453.
54. Ramsey ML, Fenlin JM Jr. Use of an antibiotic-impregnated bone cement block in the revision of an infected shoulder arthroplasty. *J Shoulder Elbow Surg* 1996;5:479–482.
55. Steinbrink K, Mella-Schmidt C. Stellenwert der Spül-Saugdrainage bei der Behandlung des Frühinfekts von Gelenkimplantaten. *Chirurg* 1989;60:791.
56. Coste, JS, Reig S, Trojani C, et al. The management of infection in arthroplasty of the shoulder. *J Bone Joint Surg Br* 2004;86:65–69.
57. Marculescu CE, Berbari EF, Hanssen AD, et al. Outcome of prosthetic joint infections treated with debridement and retention of components. *Clin Infect Dis* 2006;42:471–478.
58. Thomas P, Thomsen M. Allergy diagnostics in implant intolerance [in German]. *Orthopäde* 2008;37:131–135.
59. Mileti J, Sperling JW, Cofield RH. Shoulder arthroplasty for the treatment of postinfectious glenohumeral arthritis. *J Bone Joint Surg Am* 2003;85:609–614.
60. Neer CS II, Craig EV, Fukuda H. Cuff-tear arthropathy. *J Bone Joint Surg Am* 1983;65:1232–1244.
61. Heitmann C, Higgins LD, Levin LS. Treatment of deep infections of the shoulder with pedicled myocutaneous flaps. *J Shoulder Elbow Surg* 2004;13:13–17.
62. Ince A, Seemann K, Frommelt L, et al. One-stage exchange shoulder arthroplasty for periprosthetic infection. *J Bone Joint Surg Br* 2005;87:814–818.
63. Ince A, Seemann K, Frommelt L, et al. One-stage revision of shoulder arthroplasty in the case of periprosthetic infection. *Z Orthop Ihre Grenzgeb* 2004;142:611–617.
64. Loebenberg MI, Zuckermann JD. An articulating interval spacer in the treatment of an infected total shoulder arthroplasty. *J Shoulder Elbow Surg* 2004;13:476–478.
65. Buchholz HW, Engelbrecht H. Über die Depotwirkung einiger Antibiotika bei Vermischung mit dem Kunstharz Palacos. *Chirurg* 1970;41:511–515.
66. Proubasta IR, Itarte JP, Lamas CG, et al. Permanent articulated antibiotic-impregnated cement spacer in septic shoulder arthroplasty: a case report. *J Orthop Trauma* 2005;19:666–668.
67. Themistocleous G, Zalavras C, Stine I, et al. Prolonged implantation of an antibiotic cement spacer for management of shoulder sepsis in compromised patients. *J Shoulder Elbow Surg* 2007;16:701–705.
68. Grammont PM, Trouilloud P, Laffay JP, et al. Etude et realisation d'une nouvelle prothèse d'èpaule. *Rhumatologie* 1987;10:407–418.
69. Grammont PM, Baulot E. Delta shoulder prosthesis for rotator cuff rupture. *Orthopedics* 1993;16:65–68.
70. Sanchez-Sotelo J, Cofield RH, Rowland CM. Shoulder hemiarthroplasty for glenohumeral arthritis associated with severe rotator cuff deficiency. *J Bone Joint Surg Am* 2001;83:1814–1822.
71. Willams GR Jr, Rockwood CA Jr. Hemiarthroplasty in rotator cuff-deficient shoulders. *J Shoulder Elbow Surg* 1996;5:362–367.
72. Worland RL, Jessup DE, Arredondo J, et al. Biopolar shoulder arthroplasty for rotator cuff arthropathy. *J Shoulder Elbow Surg* 1997;6:512–515.
73. Gerber C. Latissimus dorsi transfer for the treatment of irreparable tears of the rotator cuff. *Clin Orthop Relat Res* 1992;275:152–160.
74. Frankle M, Siegal S, Pupello D, et al. The reverse shoulder prosthesis for glenohumeral arthritis associated with severe rotator cuff deficiency: a minimum 2-year follow-up study of 60 patients. *J Bone Joint Surg Am* 2005;87:1697–1705.
75. Wirth MA, Rockwood CA Jr. Complications of shoulder arthroplasty. *Clin Orthop Relat Res* 1994;307:47–69.
76. Seitz WH Jr, Damacen H. Staged exchange arthroplasty for shoulder sepsis. *J Arthroplasty* 2002;17(4 suppl 1):36–40.
77. Zimmerli W, Trampuz A, Ochsner P. Prosthetic infections. *N Engl J Med* 2004;16:39–48.
78. Goutallier D, Postel JM, Bernageau J, et al. Fatty muscle degeneration in cuff ruptures: pre- and postoperative evaluation by CT scan. *Clin Orthop Relat Res* 1994;304:78–83.
79. Boileau P, Watkinson DJ, Hatzikadis AM, et al. Neer Award 2005: the Grammont reverse shoulder prosthesis: results in cuff tear arthritis, fracture sequelae, and revision arthroplasty. *J Shoulder Elbow Surg* 2006;15:527–540.
80. Braman, JP, Sprague M, Bishop J, et al. The outcome of resection shoulder arthroplasty for recalcitrant shoulder infections. *J Shoulder Elbow Surg* 2006;15:549–553.
81. Debeer P, Plasschaert H, Stuyck J: Resection arthroplasty of the infected shoulder: a salvage procedure for the elderly patient. *Acta Orthop Belg* 2006;72:126–130.
82. Rispoli DM, Sperling JW, Athwal GS, et al. Pain relief and functional results after resection arthroplasty of the shoulder. *J Bone Joint Surg Br* 2007;89:1184–1187.
83. Clare DJ, Wirth MA, Groh GI, et al. Shoulder arthrodesis. *J Bone Joint Surg Am* 2001;83:593–600.
84. Wick M, Muller EJ, Ambacher T, et al. Arthrodesis of the shoulder after septic arthritis: long-term results. *J Bone Joint Surg Br* 2003;85:666–670.
85. Flick AB, Herbert JC, Goodell J, et al. Noncommercial fabrication of antibiotic-impregnated polymethylmethacrylate beads: technical note. *Clin Orthop* 1987;223:282–286.
86. Lodenkämper H, Lodenkämper U, Trompa K. Über die Ausscheidung von Antibiotika aus dem Knochenzement Palacos (Eigene Erfahrungen aus bakteriologischer Sicht nach 10 jähriger Anwendung in der Gelenkersatzchirurgie). *Z Orthop* 1982;120:801–805.
87. Zimmerli W. Role of antibiotics in the treatment of infected joint prosthesis. *Orthopäde* 1995;24:308–313.
88. Cofield RH, Edgerton BC. Total shoulder arthroplasty: complications and revision surgery. *Instr Course Lect* 1990;39:449–462.
89. Post M. Constrained arthroplasty of the shoulder. *Orthop Clin North Am* 1987;18:455–462.
90. Boileau P, Watkinson DJ, Hatzikadis AM, et al. Grammont reverse prosthesis: design, rationale, and biomechanics. *J Shoulder Elbow Surg* 2005;14(1 suppl S):147–161.
91. De Wilde L, Mombert M, Van Petegem P, et al. Revision of shoulder replacement with a reversed shoulder prosthesis (Delta III): report of five cases. *Acta Orthop Belg* 2001;67:348–353.
92. Rockwood CA Jr. The reverse total shoulder prosthesis: the new kid on the block. *J Bone Joint Surg Am* 2007;89:233–235.
93. Wall B, Nové-Josserand L, O'Connor DP, et al. Reverse total shoulder arthroplasty: a review of results according to etiology. *J Bone Joint Surg Am* 2007;89:1476–1485.
94. Constant CR, Murlay AH: A clinical method of functional assessment of the shoulder. *Clin Orthop Relat Res* 1987;214:160–164.

Duong Nguyen
Matt Kippe
Louis U. Bigliani
William N. Levine

CHAPTER

21

Failed Hemiarthroplasty

INTRODUCTION

Humeral head replacement has been shown to produce satisfactory results in patients with glenohumeral arthritis,[1–6] as well as for fractures of the proximal humerus.[9–16] Many surgeons still prefer to perform humeral head replacement instead of total shoulder arthroplasty for osteoarthritis, especially in younger, active patients, to prevent early glenoid loosening. Initial published reports suggested encouraging results with hemiarthroplasty, but in recent years, several authors have reported unsatisfactory results, often necessitating revision surgery in patients undergoing humeral head replacement for osteoarthritis.[5,17,18] Neer[2,3] recognized early on that a subset of patients had prolonged discomfort, slow recovery of adequate strength, and continuing fatigability after humeral head replacement.[1]

Reasons for failure of a hemiarthroplasty can include prosthetic malposition, poor rehabilitation, tuberosity nonunion and malunion, periprosthetic fracture, instability, glenoid arthrosis, neurological injury, aseptic loosening, infection, impingement, and component failure. Most patients tend to have a combination of these factors as the underlying causes of failure.[9]

Component malposition tends to be underreported in the literature because it is often an underlying cause of other more easily detected complications, such as tuberosity failure, impingement, rotator cuff insufficiency, and instability.[9,19–22]

Poor compliance with postoperative rehabilitation is another source of failure.[9,12,13,23,24] This is often linked to increasing age and associated medical problems.[12,13,20,23]

Failure of tuberosity healing is a major factor in poor outcome following hemiarthroplasty.[12,13,21,22,24–28] This complication is usually related to poor tuberosity fixation, nonunion, malunion, tuberosity resorption, or rotator cuff insufficiency. The variable rates (0% to 50%) of this complication are due to the lack of a clearly accepted radiographic or clinical definition of tuberosity failure.[29]

Periprosthetic fractures can occur from trauma after the index shoulder hemiarthroplasty but arise more commonly during the revision procedure.

Instability tends to occur more frequently following hemiarthroplasty performed on a delayed basis.[30,31] It is associated with rotator cuff insufficiency, failure of tuberosity fixation, improper component position or size, and neurological injury.[29] The pattern seen is one of anterosuperior subluxation of the humeral head and adversely affects outcomes.[21,24,26]

The most common cause for revision of a humeral head replacement is glenoid arthrosis. Glenoid erosion is, however, infrequently cited as a source of failure because quantifying glenoid erosion is often difficult.[9,12,21] It is also unclear whether glenoid erosion occurs without the influence of component malposition or instability and may be part of the natural history of hemiarthroplasty.[29] Glenoid erosion usually manifests itself in the form of radiographic glenoid arthritis, many years after the index hemiarthroplasty.[13,22,24] Levine et al[18] also emphasized the importance of glenohumeral congruence for good outcomes.

Although nerve injury is a relatively common complication of comminuted proximal humerus fractures,[32] the incidence is much lower after hemiarthroplasty for proximal humeral fractures.[13,26,28]

Symptomatic aseptic loosening is not commonly reported in the failed hemiarthroplasty population, partially because of the relative short-term follow-up periods of most published series.[9,22] Many authors have reported radiolucent lines adjacent to both cemented and cementless humeral prostheses.[12,13,21,22,24,26,33] There is currently no proven relationship between radiolucency and symptomatic loosening.[29]

Infection most likely results from bacterial contaminants at the time of original surgery.[22] Common organisms include *Staphylococcus aureus, S. epidermidis,* and *Propionibacterium acnes.* Patients undergoing hemiarthroplasty for proximal humeral fractures are especially at risk for infections because they are often elderly and debilitated, have a poor nutritional status, and have multiple medical problems. They often have other concomitant infections such as in the upper respiratory and urinary tracts. Moreover, joint replacement in the setting of acute fracture hematoma and associated soft tissue injury presents an environment that may be favorable to bacterial growth.[29]

Lastly, subacromial impingement is multifactorial and relates to the other complications listed earlier, that is, failure of tuberosity fixation and/or reduction, inappropriate component height, and heterotopic ossification.[19,22,26,29] Ectopic bone formation is associated with fracture-dislocation, repeated attempts at reduction, and delayed fracture treatment.[15] Although heterotopic ossification has been frequently reported,[11,20,24,26,28] it rarely affects outcomes.[9,15,19–24,26,28,30,31,33–37,39]

In this chapter, we will sequentially address the preoperative evaluation of the patient with a failed hemiarthroplasty, the indications for revision surgery, the surgical techniques, the pitfalls of this challenging type of surgery, the rehabilitation protocol, and the outcomes of revision surgery.

HISTORY AND PHYSICAL EXAMINATION

A good history is critical in evaluating a patient's failed shoulder hemiarthroplasty. It is especially important to determine whether the patient had a pain-free interval after the index procedure. This would suggest the causative factors for failure may not be related to technical errors, intraoperative complications, or missed concomitant diagnoses related to the initial surgery. The surgeon should determine the exact location of the pain and whether it is of recent onset, suggesting a traumatic etiology or medical illness.

Painful glenoid arthrosis is usually the most common reason for revision of a hemiarthroplasty. However, one must rule out stiffness, instability, impingement, rotator cuff pathology, nerve injury, infection, acromioclavicular pathology, biceps pathology, and cervical causes as the source of pain.[40]

The number and nature of prior surgical procedures are important to know because they will often predict the quality of the soft tissues and potentially modify the planned revision procedure. The initial fracture type or diagnosis, the surgical approach, the type and size of the components, the method of implant fixation (cement versus press-fit), and the postoperative rehabilitation protocol are all important points of information to consider. The management of a failed hemiarthroplasty for fractures of the proximal humerus requires special attention to the quality of the previous tuberosity fixation.

Operative reports of previous procedures are also essential to determine the quality of the soft tissues and presence or absence of prosthetic modularity. This facilitates preoperative planning, ensuring that the appropriate instrumentation for implant extraction, components for modular replacement, custom prostheses, and necessary bone or soft tissue grafts are available for the revision surgery.[41]

A comprehensive physical examination is critical in the preoperative evaluation of the patient with a failed hemiarthroplasty. The site of the previous incision is important to identify because this will affect the approach used for the revision surgery. Skin changes can represent a possible acute or chronic infection. Weakness and muscle atrophy may indicate mechanical problems, such a rotator cuff tear, or neurological deficits. The strength examination should include assessment of the integrity of the deltoid and the rotator cuff, which may have been injured in previous surgeries. Particular attention is paid to the status of the deltoid because deltoid dehiscence or severe dysfunction is a devastating complication with limited salvage options. The function of the subscapularis is important to assess with the belly-press, lift-off, and internal rotation lag tests. This is important because a reverse type shoulder prosthesis may be indicated in the rotator cuff deficient shoulder with an intact deltoid.[42–44] An electromyelographic nerve conduction velocity study should be obtained if the examination suggests a neurological injury.[31]

Active and passive ranges of motion (ROM) are also important to document preoperatively because contractures of the glenohumeral joint and particularly the subscapularis are common in the failed hemiarthroplasty. This may simply be due to

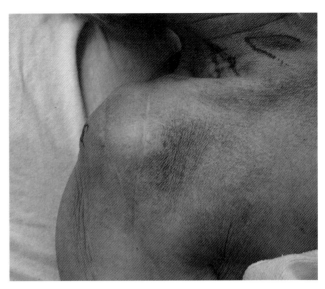

Figure 21.1. Preoperative photograph of a patient with anterosuperior instability after hemiarthroplasty.

soft tissue contractures or may be indicative of oversized or malpositioned components. Discrepancies between active and passive ROM may be indicative of pain, tuberosity nonunion or malunion, neurological dysfunction, and instability.[29]

Instability on physical examination may suggest component malposition, as well as soft tissue inadequacy. Anterosuperior instability is a common presentation in failed hemiarthroplasty (Fig. 21.1).

RADIOGRAPHIC FEATURES

Serial radiographs are often helpful to determine accurately whether the prosthesis was placed incorrectly at the time of surgery or shifted in the postoperative period with development of radiolucent lines.[40] Radiographs should include true anteroposterior images of the scapula in neutral, internal, and external rotation, as well as axillary and outlet views. Implant size and position, tuberosity integrity and reduction, evidence of implant loosening, bony or prosthetic fracture, and condition of the glenoid are also noted.

In cemented prostheses, radiolucencies are usually located at the bone-cement interface. The extent of radiolucency around the prosthesis is graded as 0 if there is no radiolucent line, grade 1 if the line is 1 mm wide and incomplete, grade 2 if the line is 1 mm wide and complete, grade 3 if the line is 1.5 mm wide and incomplete, grade 4 if the line is 1.5 mm wide and complete, and grade 5 if the line is 2 mm wide and complete (Fig. 21.2).[39]

Glenohumeral instability can be detected on a good axillary radiograph by measuring the amount of translation of the center of the humeral head with respect to the center of the glenoid component. Subluxation can be graded as none, mild (<25% translation), moderate (25% to 50% translation), or severe (>50% translation).[39]

Glenoid arthrosis can often be detected as progressive loss of joint space as well as posterior and superior bone erosion (Fig. 21.3). This is best seen on the axillary radiograph (Fig. 21.4).

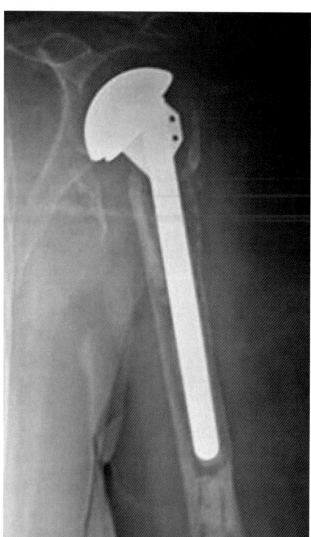

Figure 21.2. Anteroposterior radiograph of a failed hemiarthroplasty with extensive loosening. In this case, the shoulder was infected.

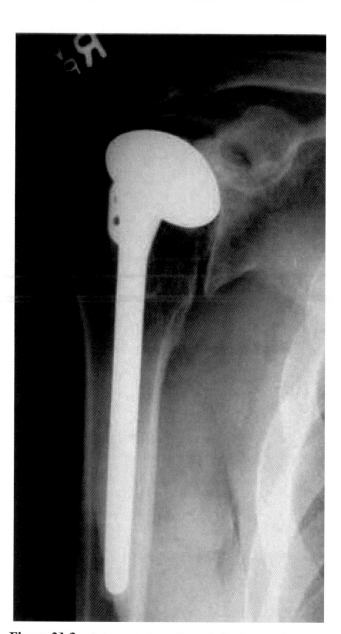

Figure 21.3. Anteroposterior radiograph showing superior glenoid erosion.

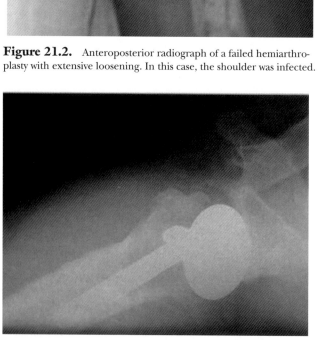

Figure 21.4. Axillary radiograph showing posterior glenoid erosion.

A metal-subtracting computed tomography (CT) scan preoperatively is often helpful for determination of glenoid bone stock, glenoid version, and the depth of the vault and to better assess glenoid arthrosis with decreased interference from the metallic humeral stem.

A magnetic resonance imaging (MRI) scan can help the revision surgeon rule out other soft tissue pathology such as rotator cuff tears and atrophy.

PREOPERATIVE CONSIDERATIONS

Laboratory investigations to rule out infection are essential in the pre-revision evaluation. White blood cell count with differential, erythrocyte sedimentation rate, and C-reactive protein are markers for inflammation. They serve as a baseline as well as an indicator of improvement following the treatment of an infected hemiarthroplasty.

If infection is suspected based on the history, physical examination, and laboratory results, the surgeon should proceed with a combination of an indium-labeled white blood cell scan as well as aspiration of the glenohumeral joint. Caution is necessary because some causative organisms require a longer period of incubation for diagnosis. If in doubt, the patient should be taken back to the operating room for a formal irrigation and debridement with intraoperative frozen section and assessment. The surgeon should err toward a two-stage revision arthroplasty if there is any suspicion of an infection. Irrigation and debridement with retention of the components can be performed in select cases in which the infection occurs in the early postoperative period (<6 weeks). A resection arthroplasty is indicated in cases of persistent, life-threatening infection.

Shoulder arthroscopy can occasionally be a useful adjunctive tool for the failed shoulder hemiarthroplasty. In complicated cases, evaluation of the glenoid, rotator cuff musculature, and capsular contractures can be performed with the arthroscope.[45] In addition, therapeutic interventions such as subacromial decompression (acromioplasty and/or tuberoplasty) for tuberosity malunion resulting in impingement, acromioclavicular joint resection, synovectomy, and contracture release can be performed without the need for a big open revision operation.[41]

INDICATIONS FOR SURGERY

Patients should be carefully screened and selected before proceeding with a major revision surgery for failed hemiarthroplasty. They should undergo revision surgery only if their pain level is not controlled with adequate pain medication (anti-inflammatory and narcotic medications) and their level of function is deteriorating. Nonsurgical modalities such as physical therapy and corticosteroid injections should be optimized. Patients should understand that the risks and complications of surgery are greater in the revision setting and that the exact procedure performed will vary greatly on the intraoperative findings. Moreover, the revision surgeon should educate the patient about the limited goals of treatment in these situations so that realistic expectations can be achieved with either nonsurgical or surgical treatment. For instance, limited preoperative ROM is often a negative predictive factor for good postoperative ROM.[46]

The indications for surgical treatment of neurological dysfunction are unclear.[29] The role and effectiveness of nerve exploration and grafting are also uncertain. Tendon or muscle transfers may be helpful in select cases, but generally nonsurgical management is recommended.

SURGICAL APPROACH

Revision of the failed hemiarthroplasty is fraught with technical challenges. Soft tissue contractures are common and may distort the normal anatomy, placing neurovascular structures such as the musculocutaneous and axillary nerves at risk. The surgeon can no longer rely on landmarks such as the coracoid or the acromion to find safe tissue planes. The dissection should therefore start as laterally and distally as possible (over the humeral shaft near the deltoid insertion) and must proceed in a slow, meticulous fashion. Rotating the humerus can sometimes help identify intermuscular planes.

An extended deltopectoral skin incision is typically used, incorporating the previous incision if possible. The vascularity of the subcutaneous tissue around the shoulder is excellent, and skin necrosis has been a rare problem in our practice.[41] Previous injury to the cephalic vein and obliteration of fascial planes from scarring are common. Therefore blunt finger dissection or use of a Cobb elevator can be used to separate tissue planes through the deltopectoral interval and clavipectoral fascia, staying lateral to the conjoined tendon. The topmost aspect of the pectoralis major insertion can be released to augment exposure to the glenoid.

In the non–cuff-deficient shoulder, the anterior portion of the coracoacromial ligament can be excised next to facilitate superior exposure. This is then followed by the release of all adhesions in the subdeltoid and subacromial spaces with an elevator with care to avoid injury to branches of the axillary nerve that travel on the surface of the subdeltoid fascia. This step is essential to optimize glenoid exposure and increase postoperative ROM.

Further releases can also be performed between the strap muscles and the pectoralis major and the subscapularis to allow adequate muscular excursion. This allows for increased external rotation and maximizes the joint volume available for certain reconstructive options, such as larger humeral head sizes and prosthetic glenoid insertion. Care should be taken at this point to identify and protect the axillary nerve (by adducting and externally rotating the arm, which moves the nerve away from the operative field), which courses on the inferior aspect of the subscapularis on its way posterior to the quadrangular space. It is often necessary to release the coracohumeral ligament to improve the excursion of the superior aspect of the subscapularis. At our institution, the tendon is typically released off the lesser tuberosity, leaving a small cuff of tissue for later repair.[41,47] The release is continued inferiorly onto the shaft of the humerus in a subperiosteal fashion to avoid damaging the axillary nerve and posteriorly above the latissimus dorsi tendon along the medial neck of the humerus. The upper portion of the latissimus dorsi can also be released in tight shoulders. Scar tissue around the humeral head and neck must be cleared to externally rotate the arm for exposure.

Modular components allow the surgeon to leave the humeral stem undisturbed, and therefore the head of the modular prosthesis can be removed for better exposure. The often obliterated interval between the subscapularis and the anterior capsule is developed at the level of the glenoid with blunt dissection to prevent denervation of the muscle. The anterior capsule is then completely excised, and the subscapularis muscle is released circumferentially.

To further improve exposure, the capsule can be released superiorly and inferiorly as needed and the contracted long head of the biceps can be released with subsequent tenodesis at the conclusion of the operation.

In very rare situations in which exposure is still limited, the deltoid can be detached, leaving a stout periosteal sleeve for later repair.[41] The split is at the raphe between the anterior and middle thirds of the deltoid in a longitudinal fashion, with care not to extend it more than 4 cm lateral to the acromion to avoid injury to the axillary nerve. The postoperative rehabilitation should then also focus on protection of this repair because dysfunction of the anterior deltoid is a disastrous complication.

COMPONENT REMOVAL

Indications for removal of components often include loosening, malposition, instability, inadequate cement mantle, infection, and mechanical failure.[41] Prosthetic loosening is assessed by removing soft tissues circumferentially from the cement-bone, prosthesis-cement or prosthesis-bone interface, and impacting gently the proximal aspect of the implant to rule out micromotion. In the absence of significant wear or infection, the humeral stem may be preserved and an extended humeral osteotomy and removal of the cement can be avoided.

Revision arthroplasty requires both patience and special instrumentation to avoid intraoperative fractures or the creation of unnecessary bony defects.[41] The tools used can be either system-specific or universal. Flexible osteotomes are helpful both at the implant/cement and bone/cement interfaces. Special extraction devices that hook under the collar and attach to a slap hammer or a heavy chisel to create a vertical, in-line force under the collar are usually successful at removing the humeral component (Fig. 21.5A,B).

Cement removal can then be performed, if needed, with hooks, curettes, flexible reamers, or the special long chisels often found in the revision hip instrument set. In difficult cases, some surgeons have had success with ultrasonic wave devices that melt the cement and therefore facilitate its removal. The risk of neurovascular injury with these devices is a concern to consider.

In cases in which visualization of the cement is poor, an anterior humeral osteotomy can be performed to gain exposure to the entire length of the humeral stem.[41,47,48] The skin incision is then extended distally, and the deltopectoral approach is extended to an anterior approach to the humerus with splitting of the lateral one third of the brachialis. Care should be taken to identify and protect the musculocutaneous nerve medially and the radial nerve more distally. Predrilling the humerus can be helpful to allow for a controlled osteotomy. An anterior L-shaped window of the humerus is then created with a sagittal saw, high-speed burr, or osteotomes, starting from the lateral aspect of the bicipital groove, extending down distally between the pectoralis major and deltoid insertions, and ending several centimeters proximal to the tip of the prosthesis (Fig. 21.6). The horizontal limb of the osteotomy enables a window of cortex to be hinged open, creating excellent access to the cement mantle and the entire humeral prosthesis. Care is exercised proximally to prevent a fracture of the tuberosities, especially in the failed hemiarthroplasty for a fracture of the proximal humerus. The anterior window is closed once all the cement is removed and secured in place with cerclage wires before insertion of the new revision prosthesis (Fig. 21.7).

HUMERAL COMPONENT INSERTION

The goals of proximal humerus reconstruction are to restore the humeral height, offset, and version; achieve secure fixation of the humeral component; and securely repair the rotator cuff muscles to the tuberosities.

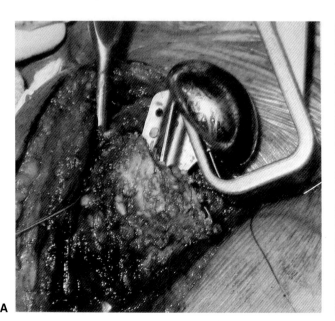
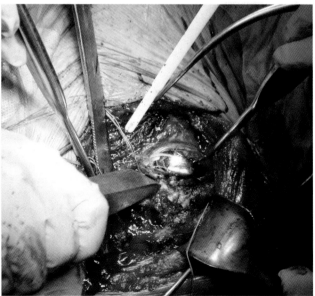

A   B

Figure 21.5.   Humeral component removal devices. **(A)** Hook. **(B)** Chisel.

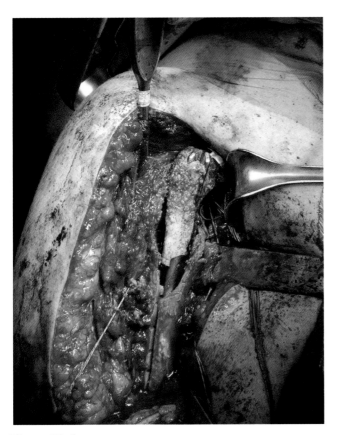

Figure 21.6. Humeral osteotomy.

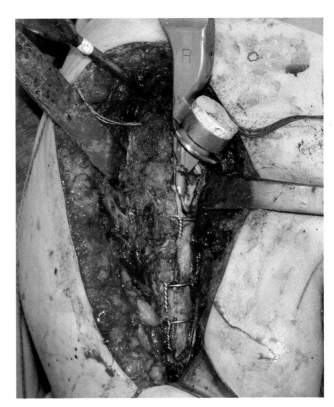

Figure 21.7. Cerclage wiring of the humerus around the osteotomy and the cemented prosthesis.

Determining the appropriate humeral height can be a challenging task in the revision setting with the loss of anatomic landmarks. This is a common problem in the setting of hemiarthroplasty for fracture. Implant-specific instruments such as sponges and jigs can be helpful to determine the optimal height for reconstruction (Fig. 21.8A,B). Ideally, the top of the humeral head should be 4 to 6 mm superior to the top of the greater tuberosity to optimize the tension on the rotator cuff and to avoid mechanical impingement beneath the coracoacromial arch. The humeral head should interact concentrically with the glenoid surface such that the superior tip of the metallic head is roughly equivalent to the top of the glenoid.[49] On the other hand, placing the prosthesis too low alters the tension in the rotator cuff and the deltoid myofascial sleeve and weakens the lever arm of the shoulder.[37] This results in limitation of active motion, weakness, erosion of the inferior aspect of the glenoid component, and impingement of the tuberosities onto the acromion.

The humeral component also needs to be fixed into the canal in appropriate version, with the humeral head centered in the glenoid after gentle traction on the arm is applied. The traction is important to restore the normal myofascial tension around the shoulder. In most instances, the humeral component should be inserted in 20 to 40 degrees of retroversion. Inappropriate version of the humeral component may lead to instability of the shoulder and eccentric wear over time.

Instability is more likely to occur in the revision of the failed hemiarthroplasty for a previous fracture-dislocation.[29] In this situation, soft tissues are contracted or redundant to accommodate the deformity and the surgeon may have to adjust the final version of the humeral component accordingly. The use of surgical instrumentation that allows assessment of intraoperative version in this setting can be extremely helpful (Fig. 21.9A,B). At the conclusion of the operation, the subscapularis is typically repaired with the arm in 30 to 40 degrees of external rotation, 30 degrees of abduction, and neutral alignment in the coronal plane. Soft tissues, usually the posterior capsule, should be assessed for residual laxity, which may require capsular plication or cuff tensioning procedures.[29] Hamstring tendon graft augmentation, Achilles-calcaneal allograft fixation to the scapular neck and humerus, or a subcoracoid pectoralis major transfer can be performed if the subscapularis tendon is deficient, causing anterior instability.[41,50]

The size of the final prosthetic humeral head is another technical consideration. An excessively large humeral head component overstuffs the joint and often will lead to limited motion, persistent pain, and possibly subscapularis failure. Undersizing the head decreases humeral offset and weakens the functional lever arm of the shoulder, which may cause glenohumeral instability.[37] The use of modular designs is recommended, which allows the revision surgeon to try various head heights, diameters, and degrees of eccentricity of the head shape (Fig. 21.10). Proper soft tissue tension is achieved when the humeral head translates approximately 50% of the glenoid articular diameter in both the anteroposterior and superoinferior directions.[29,51] The patient's hand should also be adducted to the contralateral axilla without excessive tension.

If the tuberosities are detached, repair of the tuberosities with heavy nonabsorbable sutures is performed and autoge-

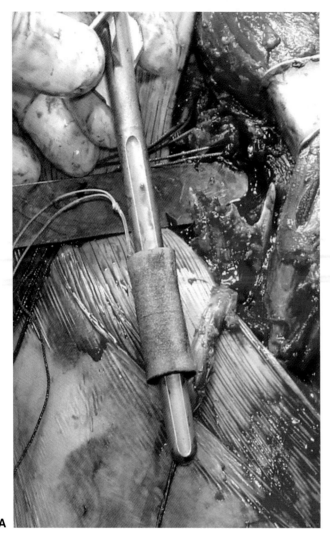

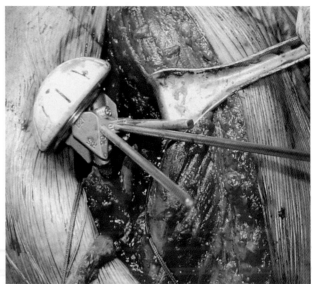

Figure 21.8.   Intraoperative guides to assess height. **(A)** Sponge. **(B)** Height and version guide.

nous bone graft is placed to augment healing. Wire or cable fixation can also be added to provide additional stability of the tuberosities.

Greater tuberosity malunion and nonunion can cause unique challenges. The prevalence of tuberosity malunion can be as high as 39%.[25] The greater tuberosity can be positioned either too inferiorly (>10 mm inferior to the top of the humeral head) or too superiorly (<5 mm to the top of the humeral head). Patients typically complain of pain, stiffness, and limited ability to actively move the arm. These symptoms are due to either the nonfunctional rotator cuff or displacement of the tuberosities creating a mechanical block to motion beneath the acromion or against the glenoid rim.[29] If the superior displacement of the greater tuberosity is mild, anterior acromioplasty may provide adequate decompression of the subacromial space. More severe displacement may necessitate tuberosity osteotomy and repair.

Tuberosity nonunion is usually due to inadequate reduction and fixation or excessive tuberosity resection and tension overload of the rotator cuff tendons at the time of initial surgery.[29] This can lead to loss of motion and weakness, as well as superior migration from compromised rotator cuff function.[25] Achieving bony union is often a challenge and may require au-

tograft or allograft bone, bone morphogenic proteins, or special porous in-growth components such as trabecular metal.

PERIPROSTHETIC FRACTURE

Treatment of periprosthetic fractures is based on the stability of the prosthesis. No revision of the prosthesis is needed if the fracture is distal to the tip of the prosthesis, because the entire construct remains stable. However, if the fracture occurs at or proximal to the tip, revision to a long-stemmed component that bridges the fracture by 2.5 cortical diameters is typically required.[47] The type of reconstruction used will depend on the type of fracture. Options include open reduction and internal fixation with plates and screws and cerclage wiring with or without bone grafting (Fig. 21.11).[52]

BONE DEFICIENCY

Revision of the failed hemiarthroplasty will depend on the specific issues particular to that case. Bone deficiency on either the humeral or glenoid side can be due to abnormal or eccentric

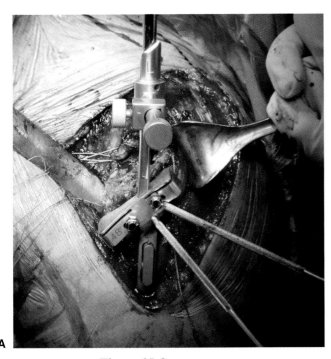
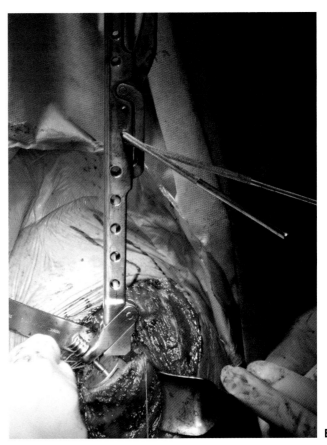

A   B

Figure 21.9. Intraoperative guides to assess humeral version. (**A**) Cutting guide. (**B**) Stem inserter.

wear, instability, infection, malaligned components, tuberosity resorption, and intraoperative bone loss during component removal. Several options are available to the revision surgeon, including resection arthroplasty, arthrodesis, osteotomy, and restoration of the proximal humerus with autograft, allograft, a

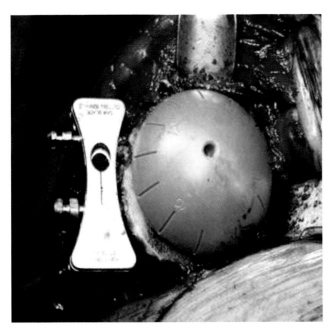

Figure 21.10. Offset humeral head trial.

custom prosthesis, an allograft-prosthetic composite, or special porous in-growth stems.

Bone grafting can be performed using either autograft from the proximal humerus osteotomy or autograft from the iliac crest. Alternatively, allograft bone chips or strut allografts can be used to reconstruct the proximal humerus. The graft can be placed at the junction of the proximal part of the humerus and the prosthesis, at the site of the tuberosities nonunion, in defects created during removal of the humeral component or in the medullary canal to improve bone stock.[39]

When bone deficiency is extensive, as often is the case after component removal, the tuberosities cannot be approximated to the shaft of the humerus. In these cases, cortical strut allograft in combination with autograft can be used. Cerclage wires are used to achieve fixation of the strut allograft to the shaft of the humerus distally and to the prosthesis proximally.[41]

Because of the compromised bone stock often seen in these settings, the use of cemented prostheses with modern cementing techniques is preferred by the authors to maintain proper positioning and provide rotational stability. Cementing the humeral component may decrease the rate of loosening seen with uncemented press-fit or porous-coated humeral prostheses.[39,53–55]

In cases of tuberosity nonunion or proximal humerus bony insufficiency, trabecular metal implants represent an emerging technology that might allow for bone and even soft tissue in-growth. Trabecular metal has great potential for achieving firm reattachment of the tuberosities around the proximal part of the humeral stem (Fig. 21.12A,B).[41] Other alternatives

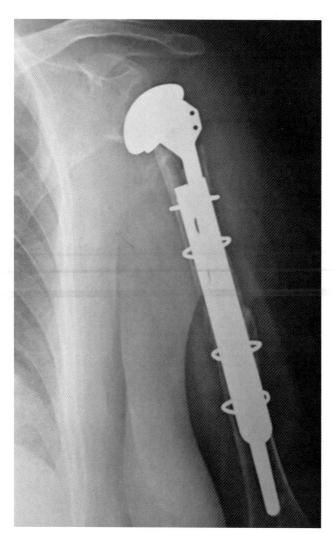

Figure 21.11. Revision of a periprosthetic fracture around a failed hemiarthroplasty with a long-stemmed prosthesis augmented with a cable-plate construct.

include osteoarticular allografts and allograft-prosthetic composites that allow for reconstruction of the proximal humerus. However, anatomic healing of the tuberosities onto the allografts and therefore adequate rotator cuff function can be difficult in these tumor-like cases.

In other select cases in which the tuberosities cannot be reconstructed and the rotator cuff has become nonfunctional, anterosuperior instability develops, especially if the coracoacromial arch is incompetent. This is a very difficult situation with no consistently reliable surgical options. Static reconstructions of the coracoacromial arch with an Achilles allograft have previously been described to have limited success.[56,57] Some other authors have had some success using dynamic reconstructions with transfer of the pectoralis major tendon.[50,58] Both static and dynamic reconstructions are, however, salvage operations that are mainly indicated to relieve pain.

The reverse ball-and-socket prosthesis (Fig. 21.13) is a newer alternative and can then be implanted if deltoid function is intact.[42,43,57] This is also a salvage operation but may allow the patient to have return of forward elevation. This option has

become increasingly popular with the advent of newer designs and as we gain more understanding of the biomechanics behind the success of this prosthesis in rotator cuff arthropathy. European reports have shown successful outcomes with the use of this prosthesis, although clinical experience is limited in the United States, especially in the setting of revision surgery.[42,43,59] Adequate glenoid bone stock is necessary to provide support for the screws going through the baseplate of the reverse prosthesis.

GLENOID BONE DEFICIENCY

The key issue in revision of the failed hemiarthroplasty is to determine whether implantation of a glenoid component is technically feasible.[41] Resurfacing the glenoid is important because the literature suggests that total shoulder arthroplasty provides better pain relief than hemiarthroplasty alone.[17,60,61] The integrity and reparability of the rotator cuff, the availability of sufficient bone stock, and the presence of adequate joint volume all affect the feasibility of glenoid implantation. Insufficient bone stock to achieve secure fixation of the glenoid component also prohibits implantation. Massive rotator cuff deficiency precludes the use of a glenoid component to avoid the creation of a rocking horse glenoid.[62] In these cases, the shoulder should be revised only to a hemiarthroplasty.[57,63]

If glenoid arthrosis is present, the glenoid can be resurfaced with a cemented polyethylene glenoid component using modern cementing techniques, which include the use of glenoid implant–specific instrumentation, a variety of component sizes, pulsatile lavage, thrombin-soaked gauzes, vacuum-mixed cement, pressurization of the cement, and firm impaction of the component. In challenging cases with inadequate bone stock, management will depend on whether the defect is central (peripheral rim of bone intact) or peripheral or a combination of the two.[64] Another consideration is whether the deficiency is mild, moderate, or severe. In the instance in which there is mild to moderate central deficiency, cancellous bone grafting of the glenoid vault can be performed with either autograft or allograft and the glenoid component can then be cemented in place. We prefer using allograft bone chips to avoid creating another painful incision at the iliac crest. In cases of severe central deficiency or unreconstructable glenoid, a two-stage procedure with bone grafting and glenoid implantation at a later time may be necessary.

Eccentric posterior wear and abnormal version are often present in failed hemiarthroplasty (Fig. 21.14). In these difficult cases, the native glenoid can be preferentially reamed anteriorly to restore appropriate version. The glenoid bone remaining is often small, and the use of a glenoid prosthesis that offers two radii of curvature can be helpful in dealing with these challenging cases.[41] The shoulder system used at our institution has the versatility to go up or down one size on the articulating surface compared with the nonarticular surface (Fig. 21.15). This feature is helpful when glenoid bone stock is limited and the size of the humeral head is large. For example, a glenoid component with a 40-mm radius of curvature on the nonarticular side and a 46-mm curvature on the articular side can be implanted to match a humeral head size of 46 mm.

However, if the defect is uncontained, a structural wedge autograft from the iliac crest may be used to reconstruct the

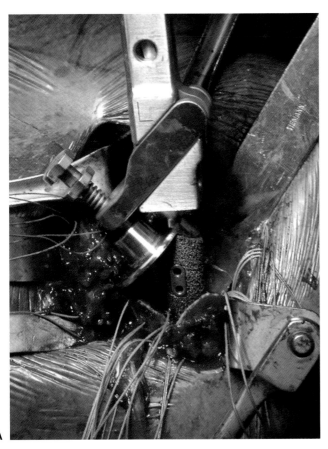

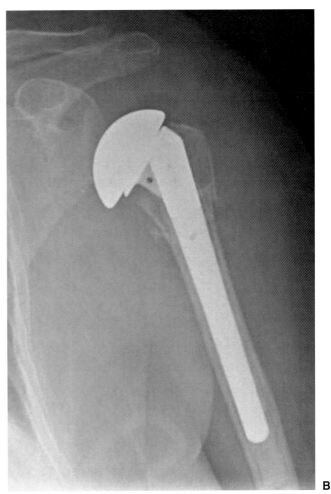

A   B

Figure 21.12.   Trabecular metal as an ingrowth surface for tuberosities. **(A)** Trabecular metal humeral stem. **(B)** Radiograph of healed tuberosities onto trabecular metal surface.

glenoid vault to allow for a second-stage glenoid resurfacing once the bone graft unites.[36] A posterior approach or percutaneous technique can be used to achieve fixation of structural bone graft for posterior glenoid deficiency. After secure fixation of the graft, reaming is performed to achieve a concentric glenoid in appropriate version.

Alternatively, a local bone transfer in the form of a coracoid transfer can be performed (Latarjet procedure).[65,66] An osteotome or sagittal saw is used to perform an osteotomy of the coracoid distal to the coracoclavicular ligaments. Care is exercised not to damage neurovascular structures medial to the coracoid. The coracoid is shaped to fit the anterior glenoid defect and secured in place with two 3.5-mm cortical screws.

The use of structural bone allograft is not recommended by the authors because these tend to resorb over time. In very select cases in which the uncontained defect is minimal, a metal-backed[67] or trabecular glenoid component can be implanted, although our experience with this technology is limited at this point (Fig. 21.16).

In failed hemiarthroplasty cases involving younger patients (under 40 years of age), a soft tissue interposition with Achilles or meniscal allograft and resurfacing of the glenoid can be performed, which may decrease the incidence of postoperative pain.[68] Bioabsorbable anchors are placed in the glenoid face,

and the allograft tissue is secured to the glenoid and surrounding tissue.

REHABILITATION

The postoperative rehabilitation protocol is individualized depending on the associated injuries, the quality of the soft tissues, the type of prosthesis used (total shoulder arthroplasty versus reverse prosthesis), confidence in tuberosity fixation, and patient compliance.[34] A fine balance between achieving stability and healing of soft tissues while avoiding stiffness should be sought. Regular interaction with the therapist is helpful for adjustments in the protocol, monitoring progress, and answering questions. In patients with severe bony or soft tissue defects, the goals of rehabilitation are more limited.

Therapy typically begins on postoperative day 1 and consists of pendulum exercises and, in the supine position, passive forward elevation and external rotation. The allowed ROM is gradually increased during the first 6 weeks, and pulley exercises are avoided until radiographic evidence of tuberosity healing is demonstrated or confidence in healing of the repaired soft tissues is achieved.

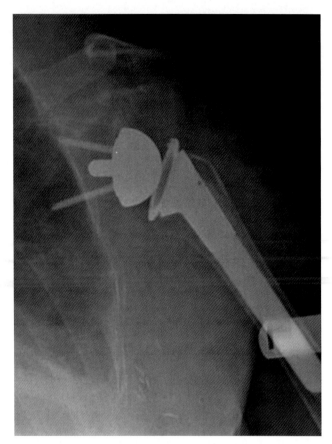

Figure 21.13. Postoperative radiograph of the trabecular metal reverse prosthesis.

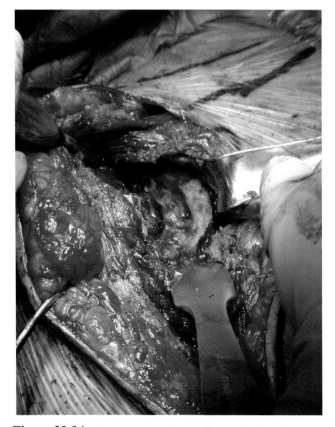

Figure 21.14. Intraoperative picture of posterior glenoid wear.

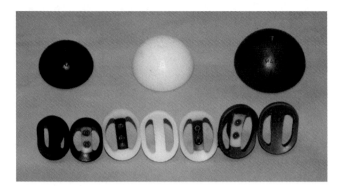

Figure 21.15. Various size selections of dual radius polyethylene glenoid components.

At 6 to 8 weeks, the patient begins pulley exercises, deltoid isometrics, and active exercises in the supine and erect positions. Light resistance exercises and stretching are then started at 12 weeks.

If a reverse prosthesis is implanted, the rehabilitation protocol should be more conservative. A shoulder immobilizer is worn for 6 weeks. Passive ROM exercises (pendulum), under the supervision of a physical therapist, is usually started 2 to 4 weeks postoperatively to avoid instability. Gentle active and active-assisted exercises are begun at 6 weeks, and resistive exercises are delayed until 12 weeks.

OUTCOMES

A review of the Columbia experience with humeral replacement for osteoarthritis revealed unacceptably high rates of unsatisfactory results (39%) and revision (14%) for persistent pain and glenoid arthrosis.[69] This rate of revision is significantly higher than the failure rate of patients after total shoulder replacement for osteoarthritis.[1,3,70,71,72,73,74] In the special case of revision total shoulder arthroplasty for a failed hemiarthroplasty, pain relief is usually provided. However, it is often unpredictable and does not always meet patients' expecta-

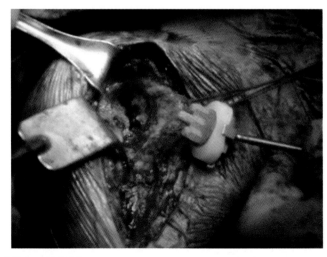

Figure 21.16. Intraoperative picture of a trabecular metal glenoid component before implantation.

tions.[40] There are few data available on revision surgery for failed humeral head replacement.[19,36,39,40,42,43,63,75–79]

The introduction of humeral component modularity was intended to facilitate the conversion of failed hemiarthroplasty to total shoulder replacement.[80–82] Theoretically, the modular head could be removed, the glenoid implanted, and the head replaced while avoiding the often difficult task of removing the humeral stem. However, this is a technically challenging procedure. The surgeon is often confronted with asymmetrical glenoid wear as well as a scarred and contracted subscapularis tendon that increases the surgical complexity.

Carroll et al[40] demonstrated that revision of a humeral head replacement to a total shoulder arthroplasty is indeed a salvage procedure and that the results are inferior to those of a primary total shoulder arthroplasty. They have shown that at a mean of 5.5 years (range, 2–14 years) postoperatively, 47% of their study group had unsatisfactory results based on the Neer criteria.[40] Five of seven patients with unsatisfactory results (71%) had inadequate pain relief after the revision procedure.

These authors found that humeral head replacement may not preserve glenoid bone stock for later revision because a significant number of their patients had glenoid wear that altered the revision surgery. This asymmetrical glenoid wear was usually posterior and superior and required reaming of the existing bone stock anteriorly to allow placement of the glenoid component. The anterior capsule and subscapularis were often contracted while the posterior capsule was stretched. In addition, humeral component malposition contributed to glenoid wear and soft-tissue contractures. The combination of soft-tissue imbalance, glenoid bone loss, and humeral component malposition increased the surgical complexity. In several cases, the humeral stems required revision for optimal reconstruction but could not be removed without substantial structural damage to the proximal humerus. The authors would often perform an extended humeral osteotomy between the pectoralis major and deltoid insertions when humeral component revision is necessary and stem extraction is difficult. Despite the modest outcomes, 73% of the patients in their series were satisfied with the revision procedure and would undergo this surgery again.

Sperling and Cofield[39] have also reported inferior outcomes to primary total shoulder arthroplasty, with unsatisfactory results in seven of 18 shoulders in a report on revision total shoulder arthroplasty of failed hemiarthroplasties for glenoid arthrosis. The poor results were attributed to poor postoperative ROM. In ten of the patients, the humeral head replacement was performed after a displaced fracture.

The patient demographics between the two study groups above are quite different. The majority of Carroll's patients had osteoarthritis before humeral head replacement, whereas Sperling and Cofield[39] had a preponderance of posttraumatic humeral head replacements. Nonetheless, the rate of unsatisfactory results in both studies is quite alarming. Conversion of the failed hemiarthroplasty to a total shoulder arthroplasty is a technically difficult revision procedure that does not have the same success rate as primary total shoulder arthroplasty for osteoarthritis of the glenohumeral joint.

In yet another series, Ramappa et al[79] reported on a similar group of patients undergoing revision total shoulder arthroplasty for painful humeral head replacement. At a mean of 6.4 years, four of 17 patients had undergone a subsequent revision surgery. Kaplan-Meier survivorship analysis estimated the rate of freedom from revision in this population to be 81% at 5 years

and 68% at 10 years. These survivorship data compare poorly with the estimated survivorship of primary total shoulder arthroplasty, which has been reported to be 93% at 10 years.[75]

A more recent review of revision total shoulder arthroplasty by Dines et al[77] has shown slightly better outcomes for conversion of a hemiarthroplasty to a total shoulder arthroplasty in 11 of 16 patients. They were able to obtain good to excellent outcomes in this subset of patients using the University of California–Los Angeles shoulder rating scales, the L'Insalata shoulder rating questionnaire, and a self-assessment satisfaction scale questionnaire. A potential explanation offered by the authors for the difference in the outcomes was the lack of postoperative infections in this subgroup compared to those in the other two studies.[77] An alternative explanation could be that different outcome measures were used in the studies, with Neer's criteria being stricter with respect to pain relief and ROM. Seventy-three percent of the patients in Carroll's study[40] said they were satisfied with the revision surgery and would undergo the procedure again.

In conclusion, revision of the failed hemiarthroplasty is a salvage operation. The need for glenoid revision after total shoulder arthroplasty is less common than the conversion of humeral head replacement to total shoulder arthroplasty for secondary glenoid arthritis. We currently recommend total shoulder arthroplasty for the primary treatment of glenohumeral arthritis. The specific type of reconstruction used in the revision of the failed hemiarthoplasty will ultimately depend on the patient's demands, the quality of soft tissues available, the adequacy of the bone stock of the proximal humerus and the glenoid, and the function of the neuromuscular envelope around the glenohumeral joint.

REFERENCES

1. Cofield RH. Total shoulder arthroplasty with the Neer prosthesis. *J Bone Joint Surg Am* 1984;66:899–906.
2. Neer CS II. Replacement arthroplasty for glenohumeral osteoarthritis. *J Bone Joint Surg Am* 1974;56:1–13.
3. Neer CS II. Revision of humeral head and total shoulder arthroplasties. *Clin Orthop Relat Res* 1982;170:189–195.
4. Norris TR, Iannotti JP. Functional outcome after shoulder arthroplasty for primary osteoarthritis. *J Shoulder Elbow Surg* 2002;11:130–135.
5. Sperling J, Cofield R, Rowland C. Neer hemiarthroplasty and Neer total shoulder arthroplasty in patients 50 years old or less: long-term results. *J Bone Joint Surg Am* 1998;80:464–473.
6. Zuckerman JD, Cofield RH. Proximal humeral prosthetic replacement in glenohumeral arthritis. *Orthop Trans* 1986;10:231–232.
7. Bigliani LU, McCluskey GM. Prosthetic replacement in acute fractures of the proximal humerus. *Semin Arthroplasty* 1990;1:129–137.
8. Cofield RH. Comminuted fractures of the proximal humerus. *Clin Orthop Relat Res* 1988;230:49–57.
9. Compito CA, Self EB, Bigliani LU. Arthroplasty and acute shoulder trauma: reasons for success and failure. *Clin Orthop Relat Res* 1994;307:27–36.
10. Connor PM, D'Alessandro DF. Role of hemiarthroplasty for proximal humeral fractures. *J South Orthop Assoc* 1995:9–23.
11. Goldman RT, Koval KJ, Cuomo F, et al. Functional outcome after humeral head replacement for acute three- and four-part proximal humeral fractures. *J Shoulder Elbow Surg* 1995;4:81–86.
12. Green A, Barnard L, Limbird RS. Humeral head replacement for acute, four-part proximal humerus fractures. *J Shoulder Elbow Surg* 1993;2:249–254.
13. Hawkins RJ, Switlyk P. Acute prosthetic replacement for severe fractures of the proximal humerus. *Clin Orthop Relat Res* 1993;289:156–160.
14. Levine WN, Connor PM, Yamaguchi K. Humeral head replacement for proximal humeral fractures. *Orthopedics* 1998;21:68–75.
15. Neer CS II. Displaced proximal humeral fractures: Part II. Treatment of three- and four-part displacement. *J Bone Joint Surg Am* 1970;52:1090–1103.
16. Neer CS II. Recent results and techniques of prosthetic replacement for four-part proximal humeral fractures. *Orthop Trans* 1986;10:475.
17. Gartsman GM, Roddey TS, Hammerman SM. Shoulder arthroplasty with or without resurfacing of the glenoid in patients who have osteoarthritis. *J Bone Joint Surg Am* 2000;82:26–34.

18. Levine WN, Djurasovic M, Glasson JM, et al. Hemiarthroplasty for glenohumeral osteoarthritis: results correlated to degree of glenoid wear. *J Shoulder Elbow Surg* 1997;6:449–454.

19. Bigliani LU, Flatow EL, McCluskey GM et al. Failed prosthetic replacement for displaced proximal humerus fractures. *Orthop Trans* 1991;15:747–748.

20. Dimakopoulos P, Potamitis N, Lambiris E. Hemiarthroplasty in the treatment of comminuted fractures of the proximal humerus. *Clin Orthop Relat Res* 1997;341:7–11.

21. Moeckel BH, Dines DM, Warren RF, et al. Modular hemiarthroplasty for fractures of the proximal part of the humerus. *J Bone Joint Surg Am* 1992;74:884–889.

22. Muldoon MP, Cofield RH. Complications of humeral head replacement for proximal humeral fractures. *Instr Course Lect* 1997;46:15–24.

23. Kraulis J, Hunter G. The results of prosthetic replacement in fracture-dislocation of the upper end of the humerus. *Injury* 1976;8:129–131.

24. Tanner MW, Cofield RH. Prosthetic arthroplasty for fractures and fracture-dislocation of the proximal humerus. *Clin Orthop Relat Res* 1983;179:116–128.

25. Boileau P, Krishnan SG, Tinsi L, et al. Tuberosity malposition and migration: reasons for poor outcome after hemiarthroplasty for displaced fractures of the proximal humerus. *J Shoulder Elbow Surg* 2002;11:401–412.

26. Bosch U, Skutek M, Fremery RW, et al. Outcome after primary and secondary hemiarthroplasty in elderly patients with fractures of the proximal humerus. *J Shoulder Elbow Surg* 1998;7:479–484.

27. Norris TR, Green A, McGuigan FX. Late prosthetic shoulder arthroplasty for displaced proximal humeral fractures. *J Shoulder Elbow Surg* 1995;4:271–280.

28. Zyto K, Wallace WA, Frostick SP, et al. Outcome after hemiarthroplasty for three- and four-part fractures of the proximal humerus. *J Shoulder Elbow Surg* 1998;7:85–89.

29. Lervick GN, Carroll RM, Levine WN. Complications after hemiarthroplasty for fractures of the proximal humerus. *Instr Course Lect* 2003;52:3–12.

30. Boileau P, Trojani C, Walch G, et al. Shoulder arthroplasty for the treatment of the sequelae of fractures of the proximal humerus. *J Shoulder Elbow Surg* 2001;10:299–308.

31. Frich LH, Sojbjerg JO, Sneppen O. Shoulder arthroplasty in complex acute and chronic proximal humeral fractures. *Orthopedics* 1991;14:949–954.

32. Stableforth PG. Four-part fractures of the neck of the humerus. *J Bone Joint Surg Br* 1984;66:104–108.

33. Kay SP, Amstutz HC. Shoulder hemiarthroplasty at UCLA. *Clin Orthop Relat Res* 1988;228:42–48.

34. Hughes M, Neer CS II. Glenohumeral joint replacement and postoperative rehabilitation. *Phys Ther* 1975;55:850–858.

35. Neer CS II. Displaced proximal humeral fractures: Part I. Classification and evaluation. *J Bone Joint Surg Am* 1970;52:1077–1089.

36. Neer CS II, Watson KC, Stanton FJ. Recent experience in total shoulder replacement. *J Bone Joint Surg Am* 1982;64:319–337.

37. Rietveld AB, Daanen HA, Rozing PM, et al. The lever arm in glenohumeral abduction after hemiarthroplasty. *J Bone Joint Surg Br* 1988;70:561–565.

38. Schai P, Imhoff A, Preiss S. Comminuted humeral head fractures: a multicenter analysis. *J Shoulder Elbow Surg* 1995;4:319–330.

39. Schai P, Imhoff A, Preiss S. Comminuted humeral head fractures: a multicenter analysis. *J Shoulder Elbow Surg* 1995;4:319–330.

40. Carroll RM, Izquierdo R, Vazquez M, et al. Conversion of painful hemiarthroplasty to total shoulder arthroplasty: long-term results. *J Shoulder Elbow Surg* 2004;13:599–603.

41. Voloshin I, Setter KJ, Bigliani LU. Revision shoulder arthroplasty and related tendon transfers. In: Bigliani LU, Flatow EL, eds. *Shoulder Arthroplasty*. New York: Springer; 2005: 117–148.

42. Levy J, Frankle MA, Mighell M, et al. The use of the reverse shoulder prosthesis for the treatment of failed hemiarthroplasty for proximal humeral fracture. *J Bone Joint Surg Am* 2007;89:292–300.

43. Levy JC, Virani N, Pupello D, et al. Use of the reverse shoulder prosthesis for the treatment of failed hemiarthroplasty in patients with glenohumeral arthritis and rotator cuff deficiency. *J Bone Joint surg Br* 2007;89:189–195.

44. Nicholson GP. Treatment of anterior superior shoulder instability with a reverse ball-and-socket prosthesis. *Oper Tech Orthop* 2003;13:235–241.

45. Tytherleigh-Strong GM, Levy O, Sforza G. The role of arthroscopy for the problem shoulder arthroplasty. *J Shoulder Elbow Surg* 2002;11:230–234.

46. Cofield RH. Revision procedures for shoulder arthroplasty. In: Morrey BF, ed. *Reconstructive Surgery of the Joints*. New York: Churchill Livingstone; 1996:789–799.

47. Ankem HK, Blaine TA. Revision shoulder arthroplasty. *Tech Shoulder Elbow Surg* 2005;6:189–198.

48. Sperling JW, Cofield RH. Humeral windows in revision shoulder arthroplasty. *J Shoulder Elbow Surg* 2005;14:258–263.

49. Plausinis D, Kwon YW, Zuckerman JD. Complications of humeral head replacement for proximal humeral fractures. *J Bone Joint Surg Am* 2005;87:204–213.

50. Klepps SJ, Galatz L, Yamaguchi K. A salvage procedure for irreparable subscapularis deficiency. *Tech Shoulder Elbow Surg* 2001;2:85–91.

51. Neer CS II. *Shoulder Reconstruction*. Philadelphia: WB Saunders; 1990:143–271.

52. Wright TW, Cofield RH. Humeral fractures after shoulder arthroplasty. *J Bone Joint Surg Am* 1995;77:1340–1346.

53. Klimkiewicz JJ, Iannotti JP, Rubash HE, et al. Aseptic loosening of the humeral component in total shoulder arthroplasty. *J Shoulder Elbow Surg* 1998;7:422–426.

54. Torchia ME, Cofield RH, Settergren CR. Total shoulder arthroplasty with the Neer prosthesis: long-term results. *J Shoulder Elbow Surg* 1997;6:495–505.

55. Wirth MA, Agrawal CM, Mabrey JD. Isolation and characterization of polyethylene wear debris associated with osteolysis following total shoulder arthroplasty. *J Bone Joint Surg Am* 1999;81:29–37.

56. Dines D, Warren RF, Font-Rodriguez D. Revision shoulder arthroplasty. *Tech Shoulder Elbow Surg* 2001;2:26–37.

57. Flatow EL, Connor PM, Levine WN, et al. Coracoacromial arch reconstruction for anterosuperior subluxation after failed rotator cuff surgery: a preliminary report. *J Shoulder Elbow Surg* 1997;6:228.

58. Wirth MA, Rockwood CA. Complications of total shoulder replacement arthroplasty. *J Bone Joint Surg Am* 1996;78:603–616.

59. Rittmeister M, Kerschbaumer F. Grammont reverse total shoulder arthroplasty in patients with rheumatoid arthritis and nonreconstructable rotator cuff lesions. *J Shoulder Elbow Surg* 2001;10:17–22.

60. Edwards TB, Kakakia NR, Boulahia A. A comparison of hemiarthroplasty and total shoulder arthroplasty in the treatment of primary glenohumeral osteoarthritis: results of a multicenter study. *J Shoulder Elbow Surg* 2003;12:207–213.

61. Orfaly RM, Rockwood CA, Esenyel CZ, et al. A prospective functional outcome study of shoulder arthroplasty for osteoarthritis with an intact rotator cuff. *J Shoulder Elbow Surg* 2003;12:214–221.

62. Franklin JL, Barrett WP, Jackins SE, et al. Glenoid loosening in total shoulder arthroplasty: association with rotator cuff deficiency. *J Arthroplasty* 1988;3:39–46.

63. Boyd AD, Thomas WH, Scott RD. Total shoulder arthroplasty versus hemiarthroplasty: indications for glenoid resurfacing. *J Arthroplasty* 1990;5:329–336.

64. Antuña S. Sperling JW, Cofield RH. Reimplantation of a glenoid component after component removal and allograft bone grafting: a report of 3 cases. *J Shoulder Elbow Surg* 2002;11:637–641.

65. Allaine J, Goutallier D, Glorio C. Long-term results of the Latarjet procedure for the treatment of anterior instability of the shoulder. *J Bone Joint Surg Am* 1998;80:841–852.

66. Latarjet M. Techniques chirurgicales dans le traitement de la luxation anteriointerne recidivante de l'epaule. *Lyon Chir* 1965;61:313–318.

67. Antuña SA, Sperling JW, Cofield RH. Glenoid revision surgery after total shoulder arthroplasty. *J Shoulder Elbow Surg* 2001;10:217–224.

68. Burkhead WZ, Hutton KS. Biologic resurfacing of the glenoid with hemiarthroplasty of the shoulder. *J Shoulder Elbow Surg* 1995;4:263–270.

69. Bauer GS, Levine WN, Blaine TA, et al. Hemiarthroplasty for glenohumeral arthritis: long term results. In: Specialty Day (American Shoulder and Elbow Surgeons). Edited, Dallas, Tex; 2002.

70. Barrett WP, Franklin JL, Jackins SE, et al. Total shoulder arthroplasty. *J Bone Joint Surg Am* 1987;69:865–872.

71. Barrett WP, Thornhill TS, Thomas WH, et al. Nonconstrained total shoulder arthroplasty in patients with polyarticular rheumatoid arthritis. *J Arthroplasty* 1989;4:91–96.

72. Boyd AD Jr, Aliabadi P, Thornhill TS. Postoperative proximal migration in total shoulder arthroplasty: incidence and significance. *J Arthroplasty* 1991;6:31–37.

73. Figgie HE III, Inglis AE, Goldberg VM. An analysis of factors affecting the long-term results of total shoulder arthroplasty in inflammatory arthritis. *J Arthroplasty* 1998;3:123–130.

74. Hawkins RJ, Bell RH, Jallay B. Total shoulder arthroplasty. *Clin Orthop Relat Res* 1989;242:188–194.

75. Caldwell GL, Dines D, Warren R, et al. Revision shoulder arthroplasty. *Orthop Trans* 1993;17:140–141.

76. Cofield RH, Edgerton BC. Total shoulder arthroplasty: complications and revision surgery. *Instr Course Lect* 1990;39:449–462.

77. Dines JS, Fealy S, Strauss EJ, et al. Outcomes analysis of revision total shoulder replacement. *J Bone Joint Surg Am* 2006;88:1494–1500.

78. Neer CS II, Kirby RM. Revision of humeral head and total shoulder arthroplasties. *Clin Orthop Relat Res* 1982;170:189–195.

79. Ramappa AJ, Gomoll A, Thornhill TS. Failed shoulder hemiarthroplasty: pattern of failure and outcomes of revision surgery. Presented at the Open American Shoulder and Elbow Surgeons Meeting; March 16, 2000; Orlando, Fla.

80. Flatow EL. Prosthetic design considerations in total shoulder arthroplasty. *Semin Arthroplasty* 1995;6:233–244.

81. Gartsman GM, Russell JA, Gaenslen E. Modular shoulder arthroplasty. *J Shoulder Elbow Surg* 1997;6:333–339.

82. Skirving AP. Total shoulder arthroplasty: current problems and possible solutions. *J Orthop Sci* 1999;4:42–53.

Brent B. Wiesel
Gerald R. Williams

The Reverse Prosthesis for Failed Anatomic Shoulder Arthroplasty

INTRODUCTION

Reverse shoulder arthroplasty (RSA) is primarily used for the treatment of combined glenohumeral arthritis and rotator cuff tears. Rotator cuff arthropathy is the hallmark indication for RSA. However, failed anatomic arthroplasty is an increasingly common indication. This condition is especially challenging because it is often characterized not only by rotator cuff deficiency but also by glenohumeral instability and bone loss. The unique geometry of RSAs can allow the surgeon to compensate for severe soft tissue deficiency that can be encountered during revision shoulder arthroplasty.

Reverse shoulder arthroplasty is associated with a substantial complication rate, and this complication rate is highest when the procedure is used for revision of failed anatomic prostheses. In many of these cases, however, RSA is the only surgical option that is likely to both maintain or improve function and improve pain level.

BIOMECHANICAL PRINCIPLES OF THE CURRENT REVERSE SHOULDER ARTHROPLASTY DESIGNS

Early attempts to provide increased stability via greater constraint or reverse ball-and-socket design for rotator cuff deficient shoulders failed, possibly because the prosthetic design attempted to maintain the shoulder's center of rotation in its anatomic, lateralized position. In the normal shoulder, the rotator cuff muscles provide a compressive force that keeps the humeral head centered in the glenoid and resists the sheer forces generated by the deltoid, especially with elevation of the arm from 0 to 60 degrees. The original nonanatomic designs attempted to compensate for the loss of rotator cuff function through increased conformity of the articulation. Attempting to control the sheer forces across the glenohumeral joint with increased conformity leads to significant stress within the prosthesis and at the bone-implant interface. This resulted in either loosening or breakage of the implant in an unacceptably large number of cases.

Most current RSAs are based on the novel 1985 design of professor Paul Grammont that shifted the center of rotation medially to a point on the interface between the glenoid component and the host bone.[1] Medializing the center of rotation converts a greater portion of the force generated by the deltoid into rotational movement instead of sheer stress. This medialization presumably allows for enough conformity within the prosthesis to provide a stable fulcrum for elevation of the arm without generating excessive stress at the bone-prosthesis interface. The new center of rotation also increases the moment arm of the deltoid muscle, allowing it to become a more efficient elevator of the arm. Not all current RSA designs incorporate the same degree of medialization as Grammont's design. However, all current designs incorporate some medialization compared to the early, failed constrained designs. The ideal degree of medialization is currently unknown.

In addition to establishing a stable, medialized fulcrum for elevation of the arm, the increased conformity of the Grammont prosthesis provides potentially increased anterior and posterior stability compared to that with anatomic shoulder arthroplasties. Prosthetic stability is likely further enhanced by the increase in the angle between the humeral shaft and articular surface to 155 degrees. When properly inserted, RSAs lower the deltoid insertion, which leads to increased tension within the muscle. The higher tension generates increased compressive force across the glenohumeral joint, which theoretically results in enhanced stability of the articulation. It should be noted, however, that the incidence of instability following RSA is higher than after anatomic arthroplasty. This likely reflects the importance of the rotator cuff in maintaining prosthetic shoulder stability.

INDICATIONS

The primary indication for reverse prostheses following failed anatomic shoulder arthroplasty is refractory instability. This includes superior, anterior, and posterior instability, each of which typically occurs when there is insufficiency of various portions of the rotator cuff. This instability is also often accompanied by asymmetrical bone loss, making reconstruction even more challenging.

Anterosuperior escape can occur following anatomic shoulder arthroplasty when there is loss of the posterosuperior rotator cuff and disruption of the coracoacromial arch—especially when the rotator cuff tear extends into the rotator interval and upper subscapularis (Fig. 22.1). When anterosuperior escape occurs following arthroplasty, attempts to restore superior stability through cuff repair or muscle transfers are generally unsuccessful. These patients typically have significant pain and minimal ability to actively elevate their arm. For these patients, the reverse prosthesis offers the most effective means of restoring a stable fulcrum and improving the ability to elevate the arm.

Anterior instability following total shoulder arthroplasty is difficult to treat. Revision surgery with anatomic implants has been reported to have a failure rate greater than 50%.[2] The instability is typically due to subscapularis deficiency with or without component malposition. In younger patients or when the causes of the instability can be clearly identified and corrected, we recommend continued use of anatomic arthroplasty components. However, in older individuals with anterior instability resulting from a problem that is not easily corrected, such as complete attenuation of the subscapularis tendon, the reverse prosthesis provides the best possibility of restoring stability and function.

Although less common than anterior instability, posterior instability following anatomic arthroplasty is often due to inappropriate version of either the humeral or glenoid components.[3] When this cannot be addressed by traditional surgical techniques or there is irreparable deficiency of the rotator cuff, the reverse prosthesis can be used to create a stable joint.

CONTRAINDICATIONS

As with all revision arthroplasties, active infection is an absolute contraindication to implantation of a RSA. Given the fact that RSA relies almost exclusively on the deltoid muscle for stability and movement of the joint, complete lack of deltoid muscle

function is also a contraindication to the use of a reverse arthroplasty. Patients with isolated loss of the anterior deltoid from partial deltoid dehiscence or injury to the anterior portion of the axillary nerve may still benefit from RSA, although the functional outcome may be inferior to results obtained with complete deltoid function. If there is loss of the middle deltoid, the patient will likely not experience significant functional gain from the surgery and it may be difficult to maintain stability of the implant; therefore the use of a reverse prosthesis is probably not indicated under these circumstances.

Implantation of a RSA requires sufficient glenoid bone stock to support the metaglene (i.e., glenoid baseplate) component. In cases of glenoid bone deficiency, the central peg and peripheral screws of the glenoid baseplate can be used to secure the bone graft to the native scapula during a one-stage or two-stage revision procedure. However, there must be enough host bone to secure at least a portion of the central peg and at least two or three peripheral screws or it is unlikely that the glenoid component will achieve lasting, stable fixation. Under these circumstances, the use of RSA is contraindicated. If the bone defect is reconstructable, RSA may be possible at a later date, after successful incorporation of the graft.

PREOPERATIVE EVALUATION

When evaluating a patient for possible revision to RSA it is important to consider any factors in the history that may indicate the possibility of latent infection. We routinely obtain erythrocyte sedimentation rate (ESR) and C-reactive protein levels on all patients being evaluated for revision arthroplasty. If either value is elevated, we proceed with a further workup, including aspiration of the joint.

Many patients undergoing revision shoulder arthroplasty are elderly and have multiple medical comorbidities. Preoperative medical consultation should be requested when appropriate. In addition, perioperative transfusion is often necessary. Therefore

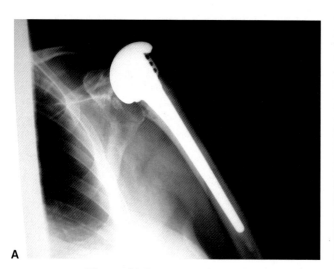
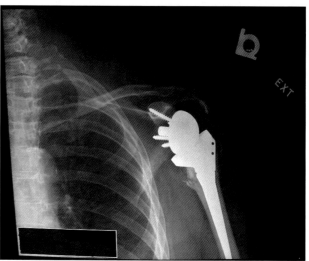

A

B

Figure 22.1.   **(A)** A 58-year-old right-hand dominant woman presented with pain and a flail left upper extremity secondary to rotator cuff insufficiency and anterior superior escape following a hemiarthroplasty. **(B)** The patient regained 150 degrees of active forward elevation following revision to a reverse shoulder arthroplasty.

arrangements for preoperative autologous blood donation or routine type and crossmatch should be performed.

On physical examination it is important to note the location of the patient's previous incision, as well as the overall condition of the soft tissues about the shoulder girdle. It is usually possible to use the previous incision. However, if using the previous incision might compromise exposure, a long deltopectoral incision with minimal subcutaneous dissection should be used. As noted above, some loss of anterior deltoid function can be tolerated, but complete loss of deltoid function, whether neurogenic or structural, is a contraindication to RSA.

Simovitch et al[4] has recently demonstrated the importance of teres minor function following RSA for patients with cuff tear arthropathy. It is important to evaluate teres minor function by testing external rotation strength with the arm at 90 degrees of abduction as described by Walch et al.[5] Patients who are unable to resist gravity in this position may have difficulty elevating the arm above 90 degrees following RSA because they will not be able to prevent internal rotation of the arm with increasing elevation. Gerber et al described favorable results with simultaneous RSA and latissimus dorsi transfer in patients with a positive hornblower sign.[6] Boileau et al[7] described transfer of the latissimus dorsi and teres major for this same patient population. Neither of these studies had a control group that did not undergo transfer. Moreover, in most cases, patients will be satisfied following successful revision to RSA without an accompanying transfer because of improved stability and modest improvements in function. Therefore indications for transfer are evolving and should be individualized.

A complete set of radiographs (anteroposterior in internal and external rotation, scapular Y, and axillary view) is used to evaluate the current prosthesis and the condition of the native bone. The humeral bone stock can usually be evaluated on plain radiographs. In general, a revision stem length is selected that will bypass the tip of the previous prosthesis by at least two cortical diameters. However, in many cases of a previously cemented humeral component, most if not all of the cement mantle remains in the humerus after removal of the previous stem. Under these circumstances, cementing a smaller, standard-length stem into the previous cement mantel may prevent intraoperative fracture.

Although the remaining glenoid bone stock can be evaluated on plain radiographs, axial computed tomography (CT) scans provide better assessment of the condition of the host bone surrounding the original glenoid component. Although metallic artifact can make visualization of the glenoid bone difficult, with the appropriate windows, adequate bone analysis is often possible. If there is a question as to whether there is sufficient bone to support the glenoid baseplate, the patient is counseled that a two-stage revision as described later in the chapter may be necessary.

PREOPERATIVE PLANNING

Familiarity with the failed implant is helpful. Many humeral implants have porous coating or other surface treatments that encourage bone in-growth. This can make removal difficult. Moreover, many shoulder implant systems have specialized instruments that facilitate component removal. If the surgeon is not familiar with the failed implant on the basis of its radiographic appearance, review of the original operative report may prove extremely valuable. If possible, the manufacturer's instruments should be available intraoperatively.

Regardless of the specific type of failed implant, a specialized set of revision instruments is critical. There are revision instrument sets commercially available. However, most are designed for hip revision and are not ideal for shoulder revision. Important revision instruments include a full set of both rigid and flexible osteotomes; a heavy mallet; a bone tamp; a full set of intramedullary reamers, including at least one that is end-cutting; reverse-cutting osteotomes; a burr; and long-handled graspers. An ultrasonic cement removal device is also useful in the case of failed cemented humeral stems. Finally, in any revision situation, one should be prepared for intentional or accidental intraoperative humeral fracture. Adequate preparation includes a microsagittal saw, standard and long-stemmed implants, a cerclage wire or cable set, standard osteosynthesis implants such as plates and screws, and intraoperative radiographs or C-arm.

Both humeral and glenoid bone deficiencies are often encountered in revision arthroplasty. If either has been identified during preoperative evaluation, arrangements should be made to have bone graft available in the operative setting. This might include both allograft cancellous chips and structural allograft.

OPERATIVE TECHNIQUE

POSITIONING AND SKIN INCISION

Revision shoulder arthroplasty is performed in the beach chair position with the patient's back elevated 30 to 45 degrees relative to the plane of the floor. Although the superior approach may be acceptable for implantation of a RSA for primary cuff tear arthropathy, the extended deltopectoral approach is used in the revision situation. Prophylactic antibiotics are administered at least 30 minutes before skin incision. The extended deltopectoral approach exploits an internervous plane and is, therefore, extensile. In addition, this approach generally allows for use of the patient's previous skin incision and provides necessary access to the humeral shaft for removal of the old component.

SUPERFICIAL DISSECTION

Identification of the deltopectoral interval in revision arthroplasty can be difficult. The cephalic vein is often diminutive or absent. If it can be identified, it is retracted laterally with the deltoid. If it cannot be identified, the tip of the coracoid process is used as a reference for the deltopectoral interval. This interval is developed down to the tip of the coracoid. There are often dense adhesions between the deep surface of the pectoralis major and the superficial surface of the conjoined tendon of the coracobrachialis and the short head of the biceps. These adhesions are safely released as long as the dissection remains superficial to the obvious superiorly to inferiorly running fibers of the conjoined tendon. The deep surface of the pectoralis major is freed all the way to its insertion on the humerus.

The undersurface of the deltoid is often scarred to the underlying humerus. However, if the greater tuberosity or any portion of the metaphyseal flare of the humerus is present, a natural plane can be developed at this transitional area between the humerus and overlying deltoid with minimal blunt dissection. A blunt Homan retractor can then be safely placed between the deltoid and humerus, taking care to place the retractor directly on bone to avoid injury to the axillary nerve. This interval can then be extended distally to the deltoid insertion and proximally to the subacromial space.

The subacromial space is also frequently filled with scar and adhesions. These should be removed. In addition, any soft tissue that spans from the superior glenoid to the greater tuberosity may prevent external rotation and posterior translation of the humerus required for glenoid exposure. In many cases, this tissue may even include a portion of the supraspinatus. However, if the decision to convert to a reverse prosthesis has already been made, absence of the supraspinatus will likely not affect postoperative function. Therefore we routinely clear the subacromial space of all soft tissue when revising a failed anatomic prosthesis to a reverse prosthesis, even if this requires excision of some remnants of the supraspinatus. Care is taken to preserve portions of the infraspinatus or teres minor that remain.

DEEP DISSECTION

In most cases of failed anatomic arthroplasties, the subscapularis is deficient. However, complete absence of anterior soft tissue is uncommon. Often, a sheet of anterior soft tissue including some portion of the subscapularis (usually the inferior third), the anterior capsule, and scar tissue covers the anterior aspect of the joint. The interval between the deep surface of the conjoined tendon and these anterior soft tissues is dissected at the most inferior portion of the joint to identify the axillary nerve so that it can be protected throughout the procedure. Complete separation of the conjoined tendon from the deep anterior soft tissue envelope must be undertaken carefully because one may be left with extremely poor-quality tissue for repair. If preoperative passive external rotation is less than 30 degrees, the anterior soft tissue envelope should be completely released from the overlying conjoined tendon.

The anterior soft tissue structures are preserved by elevating them subperiosteally, starting at the medial lip of the bicipital groove. Superiorly, the entire anterior soft tissue sleeve is released to the base of the coracoid. Inferiorly, as the humerus is externally rotated, the subperiosteal elevation is continued medially and posteriorly to the medial neck, taking care to protect the axillary nerve. The humerus is then delivered into the wound with simultaneous adduction, extension, and external rotation. Exposure is facilitated by placing a Brown deltoid retractor or modified Taylor retractor between the deltoid and humerus superiorly, a large Darrach retractor medially between the glenoid and the humerus, and a blunt Homan retractor inferiorly along the medial neck of the humerus. The blunt Homan retractor must be carefully placed directly on bone so as to avoid injury to the axillary nerve.

HUMERAL COMPONENT EXTRACTION

The key to humeral component extraction is gaining access to the most medial and inferior aspect of the prosthesis and native humeral neck. This requires adequate subperiosteal release and external rotation, adduction, and extension as described above. Although many implants have specific extraction devices, none work any better than a well-placed tamp under

the medial lip of the humeral prosthesis. This requires that a small gap exists between the collar of a modular prosthesis or the head of a monoblock prosthesis and the native humeral bone. If there has been no erosion in this area, the gap must be created by removing a small area of the medial neck with a rongeur or a burr. If access to the medial aspect of the prosthesis is not adequate or the prosthesis does not have a collar or lip to support the bone tamp, an extractor attached to the implant may be required. Under these circumstances, specialized extraction devices designed by the specific manufacturer may be critical.

Before attempting to remove the humeral prosthesis by hitting the tamp with a mallet, every attempt should be made to interrupt any areas where the bone and prosthesis may be bonded together. If the prosthesis is a monoblock, an osteotome can be passed parallel to the undersurface of the head, between it and the humeral bone. This is especially helpful if the undersurface of the head contains a surface treatment to encourage biological in-growth. If the prosthesis is modular, the humeral head should be removed and a small osteotome should be passed along the prosthesis-bone interface circumferentially. A flexible osteotome may be required with components with a large collar. The osteotome should be passed only to the level of the metaphyseal/diaphyseal junction. This decreases the likelihood of fracturing the tuberosities. In addition, even in implants that have a surface coating to encourage biological in-growth, this surface treatment rarely extends beyond the metaphysis. When extracting a humeral component that was placed for fracture, it is especially important to release all nonabsorbable sutures attached to the prosthesis.

Once the metaphyseal portion of the prosthesis has been separated from the native bone as much as is possible, the tamp is placed at the inferior aspect of the prosthesis and is hit firmly with a mallet. If the prosthesis cannot be removed after several mallet blows, one can attempt removal with any specialized instruments, such as extraction handles. If this still does not work, which is uncommon unless the prosthesis is cemented, a single relaxing osteotomy in the humerus may be required.

Single Osteotomy

A microsagittal saw is used to make an osteotomy in the humerus approximately 2 to 3 mm posterior to the bicipital groove. The osteotomy should begin at the most superior extent of the greater tuberosity and extend inferiorly to the level of the superior extent of the deltoid insertion. A small drill hole (2 mm) is placed at the distal extent of the osteotomy to discourage distal propagation. A large osteotome is passed into the osteotomy and tapped with a mallet until it makes contact with the metal of the prosthesis. This is done throughout the entire length of the osteotomy. Another attempt is then made to extract the prosthesis with a tamp and mallet or any specialized extraction devices. In 90% or more of cases, this will be sufficient to extract the prosthesis.

Cortical Window

If a single osteotomy is unsuccessful in removing the failed prosthesis, a cortical window is required. At the most inferior extent of the previous osteotomy, a microsagittal saw is used to make a transverse cut in the humeral shaft starting anteriorly and moving posteriorly for a distance equal to approximately one third of the circumference of the shaft (Fig. 22.2). A large (2-inch) straight osteotome is then placed within the previously placed longitudinal osteotomy and is carefully twisted about its long axis to open the osteotomy slightly. This may require placing it at multiple sites along the longitudinal osteotomy. A large Cobb elevator is then placed in the longitudinal osteotomy at multiple levels and twisted about its long axis. The osteotomy is opened just enough to allow adequate access to the humeral canal to loosen the prosthesis. If one has been careful, the humerus will crack longitudinally, starting inferiorly at the most posterior extent of the transverse osteotomy and extending superiorly. The anterolateral humeral shaft will then hinge open on the posterior crack to allow access to the implant. The failed prosthesis can almost always be removed with this technique.

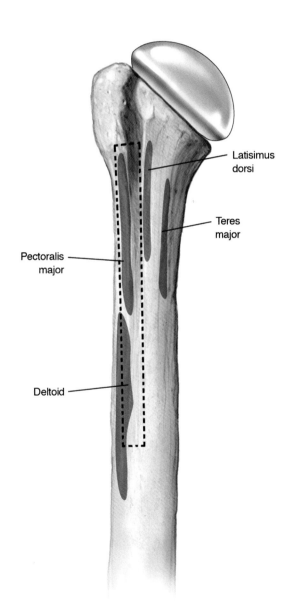

Figure 22.2.   Creation of a cortical window for removal of a well-fixed stem.

Latissimus dorsi

Teres major

Pectoralis major

Deltoid

Cement Removal

As mentioned previously, if the failed implant can be removed without creating a window and without removing a well-fixed cement mantle, cementing a smaller stem into the previous cement mantle is often desirable. This may require partial ultrasonic cement removal to seat the reverse component to the appropriate level. However, it is often possible to avoid complete cement removal, especially the distal cement plug.

If a cortical window or a single osteotomy had to be performed and the decision was made to bypass the defect by at least two cortical diameters, any obstructing cement will need to be removed. An ultrasonic cement remover can facilitate this process. However, if it is used distal to the deltoid insertion, periods of application of the ultrasonic energy should be minimized to prevent heat injury to the radial nerve.[8] Intraoperative radiography is helpful in confirming complete cement removal and distal intramedullary placement of the humeral reamer.

Once the humeral prosthesis and cement have been removed, the very next step is to fix the humeral osteotomy or window with two or three cerclage wires. A long-stemmed trial (if the system you are using has one) or the real long-stemmed implant is placed within the intramedullary canal to protect the humerus and to aid in reduction of the cortical window, if one has been made. Alternatively, the intramedullary reamer may be used. Two or three cerclage wires or cables are passed around the humeral shaft and tightened, thereby fixing the humeral osteotomy or window. Care must be taken to place the cerclage wires or cables subperiosteally to avoid capturing the axillary or radial nerves. Attention can then be turned to exposing the glenoid.

GLENOID EXPOSURE

The humerus is retracted posteriorly with a ring, Carter Rowe, or blunt Homan retractor. An incision is made between the anterior capsule and the anterior glenoid rim, starting superiorly at the base of the coracoid and extending inferiorly to the 5:30 to 6 o'clock position (right shoulder). The location of the axillary nerve must be known and the nerve protected during this portion of the procedure. A large Darrach or reverse double-prong Bankart retractor is then placed through this anterior capsulotomy onto the anterior neck of the scapula.

In the absence of an anatomic glenoid component, the surface of the native glenoid must be exposed adequately for placement of the glenoid baseplate and glenoid sphere. The glenohumeral space typically contains a substantial amount of scar tissue, which should be excised. When revising failed anatomic arthroplasties, particularly if there is fixed superior humeral migration, a band of scar tissue traversing the most inferior extent of the glenoid from anterior to posterior is often found. This inferior band may prevent adequate inferior displacement of the humerus and may also cause dislocation of the RSA when the arm is adducted. Therefore this entire fibrous band, along with the entire inferior capsule, is excised. To accomplish this safely, the axillary nerve must be identified and protected. Finally, the entire labrum and any remnant of the long head of the biceps should be excised. The distal portion of the long head of the biceps can be tagged with a suture so that it can be identified later and tenodesed, if so desired.

GLENOID PREPARATION AND BASEPLATE PLACEMENT

Hemiarthroplasty to Reverse Shoulder Arthroplasty

The exposed glenoid must be prepared to accept the glenoid baseplate. This is easiest when the revision is being performed for hemiarthroplasty. In most RSA systems, a central guide pin is placed that dictates reaming and baseplate placement. This guide pin must be positioned so that the most inferior extent of the glenoid baseplate coincides with the most inferior extent of the native glenoid. In addition, it should be perpendicular to both the superoinferior and anteroposterior axes of the glenoid. In many systems, a specific guide is used to facilitate proper pin placement. Appropriate placement of this guide pin is critical because it dictates the remainder of the procedure. Therefore extra time taken to ensure proper placement is time well spent.

The glenoid is reamed over the previously placed guide pin to ensure maximum conformity between the back of the glenoid baseplate and the surface of the glenoid. Multiple types of glenoid baseplates exist. Components with a convex medial surface require less reaming than those with a flat back. In either case, the subchondral bone of the glenoid should be preserved as much is possible. The periphery (superior) of the glenoid is also reamed to allow adequate seating of the glenoid sphere. The central drill hole for the central peg of the glenoid baseplate is made over the central guide pin and the pin is removed.

The glenoid baseplate is then placed. It is important to align the component so that the superior and inferior holes allow placement of screws into the base of the coracoid superiorly and the lateral angle/pillar of the scapula inferiorly. This usually requires that the component be turned approximately 15 to 20 degrees clockwise (right shoulder). It is also helpful to have screws that can be inserted at varying angles and then locked to the baseplate. This allows the surgeon to alter the angle of insertion to maximize bone contact while still capturing the benefits of added rigidity from locking the screws to the plate. We typically place the inferior and superior locking screws first, followed by nonlocking screws anteriorly and posteriorly. However, if the bone quality is poor, locking screws can be placed in all four holes.

Total Shoulder Arthroplasty to Reverse Shoulder Arthroplasty

If a failed anatomic total shoulder arthroplasty is being revised, the anatomic glenoid component must be removed. If the anatomic glenoid component is loose, its removal is easy. If it is well fixed and all polyethylene, it can usually be removed by levering it out with a Cobb elevator or by passing a thin, curved osteotome between the back of the component and the glenoid surface. In rare cases, the polyethylene surface must be sectioned and removed from the anchoring points, which are then removed with a burr or drill. Any cement that is loose is removed, but any portion of the cement mantle that remains stably fixed to the glenoid vault is left in place.

Failed anatomic glenoid components that are metal-backed and biologically fixed to the native glenoid bone can be very difficult to remove without causing substantial damage to the remaining glenoid bone stock. If the patient is sedentary and

the metal tray is very well fixed, one potential option is to leave the tray in place and have a custom reverse glenoid component made to fix to the tray (Fig. 22.3). This will require a second procedure. Under most circumstances, the well-fixed metal tray from the anatomic component will have to be removed. This is most easily done by passing a small osteotome under as much of the tray as is possible in order to break the biological bond between the tray and the glenoid before levering or malleting it out. Access to the interface between the posterior portion of the glenoid and the metal tray can be difficult. One solution is to pass a small osteotome percutaneously from posterolaterally into the glenohumeral joint, as if one were establishing a posterolateral arthroscopic portal. Obviously, the entry site must be superior enough to avoid the axillary nerve.

Once the failed anatomic glenoid component has been removed, the native glenoid is prepared for installation of the glenoid baseplate and glenoid sphere. The main challenge, of course, is managing the bone loss resulting from the previous failed component. Glenoid preparation and instrumentation in the presence of bone loss is such a prominent part of revision RSA that we have chosen to discuss it as a separate topic for both failed hemiarthroplasty and total shoulder arthroplasty.

GLENOID BONE LOSS

Classification

Glenoid defects can be classified as follows: I: central—contained and uncontained; II: peripheral—symmetrical and asymmetrical; and III: combined—symmetrical and asymmetrical (Fig. 22.4).[9,10] Each clinical situation must be individualized, and the decision to graft is ultimately made intraoperatively. However, some generalizations can be made. Mild and most moderate central defects can be handled with cancellous chips. Severe central defects often require structural grafts for one-stage revisions. Mild and most moderate, symmetrical peripheral and combined defects usually require only nonstructural (i.e., cancellous) grafting. Mild and most moderate asymmetrical peripheral and combined defects, especially if they are superior, can often be handled with asymmetrical reaming with or without cancellous or nonstructural graft. Severe peripheral and combined defects, both symmetrical and asymmetrical, most often will require structural grafts to support the glenoid baseplate (Table 22.1). In some cases, the bone loss may be so severe that revision to RSA is not possible or must be accomplished in two stages.

Hemiarthroplasty to Reverse Shoulder Arthroplasty

Glenoid bone loss severe enough to require structural bone graft is uncommon when revising failed anatomic hemiarthroplasties. When glenoid bone loss is present, it most often is peripheral, asymmetrical (e.g., superior), and mild to moderate. Because the glenoid baseplate should be placed on the inferior glenoid surface such that the most inferior portion of the baseplate aligns with the inferior border of the glenoid, very little if any of the baseplate will rest in the glenoid defect. If any bone graft is required, cancellous allograft chips are often sufficient. The graft is placed between the baseplate and the native glenoid before the baseplate is impacted into position; the baseplate is fixed in the usual fashion as described above.

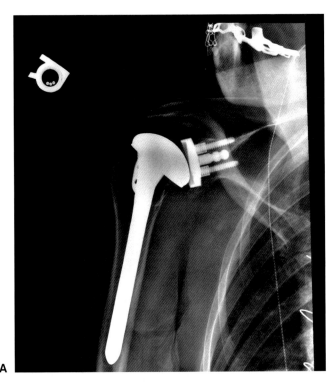

A

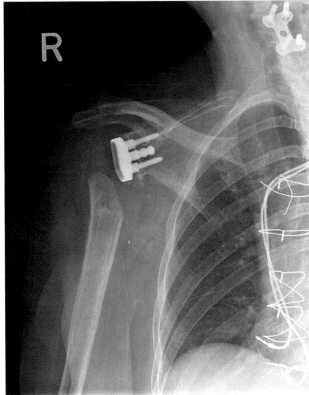

B

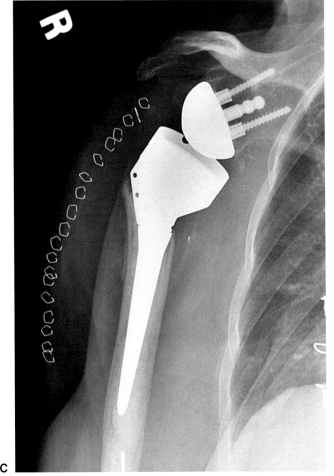

C

Figure 22.3.   When revising a shoulder with a well-fixed metal-backed glenoid component (**A**), one option is to leave the tray in place and have a custom reverse glenoid component created to fit the tray. In stage one of the procedure, the humeral component and plastic glenoid portion of the original prosthesis are removed, and, after confirming that the metal glenoid component is well fixed, measurements are made for creation of the custom component (**B**). Once the custom glenosphere has been created, it is implanted during a second procedure along with the humeral portion of the reverse shoulder arthroplasty (**C**).

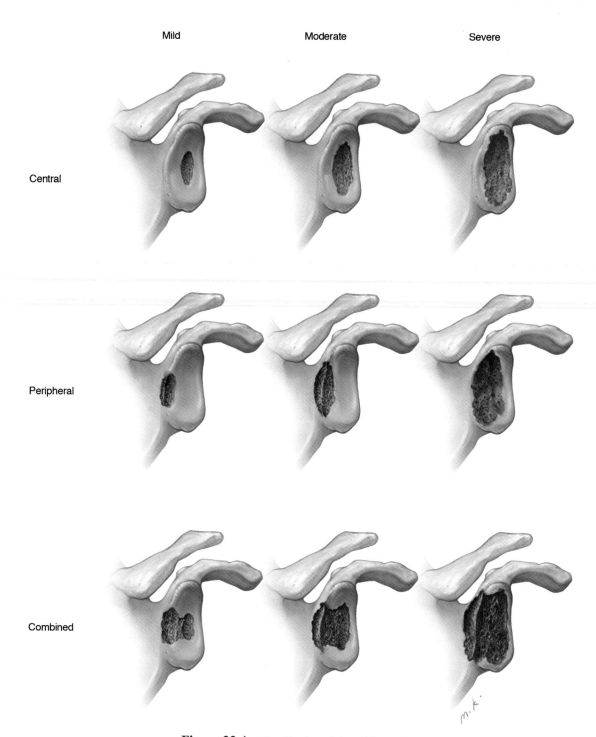

Figure 22.4. Classification of glenoid bone defects.

If preoperative radiographs reveal a moderate to severe asymmetrical peripheral defect, a humeral head allograft can be used to interpose between the native glenoid and the glenoid baseplate. Often, because the humeral head created the defect, a graft can be fashioned from the humeral head allograft that contours to the defect quite well. Although exact size matching is difficult, one can estimate whether the allograft should be small, medium, or large.

The guide pin should be placed in the appropriate position and inclination, as if the defect were not present. The glenoid

is reamed, the central hole for the central peg of the baseplate is drilled, and the central pin is removed. The graft is fashioned to fit the peripheral defect, placed into the defect with the articular side pointing toward native glenoid, and provisionally held with two Kirchner wires that are placed as peripherally as possible. A burr is used to contour the surface of the graft so that it approximates the surface of the remaining, reamed, native glenoid. If any of the graft covers the central hole, the burr is used to remove it. The baseplate is then inserted and impacted into position. Usually, at least one of the provisional

TABLE 22.1	Guidelines for Glenoid Bone Grafting During Revision to Reversed Shoulder Arthroplasty
Glenoid Bone Defect	*Type of Bone Graft*
Central	
Mild	Cancellous chips
Moderate	Cancellous chips
Severe	Structural (especially one-stage revision)
Peripheral	
Symmetrical	
Mild	Cancellous chips
Moderate	Cancellous chips or structural
Severe	Structural
Asymmetrical	
Mild	Asymmetrical Reaming
Moderate	Asymmetrical reaming or structural
Severe	Structural
Combined	
Symmetrical	
Mild	Cancellous chips
Moderate	Cancellous chips or structural
Severe	Structural
Asymmetrical	
Mild	Asymmetrical reaming
Moderate	Asymmetric reaming or structural
Severe	Structural

Kirchner wires can be left in place until screws have been placed. The first screw should capture the graft and have good purchase in the native glenoid. Variable-angle locking screws can be used but should not be locked to the plate until all screws have been placed and the baseplate maximally compressed. When all of the screws have been placed and locked, the provisional Kirchner wire(s) is removed. It is important to recess the graft that is peripheral to the baseplate to allow complete seating of the glenoid sphere. This can be confirmed with the glenoid sphere trial.

Total Shoulder Arthroplasty to Reverse Shoulder Arthroplasty

By definition, revision of a failed anatomic total shoulder arthroplasty to a RSA always requires reconstruction of at least a central glenoid defect. If the glenoid rim is intact and at least 50% of the glenoid subchondral surface remains, most defects can be reconstructed with minimal reaming and cancellous or nonstructural graft. The guide pin is placed in the appropriate location and inclination, as if the defect were not present. The glenoid surface is reamed just enough to create a conforming surface on the remaining subchondral bone; overreaming should be avoided. The central hole for the central peg of the glenoid baseplate is drilled, and the drill is left in place as a post around which cancellous bone graft is packed into the central defect. The drill and guide pin are then removed, and the glenoid baseplate is inserted and fixed as described earlier.

Severe central defects may also be managed with nonstructural grafts but may require a custom component with a longer central peg. The need for this component can be suspected on the basis of preoperative radiographs or CT scans in many cases. The goals are to obtain some fixation (e.g., 0.5 to 1.0 cm) of the central peg in the native glenoid, achieve stable seating of the periphery of the baseplate on the remaining rim, and place four screws through the baseplate with excellent purchase in the native bone. At least two of these screws should be locking. If, before locking the first two screws, it is determined that the purchase is suboptimal, the remaining screws can be made locking screws. To avoid catastrophic failure of the initial glenoid fixation when the humerus is articulated with the glenoid sphere, bone quality and initial fixation strength must be considered. In general, if the central peg is contained within native bone and at least three screws have excellent purchase (with at least two of them being locking screws), a one-stage revision is safe. These are, of course, merely guidelines, and each case should be individualized.

The guide pin is again placed in the location and inclination that will allow the inferior aspect of the glenoid component to coincide with the inferior aspect of the remaining glenoid rim in neutral inclination. No reaming of the rim or subchondral surface of the glenoid is required. The standard glenoid baseplate is passed over the guide pin to confirm that the central peg contacts the base of the glenoid vault before the periphery contacts the glenoid rim. If it does not, a custom component with a longer central peg will be required. The drill for the central peg of the baseplate is passed over the guide pin, and a hole is drilled into the remaining glenoid bone for a distance of approximately 0.5 to 1.0 cm. Cancellous bone is packed around the drill, the drill and guide pin are removed, and the glenoid base plate is inserted and fixed as described previously. Penetration of the vault is generally well tolerated in this older, sedentary population. However, if bone quality is poor and there is concern for stress fracture, conversion to a two-stage revision is considered.

If the central peg of a standard baseplate does not contact the base of the glenoid before the periphery contacts the remaining glenoid rim and a custom component with an elongated central peg is not available, at least two choices remain. First, one can insert the standard component such that the central peg is impacted into firmly packed cancellous graft and the periphery of the component rests against the remaining rim. Second, a structural allograft containing the baseplate can be placed within the glenoid vault as described later. In either case, the screws are passed through the baseplate and into native bone as described previously. Because the central peg is not contained within native bone, strong consideration should be given to placing the glenoid sphere and the humeral component at a second stage.

If the glenoid rim is deficient, in addition to the central defect, a combined glenoid deficiency exists and reconstruction is even more challenging. Symmetrical combined defects are almost always characterized by a severe central defect and varying degrees of symmetrical, medial erosion of the glenoid rim. In cases of mild to moderate medial erosion (e.g., the remaining rim is equal or lateral to the most lateral extent of the base of the coracoid process), it is often possible to reconstruct the defect with cancellous graft and a RSA in a single sitting. The technique is similar to that described earlier for severe central defects.

Severe symmetrical and moderate to severe asymmetrical combined defects are most often reconstructed using structural bone grafting combined with RSA. Debate exists with regard to the use of allograft or autograft and which bone to use. We have had success using glenoid allografts. An entire scapula allograft is obtained. Although we do not exactly match the allograft size to the native glenoid, we attempt to judge whether a small, medium, or large graft is required. In general, we prefer an undersized allograft so that it fits easily within the remaining, native glenoid vault. Cancellous chips can be added to improve the fit of an undersized graft.

On the back table, the glenoid surface of the allograft is instrumented with a central guide pin so that the inferior aspect of glenoid component coincides with inferior aspect of the glenoid allograft in neutral inclination. The allograft glenoid is then reamed and drilled to accommodate the central peg of the glenoid baseplate. The baseplate is then implanted onto the allograft glenoid surface, without placing the peripheral screws. Care should be taken to align the baseplate so that the superior and inferior holes coincide with the base of the coracoid and the lateral angle of the scapula, respectively. The glenoid process is then detached from the remaining scapular allograft. A burr and rongeur are used to remove bone from the base of the glenoid allograft so that it fits into the native glenoid vault and 0.5 to 1.0 cm of the central peg protrudes from the allograft (Fig. 22.5).

The glenoid allograft is then inserted into the remaining native glenoid so that the inferior aspect of the glenoid baseplate coincides with the projected inferior border of the native glenoid. While the allograft is held in position, the central guide pin is passed through the hole in the glenoid baseplate and into the

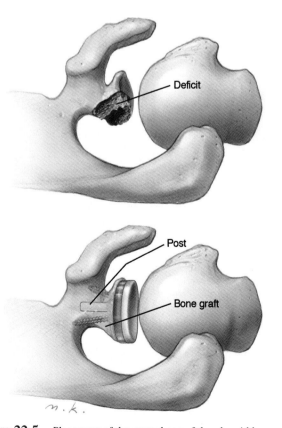

Figure 22.5. Placement of the central peg of the glenoid baseplate in a scapular allograft, removal of the allograft so that 0.5 to 1.0 cm of central peg is exposed and then the prosthetic-allograft composite is impacted into the glenoid bone defect.

native glenoid in neutral inclination. The allograft is then removed, and the drill for the central peg of the glenoid baseplate is used to make a hole 0.5 to 1.0 cm in depth. With the drill in place, cancellous graft is packed into the glenoid vault to ensure that, when the allograft is reinserted, it will have maximum peripheral contact. The drill is removed; the allograft is impacted into the glenoid vault with the central peg in the previously drilled hole. The allograft is provisionally fixed by passing Kirchner wires through the anterior and posterior holes of the glenoid baseplate and into the native glenoid. The inferior and superior screws are then placed. The use of variable-angle locking screws facilitates gaining good purchase within bone. In addition, it is helpful to place both screws in compression mode before locking them. The two provisional Kirchner wires are removed, and the two remaining screws are placed.

Norris (personal communication) has described a similar technique using bicortical iliac crest autograft instead of scapular allograft. The potential advantage of better incorporation must be weighed with the quality of the bone obtained and the morbidity of iliac crest harvest in this often-elderly patient population. In either technique, the principle of fixation in native bone is important.

A decision must be made regarding whether the reconstructed glenoid is strong enough to immediately load with a reverse humeral component. Although no generally accepted guidelines exist, a one-stage revision can probably be performed if overall bone quality is good, a portion of the central peg is contained within native bone, the glenoid allograft is supported throughout 70% to 75% of its circumference by the native glenoid vault, and at least three peripheral screws (at least two of which are locking) have good purchase in native bone. Should these criteria not be filled, it may be safer to allow the glenoid reconstruction to mature for 3 months and return to place the glenoid sphere and humeral component at a second stage (Fig. 22.6).

GLENOID SPHERE AND HUMERAL COMPONENT PLACEMENT

If the glenoid reconstruction has been deemed to be sufficiently stable to allow a one-stage revision, a trial glenoid sphere is placed for later trial reduction. In general, stability will be enhanced if the largest glenoid sphere is used (e.g., 42-mm diameter). However, if the glenoid is small and too much of the glenoid sphere is unsupported by bone, an excessive rocking moment may cause premature loosening of the glenoid component. Under these circumstances, the smaller glenoid sphere is indicated (e.g., 38 mm). If there is any question about whether the inferior portion of the sphere is aligned with or slightly inferior to the inferior glenoid rim, an inferiorly eccentric glenoid sphere component can be used.

The humerus is redelivered into the wound with simultaneous adduction, extension, and external rotation. The trial humeral component is placed in 0 degrees of retroversion. A long-stemmed trial may be used if a cortical defect must be bypassed or if the entire cement mantle, including the distal plug, of a previously cemented prosthesis was removed and created a stress riser. Trial liners of 3-, 6-, and 9-mm are sequentially tested for stability. This test is a rough trial intended to determine whether a 9-mm spacer is required. If the 9-mm liner provides insufficient tension, a 9-mm spacer is added to

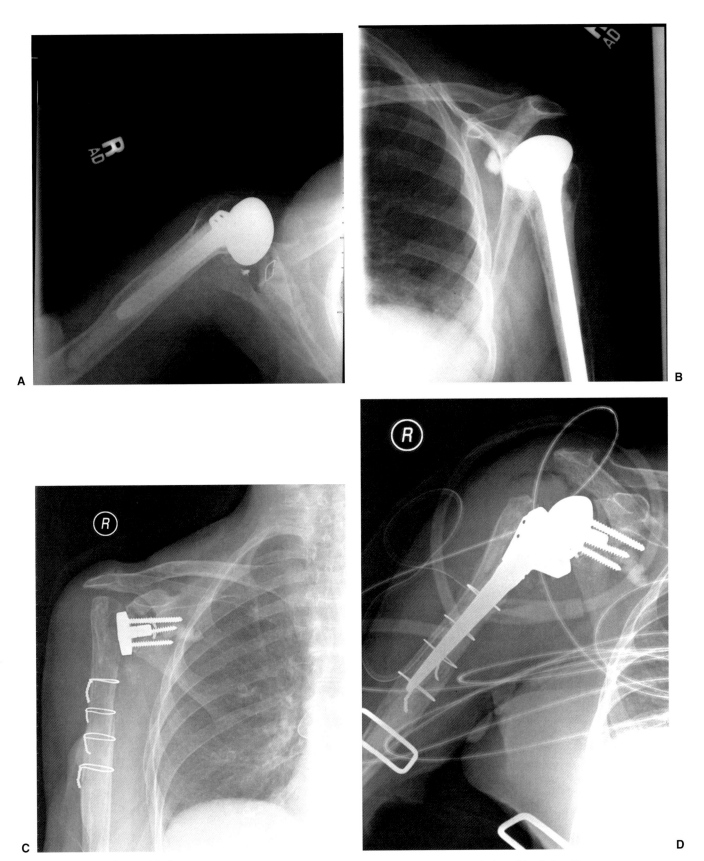

Figure 22.6.   For cases of severe symmetrical and moderate to severe asymmetrical combined glenoid bone defects, the glenoid baseplate can be implanted onto a structural bone graft. The graft prosthetic composite is then fixed into the defect. This 80-year-old woman had severe bone loss following removal of a failed total shoulder arthroplasty (**A,B**). Revision required a two-stage procedure with initial placement of a baseplate allograft composite (**C**). After allowing 3 months for graft incorporation, the glenosphere and humeral components were inserted (**D**).

the trial stem and the 3-, 6-, and 9-mm trial liners are again tested. Through these various combinations, 18 mm of overall humeral length can be recreated. This is usually sufficient, unless circumferential humeral bone loss is present.

The management of humeral bone loss is even more controversial than glenoid bone loss, and there are even fewer guidelines. A detailed discussion of techniques used to manage humeral bone loss is not possible in this chapter. However, in general, we do not reconstruct bone loss during revision of an anatomic arthroplasty to a RSA unless it involves the entire humeral metaphysis or extends into the humeral shaft. Onlay humeral allograft struts are used if the bone loss involves greater than 25% of the circumference of the shaft. A complete proximal humeral allograft is considered if the entire circumference of the shaft or the entire metaphysis is deficient. If any humeral allograft is required, it is performed at this time.

The trial humeral component and glenoid sphere are removed, and the final glenoid sphere is implanted. The humerus is redelivered into the wound, the canal is irrigated, and the final stem is implanted in 0 degrees of retroversion. The stem almost always requires cement. Antibiotic-impregnated cement is routinely used with RSA in our hospital. Once the cement has hardened, the liners are re-trialed. Optimal soft tissue tension is difficult to judge, especially during revision RSA. To accurately judge stability and soft tissue tension, all retractors should be removed. There should be no more than 1 to 2 mm of gapping with distal traction in neutral rotation and 1 to 2 mm of anterior gapping with external rotation. The conjoined tendon should be palpably taught.

Once the appropriate liner has been selected, the humerus is re-dislocated, the trial liner is removed, and the final liner is placed. The humerus is then reduced. Pulse irrigation is used throughout the procedure to help prevent infection. Any portion of the anterior soft tissue envelope that can be reattached to the anterior humeral metaphysis is repaired through drill holes. It may be easier to place these drill holes and fill them with passing sutures before placing the final humeral component. The wound is closed over a closed suction drainage system placed deep to the deltoid and brought out through a separate stab wound.

POSTOPERATIVE CARE

Patients generally are discharged from the hospital on the second postoperative day. They are instructed to keep the operative extremity supported in a sling with a small abduction pillow for the first month to allow the incision to heal and the deltoid to adjust to its new resting length. After the first month, patients are gradually weaned from the sling and instructed to begin using their arms for waist-level activities. Over the following months, patients are permitted to gradually increase the use of their arms as dictated by their comfort level. Maximal function improvement is generally achieved by 4 to 6 months. Unlike in anatomic shoulder arthroplasty, we have found that these patients typically do not benefit from a structured physical therapy program.

RESULTS

The use of RSA for revision arthroplasty is associated with inferior functional results and a higher complication rate when

compared to its use for the treatment of cuff tear arthropathy or massive rotator cuff tears.[11–13] Wall et al reported the results of 191 RSAs at an average of 39.5 months performed at the Clinique Sainte Anne Lumiere in France.[14] For all patients, the Constant score improved from 22.8 to 59.7 and active elevation improved from 86 to 137 degrees. This series included 30 patients who underwent revision from a hemiarthroplasty to a RSA and 24 patients who were converted from a total shoulder arthroplasty to a RSA. For these 54 patients, the average Constant score improved from 19.7 to 52.2 and forward elevation improved from 58 to 118 degrees. The complication rate for patients undergoing revision surgery was 36.7%, compared to 13.3% for primary surgery.

In a multicenter study, Wall et al reported the results for 24 RSAs performed for revision after failed total shoulder arthroplasty.[15] These patients were part of a series of 457 RSAs performed at five institutions in France between 1992 and 2003. Twenty patients were available at an average of 38.3 months after their revision procedure. Active elevation improved from 61 degrees to 113.5 degrees with no significant change in internal rotation and eternal rotation, with the arm at the side or external rotation in 90 degrees of abduction. The Constant score improved from 23.3 to 51.2 with the adjusted Constant score improving form 36.6% to 71.3%. Of the 20 patients, 17 were very satisfied or satisfied with the results of the procedure. There were ten postoperative complications (50%) requiring 6 re-operations. Dislocation accounted for five of the ten complications. The authors concluded that despite the high complication rate, RSA is a valuable tool for the treatment of failed total shoulder arthroplasty with glenohumeral instability or rotator cuff dysfunction.

COMPLICATIONS

The most common serious complication following RSA for revision of failed total shoulder arthroplasty is instability. This can be addressed by increasing the length of the humeral component through the addition of polyethylene or metallic spacers. If additional length fails to improve stability, conversion to a hemiarthroplasty or resection arthroplasty is the only option. Although this may improve that patient's comfort level, it is likely to result in minimal function of the shoulder.

Infection in this situation is a devastating complication. Standard treatment involves removal of the prosthesis and an extended course of intravenous antibiotics. If sufficient bone remains, attempts can be made to reimplant a RSA once the patient is thought to be infection free; however, often there is insufficient bone stock and resection arthroplasty is the only option.

Humeral fractures following RSA can be addressed with the same techniques used following fractures after anatomic arthroplasty. These fractures often occur at areas of bone loss caused by loosening of the previous implant or removal of the old cement mantle.

CONCLUSION

Revision of failed anatomic total shoulder arthroplasty is one of the most difficult problems in shoulder surgery. When these patients have instability resulting from rotator cuff deficiency, it is often impossible to restore stability or significant function with revision to another anatomic prosthesis. The increased conformity and unique biomechanical principals of RSA provide the surgeon with a powerful tool for re-establishing a stable, functional glenohumeral articulation in these patients. Although revision to a RSA represents the best opportunity for functional improvement, it is important for both the surgeon and the patient to appreciate that it is a technically difficult operation, and, even in the most experienced hands, associated with a significant complication rate. As our experience continues to grow, hopefully our ability to identify which patients are at greatest risk for complications and better techniques to avoid them will also improve.

REFERENCES

1. Boileau P, Watkinson DJ, Hatzidakis AM, et al. Grammont reverse prosthesis: design, rationale and biomechanics. *J Shoulder Elbow Surg* 2005;14(1 suppl S):147S–161S.
2. Sanchez-Sotelo J, Sperling JW, Rowland CM, et al. Instability after shoulder arthroplasty: results of surgical treatment. *J Bone Joint Surg Am* 2003;85:622–631.
3. Bohsali KI, Wirth MA, Rockwood CA Jr. Complications of total shoulder arthroplasty. *J Bone Joint Surg Am* 2006;88:2279–2292.
4. Simovitch RW, Helmy N, Zumstein MA, et al. Impact of fatty infiltration of the teres minor muscle on the outcome of reverse total shoulder arthroplasty. *J Bone Joint Surg Am* 207;89:934–939.
5. Walch G, Boulahia A, Calderone S, et al. The "dropping" and "hornblower's" sign in evaluation of rotator cuff tears. *J Bone Joint Surg Br* 1998;80:624–628.
6. Gerber C, Pennington SD, Lingenfelter EJ, et al. Reverse delta III total shoulder replacement combined with latissimus dorsi transfer. *J Bone Joint Surg Am* 2007;89:940–947.
7. Boileau P, Chuinard C, Roussanne Y, et al. Modified latissimus dorsi and teres major transfer through a single deltopectoral approach for external rotation deficit of the shoulder: as an isolated procedure or with a reverse arthroplasty. *J Shoulder Elbow Surg* 2007;16: 671–682.
8. Goldberg SH, Cohen MS, Young M, et al. Thermal tissue damage caused by ultrasonic cement removal from the humerus. *J Bone Joint Surg Am* 2005;87:583–591.
9. Antuña SA, Sperling JW, Cofield RH, et al. Glenoid revision surgery after total shoulder arthroplasty. *J Shoulder Elbow Surg* 2001;10:217–224.
10. Williams GR Jr, Iannotti JP. Options for glenoid bone loss: composites of prosthetics and biologics. *J Shoulder Elbow Surg* 2007;16(5 suppl):S267–S272.
11. Werner CML, Steinmann PA, Gilbart M, et al. Treatment of painful pseudoparesis due to irreparable rotator cuff dysfunction with the delta III reverse-ball-and-socket total shoulder prosthesis. *J Bone Joint Surg Am* 2005;87:1476–1486.
12. Boileau P, Watkinson D, Hatzidakis AM, et al. Neer award 2005: the Grammont reverse shoulder prosthesis—results in cuff tear arthritis, fracture sequelae, and revision arthroplasty. *J Shoulder and Elbow Surg* 2005;15:527–540.
13. Frankle M, Siegal S, Pupello D, et al. The reverse shoulder prosthesis for glenohumeral arthritis associated with severe rotator cuff deficiency. *J Bone Joint Surg Am* 2005;87: 1697–1705.
14. Wall B, Nové-Josserand L, O'Connor DP, et al. Reverse total shoulder arthroplasty: a review of results according to etiology. *J Bone Joint Surg Am* 2007;89:1476–1485.
15. Wall B, Walch G, Jouve F, et al. The reverse shoulder prosthesis for revision of failed shoulder arthroplasty. In: Walch G, Boileau P, Molè D, et al, eds. *Nice Shoulder Course: Reverse Shoulder Arthroplasty.* Paris: Sauramps Medical; 2006:231–242.

Mark Tauber
Herbert Resch

Prosthetic Arthroplasty for Delayed Complications of Proximal Humerus Fractures

INTRODUCTION

Independent of primary fracture management, proximal humerus fractures are at risk for a variety of secondary complications. The time interval between the initial injury and the onset of symptoms is often unpredictable. One may distinguish between specific fracture-related complications and complications associated with fractures in general. Regarding the fracture, variables such as comminution, significant fragment displacement, open injuries, involvement of the articular surface, fracture dislocation, and delayed operative treatment are viewed as negative prognostic factors. General unfavorable factors include advanced age of the patient, reduced general health status, metabolic diseases such as diabetes, and nicotine or alcohol abuse. Vascular impairment through periosteal and vessel disruption represents a main reason for further complications.

Humeral head replacement is a common option for treatment[1–4] for acute proximal humerus fractures, especially in elderly patients with four-part proximal humerus fractures. The results of primary hemiarthroplasty[1,5–7] are reported to be superior to those after late prosthetic surgery.[8–13]

Possible delayed complications of proximal humerus fractures are avascular necrosis,[11] tuberosity malunion[14] or nonunion,[15] nonunion of the surgical neck,[16] or a locked chronic fracture dislocation.[17,18] Usually, all are associated with pain and restriction of shoulder motion, so that prosthetic humeral head replacement may become necessary in many of these cases. Salvage shoulder arthroplasty for the late sequelae of proximal humerus fractures is a technically demanding procedure whose main objective is to relieve pain and improve shoulder function. Distorted glenohumeral anatomy, significant soft-tissue scarring, as well as potential rotator cuff deficiency make the implantation of the prosthesis often difficult.

In the literature, several authors have reported their experience with prosthetic shoulder arthroplasty for delayed complications of proximal humerus fractures (Table 23.1). In a multicenter study including 203 patients, Boileau et al[8] proposed a novel radiographic classification of proximal humerus fracture sequelae consisting of four types. Impacted fractures with humeral head collapse or necrosis (type 1) and irreducible dislocations or fracture-dislocations (type 2) showed predictably good results after nonconstrained shoulder arthroplasty. In these groups, total shoulder arthroplasty yielded better results than humeral head replacement. Among patients with nonunion of the surgical neck (type 3) and severe tuberosity malunion (type 4), both groups in which osteotomy of the greater tuberosity was necessary, the outcome after nonconstrained prosthetic shoulder replacement was poor. They recommend peg bone grafting[19] or a low-profile fracture prosthesis for type 3 and the use of reverse arthroplasty for type 4.

Mansat et al[12] outlined the crucial role of cuff integrity, as well as avoidance of greater tuberosity osteotomy for satisfactory results after secondary shoulder arthroplasty in 28 patients. In cases with major displacement of the greater tuberosity, the results are unpredictable when osteotomy must be performed.

Norris et al[13] reviewed 23 patients with late prosthetic shoulder arthroplasty after failed treatment of three-part and four-part proximal humerus fractures. Most were treated with total shoulder arthroplasty, with the necessity for tuberosity osteotomy in 50% of patients. These results were reported to be satisfactory but inferior to those reported for acute humeral head replacement. Additionally, they emphasized that late surgery for failed early treatment is technically difficult.

Bosch et al[1] observed statistically better outcomes concerning the University of California–Los Angeles and Constant scores in acute humeral head replacement than after late (at least 4 weeks) hemiarthroplasty in elderly patients. Thus they recommended making the decision to perform prosthetic humeral head replacement as early as possible after trauma.

Frich et al[11] compared their results with primary and secondary shoulder arthroplasty after complex proximal humerus fractures. They noted better results concerning pain relief, active motion, and function in acute cases. Most of the secondary cases had total shoulder replacement. In the chronic group, the original fracture pattern did not have a statistically significant impact

TABLE 23.1	Literature Overview of Secondary Shoulder Replacement in Posttraumatic Cases with Type of Prosthesis					
Author	Cases	HHR/TSA	GT Osteotomy	Satisfactory Results (%)	Complications (%)	Revision (%)
Neer et al,[33] 1982	35	0/35	NA	56	NA	NA
Frich et al,[11] 1991	27	4/23	NA	15	26	NA
Habermayer et al,[32] 1992	18	7/11	NA	32	NA	NA
Postel et al,[34] 1995	48	19/39	9	19	12.5	12.5
Norris et al[13] (1995)	23	6/17	13	NA	26	21
Boileau et al,[9] 2001	71	46/25	13	42	27	5.6
Antuña et al,[14] 2002	50	25/25	24	50	6	14
Mansat et al,[12] 2004	28	20/8	3	64	3.5	3.5
Boileau et al,[8] 2006	203	119/84	19	88	27	12

GT, greater tuberosity; HHR, humeral head replacement; TSA, total shoulder arthroplasty.

on the results. They concluded that failed primary treatment reduces the possibility of a good result with revision arthroplasty.

Based on the literature, it can be said that late prosthetic arthroplasty in proximal humerus fractures is associated with inferior results compared to those of primary humeral head replacement. However, in our practice, primary prosthetic management is justified in elderly patients only with a comminuted fracture pattern and associated cuff deficiency. Primary implantation of a reverse shoulder prosthesis seems to be a reasonable alternative in this group of patients of advanced age and porotic bone. As the results after primary humeral head replacement are also not clearly convincing,[4] we believe that humeral head–preserving management should be the treatment of choice for this group of patients. Only those cases in which reconstruction seems to be unachievable do we opt for prosthetic replacement. Our regimen of fracture management is primary minimally invasive stabilization, even in complex proximal humerus fractures with percutaneous screw fixation of the tuberosities to achieve good alignment of the tuberosities with restored anatomy of the humeral head. Thus secondary tuberosity osteotomy can be avoided, which is reported to be the main negative prognostic factor in late prosthetic arthroplasty. Therefore initial trauma management should be directed toward anatomic reduction and, if possible, minimally invasive fracture stabilization.

Maintenance of the anatomic shape of the proximal humerus, even in cases in which some head collapse has taken place, makes implantation of the humeral component easier and contributes to preservation of the rotator cuff.

DIAGNOSTICS

CLINICAL EVALUATION

A meticulous clinical examination represents a critical part in the evaluation of patients with shoulder complaints. First, muscle atrophy at the shoulder should be assessed with careful attention directed at the integrity of the deltoid, particularly among those patients who have previously undergone attempted open reduction and internal fixation. Muscle function of the infraspinatus, supraspinatus, and subscapularis tendons should be evaluated.

However, in patients with malunion or nonunion of the tuberosities, the status of the rotator cuff can be difficult to determine because of stiffness and inhibition of muscle firing as a result of pain.

RADIOLOGICAL EVALUATION

As primary imaging diagnostics, shoulder radiographs should be obtained. Standard views are an anteroposterior view with the adducted arm in neutral position and an axillary view with the arm abducted at 90 degrees in the scapular plane. If an axillary view is not possible to obtain because of shoulder stiffness, a transscapular view can be obtained as a second view. Radiological signs vary from discreet sclerotic subchondral changes to complete collapse of the head. The early subchondral necrotic areas (Fig. 23.1), which can cause nonspecific, subtle shoulder pain, are not visible by standard radiographs. In suspicious cases, magnetic resonance imaging (MRI) is the

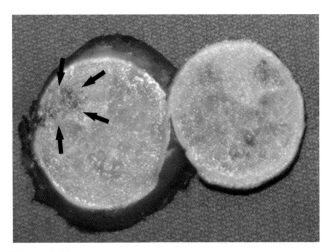

Figure 23.1. In the subchondral area of the resected articular humeral head segment, necrotic cancellous bone tissue can be seen *(arrows)*. This early stage of avascular humeral head necrosis is not visible on normal radiographs, but it can only be seen on magnetic resonance imaging.

diagnostic tool of choice. Often, the necrosis is accompanied by malunion of the tuberosities with deformity of the proximal humerus. Sometimes, posttraumatic osteoarthritis can be seen, with narrowing of the glenohumeral joint line and presence of caudal osteophytes at the humeral head and inferior glenoid pole. From the acromiohumeral distance, indirect conclusions can be drawn regarding the condition of the rotator cuff. A reduced subacromial space is almost always due to a rotator cuff defect involving at least two tendons. In the case of clinically presumed rotator cuff defects, further imaging diagnosis using MRI should be performed. On the axillary view, glenohumeral subluxation can be assessed in the anteroposterior direction, as well as inclination of the glenoid. This is important in those cases in which total shoulder arthroplasty should be performed. Bony glenoid rim defects of a certain amount represent the indication for bone grafting to restore the glenoid bone stock for implantation of the glenoid component. In primary operatively treated proximal humerus fractures, frequently osteosynthesis material such as screws, plates, or pins are still in situ, with the necessity for removal before performing prosthetic shoulder arthroplasty. A clear radiographic evaluation of the positioning and possible osseous incorporation of the implants can be very useful before humeral head replacement.

Computed tomography (CT) scanning with three-dimensional reconstruction can provide additional information about posttraumatic deformity with exact representation of the humeral head. In addition, bony defects of the glenoid are clearly visible on the axial slices of the CT scan. To evaluate nonunion of the tuberosities or the surgical neck, CT is more reliable than conventional radiographs.

Further imaging by MRI provides important information concerning the soft tissue envelope but is required only in exceptional cases. In contrast to radiography and CT, MRI can detect early stages of avascular head necrosis. Rotator cuff deficiency with secondary muscle belly changes as fatty infiltration or muscle atrophy can be shown. This is of crucial importance with regard to the final functional outcome after shoulder arthroplasty. Due to the fact that degenerative histological muscle changes are irreversible, the functional outcome to expect in patients with chronic rotator cuff deficiency is only moderate, even if hardware implantation has been performed correctly.

CLASSIFICATION

Faced with the enormous variability of secondary posttraumatic complications and their diversity of combinations, introducing a reliable and clear system of classification, from which conclusions for treatment can be drawn, is not simple. Originally, the fracture sequelae were grouped as a heterogeneous series within which various different lesions coexisted, such as malunion with avascular humeral head necrosis, nonunion, or a locked fracture-dislocation. Most studies about late shoulder arthroplasty in proximal humerus fracture reported in the literature do not take into account the heterogeneity of delayed posttraumatic complications and do not allow any conclusion regarding the treatment. However, it is obvious that different complications have to be considered individually regarding secondary prosthetic shoulder arthroplasty. Therefore, in

accordance with Boileau et al,[8] we recommend classifying late posttraumatic complications as follows:

- Posttraumatic avascular humeral head necrosis
- Tuberosity malunion
- Surgical neck nonunion
- Chronic fracture dislocation

Obviously, overlapping forms can make differentiation sometimes difficult, but generally, classification of fracture sequelae should be possible.

In this chapter, we will focus only on the posttraumatic avascular humeral head necrosis and tuberosity malunion; prosthetic shoulder arthroplasty in surgical neck nonunion and chronic fracture dislocation are dealt by with other authors (see References).

POSTTRAUMATIC AVASCULAR NECROSIS OF THE HUMERAL HEAD

The risk for development of posttraumatic avascular head necrosis is mostly determined by the type of fracture. An incidence between 3% and 14% has been reported for three-part fractures and 13% to 34% for four-part fractures.[20–22] Brooks et al[23] and Gerber et al[24] emphasized the importance of the ascending branch of the anterior circumflex artery (Fig. 23.2) and its intraosseous continuation, the arcuate artery for the blood supply of the humeral head. As in four-part fractures, the arcuate artery is disrupted and the blood supply to the humeral head is

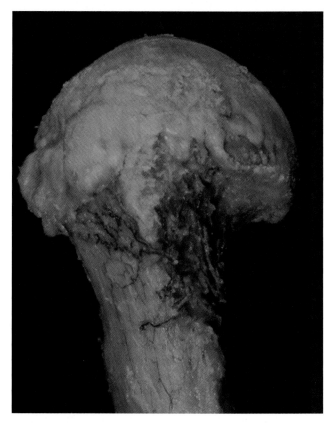

Figure 23.2. Anatomic specimen showing the anterior arterial supply of the proximal humeral head by the anterior circumflex artery.

provided only by the branches entering the head on the postero-medial side of the humeral neck.[23,25,26] Hertel et al[25] published on a diminished blood supply in cases with a medial displacement of 2 mm of the shaft. Hausberger et al[27] reported a study in which that disruption of the periosteum on the medial side of the neck displacing the shaft 6 mm to the lateral direction and 9 mm to the medial direction jeopardized the blood supply to the humeral head. Based on these observations, the quality of vascularity of a four-part fractured humeral head can be assessed roughly only by checking the radiographs at the time of injury.

The time interval between injury and the first hints of radiological changes is unpredictable and ranges from several months to several years. The patient's complaints are usually very non-specific at the beginning and may lead to severe pain and restriction of movement in the advanced stage.

Avascular necrosis has been classified by Ficat and Arlet[28] and was modified by Cruess[29] for the humeral head, as follows:

- Stage I: No radiographic evidence of necrosis
- Stage II: Presence of mottled sclerosis

- Stage III: Subchondral fracturing, crescent sign, occasionally with flattening of articular surface (Fig. 23.3).
- Stage IV: Collapse of subchondral bone, loss of humeral head sphericity (Fig. 23.4)
- Stage V: Stage IV plus glenoid arthrosis (Fig. 23.5)

Due to the collapse of the head in advanced cases (stage IV and V), the center of rotation of the humeral head is displaced medially (medialization of the center of rotation) and is associated with a restricted capsule and shortened rotator cuff muscles adapted to the changed position of the center of rotation. This has to be taken into consideration when inserting a humeral head component of normal size and even more when total shoulder arthroplasty is planned with insertion of a glenoid component. Extensive soft tissue management with capsule release on the humeral as well as on the glenoid side is of utmost importance in these cases to avoid overstuffing followed by pain and postoperative stiffness. Depending on the position of the tuberosities, two different types must be distinguished, as discussed in the following sections.

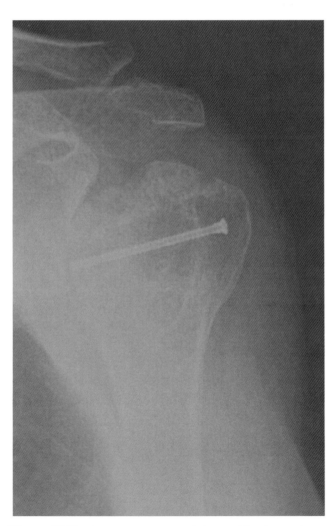

Figure 23.3. A stage III posttraumatic humeral head necrosis after operative primary fracture treatment showing subchondral fracturing (crescent sign). Note that the sphericity of the articular segment is conserved.

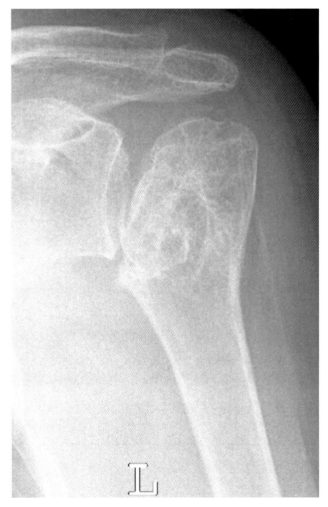

Figure 23.4. Stage IV is characterized by the collapse of subchondral bone and loss of the humeral head sphericity. The majority of patients undergoing shoulder arthroplasty for posttraumatic avascular necrosis have this stage of pathology.

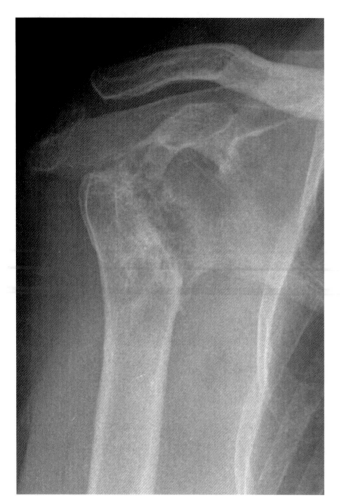

Figure 23.5. In stage V, the glenoid shows degenerative changes. In this advanced stage, the center of rotation is medialized and the surrounding soft tissue envelope has adapted to this biomechanically changed situation.

Avascular Necrosis with Good Alignment of the Tuberosities

In cases with good alignment of the tuberosities, the bony conditions for insertion of the humeral component are similar to that found in idiopathic arthrosis. Two features make arthroplasty in this setting slightly different. First, bone at the resection and preparation of the humerus can be more challenging because of callus formation, and quite often the canal for the stem has to be prepared in the metaphyseal region by means of a high-speed drill. In these cases, a stemless component can be considered if there is distortion of the shaft and the proximal bone quality is good. Second, focus has to be laid on soft tissue management. Because of the change of the position of the center of rotation in advanced cases, the soft tissue around the joint has adapted to the medialized head position. Elasticity of the soft tissue has been lost by preoperative restriction of motion and stiffness. Capsule release has to be performed first on the humeral side where the capsule is stripped off from the humeral neck. This allows better external rotation of the humeral head and gives better access to the glenoid. After the head is resected, the capsule surrounding the glenoid is released from the glenoid rim (circular capsule release). Gentle mobilization of the subscapularis

muscle on both sides between scapula and muscle and between muscle and conjoint tendon is performed, the latter by blunt dissection. Insertion of a normal-size head component might cause a so-called relative overstuffing followed by restriction of range of motion. A smaller head size might be indicated in such cases.

Avascular Necrosis with Malunion of the Tuberosities

These cases usually present with severe pain, a collapsed and distorted head, and severe glenohumeral joint stiffness. Extensive soft tissue releases, as described previously, are mandatory. CT examination with three-dimensional reconstruction is very useful in these cases for preoperative planning. Because of the pull of the infraspinatus and supraspinatus muscles during fracture healing, the greater tuberosity frequently heals in the posterior and sometimes the cranial position. The posterior displacement of the greater tuberosity creates a huge posterior offset. The center of rotation is determined by the insertion of the rotator cuff, so this also changes its position in a posterior direction. The humeral component has to adapt to this position to cover the resection area as much as possible.

It has been reported in the literature that correction osteotomy of the greater tuberosity has shown disappointing results and therefore should be avoided.[9,21] We agree with this conclusion except in those cases in which the posterior displacement is too excessive and exceeds 1 cm because such a significant displacement cannot be dealt with by a prosthesis, even a third-generation design. Cranial displacement is easier to handle by the length of the prosthesis, and osteotomy is rarely necessary. In the case of osteotomy, fixation of the osteotomized tuberosity with circular wire cerclage is recommended (Fig. 23.6).

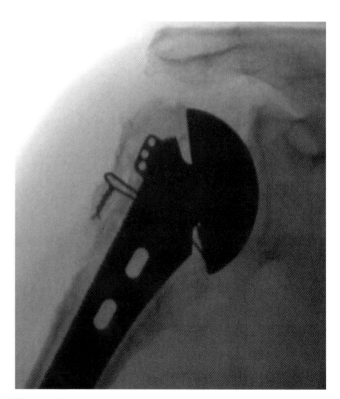

Figure 23.6. Cerclage fixation of the osteotomized greater tuberosity after implantation of the humeral component. Note the anatomic alignment from the tip of the greater tuberosity to the head component of the prosthesis.

Arthritis of Glenoid

Surprisingly, no arthritic changes of the glenoid are seen in most cases with posttraumatic head necrosis, even in advanced cases. Therefore total shoulder arthroplasty is rarely necessary. It is our experience that more often we have had to insert a glenoid component because of destruction of the glenoid by penetration or protrusion of screws rather than by arthritic changes. In contrast to what is seen in idiopathic arthritis, the version of the glenoid is almost never changed and the bone stock is of good quality. Yet, insertion of the glenoid component might be a challenge because of scarring and glenoid exposure might be difficult. Extended soft tissue release is crucial and is a prerequisite for total shoulder replacement.

Condition of the Rotator Cuff

Although discussed in the literature, large rotator cuff tears are rarely seen. This might be explained by the relatively young age of the patients and by the restricted movement in the posttraumatic time period.

Because existing tears are usually small, tendon repair back to the footprint is recommended at the time of prosthetic replacement and hemiarthroplasty is performed. To lower the tension on the repaired tendon, a smaller head size might be used. In the rare case of a large tear, insertion of a reverse prosthesis might be taken into consideration.

Absorption of Tuberosities

In contrast to primary arthroplasty in acute fracture cases, partial absorption or complete resorption of tuberosities is rarely seen in secondary cases. If not healed in the correct position, they are consolidated in malposition and the decision as to whether correction osteotomy should be performed is made on an individual basis (see earlier discussion). In the rare case of an absent tuberosity (Fig. 23.7), insertion of a reverse prosthesis is indicated and as with hemiarthroplasty the outcome is unsatisfying.

Type of Prosthesis

NONCONSTRAINED PROSTHESIS As in most cases, the rotator cuff is intact and hemiarthroplasty is the treatment of choice.

Stemmed Hemiprosthesis Modern design prostheses of the third generation are helpful for the adaptation of the head component to the altered anatomy. Although the variability of adaptation differs between prostheses within the third generation design, the position of the head remains connected to the orthopaedic humeral shaft axis and sets the limits of adaptability.

Stemless Prosthesis Two types of design have to be differentiated, as follows:

1. **Articular segment prosthesis:** With this type of stemless prosthesis, the entire articular segment is replaced with a cut performed at the anatomic neck. This type has proved to be very effective because positioning of the head component on the cut area can be performed independently from the orthopaedic axis of the shaft. The hard bone usually found

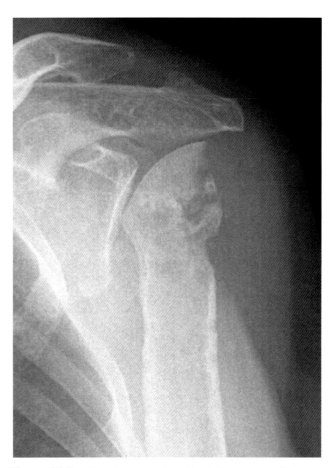

Figure 23.7. Complete resorption of both the greater and lesser tuberosity after open reduction and internal fixation of a four-segment proximal humeral head fracture. In these disastrous cases without a functional rotator cuff, the only promising solution is implantation of a reverse prosthesis.

at the level of the anatomic neck provides a good grip for the hollow screw with sufficient primary stability for the head component.

2. **Surface replacement prosthesis:** In younger patients with good bone stock and preserved sphericity of the head (stage II and III), this type of prosthesis is indicated as long as the head is not significantly distorted. In cases with severely displaced tuberosities, the position of the resurfacing cup is bound to the articular surface, not allowing adaptation to the changed anatomy.

CONSTRAINED PROSTHESIS (REVERSE PROSTHESIS) There are two indications for this type of prosthesis, as follows:

1. **Rotator cuff deficiency:** In the case of a large rotator cuff tear, involving more than one tendon, repair of the rotator cuff might not be successful. The same can be said in the case of partial tuberosity absorption or complete resorption.

2. **Severe head distortion:** In cases in which the anatomy is significantly distorted, despite adaptability of the humeral component and osteotomy of the tuberosities is not an option, a reverse prosthesis might be considered as an alternative. The older the patient, the more this type of prosthesis is indicated.

MALUNION OF TUBEROSITIES (WITHOUT HEAD NECROSIS)

Malunion after displaced humeral head fractures can be seen after conservative treatment, inadequate reduction at the time of reconstructive surgery, or re-displacement after adequate reduction in the postoperative course. Because of the distorted head, the major complaints of patients are pain and functional restriction. Meticulous analysis of the displaced fragments by CT scanning with three-dimensional reconstruction is crucial for the treatment. Basically, we have to differentiate between two indications for prosthetic replacement, as follows:

1. **Posttraumatic arthritis:** Arthritis is caused by the incongruity of the joint and altered biomechanics after a displaced humeral head fracture. According to the experience of the authors, arthritis will typically develop only if the patient has regained good movement after the trauma. As with most posttraumatic cases, the rotator cuff is usually intact; thus total shoulder arthroplasty is the treatment of choice. In cases with a major rotator cuff defect, the decision between nonconstrained or constrained (reverse) prosthesis has to be made individually.

2. **Distorted head:** For treatment, whether prosthetic replacement is indicated or not, the position of the articular fragment in relation to the shaft and to the tuberosities is important.
   - *Articular fragment in good alignment with tuberosities, but in poor alignment with the shaft:* This is an indication for correction osteotomy, not an indication for prosthetic replacement.
   - *Articular fragment in good alignment with the shaft and tuberosities in malposition:* Because the articular fragment is in good position to the shaft there is no reason to replace the articular fragment with a humeral component. Correction osteotomy of the tuberosity, which is in most cases is the greater tuberosity, may be recommended.
   - *Articular fragment in valgus position and tuberosities in almost normal position:* This type is seen as late sequelae after impacted valgus type fractures with a depressed head fragment and avulsed tuberosities. A correction osteotomy of the articular fragment, which has to be carried out at the level of the anatomic neck and may lead to head necrosis, is typically not performed. The preferred option is a cemented hemiarthroplasty with a stem.
   - *Articular fragment in poor alignment with both the shaft and the tuberosities:* This extremely distorted head is seen as a late sequela after conservative treatment of true four-part fractures in which the depressed articular fragment is severely displaced laterally, pushing away the tuberosities, which have consolidated in malposition to the shaft as well. Cemented hemiarthroplasty with stem is indicated. If possible, the tuberosities should be left in place without osteotomy. In severe cases, it might be necessary to perform osteotomy of one or both, which is fixed to the prosthesis by means of circular wire cerclage, as carried out in acute four-part fractures.

In the literature, poor outcomes are reported after osteotomy of the greater tuberosity.[9,12] Boileau et al[9] published a comparison study of cases with and without osteotomy of the greater tuberosity and found significantly better outcomes in those patients without an osteotomy. The best outcome was found in the intracapsular impacted cases (type C) because it was not nec-

essary to perform an osteotomy. The worst outcome was seen in the so-called extracapsular-disimpacted group in which osteotomy was performed because of the severe displacement. The authors conclude that osteotomy of the greater tuberosity, therefore, should be avoided. Antuna et al[14] reported a similar experience with osteotomy of the greater tuberosity. They published their findings that 42% of the osteotomized tuberosities did not heal in the correct position, resulting in nonunion, malunion, or resorption. These authors,[14] as well as Neer,[30] recommend accepting even slight varus or valgus position of the prosthesis to avoid osteotomy of the greater tuberosity. In contrast, isolated osteotomy of the lesser tuberosity had no negative influence on the outcome.[9,31]

We agree with these authors that osteotomy of the greater tuberosity should be avoided whenever possible. The prosthesis should be adapted to the distorted anatomy of the proximal humerus, accepting some minor anatomic inaccuracy. The prosthesis should be adapted to the distorted anatomy and not the proximal humerus to the prosthesis.

Despite this, in cases with severe displacement of the greater tuberosity, individual decisions have to be made depending on the amount of displacement, bone quality, experience with fixation, and so on. In our experience, in cases in which there is greater than 1 cm posterior displacement one may consider a corrective osteotomy.

To grade the malunion of the tuberosities in patients with posttraumatic avascular humeral head necrosis on the preoperative radiographs, we introduced two novel parameters that have been shown to have high intraobserver and interobserver reliability. The greater tuberosity offset describes the amount of lateral or medial displacement of the greater tuberosity in a coronal plane and is defined as the orthogonal distance between the longitudinal humeral shaft axis and the medial border of the greater tuberosity at the edge of the articular surface (Fig. 23.8).

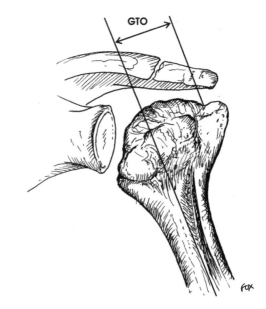

Figure 23.8. An anteroposterior drawing of stage IV humeral head necrosis shows the collapsed head with the greater tuberosity in the lateralized position and valgus malunion. For greater tuberosity offset measurement, the line of reference is given by the humeral shaft axis. The perpendicular distance from this axis to the medial edge of the greater tuberosity represents the greater tuberosity offset.

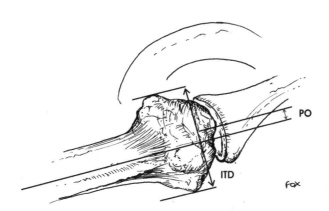

Figure 23.9. The preoperative radiographic parameters intertubicular distance (ITD) and posterior offset were measured on the axial view. The graphic shows the collapsed articular segment with a widened ITD. The distance from the midpoint of this intertubercular line to the humeral shaft axis represents the posterior offset.

This is measured on a true anteroposterior radiograph with the adducted arm in neutral position and recorded in millimeters. Posterior offset is defined as the posterior displacement of the intertubercular midpoint relative to the longitudinal axis of the humeral shaft on an axial view (Fig 23.9). A posterior offset situated anteriorly to the longitudinal shaft axis is defined as a negative value. This distance is measured in millimeters and is an indication of humeral head widening. Normal values for greater tuberosity offset (average, 10.15 mm), ITD (average, 42.24 mm), and posterior offset (average, 4.11 mm), were determined after studying 100 normal shoulder radiographs taken in two planes orthogonal to one another in patients between 50 and 80 years old.

In our own series of secondary prosthetic shoulder arthroplasty in posttraumatic avascular humeral head necrosis, we observed a statistically significant difference concerning the functional outcome and pain level in favor of those patients with good tuberosity alignment, which was quantified on the basis of the novel radiographic parameters (unpublished data).[35] Patients with severe deformity of the proximal humerus resulting from tuberosity malunion had poor midterm to long-term results after shoulder replacement. Based on our experience, we strongly recommend initial trauma management directed toward anatomic restoration of the proximal humerus using minimally invasive techniques for fracture stabilization, if possible. Thus, in the case of late prosthetic shoulder arthroplasty, the anatomic configuration of the proximal humerus allows unproblematic positioning of the humeral component, avoiding tuberosity osteotomy, providing satisfying functional results.

SURGICAL TECHNIQUE

The patient is in the half-sitting position. A deltopectoral approach is used as a standard approach. All of the adhesions in the subacromial space and between subscapularis and the conjoined tendon are removed. Implant material from reconstructive surgery, such as plates and screws, is removed. The tendon of the subscapularis muscle is incised approximately 1 cm from the insertion on the lesser tuberosity. The capsule is detached from the neck of the humerus, allowing for bet-

ter external rotation and exposure of the humeral head. The head is resected using the cutting guide instrumentation. The glenoid is exposed by means of a retractor. The capsule is incised all around the glenoid to create a circular capsule release. Beneath the subscapularis, gentle mobilization is carried out by means of an elevator to gain length of this muscle for reattachment on the lesser tuberosity. Meticulous soft tissue management is mandatory in all cases because stiffness is a dominating preoperative symptom. In patients with avascular necrosis and severe collapse of the head, soft tissue is adapted to this medialized head position. Implantation of the humeral component will require additional space. To avoid overstuffing of the joint, length has to be gained by capsule and tendon mobilization.

HINTS FOR ADAPTATION OF THE HUMERAL COMPONENT TO THE DISTORTED ANATOMY OF THE PROXIMAL HUMERUS

To obtain more flexibility for the humeral component to meet the requirements of the distorted anatomy, a thin stem that is cemented in the shaft is recommended. This gives the opportunity to position the humeral component in a varus or valgus position or permits placement with an increased posterior offset. This will help to avoid osteotomy of the tuberosity in most cases.

Osteotomy of Greater Tuberosity

Although performed rarely in severely displaced tuberosities, there are some technical aspects that will help promote the healing process. When performing the osteotomy it is important that the chisel be placed in an oblique position to create an oblique osteotomy area as large as possible. This provides a larger contact area when the fragment is shifted laterally. The periosteum connecting the tuberosity distally with the shaft should only be elevated, but not cut, to preserve blood supply via this soft tissue link. Fixation is performed with circular wire cerclage. Bone graft may be harvested from the resected head and placed to promote early bony healing.

REFERENCES

1. Bosch U, Skutek M, Fremerey RW, et al. Outcome after primary and secondary hemiarthroplasty in elderly patients with fractures of the proximal humerus. *J Shoulder Elbow Surg* 1998;7:479–484.
2. Mighell MA, Kolm GP, Collinge CA, et al. Outcomes of hemiarthroplasty for fractures of the proximal humerus. *J Shoulder Elbow Surg* 2003;12:569–577.
3. Moeckel BH, Dines DM, Warren RF, et al. Modular hemiarthroplasty for fractures of the proximal part of the humerus. *J Bone Joint Surg Am* 1992;74:884–889.
4. Zyto K, Wallace WA, Frostick SP, et al. Outcome after hemiarthroplasty for three- and four-part fractures of the proximal humerus. *J Shoulder Elbow Surg* 1998;7:85–89.
5. Goldman RT, Koval KJ, Cuomo F, et al. Functional outcome after humeral head replacement for acute three- and four-part proximal humeral fractures. *J Shoulder Elbow Surg* 1995;4:81–86.
6. Green A, Barnard L, Limbard R. Humeral head replacement for acute four-part proximal humerus fractures. *J Shoulder Elbow Surg* 1993;2:249–254.
7. Hawkins R, Switlyk P. Acute prosthetic replacement for severe fractures of the proximal humerus. *Clin Orthop* 1993;289:156–160.
8. Boileau P, Chuinard C, Le Huec JC, et al. Proximal humerus fracture sequelae: impact of a new radiographic classification on arthroplasty. *Clin Orthop Relat Res* 2006;442:121–130.
9. Boileau P, Trojani C, Walch G, et al. Shoulder arthroplasty for the treatment of the sequelae of fractures of the proximal humerus. *J Shoulder Elbow Surg* 2001;10:299–308.
10. Dines DM, Klarren RF, Altcheck DW, et al. Posttraumatic changes of the proximal humerus: malunion, nonunion, and osteonecrosis: treatment with modular hemiarthroplasty or total shoulder arthroplasty. *J Shoulder Elbow Surg* 1993;2:11–21.
11. Frich LH, Sojbjerg JO, Sneppen O. Shoulder arthroplasty in complex acute and chronic proximal humeral fractures. *Orthopedics* 1991;14:949–954.

12. Mansat P, Guity MR, Bellumore Y, et al. Shoulder arthroplasty for late sequelae of proximal humeral fractures. *J Shoulder Elbow Surg* 2004;13:305–312.

13. Norris TR, Green A, McGuigan FX. Late prosthetic shoulder arthroplasty for displaced proximal humerus fractures. *J Shoulder Elbow Surg* 1995;4:271–280.

14. Antuña SA, Sperling JW, Sanchez-Sotelo J, et al. Shoulder arthroplasty for proximal humeral malunions: long-term results. *J Shoulder Elbow Surg* 2002;11:122–129.

15. Antuña SA, Sperling JW, Sanchez-Sotelo J, et al. Shoulder arthroplasty for proximal humeral nonunions. *J Shoulder Elbow Surg* 2002;11:114–121.

16. Galatz LM, Iannotti JP. Management of surgical neck nonunions. *Orthop Clin North Am* 2000;31:51–61.

17. Cheng SL, Mackay MB, Richards RR. Treatment of locked posterior fracture dislocations of the shoulder by total shoulder arthroplasty. *J Shoulder Elbow Surg* 1997;6:11–17.

18. Sperling JW, Pring M, Antuna SA, et al. Shoulder arthroplasty for locked posterior dislocation of the shoulder. *J Shoulder Elbow Surg* 2004;13:522–527.

19. Walch G, Badet R, Novè-Josserand L, et al. Nonunions of the surgical neck of the humerus: surgical treatment with an intramedullary bone peg, internal fixation, and cancellous bone grafting. *J Shoulder Elbow Surg* 1996;5:161–168.

20. Darder A, Darder A Jr, Sanchis V, et al. Four-part displaced proximal humeral fractures: operative treatment using Kirschner wires and a tension band. *J Orthop Trauma* 1993;7:497–505.

21. Neer CS. Displaced proximal humeral fractures: II. Treatment of three-part and four-part displacement. *J Bone Joint Surg Am* 1970;52:1090–1103.

22. Sturzenegger M, Fornaro E, Jakob RP. Results of surgical treatment of multifragmented fractures of the humeral head. *Arch Orthop Trauma Surg* 1982;100:249–259.

23. Brooks CH, Revell WJ, Heatley FW. Vascularity of the humeral head after proximal humeral fractures: an anatomical cadaver study. *J Bone Joint Surg Br* 1993;75:132–136.

24. Gerber C, Schneeberger AG, Vinh TS. The arterial vascularization of the humeral head: an anatomical study. *J Bone Joint Surg Am* 1990;72:1486–1494.

25. Hertel R, Hempfing A, Stiehler M, et al. Predictors of humeral head ischemia after intracapsular fracture of the proximal humerus. *J Shoulder Elbow Surg* 2004;13:427–433.

26. Resch H, Beck E, Bayley I. Reconstruction of the valgus-impacted humeral head fracture. *J Shoulder Elbow Surg* 1995;4:73–80.

27. Hausberger K, Resch H, Maurer H. Blood supply of intraarticular fractures of the humeral head: an anatomical and biomechanical study. Presented at the 14th Congress of the European Society for Shoulder and Elbow Surgery, September 20–23, 2000; Lisbon, Portugal.

28. Ficat RP. Idiopathic bone necrosis of the femoral head: early diagnosis and treatment. *J Bone Joint Surg Br* 1985;67:3–9.

29. Cruess RL. Corticosteroid-induced osteonecrosis of the humeral head. *Orthop Clin North Am* 1985;16:789–796.

30. Neer CS II. Glenohumeral arthroplasty. In: *Shoulder Reconstruction.* Philadelphia: WB Saunders; 1990:143–269.

31. Neer CS II. Old trauma in glenohumeral arthroplasty. In: Neer CS II, ed. *Shoulder Reconstruction.* Philadelphia: WB Saunders; 1990:222–234.

32. Habermeyer P, Schweiberer L. Corrective interventions subsequent to humeral head fractures [in German]. Orthopäde 1992;21:148–157.

33. Neer CS, Watson KC, Stanton FJ. Recent experience in total shoulder replacement. *J Bone Joint Surg Am* 1982;64:319–337.

34. Postel JM, Tamanes M, Levigne C, et al. Les arthroses posttraumatiques. *Rev Chir Orthop Reparatrice Appar Mot* 1995;81(suppl II):111–115.

35. Tauber M, Karpik S, Matis N, Schwartz M, Resch H. Shoulder arthroplasty for traumatic avascular necrosis. Predicters of outcome. *Clin Orthop Relat Res* 2007;465:208–214.

Samuel A. Antuña
John W. Sperling

Prosthetic Replacement for Nonunions of Proximal Humerus Fractures

INTRODUCTION

Nonunion of a fracture of the proximal humerus is uncommon. It is more frequently seen after failed treatment of displaced two-part surgical neck fractures and some three-part and four-part fractures (Fig. 24.1).[1,2] Nonunions occur with various fracture configurations, but are more common with varus displaced two-part surgical neck fractures. The diagnosis can be made as early as 3 months after the injury, when there is no evidence of radiographic bone healing.

Several factors are associated with the formation of a surgical neck nonunion. Proximal humerus fractures are more prevalent among older patients with poor bone quality and associated medical problems that create an unfavorable healing environment. There are multiple local anatomic factors that may hinder bone healing. For example, the weight of the arm causes distraction of the fracture fragments; soft tissue such as the deltoid, biceps, tendon, or rotator cuff can become interposed between the fracture fragments; synovial fluid from the joint can communicate with the fracture site, limiting hematoma formation; and the anterior displacement of the humeral shaft by the pectoralis major may limit the stability of the fracture. Other factors associated with inadequate treatment can also be involved in the development of surgical neck nonunion—excessive distraction caused by hanging casts, overly early aggressive rehabilitation, and poor fixation of surgically treated fractures.

Nonunion of a fracture of the proximal humerus represents a challenging management problem. Although patients who are minimally symptomatic or with low functional demands can be treated nonoperatively, many patients present with significant pain and severe functional impairment. The few documented series on the surgical treatment of proximal humerus nonunions almost uniformly report that open reduction and internal fixation with bone grafting results in an unsatisfactory clinical state in approximately 50% of patients.[2–7] Slightly improved results have been obtained after fixation with tension wire and an intramedullary nail[3,6] and with the use of an intramedullary bone graft.[8] These techniques, however, are applicable only when there is good bone quality and the absence of significant glenohumeral joint damage. When nonunion of the proximal humerus occurs in an elderly patient, it commonly presents with poor bone quality, severe resorption and cavitation of the humeral head, and communication of the fracture with synovial fluid from the glenohumeral joint (Fig. 24.2). All of these factors interfere with successful healing of the fracture and may preclude attempts to achieve bone union with open reduction and internal fixation. Additionally, internal fixation of a nonunion may not be feasible in the setting of a complex fracture of the proximal humerus or those fractures with a very small proximal fragment.[9] In these two groups of patients, the most viable option is replacement of the humeral head.[10,11] A third group of patients who may be candidates for a proximal humerus replacement are those who present after failed surgical reconstruction of the nonunion, in whom the bone quality has deteriorated to the point that no fixation method can be securely used.

PATIENT EVALUATION

Patients with nonunions of the proximal humerus present with pain of a variable degree and significant loss of function. Asymptomatic or minimally symptomatic patients should be encouraged to pursue nonoperative treatment. However, patients are typically unable to perform basic tasks such as dressing and self-care activities. Lifting and carrying objects weighing more than 1 or 2 kg is commonly impossible. Pain is usually present at rest and increases significantly with daily activities.

On physical examination, motion is present at the fracture site rather than at the glenohumeral joint. Forward elevation is almost always absent, although some patients may achieve less than 40 degrees. Severe atrophy of the deltoid and parascapular muscles is noted. Skin integrity should be checked in patients who have been treated surgically, and draining sinuses, denoting active infection, should be ruled out. A thorough neurological

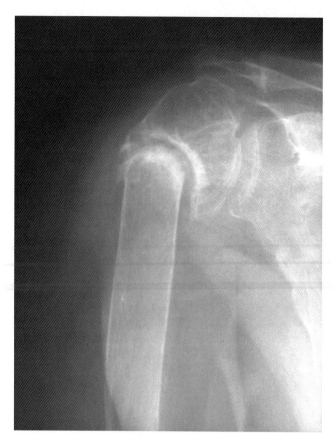

Figure 24.1. Radiograph of a 71-year-old patient who has experienced a two-part surgical neck fracture with varus displacement. Initial treatment included sling and swathe, followed by early physical therapy, resulting in a proximal humerus nonunion.

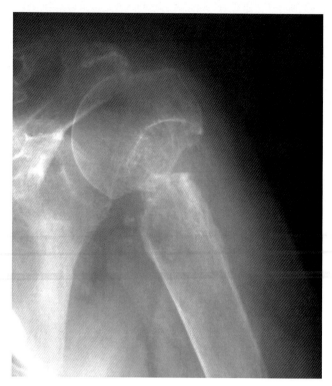

Figure 24.2. Radiograph of an 83-year-old patient with a proximal humerus nonunion. Severe resorption and cavitation of the humeral head can be noted.

SURGICAL TECHNIQUE

The patient is placed in the beach chair position with the shoulder free of the table edge. Regional or general anesthesia can be used, the latter being our preference. An extended deltopectoral incision is used. The dissection may be difficult in patients with previous open surgery because of distortion of the anatomy. If a wider exposure is necessary, an anteromedial approach (deltopectoral exposure plus release of the clavicular and anterior acromial origins of the deltoid) may be used.[12] The main landmark is the biceps tendon, which can be used as a guide to the rotator interval and to locate the subscapularis. The axillary nerve is palpated anteriorly under the inferior edge of the subscapularis or the medially retracted lesser tuberosity and posteriorly as the nerve exists from the axilla near the humeral neck.

The joint may be approached via an incision at the subscapularis insertion or by a lesser tuberosity osteotomy. Our preference now is to preserve the lesser tuberosity in continuity with the medial calcar and greater tuberosity, if possible. Once the subscapularis is retracted medially, a complete capsulectomy may be performed to help improve mobilization of the tuberosities. The nonunion site is identified and debrided by removal of any fibrous tissue or interposed soft tissue. If there is adequate bone stock in the humeral head, the greater tuberosity should not osteotomized. In these shoulders, after the articular portion of the humeral head is excised with an oscillating saw, the humeral stem is skewered through the ring-shaped portion of bone containing the greater and lesser tuberosity passing through the nonunion site (Fig. 24.3). If there is medial calcar

examination should be performed, especially if the patient had a previous operation. Deltoid and rotator cuff muscle function can be assessed by gentle contraction against minimal resistance; electromyography is mandatory when there are doubts of nerve function.

The patient's general health status should be scrutinized. Nonunions often occur in patients with metabolic bone diseases or nutritional deficits that may impede their ability to recover from surgery. Moreover, these medical issues may influence the decision made by the surgeon regarding the most appropriate treatment option for each patient. In fact, if an elderly patient appears to have a medical condition that affects bone healing, this may be an indication to consider replacement surgery instead of fixation. Blood tests should be obtained in patients treated primarily by surgical fixation to rule out an infected nonunion.

The radiographic evaluation should include at least an anteroposterior view of the shoulder in the scapular plane and an axillary view. The status of the cephalic fragment, amount of bone loss at the nonunion site, presence of avascular necrosis of the humeral head, and involvement of the joint cartilage should be carefully evaluated when a shoulder replacement is being considered. Computed tomography may be helpful in delineating a head-splitting component of the fracture and to evaluate the status of the greater tuberosity.

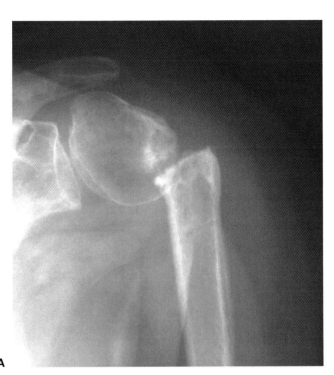
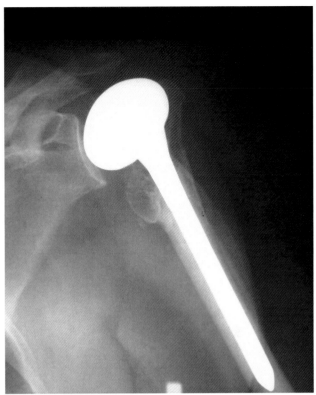

A   B

Figure 24.3. **(A)** Radiograph of a 69-year-old patient with a nonunion of the surgical neck. **(B)** The implant was inserted through both fragments and cemented in the shaft. Heavy tension band sutures were used to control rotation between the fragments, and bone graft from the humeral head was added to the nonunion site.

erosion associated with the nonunion, a C-shaped fragment containing the greater and lesser tuberosity should be preserved for later grafting of the medial calcar. If there is severe resorption of the humeral head, a small head fragment, or malunion of the greater tuberosity, it may be necessary to perform an osteotomy with removal of the head fragment (Fig. 24.4).

The glenoid is evaluated for evidence of articular damage, and a glenoid component is implanted if significant chondral damage is present. The humeral canal is prepared by use of progressively larger reamers. An appropriate-size trial stem is placed and assessed for height and version using the surgical technique similar to that used in acute fractures. After the canal is debrided and dried with peroxide-soaked gauzes, it is filled with thumb-packed cement. The final humeral component is definitively placed according to the position of the previously placed trial component. All cement at the nonunion site should be carefully removed and bone graft placed between the bone fragments. If there is a ring-shaped proximal fragment, cancellous chips from the humeral head are packed between the calcar and the shaft. If the medial calcar is deficient, a large corticocancellous bone graft from the head is wedged between the prosthetic head and the humeral shaft, according to the technique described by Lin et al[13] (Fig. 24.5). When a greater tuberosity osteotomy is performed, reconstruction follows the principles established for acute fractures.[14] The tuberosities are always repaired to each other and to the shaft with nonabsorbable sutures incorporating the rotator cuff, and the subscapularis is reattached to the lesser tuberosity.

Postoperatively, the arm is immobilized in a sling with the elbow at the site for 6 weeks. During this period, only gentle passive motion under supervision of a therapist is prescribed. Active motion is delayed until there is evidence of some bone healing on radiographs, usually at 6 weeks. Strengthening exercises are encouraged after 12 weeks.

RESULTS

Few reports in the literature exist concerning results of shoulder arthroplasty for the treatment of a proximal humerus nonunion. The majority of published series include a heterogeneous group of patients undergoing humeral head replacement for a variety of posttraumatic conditions of the shoulder[12,15–21] or a small number of cases treated with an arthroplasty in a group of surgically treated nonunions.[2–5,7]

A review of the literature for shoulder arthroplasty for surgical neck nonunions, including posttraumatic arthritis and surgical treatment of nonunions, is presented in Table 24.1. Although different scoring systems were used to express the results, information was available regarding range of motion (ROM), pain relief, and patient satisfaction for most cases. The average values for active abduction and external rotation were 93 degrees (range, 63 to 120 degrees) and 32 degrees (range, 15 to 54 degrees), respectively. The vast majority of patients achieved satisfactory pain relief and were satisfied with the result. Although there are inherent limitations to the analysis

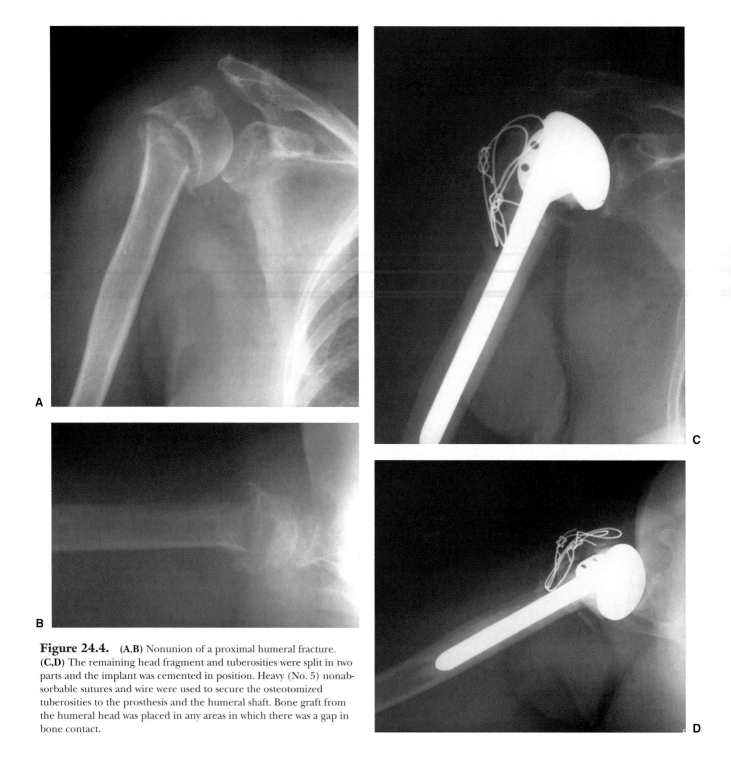

Figure 24.4. **(A,B)** Nonunion of a proximal humeral fracture. **(C,D)** The remaining head fragment and tuberosities were split in two parts and the implant was cemented in position. Heavy (No. 5) nonabsorbable sutures and wire were used to secure the osteotomized tuberosities to the prosthesis and the humeral shaft. Bone graft from the humeral head was placed in any areas in which there was a gap in bone contact.

of the results in different series, the results regarding ROM are similar in all series. The functional outcome is greatly limited because of difficulty in restoring a normal ROM. Active elevation above the horizontal should not be routinely expected. Pain relief, however, is more consistently achieved.

Complications specifically related to arthroplasties implanted for nonunions are more prevalent than in patients with osteoarthritis[22–26] and include greater tuberosity nonunion or resorption, anterior dislocation, periprosthetic humeral shaft fracture, impingement pain, axillary nerve palsy, and sympto-

matic glenoid arthritis. The most common complication found in this group of patients is related to tuberosity healing problems (Fig. 24.6). Lack of tuberosity healing may account for the limited ROM, and therefore specific attention should be paid to greater tuberosity reconstruction in these cases. When a greater tuberosity osteotomy is performed, heavy nonabsorbable sutures should be used—two placed horizontally holding the greater tuberosity to the prostheses, two figure-of-8 sutures fixing the tuberosities to the shaft, and two additional circumferential sutures around the medial aspect of the neck

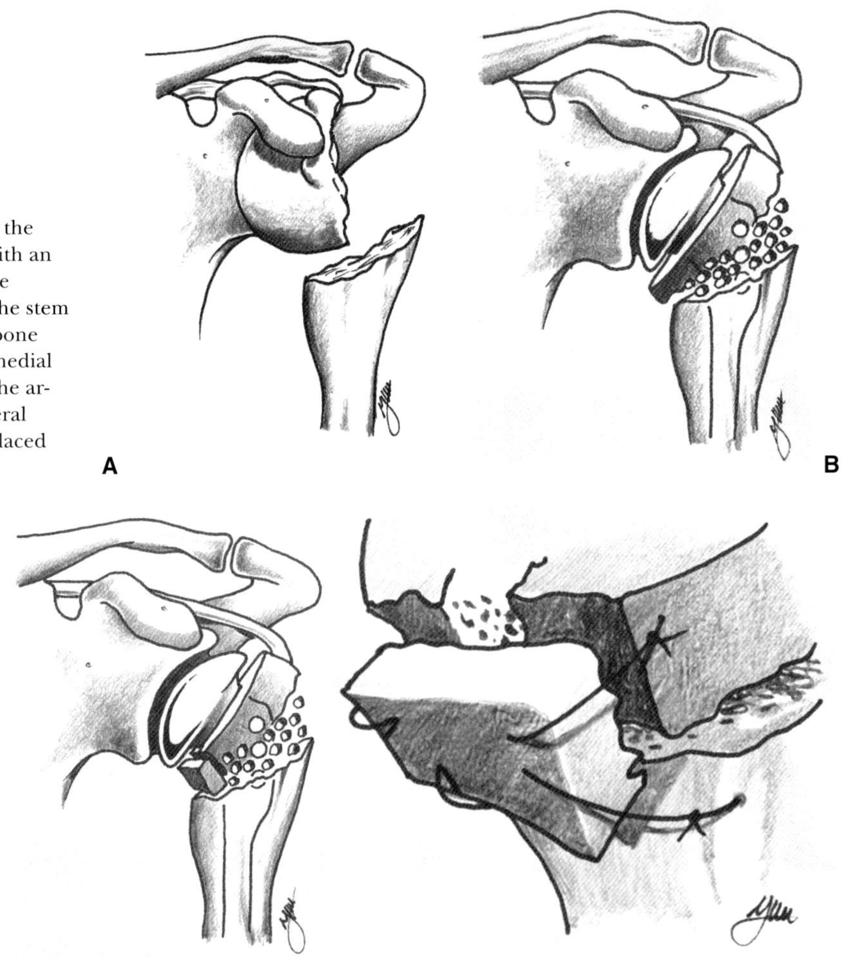

Figure 24.5. **(A)** Humeral nonunion. **(B)** After the articular portion of the humeral head is removed with an oscillating saw, a ring-shaped fragment including the greater tuberosity and medial calcar is preserved. The stem is skewed through both fragments, and cancellous bone graft is added to the nonunion site. **(C)** When the medial calcar is deficient, a C-shaped segment is left after the articular portion is removed. Restoration of the humeral contour is achieved with a corticocancellous graft placed medially.

of the prostheses, holding both tuberosities together laterally. Bone graft is placed between the tuberosity and the shaft to enhance healing. Better functional results have been reported when the proximal segment is preserved as a ring-shaped or C-shaped fragment and the prostheses is inserted through the remaining humeral neck, with either cancellous bone graft

placed at the nonunion site or a large corticocancellous graft wedged medially, substituting the absent calcar.

In those cases in which tuberosity reconstruction has been performed, active motion is delayed until there is radiographic evidence of bone healing. The relatively high incidence of instability also emphasizes the difficulty in dealing with soft tissue

TABLE 24.1	Results of Shoulder Arthroplasty for Proximal Humerus Nonunions				
Authors	*No. Cases*	*HA/TSA*	*Elevation*	*External Rotation*	*Pain Relief (%)*
Norris et al,[2] 1990	14	10/4	97	NA	100
Healy et al,[4] 1990	6	6/0	72	30	100
Frich et al,[18] 1991	7	NA	NA	NA	NA
Dines et al,[17] 1993	6	5/1	120	41	100
Norris et al,[20] 1995	3	3/0	NA	NA	100
Nayak et al,[5] 1995	7	7/0	110	20	85
Duralde et al,[3] 1996	10	9/1	86	37	NA
Boileau et al,[27] 1999	6	6/0	63	26	80
Antuña et al,[28] 2002	25	21/4	88	38	95
Mansat et al,[29] 2004	2	2/0	95	15	100
Lin et al,[13] 2006	9	8/1	113	54	100

HA, hemiarthroplasty; TSA, total shoulder athroplasty; NA, not available.

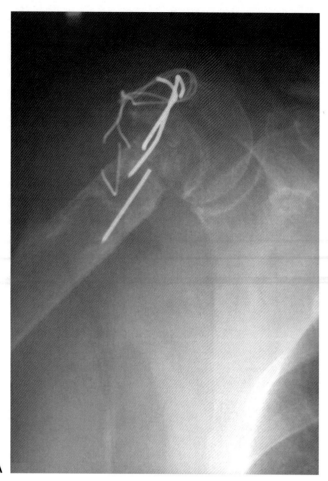

A

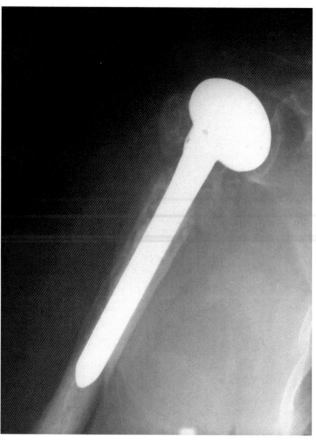

B

Figure 24.6. **(A)** Radiograph of a 66-year-old patient with a proximal humerus nonunion after a three-part fracture. **(B)** Two years after hemiarthroplasty, the patient had a poor functional result, with radiographic evidence of greater tuberosity nonunion.

deficiencies frequently seen in these cases and the necessity of performing a meticulous repair and tensioning of the musculotendinous envelope.

SUMMARY

Patients with significant pain and functional impairment secondary to a proximal humerus nonunion associated with osteoporosis, severe cavitation of the humeral head, and/or degeneration joint changes may benefit from shoulder arthroplasty. Although function is not completely restored in most patients, high levels of subjective satisfaction and pain relief can be achieved. Better functional outcome may be expected when the proximal segment containing the greater and lesser tuberosities is preserved and bone graft is used to reconstruct the deficient medial calcar.

REFERENCES

1. Cofield RH. Comminuted fractures of the proximal humerus. *Clin Orthop* 1988;230:49–57.
2. Norris TR, Turner JA, Bovill D. Nonunion of the upper humerus: an analysis of the etiology and treatment in 28 cases. In: Post M, Morrey BF, Hawkins RJ, eds. *Surgery of the Shoulder.* Chicago: Mosby-Year Book; 1990;63–67.
3. Duralde XA, Flatow EL, Pollock RG, et al. Operative treatment of nonunions of the surgical neck of the humerus. *J Shoulder Elbow Surg* 1996;5:169–180.
4. Healy WL, Jupiter JP, Kristiansen TK, et al. Nonunion of the proximal humerus: a review of 25 cases. *J Orthop Trauma* 1990;4:424–431.
5. Nayak NK, Schickendantz MS, Regan WD, et al. Operative treatment of nonunion of surgical neck fractures of the humerus. *Clin Orthop* 1995;313:200–205.
6. Neer CS II. Nonunion of the surgical neck of the humerus. *Orthop Trans* 1983;7:389.
7. Scheck M. Surgical treatment of nonunions of the surgical neck of the humerus. *Clin Orthop* 167:255–259.
8. Walch G, Badet R, Nové-Josserand I, et al. Nonunions of the surgical neck of the humerus: surgical treatment with an intramedullary bone peg, internal fixation, and cancellous bone grafting. *J Shoulder Elbow Surg* 1996;5:161–168.
9. Checchia SL, Doneux P, Miyazaki AN, et al. Classification of nonunions of the proximal humerus. *Int Orthop* 2000;24:217–220.
10. Galatz LM, Iannotti JP. Management of surgical neck nonunions. *Orthop Clin North Am* 2000;31:51–62.
11. Neer CS II. Glenohumeral arthroplasty. In: *Shoulder Reconstruction*. Philadelphia: WB Saunders; 1990;143–269.
12. Tanner MW, Cofield RH. Prosthetic arthroplasty for fractures and fractures: dislocations of the proximal humerus. *Clin Orthop* 1983;179:116–128.
13. Lin JS, Klepps SK, Miller S, et al. Effectiveness of replacement arthroplasty with calcar grafting and avoidance of greater tuberosity osteotomy for the treatment of surgical neck nonunions. *J Shoulder Elbow Surg* 2006;15:12–18.
14. Neer CS. Displaced proximal humeral fractures: Part I. Classification and evaluation. *J Bone Joint Surg Am* 1970;52:1077–1089.
15. Boileau P, Trojani C, Walch G, et al. Sequelae of fractures of the proximal humerus: results of shoulder arthroplasty with greater tuberosity osteotomy. In: Walch G, Boileau P, eds. *Shoulder Arthroplasty.* Berlin, Germany: Springer-Verlag; 1999;371–379.
16. Boileau P, Trojani C, Walsh G, et al. Shoulder arthroplasty for the treatment of the sequelae of fractures of the proximal humerus. *J Shoulder Elbow Surg* 2004;10:12–18.
17. Dines DM, Warren RF, Altchek DW, et al. Posttraumatic changes of the proximal humerus: malunion, nonunion, and osteonecrosis—treatment with modular hemiarthroplasty or total shoulder arthroplasty. *J Shoulder Elbow Surg* 1993;2:11–21.
18. Frich LH, Sojbjerg JO, Sneppen O. Shoulder arthroplasty in complex acute and chronic proximal humeral fractures. *Orthopedics* 1991;9:949–954.

19. Huten D, Duparc J. L'arthroplastie prothetique dans les traumatismes complexes récents et anciens de l'epaule. *Rev Chir Orthop* 1986;72:517–529.

20. Norris T, Green A, McGuigan F. Late prosthetic shoulder arthroplasty for displaced proximal humerus fractures. *J Shoulder Elbow Surg* 1995;4:271–280.

21. Wiater JM, Flatow EL. Posttraumatic arthritis. *Orthop Clin North Am* 2000;31:63–76.

22. Cofield RH. Total shoulder arthroplasty with the Neer prosthesis. *J Bone Joint Surg Am* 1984;66:899–906.

23. Muldoon MP, Cofield RH. Complications of humeral head replacement for proximal humeral fractures. *Instr Course Lect* 1998;47:15–24.

24. Neer CS II, Watson KC, Stanton FJ. Recent experience in total shoulder arthroplasties. *J Bone Joint Surg Am* 1982;64:319–337.

25. Sperling JW, Cofield RH, Rowland CM. Neer hemiarthroplasty and Neer total shoulder arthroplasty in patients 50 years old or less. *J Bone Joint Surg Am* 1998;80:464–473.

26. Wirth MA, Rockwood CA, Jr. Complications of shoulder arthroplasty. *Clin Orthop* 1994;307:47–69.

27. Boileau P, Walch G, Trojani C, et al. Classification and treatment for the sequelae of proximal humerus fractures: a prospective multicenter study of 71 cases. *J Shoulder and Elbow Surg* 1999;9:501.

28. Antuña SA, Sperling JW, Sanchez Sotelo J, et al. Shoulder arthroplasty for proximal humerus nonunions. *J Shoulder Elbow Surg* 2002;11:114–121.

29. Mansat P, Guity MR, Bellumore Y, et al. Shoulder arthroplasty for late sequelae of proximal humeral fracture. *J Shoulder Elbow Surg* 2004;13:12–18.

Prosthetic Arthroplasty for Arthritis after Surgery for Shoulder Instability

INTRODUCTION

The development of glenohumeral arthritis is a well-recognized complication of instability surgery.[1–8] Shoulder arthroplasty for the treatment of postcapsulorrhaphy arthritis has multiple potential challenges, including soft tissue imbalance, bone deficiency, and the young age of the patients. Although there have been a large number of reports on the outcome of shoulder arthroplasty for osteoarthritis, there is little published information available to help guide clinical decision making on postcapsulorrhaphy arthroplasty. There have been very few publications describing the specific techniques to address the distorted anatomy, the incidence, and the management of complications encountered.

The proper management of a patient who develops postcapsulorrhaphy arthritis necessitates that the surgeon obtain information in five areas. These areas include evaluating (a) the patient's occupational and recreational demands on the shoulder, (b) the instability pattern that led to the original stabilization procedure, (c) details of the stabilization surgery, (d) treatment options and planning the technical aspects of the shoulder arthroplasty, and (e) recognition of the potential benefits and limitations of the surgical procedure.

A detailed review of these areas will provide the surgeon insight into the specific problems encountered in patients with postcapsulorrhaphy arthritis. This chapter will discuss the evaluation of the patient and detail treatment planning and surgical technique. The chapter includes a literature review that addresses expected outcomes, as well as risks for revision surgery.

PATIENT EVALUATION

A careful history will allow the surgeon to determine the indication for the stabilization procedure, the type of surgical procedure performed, and whether there was recurrent instability. The answers to several questions need to be determined in regard to the procedure that was previously performed. Was the stabilization an anatomic or nonanatomic procedure? Was the instability repair a soft tissue procedure, or was there alteration of osseous anatomy? What type of instrumentation was used?

Obtaining prior surgical reports facilitates the arthroplasty by giving insight into the altered anatomy present.

The patient's primary complaint must be identified—is it pain, loss of motion, or weakness? This needs to be placed in context of the patient's demands on the shoulder. An organized examination of the shoulder, the entire upper extremity, and the cervical spine should be performed. Examination includes careful strength, range of motion (ROM), and stability testing. Frequently, there is contracture of the anterior soft tissues with subsequent posterior subluxation of the humeral head (Fig. 25.1). In theory, the reverse may be present with a prior posterior repair, but this is very uncommon. The rotator cuff is typically intact in these patients but is often distorted in association with shoulder subluxation and contractures.

At a minimum, plain radiographs of the shoulder should include a 40-degree posterior oblique view in internal and external rotation, plus an axillary view. Computed tomography (CT) can be useful for preoperative planning and allows further assessment of glenoid erosion and version. Erosion of the posterior aspect of the glenoid is also frequently present. Among patients with decreased strength, magnetic resonance imaging or electromyelography may be ordered to evaluate for a rotator cuff tear or neurological deficit.

Adjunctive tests such as C-reactive protein level, erythrocyte sedimentation rate, and white blood cell count with differential should be considered in patients in whom there is a question of infection. Paired bone scan and indium-labeled white cell radioisotope scan might be ordered to further evaluate for the possibility of a low-grade infection. If there is a higher suspicion for infection, a shoulder aspiration is performed.

After the information discussed earlier is gathered and supplemented by adjunctive tests, one is then able to better define the soft tissue and bone abnormalities that are present and proceed with treatment planning.

SURGICAL INDICATIONS

The primary indication for shoulder arthroplasty is severe pain in the setting of end-stage glenohumeral arthritis that

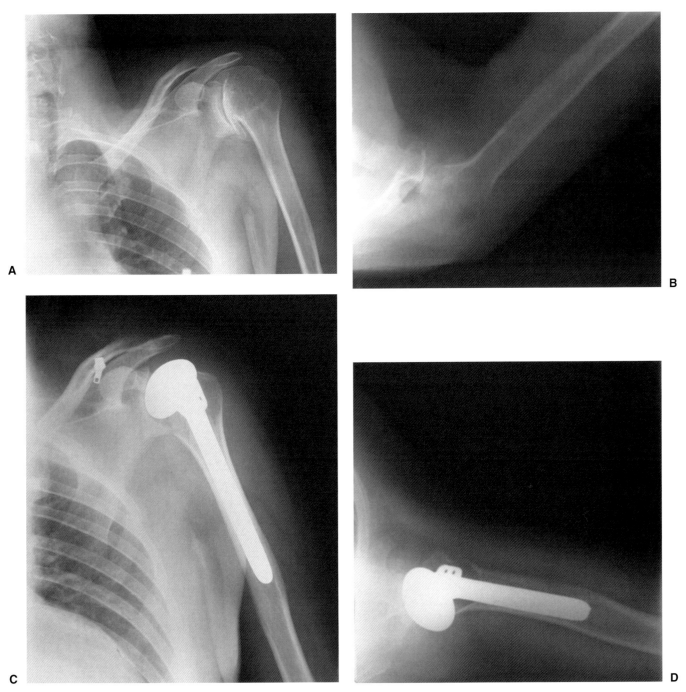

Figure 25.1. **(A,B)** Preoperative radiographs of a 43-year-old man who underwent a Putti-Platt procedure 21 years earlier for recurrent shoulder instability. He has severe pain, −10 degrees of external rotation, and active abduction of 30 degrees. The radiographs demonstrate typical posterior subluxation. **(C,D)** There is mild glenoid erosion and mild posterosuperior subluxation 8 years after hemiarthroplasty. The patient had no pain, 0 degrees of external rotation, and active abduction of 70 degrees. (From Sperling JW, Antuña SA, Sanchez-Sotelo J, et al. Shoulder arthroplasty for arthritis after instability surgery. *J Bone Joint Surg Am* 2002;84:1775–1781, with permission.)

has been unresponsive to nonoperative measures, including anti-inflammatory medications, gentle therapy, and possible cortisone injection. Patients with shoulder arthritis after instability surgery are frequently significantly younger than patients undergoing shoulder arthroplasty for osteoarthritis.

Therefore their activity level and life expectancy are higher than would be usually considered for most arthroplasty procedures. Counseling of the patient in regard to these factors when deciding between hemiarthroplasty and total shoulder arthroplasty is important.

TREATMENT PLANNING

Before undertaking the procedure, development of a problem list and determination of specific methods to address these issues is very useful in the setting of the frequently distorted soft tissue and osseous anatomy. For example, if there is significant glenoid deficiency, one should plan on glenoid bone grafting. Additionally, many patients with a history of postcapsulorrhaphy arthritis have subscapularis deficiency. It is important to be aware of this problem and plan for subscapularis reconstruction, tendon transfer, or possible soft-tissue allograft augmentation. Lastly, there may be a need for nonstandard implants or a variety of component sizes that may not be usually available; this should be included in planning.

An algorithmic approach to surgical treatment is useful. If the preoperative evaluation reveals no significant bone or soft tissue deficiency, standard arthroplasty may be performed. The decision to place a glenoid component is based on the amount of glenoid involvement, age of the patient, and activity level. If glenoid bone loss is present, placement of a glenoid component is more likely to be necessary. Glenoid bone loss may be addressed through asymmetrical glenoid reaming or augmentation (i.e., bone graft). Soft tissue deficiency can be managed with tendon transfers or allograft reconstruction. Residual shoulder instability after placement of the glenoid component can be managed with a combination of changing humeral version, humeral head size, and capsular plication.

SURGICAL TECHNIQUE

APPROACH

The standard approach is through the deltopectoral interval. The typical skin incision is over the anterior aspect of the shoulder and slightly lateral to the deltopectoral interval. In the setting of prior surgery, there are frequently one or more old surgical incisions. A prior incision can be used or incorporated into a longer incision, with approach through the deltopectoral interval. The deltopectoral interval is most easily developed just distal to the clavicle. Typically, there is a natural infraclavicular triangle of fat that separates the deltoid and pectoralis major. Exposure continues distally, leaving the cephalic vein in its bed medially.

One of the keys to restoration of motion, as well as glenoid exposure, is careful mobilization of the deltoid from the clavicle to its humeral insertion. The plane between the conjoined tendon and the subscapularis is developed medially and is frequently heavily scarred. Dissection can be facilitated in this plane by placing the arm in maximum external rotation, then progressing with the dissection from superior to inferior and from lateral to medial to develop this interval. Undoubtedly, careful dissection is required because of the close proximity to the neurovascular group. The nerves to the subscapularis are typically 1 to 0.5 cm or more medial to the glenoid rim or the medial border of the conjoined tendon group and should be carefully preserved.[9]

The rotator interval is incised along its inferior border with care to avoid injury to the long head of biceps tendon. The thickness of the anterior shoulder capsule and subscapularis by are assessed by direct evaluation of both the internal and external surfaces. In cases with severe internal rotation contracture and a thick subscapularis and anterior shoulder capsule, Z-lengthening may be considered. However, there are concerns if the tissue is too thin with resultant compromise of the integrity of the tendon.

In cases in which there is passive external rotation between 0 and 30 degrees, the subscapularis and anterior shoulder capsule are elevated from the humerus as one layer. At the completion of the arthroplasty, the subscapularis and capsule can then be advanced medially along the humerus. Typically, for every 1 cm of medial advancement, approximately 20 to 30 degrees of external rotation is gained. If passive external rotation is greater than 30 degrees, an incision is made through the subscapularis tendon and anterior shoulder capsule approximately 1 cm medial to the subscapularis insertion on the humerus. Even if there is greater than 15 degrees of external rotation, additional subscapularis and capsular length can be obtained by incising the anterior shoulder capsule at the glenoid rim from the base of the coracoid superiorly to the anterior band of the inferior glenohumeral ligament inferiorly. This results in a release of the tenodesis effect of the anterior capsule on the subscapularis and overcomes any capsular shortening that may be present, resulting in an additional 1 to 1.5 cm of length may be obtained.

In the majority of patients with postcapsulorrhaphy arthritis, there is significant contracture of the inferior capsule. To address this tightness, the inferior shoulder capsule is incised along the humeral neck from anterior to posterior. The arm is placed in adduction, with progressive external rotation as the capsule is released with electrocautery to protect the axillary nerve from damage. The inferior capsule release will usually extend past neutral to include the lower portion of the posterior capsule attachment to the humerus. This will then allow full elevation after the arthroplasty is performed and improve access to the glenoid.

HUMERAL COMPONENT

After the arthrotomy and inferior capsule release are performed, the humeral head is dislocated with extension, adduction, and gentle external rotation. Great care must be taken to avoid placing high torque on the humeral shaft to avoid fractures. Among patients with a tendency toward posterior instability, the amount of retrotorsion typically used in osteoarthritis may be decreased; for example, the retrotorsion may be decreased from 30 or 35 degrees to 15 or 20 degrees. After a trial prosthesis is placed, osteophytes should be removed and the metaphyseal bone trimmed to sit beneath the prosthetic humeral head and not extend beyond it. Humeral heads can then be trialed using the size of the patient and tension on the rotator cuff as guides.

If there is only a minor tendency for posterior subluxation with the trial head in place, it is quite likely that glenoid placement and minor adjustment of humeral head size will address the posterior shoulder capsule and rotator cuff laxity. If there is a significant amount of subluxation with the trial head, adjusting prosthetic components alone is likely not to be enough and additional attention might need to be directed toward plication of the posterior shoulder capsule. The posterior capsule can be plicated from either internally or externally. Internal plication is the most direct approach. Significant care must be taken to sequencing the repair. With the glenoid prepared before fixing the glenoid in place, plication sutures are placed through the posterior capsule and inner portion of the infraspinatus tendon. This may be performed by placing a simple figure-of-eight or horizontal mattress sutures from lateral to medial in the middle portion of the posterior capsule. Sutures are subsequently placed from superior to inferior in a sequential manner using three to five stitches. The stitches are clamped and tied after glenoid component placement. One can perform this technique through the deltopectoral exposure.

When there is extreme capsule and rotator cuff stretching, additional exposure may be necessary. There are several options available. The two most effective options are use of the anteromedial approach in which the deltopectoral incision is extended superiorly and laterally and the deltoid origin is released from the clavicle and anterior acromion. One can then internally rotate the arm and have excellent access to plicate the posterior shoulder capsule and infraspinatus tendon. If posterior shoulder capsule plication is performed, the repair must be protected so that healing may occur. Therefore the use of a gunslinger-type sling may be useful to position the arm in neutral rotation with avoidance of internal rotation.

GLENOID COMPONENT

Following preparation of the humeral component, a Fukuda type retractor is introduced and the glenoid is inspected. Patients with prior instability surgery frequently have shortening of the anterior shoulder structures, and a release of the anterosuperior shoulder capsule is performed from noon to the 4 o'clock position in the right shoulder. Elevation of these structures from the anterior scapula is performed to improve external rotation and increase the mobility of the subscapularis-anterior capsule. Glenoid exposure may be best obtained with the arm in approximately 70 to 80 degrees of abduction, neutral flexion, and extension.

In patients with glenoid cartilage loss, it is our practice to place a glenoid component for more consistent pain relief compared to hemiarthroplasty if the patient is willing to live with the restrictions of a total shoulder arthroplasty. In addition to the axillary view, a preoperative CT scan is helpful in determining the amount of bone loss present, version of the glenoid, and center point of the glenoid vault in reference to the face plate.

When the amount of posterior bone loss is less than 10 mm, a surface reamer usually can be used to asymmetrically ream the glenoid to a neutral position. Except in rare situations, this will allow enough depth in the glenoid neck to fix a glenoid component in place. However, if the bone loss is greater than 10 mm, asymmetrical reaming of the anterior glenoid is typically not sufficient to allow normalization of glenoid version. In this circumstance, a portion of the excised humeral head is used as a bone graft to correct the glenoid deficiency. This is most simply done in the following order. The glenoid surface is prepared with the circular reamer. The keel or column holes for the component are prepared. A portion of the humeral head is then tailored to fit into the defect, fixing the graft in place with two drills and replacing the drills with 3.5-mm cortical screws (Fig. 25.2). The screw heads are countersunk. The glenoid component is fixed in place using the usual fixation methods.[10]

On occasion, instrumentation from prior surgery may interfere with glenoid component replacement and might be extremely difficult to remove. In this situation, one can begin glenoid preparation in the usual manner and, when encountering these devices, remove the metal with a microsagittal instrument (Fig. 25.3).

BALANCING THE JOINT

After placing the glenoid component, humeral heads are then trialed. The specific humeral head size is based on many factors, including the size of the patient, the amount of humeral head removed, and the flexibility of the shoulder capsule and rotator cuff. This is assessed by the amount of subluxation with joint movement, ROM, and passive translation of the prosthetic humeral head against the glenoid. One would prefer to select a humeral head that would tension the supraspinatus with the arm at the side and avoid posterior humeral head subluxation when the arm is brought into elevation. One would prefer to have less than 50% of passive humeral translation posteriorly when the arm is at the side and in neutral rotation. In addition, for each head size the ability to close the anterior structures with sufficient external rotation (≥30 degrees) must be considered.

It is helpful to place the rotator interval stitches before placing the real humeral head. These stitches can then be tied after the real head is impacted in place. If the subscapularis was incised through tendon, it is closed tendon to tendon. The rotator interval area is closed to assist with support of the lateral repair and control any tendency for subluxation. If the subscapularis was taken down from the lesser tuberosity, this area and the bone medial to it on the humeral neck is roughened with a curette. Burr holes are placed through the anterior humeral neck; this is most efficaciously done before the real humeral component is seated. The subscapularis is then sutured to the bone of the humeral neck in a medialized position. After closure of the arthrotomy, the shoulder is taken through a ROM to determine the ROM that will be prescribed for passive exercises during the first 4 to 6 weeks after surgery.

In the postoperative period, if there has not been plication of the posterior shoulder capsule, the arm can be positioned in a shoulder immobilizer. Passive motion in elevation and external rotation is performed during the first 4 to 6 weeks within the safe limits determined at surgery. After this time period, active-assisted motion is performed with a pulley and wand. Strengthening exercises are typically progressed quite slowly, with isometrics beginning at the earliest at 8 to 10 weeks.

LITERATURE REVIEW

Shoulder arthroplasty in 17 patients with prior instability surgery was reported by Bigliani et al.[5] The mean age of the patients was 43 years. The mean follow-up in this study was 2.9 years. There were 13 patients with a satisfactory result and four with an unsatisfactory result. Neer et al[8] reported on a group of 18 shoulders with arthritis of dislocation. Some patients in this study had not undergone previous procedures. The author noted an excellent or satisfactory result in 17 of 18 shoulder arthroplasties. Young and Rockwood[4] reported on four patients who developed shoulder arthritis following a Bristow procedure. In this small group of patients the authors noted improvement in function and pain relief with shoulder arthroplasty.[4]

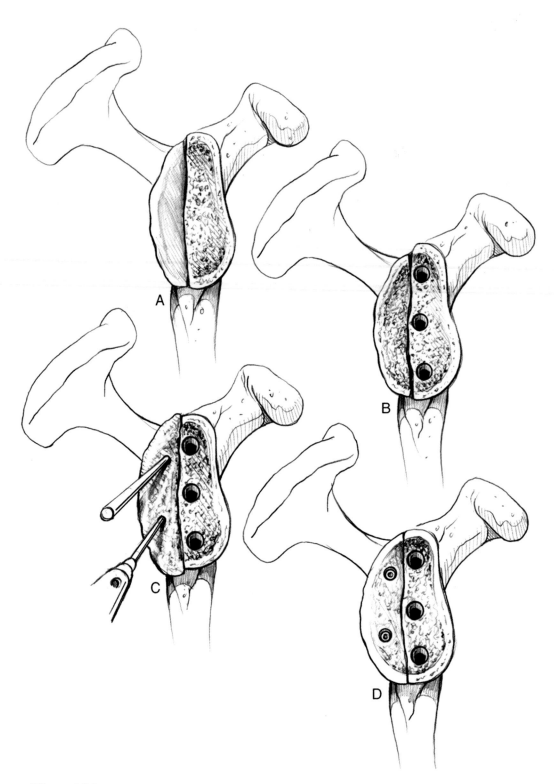

Figure 25.2.   Posterior glenoid deficiency greater than 10 mm can be managed with posterior glenoid bone grafting. **(A)** The anterior glenoid is reamed in neutral version. **(B)** The posterior glenoid is contoured with a burr, and the holes for the glenoid component are made. **(C)** The bone graft is held provisionally with two drills, and the graft is contoured to match the curvature of the anterior glenoid. **(D)** Final fixation of the graft is obtained with two cortical screws that are countersunk. The glenonid component is then implanted.

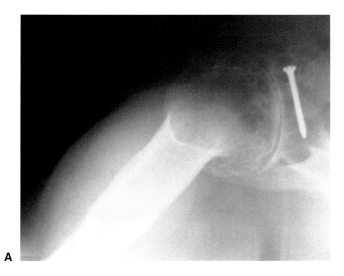

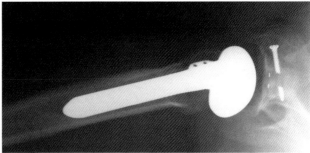

Figure 25.3. **(A)** Preoperative radiograph of a 47-year-old man who underwent stabilization surgery 27 years earlier for recurrent anterior instability. **(B)** The patient underwent placement of the total shoulder arthroplasty with drilling through the screw. (From Williams GR, Yamaguchi K, et al, eds. *Shoulder and Elbow Arthroplasty.* Philadelphia: Lippincott Williams & Wilkins; 2005, with permission.)

There have been two more recent long-term reports that appear to show significantly poorer results among these patients with postcapsulorrhaphy arthritis. Bauer et al[6] reported on the outcome of 30 patients who underwent arthroplasty after instability repairs with a mean follow-up of 8 years. There were satisfactory results in 13 of 18 total shoulder arthroplasties (72%) and four of 12 hemiarthroplasties (33%). Seven of

12 hemiarthroplasties required a revision to total shoulder arthroplasty for pain. The authors note that shoulder arthroplasty for postcapsulorrhaphy arthritis has inferior results and a higher revision rate compared to that for arthroplasty for osteoarthritis.

Sperling et al[7] published the results of 31 shoulder arthroplasties for postcapsulorrhaphy arthritis. The mean patient

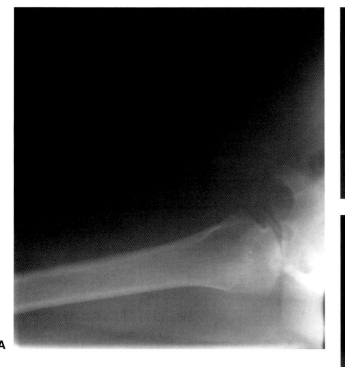

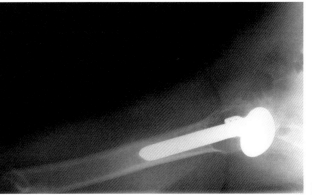

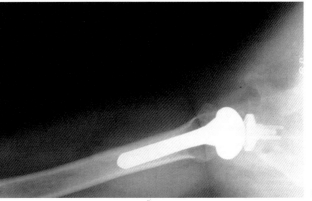

Figure 25.4. **(A)** Radiograph of a 21-year-old man who had undergone three prior instability surgeries. He had severe shoulder pain, external rotation to neutral, and elevation to 130 degrees. **(B)** Nine years after hemiarthroplasty, radiograph demonstrates posterior subluxation and glenoid arthritis. **(C)** The patient subsequently underwent revision to total shoulder arthroplasty with glenoid bone grafting and placement of an ingrowth glenoid component.

age in the study was 46 years. There were 21 total shoulder arthroplasties and 10 hemiarthroplasties. All patients were followed for a minimum of 2 years (mean, 7 years) or until the time of revision surgery. There was significant pain relief (p <0.001), improvement in active abduction from 94 to 141 degrees (p <0.001), and external rotation from 4 to 43 degrees (p <0.001). Overall, there were four excellent, two satisfactory, and four unsatisfactory results among the hemiarthroplasties. Among the total shoulder arthroplasties, there were three excellent, five satisfactory, and 13 unsatisfactory results. There were three hemiarthroplasties and eight total shoulder arthroplasties that underwent a revision procedure. The survival rate was only 61% at 10 years. The data from the study suggested that shoulder arthroplasty for postcapsulorrhaphy arthritis in this young patient group provides pain relief and improved motion. However, it is associated with a very high rate of unsatisfactory results and revision surgery because of glenoid arthritis, component failure, or instability that accrue over time in these young patients (Fig. 25.4).

CONCLUSION

Patients with postcapsulorrhaphy arthritis typically have restriction of external rotation and anterior capsular tightness. Important for shoulder arthroplasty in general, careful soft tissue balancing and adequate tissue release are very important to performing a successful arthroplasty among patients with postcapsulorrhaphy arthritis. This entails not only addressing posterior capsular laxity but also the anterior soft tissue tightness that is present.

Because of the very young age of these patients, there may be a propensity to avoid placement of a glenoid component. However, we have recognized in our practice and in a literature review, that painful glenoid arthritis represents the most common reason for revision surgery for hemiarthroplasties.[11] A methodical preoperative evaluation will allow one to predict the need for special components or bone grafting. Additionally, obtaining prior operative reports will allow one to recognize distorted anatomy and facilitate safe tissue releases.

Shoulder arthroplasty in a patient with prior instability surgery should be done with caution. It is necessary to be ready to address commonly present soft tissue contracture and bone deficiency. The literature suggests that arthroplasty after instability surgery is associated with satisfactory pain relief. However, longer term reports point to a high rate of revision surgery and unsatisfactory results from instability, implant failure, or painful glenoid arthritis.

REFERENCES

1. Hawkins RJ, Angelo RL. Glenohumeral osteoarthritis: a late complication of Putti-Platt repair. *J Bone Joint Surg Am* 1990;72:1193–1197.
2. Lombardo SJ, Kerlan RK, Jobe FW, et al. The modified Bristow procedure for recurrent dislocation of the shoulder. *J Bone Joint Surg Am* 1976;58:256–261.
3. Samilson RL, Prieto V. Dislocation arthropathy of the shoulder. *J Bone Joint Surg Am* 1983;65:456–460.
4. Young DC, Rockwood CA. Complications of failed Bristow procedure and their management. *J Bone Joint Surg Am* 1984;73:969–981.
5. Bigliani LU, Weinstein DM, Glasgow MT, et al. Glenohumeral arthroplasty for arthritis after instability surgery. *J Shoulder Elbow Surg* 1994;4:87–94.
6. Bauer GS, Freehill MQ, Masters C, et al. Glenohumeral arthroplasty for arthritis after instability surgery. Poster presented at the 69th annual meeting of the American Academy of Orthopaedic Surgeons; February 19–17, 2002; Dallas, Tex.
7. Sperling JW, Antuña SA, Sanchez-Sotelo J, et al. Shoulder arthroplasty for arthritis after instability surgery. *J Bone Joint Surg Am* 2002;84:1775–1781.
8. Neer CS, Watson KC, Stanton FJ. Recent experience in total shoulder replacement. *J Bone Joint Surg Am* 1982;64:319–337.
9. Young S-W, Lazarus MD, Harryman II DT. Practical guidelines to safe surgery about the subscapularis. *J Shoulder Elbow Surg* 1996;5:467–470.
10. Steinmann SP, Cofield RH. Bone grafting for glenoid deficiency in total shoulder replacement. *J Shoulder Elbow Surg* 2000;9:361–367.
11. Sperling JW, Cofield RH. Revision total shoulder arthroplasty for the treatment of glenoid arthrosis. *J Bone Joint Surg Am* 1998;80:860–867.

Konrad I. Gruson
Evan L. Flatow

Prosthetic Arthroplasty for Locked Shoulder Dislocations

INTRODUCTION

Chronic, locked dislocations of the glenohumeral joint are the sequelae of initially missed or misdiagnosed acute dislocations. Often, these missed dislocations are the result of late patient presentation, the lack of complete radiographic evaluation, or failure of the treating physician to include dislocation in the differential diagnosis. Although the term "chronic dislocation" of the glenohumeral joint has never been uniformly defined, most authors would agree on 3 to 4 weeks as an acceptable cutoff point between acute and chronic dislocation. It is generally not advisable to attempt a closed reduction in the emergency department of chronic dislocations because of the risk for fracture, particularly in elderly, osteoporotic individuals. Operative intervention, including closed (under anesthesia) or open reduction; open reduction with humeral or glenoid articular reconstruction; soft tissue reconstruction; or prosthetic arthroplasty is indicated in the presence of pain, functional limitations, or both. Timely diagnosis and adherence to an appropriate treatment algorithm yield superior clinical results.

CLINICAL DIAGNOSIS

Evaluation of a suspected locked glenohumeral dislocation begins with a thorough clinical history, with particular emphasis on recent or remote upper extremity trauma, its mechanism, and its timing. Anterior dislocations, for instance, result from posteriorly directed forces on the abducted, externally rotated arm. Additionally, the presence of a seizure history or electrocution provides further evidence as to a possible dislocation. Physical examination findings are often subtle, and inspection should be performed from the front and the back. Clinically, patients with a locked anterior dislocation will hold their shoulder in an extended, abducted, and, generally, neutral position. Fullness can be noted anteriorly, representing the prominent humeral head, and attempts at rotation will likely be unsuccessful and lead to significant pain. Patients with chronic anterior dislocations are more prone to functional deficits given the externally rotated posture of their glenohumeral joint, bringing their hand away from their body. With posterior dislocations, flattening of the anterior deltoid with prominence of the cora-coid process can be seen (Fig. 26.1). Compensation with truncal and scapulothoracic movements may make these patients appear to have greater glenohumeral motion and must be controlled for when evaluating the patient for the first time.

Standard radiographs include the anteroposterior, scapular lateral, and axillary views, all of which should be routinely obtained in the setting of shoulder pain or dysfunction. The latter image, when taken appropriately, provides much useful information, including the direction of dislocation, the amount of humeral head articular surface involved, and the presence of displaced glenoid or proximal humerus fractures. This view may not always be easily obtainable given patient discomfort and motion limitations, and a Velpeau view may be substituted. Posterior dislocations reportedly are missed on initial evaluation over 50% of the time, often because of inadequate radiographic evaluation. Locked posterior dislocations are often misdiagnosed as frozen shoulders, with unfortunate results if manipulation under anesthesia is attempted. Because anterior dislocations are more obvious in radiographs, chronic unreduced anterior dislocations often occur in patients without regular access to medical care or those with altered mental states, especially elderly patients in custodial institutions. The pain may seem to be normal, and thus these patients may present with new shoulder pain after a trivial injury and be mistakenly thought to have a new acute dislocation. Reviewing prior chest radiographs may help establish the long-standing nature of the dislocation. When a locked dislocation has been confirmed, computed tomography (CT) and magnetic resonance imaging (MRI) are invaluable for subsequent management, particularly in cases of mid-size humeral articular lesions (Fig. 26.2). CT allows accurate estimate of the damage to the humeral head articular arc and glenoid rim and can help establish that the dislocation is recent if anterior glenoid neck periosteal changes are seen. MRI provides information on the condition of the remaining glenohumeral articular cartilage, as well as the status of the rotator cuff. Less commonly, specialized views following joint reduction, including the West Point axillary view for evaluation of the anterior inferior glenoid rim and the Stryker Notch view for Hill-Sachs lesions have been described. The humeral defect is posterolateral with chronic anterior dislocations and anteromedial with posterior shoulder dislocations.

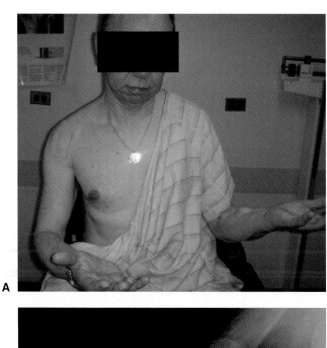

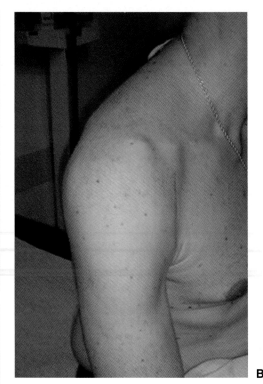

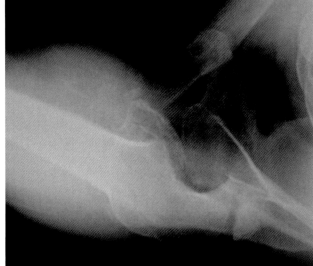

Figure 26.1. A 54-year-old right-handed man with a chronic posterior dislocation. Frontal (**A**) and side (**B**) views of a locked posterior dislocation. Note the lack of external rotation compared with the contralateral shoulder. (**C**) The axillary radiographic view demonstrates the characteristic reverse Hill-Sachs lesion.

CONSIDERATIONS FOR TREATMENT

The decision whether to proceed with surgical intervention for the treatment of chronic locked anterior or posterior dislocations, as well as the optimum technique, depends on a host of both patient-related and injury-related factors. Patients with low functional demands, including those in skilled nursing facilities or those with diminished mental capacity, may benefit from a nonoperative approach—so-called skillful neglect. Additionally, some patients, particularly with posterior dislocations, have adapted to their limited shoulder motion and do not desire surgery. On the other hand, younger patients with higher demands may wish to consider surgery. Finally, the size of the humeral head impaction injury, amount of glenoid bone deficiency, duration of the dislocation, and intraoperative status of the glenohumeral articular surface all play a significant role in the surgical decision-making process.

CLOSED VERSUS OPEN REDUCTION

Closed reduction may be attempted in the operating room under regional or general anesthesia within 3 to 4 weeks of dislocation provided that the impression fracture constitutes less than 20% of the humeral head articular surface and a concomitant proximal humerus fracture is not seen. Preoperative imaging should be examined closely for signs of chronicity. The presence of a neoglenoid or sclerosis along the impaction injury margin suggests a long-standing dislocation, and closed reduction should be avoided. The standard maneuver combines some gentle traction, a lateral pull to disengage the head, and rotation to reduce the joint, the direction of which depends on the direction of dislocation. Even when this maneuver is successful, the shoulder should be taken through a range of motion to determine stability. If unstable through a functional range, the patient should undergo planned open

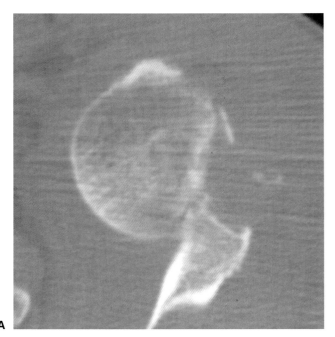

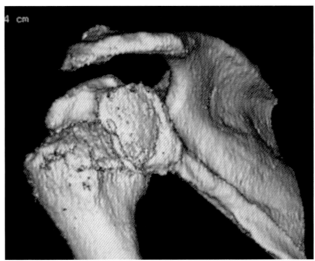

A

B

Figure 26.2. Chronic anterior glenohumeral dislocation in a 70-year-old nonverbal nursing home patient. Axial computed tomography scan **(A)** and three-dimensional reconstruction **(B)** demonstrate the chronicity of the dislocation with sclerosis along the margin of the Hill-Sachs lesion. This patient was treated with "skillful neglect."

reduction with further osseous or soft tissue reconstruction. If stable, the patient may immobilized for a period of approximately 3 weeks, as following an acute traumatic dislocation, with physical or occupational therapy for stretching and motion started thereafter. Postoperative radiographs should be obtained to confirm successful reduction.

In general, cases involving 20% to 40% humeral articular damage require both open reduction of the joint and a secondary procedure to render the impaction injury extra-articular. For anterior dislocations, an osteochondral femoral head allograft may be used, whereas for chronic posterior dislocations, the preferred method is a transfer of lesser tuberosity with attached subscapularis into the defect, fixed in place with cancellous screws.

PROSTHETIC ARTHROPLASTY

When the dislocation is of more than 6 months duration, or the size of the humeral lesion exceeds approximately 40% to 50%, arthroplasty becomes indicated. Evaluation of the humeral and glenoid osseous defects should be performed preoperatively with CT so that the appropriate implants or bone graft materials are readily available. The duration of dislocation relates to the status of the articular cartilage and subchondral bone. When the glenohumeral joint has remained dislocated for more than 6 months, arthroplasty is indicated, regardless of the size of the impaction injury. The portion of the head out of contact with the glenoid becomes soft and will usually collapse and flatten if loaded again after reduction. Whether the glenoid should also be addressed depends on the status of its

cartilage and the feasibility of obtaining a stable surface for the glenoid component. In cases more than 12 months in duration, the glenoid should probably be resurfaced. A conventional shoulder replacement may be used when the rotator cuff is intact or reconstructable. In elderly patients with massive cuff tears, a reverse arthroplasty may be required.

CONTRAINDICATIONS TO PROSTHETIC REPLACEMENT

Given the relatively uncommon nature of both chronic anterior and posterior dislocations, few strict guidelines regarding the use of arthroplasty exist. Absolute contraindications to joint replacement include the presence of an active infection within the shoulder joint and the concomitant absence of deltoid and rotator cuff function. Relative contraindications include the existence of medical comorbidities that put the patient's life at risk and poor patient nutritional status. If the patient's medical comorbidities contributed to the dislocation and late presentation thereof (e.g., seizures, alcoholism), these should be evaluated and treated during the perioperative period. Furthermore, any suggestion that a patient will be unwilling or unable to comply with postoperative activity restrictions should lead to alternative modes of treatment. Those patients who have minimal pain and/or have adapted to their functional limitations should also be considered for nonoperative treatment. Special mention should be made for young patients with large Hill-Sachs lesions and a dislocation of less than 6 months duration. Every attempt should be made to preserve the native glenohumeral joint before arthroplasty (Fig. 26.3).

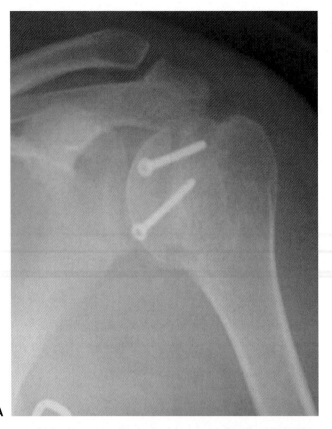

A

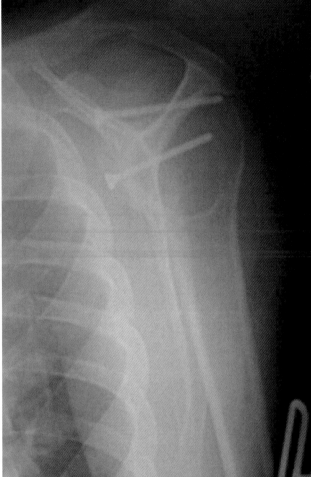

B

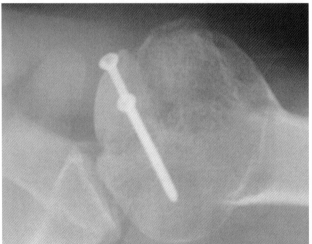

C

Figure 26.3. Allograft reconstruction in a 23-year-old man with a 9-month-old posterior glenohumeral dislocation after falling and suffering a loss of consciousness. Postoperative (**A**) anteroposterior, scapular lateral (**B**), and axillary (**C**) views demonstrate restoration of the articular surface with the allograft.

SURGICAL TECHNIQUE

PATIENT POSITIONING

Patients undergoing shoulder arthroplasty for chronic dislocations are placed in the standard beach chair position with the upper body elevated approximately 45 degrees to the horizontal. Whether to use a padded Mayo stand on which to rest the arm, or a hydraulic arm holder as in our institution, is entirely surgeon dependent. The latter reduces the number of surgical assistants needed. A head holder is employed to

maintain the neutral cervical spine alignment, and the endotracheal tube should be held firmly on the side opposite the surgical site.

LOCKED ANTERIOR DISLOCATIONS

The upper extremity and chest should be prepped widely for maximum exposure. A standard deltopectoral approach is used for anterior dislocations. Given the proximity of the brachial plexus to the anteriorly displaced humeral head, as

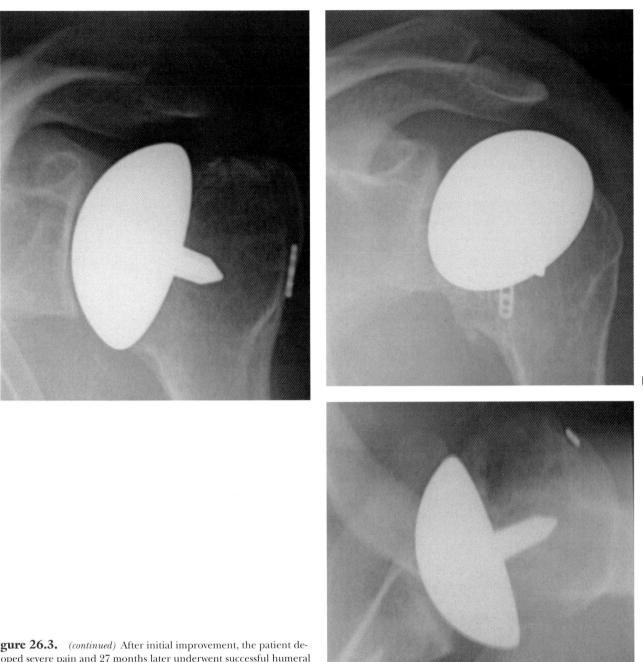

Figure 26.3. *(continued)* After initial improvement, the patient developed severe pain and 27 months later underwent successful humeral head resurfacing **(D–F)**.

well as the abnormal anatomic relationships, caution must be exercised during the approach. It is often useful to identify specific landmarks, such as the long biceps tendon and coracoid process, to help guide the initial dissection. By following the biceps proximally, the tuberosities can be located and the rotator interval opened. Routine sacrifice of the coracoacromial ligament is not recommended; however, the leading edge may be excised for better exposure. The location of the axillary nerve is critical in these cases and can be palpated along the inferior edge of the subscapularis, whereupon a tug test is performed for confirmation. After tying off the branches of the anterior circumflex humeral arteries, the inferior margin

of the subscapularis is defined. The lesser tuberosity is osteotomized and the muscle tagged with No. 2 nonabsorbable sutures at the muscle-tendon interface (Fig. 26.4). Chronic dislocations are a difficult surgical challenge, and meticulous technique is required for the extensive releases needed. There is usually granulation tissue filling the "empty" glenoid, and this must be excised to allow reduction. The humeral neck must be subperiosteally exposed and extensively released. The posterolateral defect in the humeral head can be observed with extension and external rotation of the humerus following dislocation (Fig. 26.4A). Humeral preparation technique follows the standard for total shoulders, although one should be

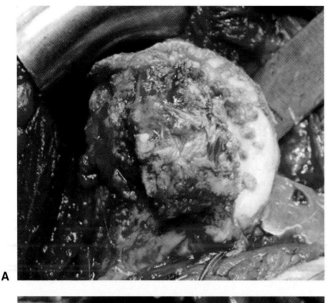

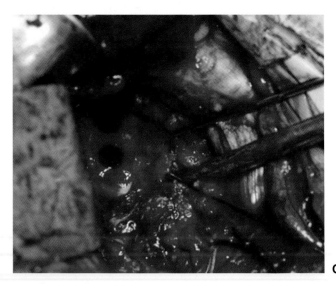

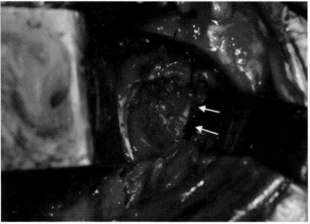

Figure 26.4. Chronic anterior dislocation in an 80-year-old woman. The lesser tuberosity was osteotomized for exposure to allow for bone-to-bone healing after repair of the subscapularis. **(A)** After dislocation, the posterolateral humeral head defect can be seen, with extension and external rotation of the humerus. **(B)** Intraoperatively, approximately 25% of the anteroinferior glenoid was noted to be deficient (*black arrows*, thickened posterior capsule; *white arrows,* articular defect), and **(C)** humeral head autograft was fashioned and definitively secured in place with suture and local soft tissue. This supported the glenoid prosthesis well.

prepared to increase the stem version (place in more retroversion) following trial implantation.

Glenoid exposure may be complicated by posterior capsular contractures, which can be dealt with through adequate release. In the presence of glenoid erosion or significant damage to the articular cartilage, resurfacing should be used. For small increases in glenoid version as measured on the preoperative CT scan and intraoperative assessment, eccentric reaming to neutral version should be performed. With significant anteversion or frank bone loss, augmentation with iliac crest bone graft, humeral head autograft, or a coracoid transfer may be indicated (Fig. 26.4C). After successful fixation to the native glenoid, this can be reamed for placement of the cemented polyethylene. A trial reduction is performed, stability assessed, and the final components placed. The axillary nerve is again located, and, if any tension is recognized, a microvascular surgeon is called to perform a neurolysis. The subscapularis is secured with nonabsorbable sutures. The wound is closed by layers in a standard fashion. Postoperative plain radiographs are obtained in the operating room to confirm component placement and concentric joint reduction (Fig. 26.4D,E). We prefer to place a suction drain for a

period of no more than 24 hours postoperatively, to lessen the chance for significant hematoma formation. Antibiotics are administered for 24 hours. Sterile dressings are maintained for 48 hours, and patients are typically discharged on the second postoperative day.

LOCKED POSTERIOR DISLOCATIONS

The deltopectoral approach may also be used for posterior dislocations. The surgeon should avoid further injury to the glenoid cartilage when unlocking the humeral head from the posterior glenoid rim. This can be accomplished with the use of a Darrach or elevator. Careful attention to the status of both the soft tissues and bony anatomy can lead to successful outcomes following arthroplasty. It may be prudent to perform a posterior capsular plication to resist further posterior instability, before or after the glenoid component has been placed. The senior author has had success with both a purse-string type capsular tightening and suture anchors placed in the posterior glenoid(Fig. 26.5). As discussed earlier, when performing a total shoulder arthroplasty, the anterior glenoid rim, or high side, may be eccentrically reamed to provide

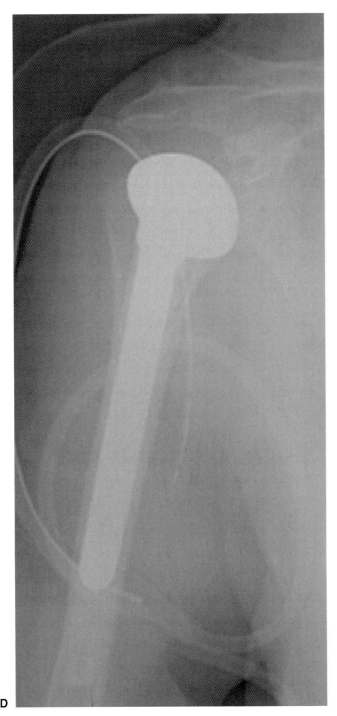

D

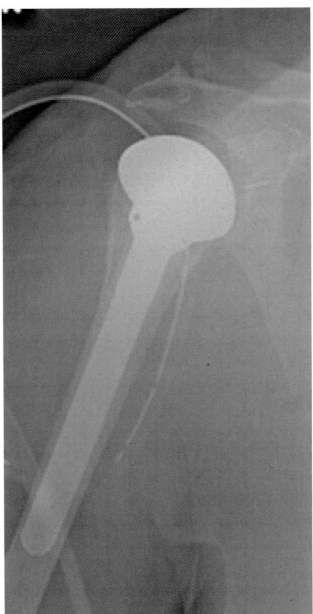

E

Figure 26.4. *(continued)* **(D,E)** Postoperative radiographs demonstrated excellent component position.

more anteversion. Bone graft can be used to augment significant glenoid deficiency, although this is far less common than with anterior dislocations. On the humeral side, either a cemented or press-fit stem may be selected based on patient age and bone quality. Our protocol dictates cement for patients above age 65 to ensure adequate fixation and prevent potential intraoperative humeral fracture from impacting an uncemented stem. The humeral stem may be anteverted to increase stability.

POSTOPERATIVE CARE

Postoperative rehabilitation begins immediately after surgery. This includes both physical therapy for ambulation training and occupational therapy for upper extremity motion and assistance with activities of daily living. Before wound closure, the surgeon should assess the amount of glenohumeral external rotation allowable without stressing the subscapularis repair. The shoulder should be maintained in a sling for the first 4 weeks after

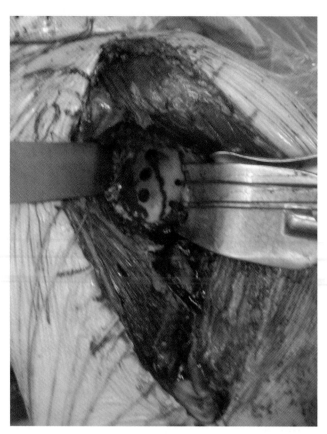

Figure 26.5.   Intra-operative photograph demonstrating the placement of Panalok (DePuy Mitek, Raynham, MA) anchors in the posterior glenoid prior to placement of the final glenoid prosthesis. This was used to plicate a patulous posterior capsule and reduce the tendency for posterior subluxation.

surgery, with the exception of therapy sessions and bathing. Gentle pendulum exercises help maintain shoulder motion in the early postsurgical period. Passive motion with progressive increase in forward flexion, internal rotation to the chest wall, and external rotation to the position determined in the operating room should be initiated. Active motion of the elbow, wrist, and digits should be started immediately as well. At 6 weeks, supine active-assisted motion and the use of a pulley can be started, with gradual progression to active motion over the following weeks. The goal is full active motion by 10 to 12 weeks, at which point early resistive strengthening may begin (Fig. 26.6).

Modifications to this protocol should be made in the event of rotator cuff repairs or capsular plication. Patients who undergo posterior soft tissue plication are placed in a gunslinger brace in neutral to slightly externally rotated position. These patients should remain in the brace for a period of approximately 2 weeks to allow for scar tissue formation. They are allowed passive forward elevation in the scapular plane with the forearm supinated. The previously described therapy protocol can then be initiated when the gunslinger sling is discontinued. Our patients return at regular intervals for postoperative checks, usually at 6 weeks, 3 months, 6 months, 12 months, and then

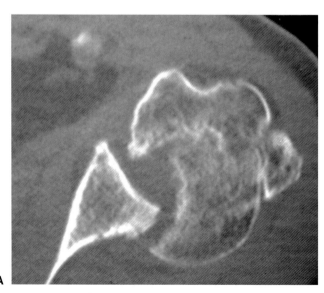

A

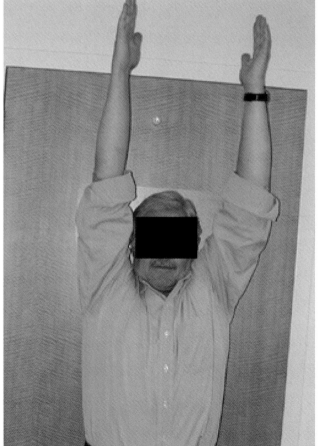

B

Figure 26.6.   Six-year clinical follow-up of a hemiarthroplasty for a locked, posterior dislocation. **(A)** Axial computed tomography demonstrates significant injury to the humeral articular surface with malunion of the greater tuberosity. Clinical images of forward elevation from the front **(B)** and from the side *(continued)*

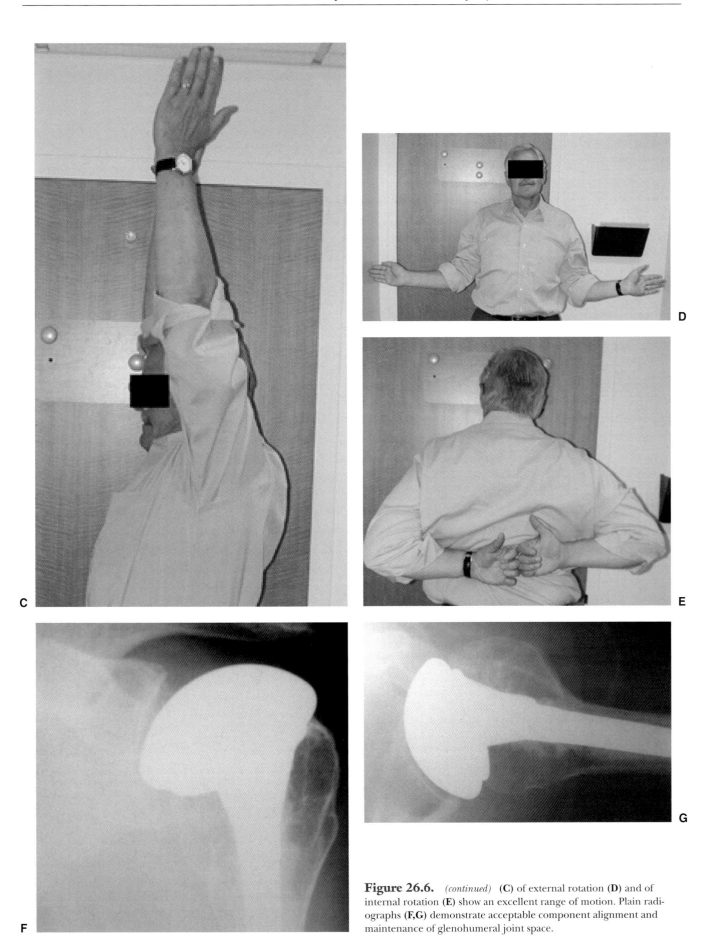

Figure 26.6. *(continued)* **(C)** of external rotation **(D)** and of internal rotation **(E)** show an excellent range of motion. Plain radiographs **(F,G)** demonstrate acceptable component alignment and maintenance of glenohumeral joint space.

TABLE 26.1	Outcomes for Prosthetic Replacement of Chronic Anterior Glenohumeral Dislocations				
Authors	No. Cases	Procedure Performed	Mean Patient Age (Range)	Mean Follow-Up (Range)	Results
Rowe et al,[1] 1982	1	1 TSR	48 years	1.8 years	Rowe and Zarins criteria: Excellent
Pritchett et al,[2] 1987	4	2 TSR 2 HHR	60 years (56–63)	2.3 years (2–3)	Rowe and Zarins criteria: 2 Good 2 Fair
Flatow et al,[3] 1993	9	8 TSR 1 HHR 3 GBG	64 years (48–73)	3.9 years (2–6)	Neer criteria: 4 Excellent 4 Satisfactory 1 LTFU (HHR at 14 months)
Matsoukis et al[4]	11	4 TSR 7 HHR 4 GBG: 3 HHR, 1 TSR	67 years (45–84)	47.7 months (24–86)	Constant score 21–46 Forward elevation 49–90 degrees External rotation 13–26 degrees

GBG, glenoid bone graft; HHR, humeral head replacement; LTFU, lost to follow-up; TSR, total shoulder replacement.

TABLE 26.2	Outcomes for Prosthetic Replacement of Chronic Posterior Glenohumeral Dislocations				
Authors	No. Cases	Procedure Performed	Mean Patient Age (Range)	Mean Follow-Up (Range)	Results
Rowe et al,[1] 1982	2	2 HHR	44.5 years (38–51)	6.5 years (3–10)	Rowe and Zarins criteria: 1 Good 1 Fair
Hawkins et al,[5] 1987	16	9 HHR (2 referrals, 1 failed McLaughlin) 7 TSR (1 failed McLaughlin)	NA	HHR (2–14 years) TSR (1–8)	HHR 6 Good 3 Failed (converted to TSR) TSR 6 Good 1 Failed (posterior dislocation)
Pritchett et al,[2] 1987	3	2 HHR 1 TSR	49 years (36–67)	2.3 years (2–3)	Rowe and Zarins criteria: HHR 2 Good TSR 1 Good
Cheng et al,[6] 1997	7	7 TSR	58 years (40–71)	27 months (13–63)	VAS pain 7.7–3.5 ROM External rotation 4–11.4 degrees Internal rotation S2 to T10 Forward elevation 77–109 degrees ASES score 20.1–55.6
Checchia et al,[7] 1998	13	8 HHR 5 TSR	HHR 47.8 years (28–79) TSR 43.2 years (31–59)	HHR 36.2 months (12–59) TSR 32.6 months (23–45)	UCLA criteria: HHR (mean 25.6 points) 3 Excellent 2 Good 1 Fair 2 Poor TSR (mean 17 points) 1 Good 1 Fair 3 Poor
Sperling et al,[8] 2004	12	6 HHR 6 TSR	56 years (36–78)	9 years (0.7–22)	Modified Neer criteria: HHR 4 Satisfactory 2 Unsatisfactory TSR 1 Excellent 2 Satisfactory 3 Unsatisfactory

HHR, humeral head replacement; NA, not available; ROM, range of motion; TSR, total shoulder replacement; VAS, visual analog scale.

annually. Radiographs are obtained at each visit. For elderly patients with massive cuff tears a reverse arthroplasty may be required.

OUTCOMES

The outcomes for the use of arthroplasty in chronic anterior and posterior shoulder dislocations are summarized in Tables 26.1 and 26.2. Most series demonstrate satisfactory patient outcomes when surgeons experienced in the use of shoulder arthroplasty are involved and careful attention is given to soft tissue and bony deficiencies (Fig. 26.5). Perhaps the most important predictors of outcome include early diagnosis, proper patient selection, thorough preoperative planning, and skillful surgical execution.

REFERENCES

1. Rowe CR, Zarins B. Chronic unreduced dislocations of the shoulder. *J Bone Joint Surg Am* 1982;64:494–505.
2. Pritchett JW, Clark JM. Prosthetic replacement for chronic unreduced dislocations of the shoulder. *Clin Orthop Relat Res* 1987;216:89–93.
3. Flatow EL, Miller SR, Neer CS II. Chronic anterior dislocation of the shoulder. *J Shoulder Elbow Surg* 1993;2:2–10.
4. Matsoukis J, Tabib W, Guiffault P, Mandelbaum A, Walch G, Nemoz C, Cortes ZE, Edwards TB. Primary unconstrained shoulder arthroplasty in patients with a fixed anterior glenohumeral dislocation. *J Bone Joint Surg Am* 2006;88(3):547–552.
5. Hawkins RJ, Neer CS II, Pianta RM, et al. Locked posterior dislocation of the shoulder. *J Bone Joint Surg Am* 1987;69:9–18.
6. Cheng SL, Mackay MB, Richards RR. Treatment of locked posterior fracture-dislocations of the shoulder by total shoulder arthroplasty. *J Shoulder Elbow Surg* 1997;6:11–17.
7. Checchia SL, Santos PD, Miyazaki AN. Surgical treatment of acute and chronic posterior fracture-dislocation of the shoulder. *J Shoulder Elbow Surg* 1998;7:53–65.
8. Sperling JW, Pring M, Antuña SA, et al. Shoulder arthroplasty for locked posterior dislocation of the shoulder. *J Shoulder Elbow Surg* 2004;13:522–527.

Emilie V. Cheung
Scott P. Steinmann

Prosthetic Arthroplasty in Shoulder Dysplasia

INTRODUCTION

Glenoid dysplasia, or hypoplasia of the scapular neck, is a rare structural anomaly. It involves decreased posterior and inferior glenoid bone, resulting in a very shallow glenoid fossa and an irregular or "dentate" glenoid articular surface.[1–5] It is believed to involve the pectoral girdle in either a symmetrical and bilateral or unilateral form.[1] There may be a familial association.[5] Rarely, shoulders with dysplasia of the glenoid develop osteoarthritis and become symptomatic enough to warrant surgical intervention.

Developmentally, most of the scapula is formed by intramembranous ossification from eight centers. The glenoid fossa develops from a proximal and distal ossification center.[7] An abnormality of one or both of these sites has been implicated in the development of glenoid hypoplasia. It is characterized by incomplete ossification of the lower two thirds of the cartilaginous glenoid and adjacent scapular neck.[8,9]

Glenoid hypoplasia is thought to be more common than previously suspected because in mild forms it is asymptomatic and frequently goes unrecognized. It has been described as an incidental finding on chest radiography in asymptomatic individuals.[6,7] Moderate to severe glenoid dysplasia was seen in a magnetic resonance imaging (MRI) study of 98 shoulders, with an incidence of 14.3%.[4] Edelson[10] found that localized hypoplasia of the posteroinferior glenoid was detected as an incidental finding in 18% of 300 shoulder computed tomography (CT) and MRI studies. He also observed localized glenoid hypoplasia in 20% to 35% of 1,150 scapular bone specimens. He concluded that this phenomenon may contribute to the posterior glenoid wear seen in osteoarthritis of the shoulder. However, he did not differentiate between posterior wear from the arthritic process and that from congenital retroversion.

Walsh et al[11] studied the morphology of the glenoid using CT in 113 shoulders with primary osteoarthritis. They found that 9% of specimens had retroversion of greater than 25 degrees, regardless of the glenoid erosion from the arthritic process, which was believed to be congenital. Retroversion in these cases was found to be primarily of dysplastic origin and may explain the etiology of osteoarthritis in this subgroup of patients.

Although there was a wide range of polymorphism in these glenoids, the authors concluded that the osteoarthritis associated with glenoid hypoplasia was distinct from that associated with advanced posterior glenoid erosion.[11] The latter phenomenon increases with age and leads to excess glenoid retroversion and humeral subluxation. The former is a result of a congenital anomaly.

ASSOCIATED FINDINGS

Associated deformities of the shoulder are variable—hypoplasia and flattening of the humeral head, varus angulation of the humeral neck,[1–3] enlargement of the acromion and increased prominence of the coracoid.[1] Hooking, or "bossing," of the distal clavicle has also been described.[3,5]

In an MRI study, posterior labral tears were detected in 64.3% of 14 shoulders with moderate to severe glenoid dysplasia.[4] There was a significantly higher association with labral tears in shoulders with moderate to severe dysplasia than those with more normal glenoids.

ASSOCIATED SYMPTOMS

Clinical findings in patients with glenoid dysplasia are varied, from severe pain to no symptoms at all. Some young patients (under the age of 40) with symptomatic glenoid dysplasia present with clicking, posterior or multidirectional instability, and/or limitation of movement, especially in abduction.[3,6] The majority of these patients respond to physical therapy.[7]

Wirth et al[7] reported on 16 patients with glenoid hypoplasia. They divided their patients into three groups—those with bilateral glenoid hypoplasia without shoulder instability, those with bilateral glenoid hypoplasia with shoulder instability, and those with unilateral glenoid hypoplasia and severe deformity of the humeral head. The majority of patients in their relatively young cohort (14 of the 16 patients) responded to conservative treatment, including activity avoidance, physical therapy, and nonsteroidal anti-inflammatories, with considerable improvement in pain ratings and activity level. In another study,[3] all patients under the age of 40 with glenoid dysplasia responded well to physiotherapy and had minimal symptoms.

RESULTS OF OPERATIVE TREATMENT

There is a paucity of published data on shoulder arthroplasty for osteoarthritis resulting from glenoid dysplasia. Sperling et al[12] reported on a series of seven shoulders, four treated with hemiarthroplasty and three with total shoulder arthroplasty, with a mean 7-year follow-up. Two of the three shoulders treated with total shoulder arthroplasty had an excellent result. The third had an unsatisfactory result because of suspected deep infection. Three of the four hemiarthroplasties had unsatisfactory results and eventually underwent revision to total shoulder arthroplasty as a result of glenoid arthrosis within the first 2.5 years (Fig. 27.1A–F). The fourth patient with hemiarthroplasty who did not undergo revision surgery had a glenoid osteotomy performed at the time of the hemiarthroplasty. The authors concluded that glenoid deficiency and cartilage wear should be addressed at the time of shoulder arthroplasty in patients with glenoid dysplasia, if possible, for the best chance of pain relief.

Edwards et al[13] studied 15 shoulder arthroplasties in patients with osteoarthritis and dysplastic glenoid morphology. A glenoid component was placed when there was at least 15 mm of glenoid bone depth at the midpoint of the glenoid as seen on axial cuts of CT scans. There were 11 total shoulders and four

hemiarthroplasties. Improvement of shoulder scores occurred in pain relief, motion, and function, reflecting favorable results overall. With the numbers available, they could not detect a significant difference between total shoulder arthroplasty and hemiarthroplasty.

Smith and Bunker[3] reported that the results of arthroplasty were disappointing in three patients, with mean pain rating score of 5 on the visual analog scale of 0 to 10. The authors warn that surgery in these patients is technically difficult and results are generally unsatisfactory. However, this may be a treatment option in patients with unremitting pain and disability.

OPERATIVE TECHNIQUE

A deltopectoral approach is used. The subacromial space, subdeltoid space, and subcoracoid space are bluntly dissected free of adhesions. The status of the rotator cuff is assessed. The biceps tendon and rotator interval are identified. The subscapularis is released from the lesser tuberosity just medial to its insertion, and this release is continued proximally and medially through the rotator interval to the level of the glenoid. Alternatively, the lesser tuberosity is osteotomized as a flake of bone with the subscapularis attached and the osteotomy site is repaired with transosseous sutures at the end of the procedure. The subscapularis may be lengthened if necessary by a Z-lengthening procedure or by a release of the anterior capsule off of the superior rolled edge of the subscapularis. If needed

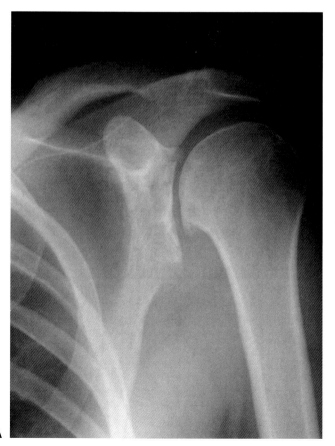

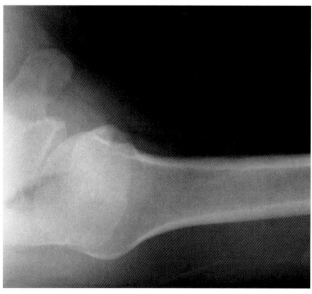

Figure 27.1. **(A,B)** Radiographs demonstrate typical posterior and inferior bone deficiency present with glenoid dysplasia.

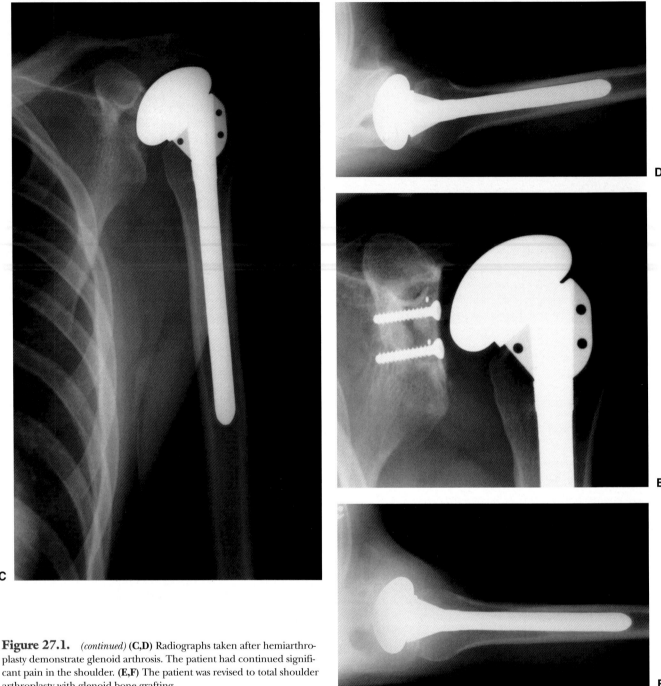

Figure 27.1. *(continued)* **(C,D)** Radiographs taken after hemiarthroplasty demonstrate glenoid arthrosis. The patient had continued significant pain in the shoulder. **(E,F)** The patient was revised to total shoulder arthroplasty with glenoid bone grafting.

in an extremely tight shoulder, transection of the superior rolled edge of the subscapularis may be performed.

The surgeon should be cognizant of proximal humeral deformity. If there is varus angulation of the humeral neck, passing a long stem down the humeral canal from the standard starting point 1 cm posterior to the bicipital groove may be technically difficult. Some shoulder prostheses are available with short or narrow stems and may be useful in these cases. The humeral component is routinely a press-fit prosthesis. It may be implanted with less retroversion to compensate for the posterior

glenoid deficiency. Consideration of a resurfacing type arthroplasty for the humerus may also be considered in such instances. However, this has not been reported in the literature.

The glenoid is often technically challenging to adequately expose. Further, there is often compromised bone stock for placement of a glenoid component. A circumferential release of the capsule around the glenoid labrum may facilitate exposure. In addition, a complete inferior release is performed directly off of the humeral neck to enhance glenoid exposure. Structural bone grafting of the dysplastic glenoid may be needed to support a glenoid component. This can be accomplished by using bone obtained from the humeral head or iliac crest. It may be performed in a fashion similar to that described for glenoid revision surgery.[14]

The center of the glenoid is identified, and a central hole is made perpendicular to neutral glenoid alignment. If the glenoid depth is shallow and cannot be shortened more than a few millimeters, segmental bone grafting may be needed. The anterior glenoid is prepared with a reamer in the normal glenoid orientation. The additional anchoring holes for the keel or pegs are prepared. The deficient posterior glenoid is prepared to receive the bone graft. Segmental bone graft from the humeral head or iliac crest is placed into the deficiency and provisionally fixed with Steinmann pins. Screws are placed across the graft into the glenoid and countersunk. The glenoid component is secured in position.

CONCLUSION

Glenoid dysplasia is a rare finding in the clinical practice of shoulder surgery and often responds to conservative management. When end-stage osteoarthritis develops, shoulder arthroplasty may be warranted. Arthroplasty for glenoid dysplasia is a technically challenging procedure, and there is little informa-

tion in the literature on this topic. The literature suggests that the glenoid should be resurfaced when technically possible.

REFERENCES

1. de Bellis U, Buarino A, Castelli F. Glenoid hypoplasia: description of a clinical case and analysis of the literature. *Chir Organi Mov* 2001:86:305–309.
2. Pettersson H. Bilateral dysplasia of the neck of the scapula and associated anomalies. *Acta Radiol Diagn (Stokh)* 1981:22:81–84.
3. Smith SP, Bunker TD. Primary glenoid dysplasia: a review of 12 patients. *J Bone Joint Surg Br* 2001:83:868–872.
4. Harper KW, Helms CA, Haystead CM, et al. Glenoid dysplasia: incidence and association with posterior labral tears as evaluated on MRI. *Am J Roentgenol* 2005:184:984–988.
5. Resnick D, Walter RD, Crudale AS. Bilateral dysplasia of the scapular neck. *Am J Roentgenol* 1982:139:387–389.
6. Weishaupt D, Zanetti M, Exner GU. Familial occurrence of glenoid dysplasia: report of two cases in two consecutive generations. *Arch Orthop Trauma Surg* 2000:120:349–351.
7. Wirth MA, Lyons FR, Rockwood CA. Hypoplasia of the glenoid: a review of 16 patients. *J Bone Joint Surg Am* 1993:75:1175–1184.
8. Currarino G, Sheffield E, Twicker D. Congenital glenoid dysplasia. *Pediatr Radiol* 1998:28:30–37.
9. Giongo F. Un caso diarticolazione coraco-clavicolare bilaterale. *Radiol Med* 1927;14:186.
10. Edelson JG. Localized glenoid hypoplasia: an anatomic variation of possible clinical significance. *Clin Orthop Relat Res* 1995:321:189–195.
11. Walch G, Badet R, Boulahia A, Khoury A. Morphologic study of the glenoid in primary glenohumeral osteoarthritis. *J Arthroplasty* 1999;14:756–760.
12. Sperling JW, Cofield RH, Steinmann SP. Shoulder arthroplasty for osteoarthritis secondary to glenoid dysplasia. *J Bone Joint Surg Am* 2002:84:541–546.
13. Edwards TB, Boulahia A, Kempf JF, et al. Shoulder arthroplasty in patients with osteoarthritis and dysplastic glenoid morphology. *J Shoulder Elbow Surg* 2004:13:1–4.
14. Cofield RH. Bone grafting for glenoid bone deficiencies in shoulder arthritis: a review. *J Shoulder Elbow Surg* 2007;16:S273–281.

Prosthetic Arthroplasty in Neuromuscular Disorders

INTRODUCTION

Shoulder replacement surgery in a patient with a coexistent neuromuscular condition is an uncommon situation but one that requires special management. Three conditions are of particular interest and have their own nuances for shoulder reconstruction. Cerebral palsy and Parkinson's disease are disorders that affect muscle tension and coordination. Neither directly results in shoulder degeneration, but the motor dysfunction complicates reconstruction. The third condition is paraplegia. Although the shoulder may not be directly affected by spinal cord injury, the injury produces a need for the shoulder to function as a weight-bearing joint. The weight-bearing status of the shoulder places it under added stress and strain, leading to ongoing deterioration. All of these patients are subject to the same ailments of age such as degenerative arthritis, and in the case of spinal cord injury are actually at increased risk. Shoulder replacement surgery may need to be considered as a treatment option because of patient symptoms, but comorbidities will challenge routine techniques for shoulder reconstruction.

CEREBRAL PALSY

Cerebral palsy is a disorder of motor function resulting from several possible insults to the brain of the fetus or young infant. In the United States, the prevalence was found to be 0.2% in children birth to 17 years of age.[1] A similar incidence is present in other developed countries.[2] Cerebral palsy can involve any or all of the extremities, leading to the use of descriptive terms such as diplegic, hemiplegic, and quadriplegic. The hallmark of cerebral palsy is motor dysfunction. Spasticity, diagnosed by an increase in muscle tone with hyperactive deep tendon reflexes, is the most common and classic physical finding. Patients may also demonstrate varying degrees of ataxia, dyskinesia, and athetosis. Ataxia is impairment in voluntary movement resulting from a loss of coordination and thus produces difficulties with fine motor skills and gait. Dyskinesias are alterations of voluntary movements resulting from fragmented or erratic motions, whereas athetosis is marked by continual slow movements. The consequences of these dysfunctions can be twisting, jerking, or

flailing motions by the patient. However, the degree of the resultant impairment varies among patients and must be individually assessed.[3] Although no means currently exist to repair the central nervous system damage responsible for the symptoms in cerebral palsy, several interventions have been tried to diminish the sources of impairment.[4,5] These modalities include medication to reduce spasticity, physical and occupational therapy, bracing, intrathecal baclofen, and selective dorsal rhizotomy. Of particular interest to the shoulder surgeon, botulinum toxin has become widespread in the treatment of cerebral palsy to reduce isolated muscle spasticity or dystonia.[5] It offers some potential advantages in the perioperative period after shoulder arthroplasty.

There are several factors to consider in the patient with symptomatic shoulder arthritis and cerebral palsy. Mental retardation may coexist with cerebral palsy. An ability to understand the postoperative activity restrictions and physical therapy is crucial for all patients and can be especially critical with the uncontrolled movements potentially present in cerebral palsy. The surgeon must be comfortable these patients are able to cooperate to the best of their physical ability with the proposed surgery. Additionally, the surgeon must carefully assess both the static posture and dynamic movements of the shoulder. Chronic spasticity of the shoulder girdle muscles may have resulted in unusual contractures differing from the patterns normally seen with shoulder arthrosis.[5] Severe rotation, extension, abduction, or other deformities can be found. The surgeon needs to be prepared to release the contractures adequately for proper intraoperative soft tissue balancing. Finally, after delineating the patient's dynamic motor dysfunctions, it is necessary to consider how to minimize the impact of the abnormal movements and motor function on the postoperative rehabilitation regimen.

Motor dysfunction has two potential influences on postoperative therapy. The central finding of cerebral palsy is spasticity, and this increased muscle tone causes resistance to passive range of motion (ROM). Although obtaining functional ROM important, the cuff repair cannot be jeopardized. Failure of the patient's therapist to accept this limitation can lead to excessive stress placed on the shoulder reconstruction and failure of cuff integrity. The soft tissue repair can also be at risk from uncontrolled dyskinetic movements. If dyskinesia or athetosis is present, prolonged protection of the shoulder in an immobilizer is necessary. Finally, as in all patients who are candidates for shoulder arthroplasty, the bone stock and preoperative integrity of the rotator cuff must be considered. Absent prior surgery, these areas do not usually present any impediment to replacement surgery.

Depending on the severity and pattern of involvement of their cerebral palsy, these patients may rely on the upper extremity for assistance in overall mobility. Conflicting demands can arise between the patient's need to use the extremity for mobilization and the importance of protecting the rotator cuff arthrotomy. If the patient is reliant on the extremity for transfers or ambulation, postoperative disposition needs to be discussed. The patient may require transfer to an acute rehabilitation hospital or skilled nursing facility until ready to return home. When the situation is unclear, referral to physical and occupational therapy preoperatively to work on adaptive measures will make disposition smoother.

Botulinum toxin has become commonly used in the treatment of spastic muscles. It can be of considerable benefit in postoperative management of the motor abnormalities with cerebral palsy. Produced by *Clostridium botulinum,* there are seven different serotypes of the neurotoxin. These are subtyped A through G.[6,7] Botulinum toxin A (BTX-A) is most commonly used in clinical practice.[8,9] BTX-A binds to receptors on the cellular membranes of cholinergic membranes and is then internalized by endocytosis.[7,8] The toxin then cleaves specific protein complexes, known as SNARE proteins, involved in the release of acetylcholine. The various subtypes cleave one or more of these proteins at distinct peptide bonds, such that no serotype acts at the same site. The result is a dose-dependent reduction in the acetylcholine at the neuromuscular junction and thus diminished muscular tension. Ultimately a sufficient dosage of botulinum toxin produces a flaccid paralysis. The various sites of action of the serotypes are believed to underlie the differing durations of efficacy. Recovery from botulinum toxin–produced neuroblockade requires restoration of the protein complexes for acetylcholine release. Initially, reduction in acetylcholine release prompts the growth of axonal sprouts at the neuromuscular junction. These new axonal sprouts release acetylcholine but appear to be temporary and retract as neurotransmitter release is re-established at the original nerve ending.[10,11] Motor function and activity are thus restored. Although evidence of muscle relaxation can persist for 4 to 6 months, the clinical usefulness seems to be a shorter 12 to 16 weeks.[4,7,12,13]

Of interest, there is some evidence of an additional benefit of pain relief from the use of botulinum toxin.[7] Laboratory studies have shown an inhibition of the release of substance P from cultured dorsal root ganglion neurons.[14] Substance P is a neurotransmitter released by nocioreceptor afferents. Another study has shown reduction in the stimulated release of calcitonin gene–related peptide (CGRP) from cultured trigeminal ganglia neurons.[15] CGRP is an inflammatory neuropeptide colocalized with substance P. In a prospective study of 60 patients with spasticity-related pain, a reduction in the level of pain was found in 90% of the patients.[16] Despite this laboratory evidence, clinically the analgesic affect may still be due primarily to a reduction in muscle spasticity.[17]

It is important to recognize that problems such as fixed joint contracture or arthrosis are not improved by the use of botulinum toxin. The use of the toxin simply provides a period of time during which additional treatments such as physical therapy or surgery can address the static disorders and thus improve activities of daily living and quality of life. A recent meta-analysis failed to show conclusive demonstration of the efficacy of BTX-A in the treatment of cerebral palsy; however, this was due to the limited number of randomized, controlled studies.[13] Additionally, weakness and poor coordination of the extremity may produce limited functional improvement after injection alone. However, the reduction in muscle tone can allow easier protected mobilization after surgical releases in arthroplasty.[18] Botulinum toxin does reproducibly reduce muscle tone and spasticity and potentially opens a valuable window for the postoperative recuperation of the patient undergoing arthroplasty.[19]

Clinical use of botulinum toxin requires particular circumstances to be effective.[9] These include use of a sufficient dose of the preparation to produce the desired muscle relaxation, dilution into a large enough fluid volume to reach all pertinent motor end plates, and accurate injection of the preparation into the fascial compartment of the spastic muscle. BTX-A is currently available in the United States in a single preparation, Botox® (Allergan Inc., Irvine California). A second preparation, Dysport® (Ipsen Ltd., Slough, United Kingdom), has a Food and Drug Administration application pending at the time of writing and is available outside the United States.[20] Botulinum toxin B is available for clinical use under the trade name Myobloc® (Elan Pharmaceuticals, San Francisco, California). Although all three preparations are measured in international units for potency, the relative potencies of the products differ. Fixed-dose ratios cannot be used between subtypes A and B or even between the two commercially available botulinum type A sources.[8,20,21] An individual assessment of the proper dosage of each product must be performed.[5]

At our institution, the patient is treated in conjunction with a neurologist conversant with the use of botulinum toxin. The patient is assessed by the orthopaedic surgeon for the severity and symptoms of the shoulder arthrosis. Particular attention is given to fixed contractures and dynamic posturing, which could influence the procedure and rehabilitation. If the patient is considered a potential surgical candidate, the patient is reviewed with the neurologist. The goal is to devise a treatment regimen that relaxes deforming muscles around the shoulder and minimizes dyskinetic movements that would disrupt a shoulder reconstruction. A trial series of injections is carried out and the patient's response evaluated. Fixed deformities that will require surgical release and the ability of the patient to engage in appropriate postoperative physical therapy are clarified. The final decision regarding the advisability of shoulder arthroplasty is then made. The proposed injection regimen is fine-tuned to optimize reduction of spasticity in the shoulder girdle.

If the decision is made to proceed with surgery, the finalized injection course of therapy is timed to maximize its postoperative benefit. Our experience is limited to the usage of Botox®. A total of 200 units is used around the shoulder girdle, diluted into a concentration of 100 units/mL. Under electromyographic guidance, the toxin is injected into multiple sites in the chosen muscles. The duration of the injections may not extend the desired length of the rehabilitation, and an additional series of injections may be necessary to protect the healing reconstruction. The duration of treatment needs to extend to the period of time sufficient to allow soft tissue reconstruction to heal. This typically will be a period of 3 to 6 months.

There are several contraindications to the use of botulinum toxin.[9,12] Patients with preexisting pseudobulbar involvement are at risk for aspiration pneumonia if there is any systemic spread of even small amounts of the toxin.[12] The presence of pseudobulbar involvement, gastroesophageal reflux, or recurring chest infections should be considered before use of botulinum toxin. Safety in pregnant or nursing women has not been established. Other potential sources of concern would be the exacerbation of its effect by muscle relaxants, the concurrent use of aminoglycoside antibiotics, or a history of a disease of the neuromuscular junction such as myasthenia gravis.

The surgical plan must include release of all articular contractures and secure repair of the arthrotomy to withstand postoperative tension during mobilization. Anterior contracture is dealt with in the familiar way, with excision of the anterior capsule off of the subscapularis tendon. The tendon is released off the anterior labrum and glenoid margin and circumferentially mobilized (Fig. 28.1A). Only on rare occasions should Z-lengthening of the tendon be considered, because this will weaken the tendon and subsequent repair. Inferiorly, the capsule is also routinely freed from the humeral neck and inferior osteophytes to approximately the 6 or 7 o'clock position. If further inferior capsulotomy is necessary because of joint tightness, this should be carried out in the direction of the inferior glenoid (Fig. 28.1B). This lessens risk to the axillary nerve. Release of the superior and posterior capsule is performed along the glenoid margin for abduction and external rotation contractures, respectively (Fig. 28.1C,D). Additionally, the bicipital tendon is often a deforming force. It is routinely tenodesed in the bicipital groove and resected intra-articularly. The objective of soft tissue release is the same as for all other patients—a stable but mobile joint with approximately 50% translation of the humeral head possible on the glenoid.

Postoperatively, the major consideration is the avoidance of damage to the soft tissue repair. This begins intraoperatively with a secure subscapularis repair. Heavy, nonabsorbable suture (no. 2 or 5) should be used and placed through both bone and tendon for the repair. Alternatively, a lesser tuberosity osteotomy may be used to improve the security of the repair by incorporating bone and tendon tissue on both sides of the repair.[27] The superior medial extension of the arthrotomy should be kept as inferior as possible to minimize anterior superior instability or escape patterns if the subscapularis still fails to heal. The progression of the rehabilitation program is slowed to emphasize soft tissue healing rather than maximal ROM. The upper extremity is supported in slight flexion and abduction for the first 6 weeks. Passive ROM is permitted initially but only within the limits established by intraoperative assessment of the soft tissue repair and the patient's residual muscle tension. Elevation is emphasized in forward flexion, and external rotation is avoided much past the neutral position. The physical therapist must understand the objectives of the procedure and the limitations placed on rehabilitation by the motor dysfunction. Frustration or overeagerness must not lead the therapist or patient to place the stability of the prosthesis at risk in an ill-advised attempt to gain excessive passive ROM.

Three patients with cerebral palsy and shoulder degenerative arthritis who had undergone shoulder arthroplasty at the Mayo Clinic were recently reported.[23] All patients had relief from severe preoperative pain and were satisfied with the procedure. However, two of the three had evidence of failure of the rotator cuff repair, which led to various degrees of weakness and limitation of motion postoperatively. Neither of these two patients had been treated with botulinum toxin. In the third patient, who was treated with BTX-A, the rotator cuff clinically healed satisfactorily, with good strength in the shoulder. The prosthesis had a stable radiographic appearance, although the shoulder was somewhat stiff. In subsequent patients the duration of treatment with botulinum toxin has been extended toward 6 months with improved ROM.

PARKINSON'S DISEASE

The interplay of Parkinson's disease and the degenerative shoulder have many of the same challenges as cerebral palsy. Parkinson's disease, however, is a progressive malady primarily in the older patient. It is linked to diminished dopamine production in the substantia nigra. The rate of progression of Parkinson's disease, although inevitable, varies and cannot be predicted at the time of diagnosis. This disease becomes more frequent with age and is considered the most common disabling movement disorder.[24] The overall prevalence is estimated at 0.3% in the American population and increases to 4% to 5% after the age of 85 years.[25] In Olmsted County, Minnesota, the lifetime risk for developing Parkinson's disease is estimated at 2.0% for men and 1.3% for women.[26]

The cardinal symptoms of Parkinson's disease are tremor, bradykinesia, rigidity, and impaired postural stability.[27–29] The tremor associated with Parkinson's disease is a resting tremor. It is most evident when the extremity is relaxed and lessened during activity. It is often described as a "pill-rolling" motion. Rigidity is an increase in muscle tone causing resistance to any passive movement of the joint. It differs from the spasticity associated with cerebral palsy in that the spastic limb has increased active muscle tone in a constant direction. Bradykinesia is defined simply as slowed movements, but it may result in a sensation of weakness for the patient because of the difficulties in activation of the specific muscle groups. Because of the rigidity and bradykinesia the patient may have difficulty adjusting to the changes in the center of gravity and thus suffer from postural instability. Additionally, these motor dysfunctions can result in difficulty with rapid and sequential activities, gait initiation, and handwriting. Dyskinesias, which are involuntary movements of the extremities, may present later in the course of the disease as a result of dopaminergic treatment.[24,30,31]

The patient with Parkinson's disease can develop nonmotor symptoms, including autonomic disturbances. The symptom that perhaps can add most to the challenge of the orthopaedic management of these patients is the development of dementia. Dementia that develops 1 year or more after the onset of the motor symptoms is classified as Parkinson's disease dementia.[32] Symptoms can include reduced mental speed, inattention, and memory and language problems.[33] Neuropsychiatric symptoms occur as well and most commonly include depression, hallucinations, and anxiety.[34] A review of prevalence studies found that dementia was diagnosed in up to 31% of the Parkinson's disease patient population.[25] Cooperation with perioperative instructions and restrictions will obviously be limited with increasing degrees of dementia.

Treatment of Parkinson's disease is usually instituted at the onset of functional impairment, and establishment of the

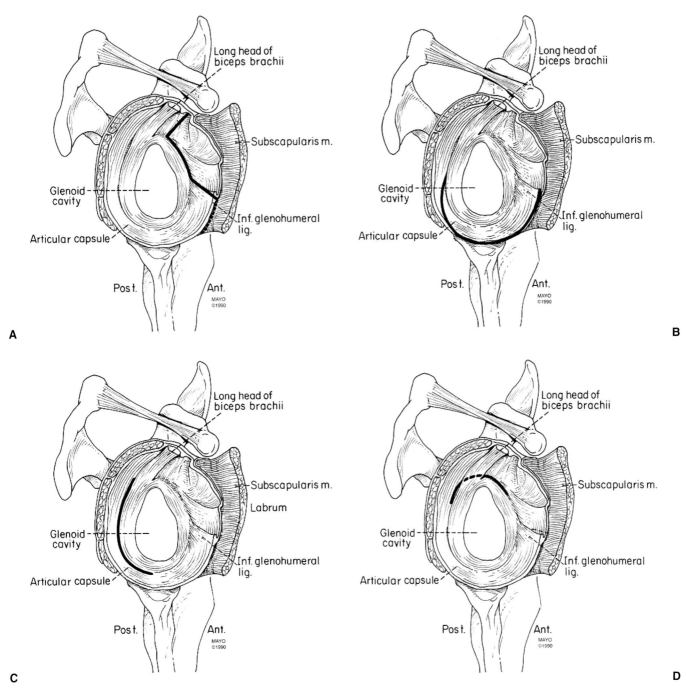

Figure 28.1. Anterior capsular release is routinely performed with shoulder arthroplasty. After arthrotomy, the capsule is identified medial to its confluence with the subscapularis and excised. **(A)** The inferior capsule is released on the humeral side to approximately the 6 o'clock position as part of exposure. It can readily be released off of the glenoid margin inferiorly after excision of the labrum. On rare occasions, the inferior capsule remains excessively tight. It must then be incised from the glenoid to humeral release after careful protection of the axillary nerve. **(B)** Less commonly, the soft tissues are so contracted that circumferential release is necessary. The capsule is then directly incised along the remaining posterior and superior glenoid margins to improve rotator cuff excursion. **(C,D)** The bicipital tendon will typically have been excised after tenodesis.

conclusive diagnosis requires substantial improvement with dopamine replacement therapy.[24] Unfortunately, there is no therapy that will slow or prevent the course of Parkinson's disease. Levodopa is the most effective medication for treatment. It is combined with carbidopa (Sinemet®) to increase central levodopa bioavailability by blocking peripheral conversion of

levodopa to dopamine by dopa decarboxylase. This also has the advantage of decreasing stimulation of the emetic center and resultant nausea. Unfortunately, dyskinesias may develop and become troublesome after years of therapy.[24,30,31,36] Dopamine agonists may cause fewer motor complications than levodopa, but they also are less effective. These medications directly stimulate dopamine receptors and include pramipexole (Mirapex®) and ropinirole (Requip®). Either levodopa/carbidopa or a dopamine agonist may be chosen as initial therapy.[37] Many other potential treatment options exist and include monoamine oxidase inhibitors, anticholinergic agents, the N-methyl-D-aspartate receptor inhibitor amantidine, catechol O-methyltransferase inhibitor, and surgery.[38] Botulinum toxin has been tried for the treatment of several of the motor and nonmotor symptoms of Parkinson's disease, including limb dystonia.[39] However, there is no literature on the use of botulinum toxin in conjunction with surgery and we similarly have no experience with its use in shoulder arthroplasty in the patient with Parkinson's disease.

With treatment, many or most patients can experience significant improvement in function, often for years. However, as noted previously, Parkinson's disease is a progressive disorder. Treatment typically becomes less effective over time. The period of time during which medication is controlling the patient's symptoms—the "on" time—diminishes or even becomes unpredictable.[36,40] Dose failures, akinesia, and dyskinesias can develop. Dyskinesias can be as frequent as 30% to 80% after several years of levodopa therapy.[41] In a meta-analysis of the literature, Ahlskog and Muenter[4] found that at 4 to 6 years of follow-up both motor fluctuations and dyskinesias occurred in approximately 40% of patients. The rate of dyskinesias was almost 60% at 10 years in an Olmsted County epidemiology study.[31] Akinesia can occur as well and extend for hours during the patient's "off" time. These motor changes frequently result in the need for increase in dosing regimens or use of adjunctive medications. Although with the increasing severity of Parkinson's disease, on and off times become more difficult to predict, the on periods are more conducive to effective physical therapy.

The ability of the patient with Parkinson's disease to withstand a surgical procedure, especially an elective one, is a significant concern. Although the life expectancy of patients is improved with modern therapy, it is clear that these patients have a shortened life expectancy compared to that in the general population.[42] They have been reported to be at an increased risk for death over 2.5 times higher than that of individuals who do not have Parkinson's disease.[43] Perioperatively, the patient's symptoms such as increased rigidity, akinesia, and cognitive impairment can challenge recovery from any surgical procedure because of problems with mobilization and pulmonary toilet. Prior orthopaedic literature studying lower extremity surgery have shown disturbing frequencies of pneumonia, decubitus ulcers, urinary tract and wound infections, and even death in patients with Parkinson's disease.[44–46] Some authors think that the prognosis of the patient with a hip fracture and Parkinson's disease is particularly poor because of these factors. Turcotte et al,[47] however, found that the overall mortality rate after hip fracture was comparable to that in the population without Parkinson's disease and was more a reflection of other medical comorbidities. Similarly, Koch et al[48] did not find a high level of medical complications after shoulder replacement in the patient with Parkinson's disease.

The salient issues the orthopaedic surgeon faces in the patient with Parkinson's disease and entertaining shoulder replacement are motor disorders, progression, and cognitive impairment. The motor disorders challenge hospital care and rehabilitation. Rigidity makes it difficult to range the shoulder postoperatively in therapy without jeopardizing the cuff repair.

Dyskinesias are potentially disruptive to the repair because of uncontrolled movements. Akinesia can limit pulmonary toilet and mobilization, risking pneumonia and skin breakdown. Additionally, the disease is inevitably progressive. Akinesia, or off time, becomes increasingly more likely, as does dyskinesia. When discussing treatment options with the patient with a symptomatic arthritic shoulder, the surgeon needs to keep in mind that future reconstruction will probably become more challenging. A decision may need to be made to proceed with surgery earlier than otherwise would be chosen to avoid the problems encountered with progression. Finally, the prevalence of Parkinson's disease dementia increases with time. The patient may lose the capacity to cooperate with the rehabilitation program. Because arthroplasty is typically an elective procedure, the patient may simply not be a candidate for replacement in advanced Parkinson's disease. The decision on proper timing for reconstruction can be difficult.

The indication for shoulder arthroplasty in these patients is the same as for all other individuals—the presence of a sufficiently symptomatic degenerated shoulder. Parkinson's disease is a comorbidity to be considered among others and may move the patient and physician to either elect earlier surgery before the progression of the Parkinson's disease or decline surgery in advanced stages. Once chosen, the technique of the surgery is fairly straight-forward because the patients will not have the atypical contractures present in cerebral palsy or rotator cuff disease seen with paraplegia (Fig. 28.2). The challenge of surgery in the patient with Parkinson's dsease is in perioperative care and postoperative rehabilitation.

Preoperatively patients should be reviewed by their neurologist. It is essential that their medication regimen be optimized and continued through the hospitalization. Rigidity and akinesia will reduce the ability of the patient to comply with pulmonary toilet regimens after surgery. A proactive approach with involvement of respiratory therapy can help minimize complications. Additionally, meticulous nursing care and early mobilization can help reduce the operative morbidity. Physical therapy for transfer and gait instruction and occupational therapy for activities of daily living are valuable. Prolonged protection of the soft tissue repair in shoulder arthroplasty is necessary to reduce subsequent failure. As in cerebral palsy, the therapists treating the operative shoulder must understand the goal of surgery—a relatively pain-free shoulder with functional motion that works within the limits of the patient's disease. Excessive stretching, especially against the rigidity likely present in the shoulder, is counterproductive. The disease may fluctuate in severity through the day, so physical therapy should be scheduled to take advantage of the patient's on time. Finally, use of the extremity for transfers should be deferred for a minimum of 3 months and preferably 6 months.

Despite a cautious approach to the management of the soft tissues, the results of shoulder arthroplasty in this setting can be disappointing. In a review of the patients treated at the Mayo Clinic, Koch et al[48] found patients achieved fairly consistent pain relief but often poor motion. At an average follow-up of 5.3 years, there were four excellent, two satisfactory, and ten unsatisfactory results. This was accompanied by an average decrease in postoperative active forward flexion of 8 degrees from the preoperative measurement. Three shoulders required revision surgery—two for painful subluxation and one for glenoid loos-

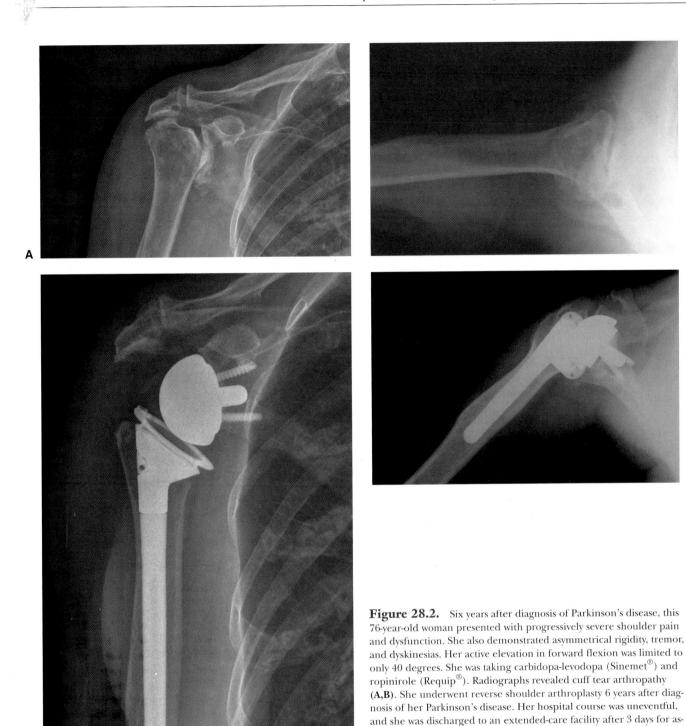

Figure 28.2. Six years after diagnosis of Parkinson's disease, this 76-year-old woman presented with progressively severe shoulder pain and dysfunction. She also demonstrated asymmetrical rigidity, tremor, and dyskinesias. Her active elevation in forward flexion was limited to only 40 degrees. She was taking carbidopa-levodopa (Sinemet®) and ropinirole (Requip®). Radiographs revealed cuff tear arthropathy **(A,B)**. She underwent reverse shoulder arthroplasty 6 years after diagnosis of her Parkinson's disease. Her hospital course was uneventful, and she was discharged to an extended-care facility after 3 days for assistance in mobility. **(C,D)** At last follow-up she had occasional minimal pain and active elevation to 150 degrees.

ening. A total of nine shoulders were found to have subluxation of the prosthesis on follow-up radiographs, and these subluxations were progressive. The joint malpositions were thought to be due to gradual stretching of the arthrotomy site and difficulties with postoperative rehabilitation with increased muscle tone. Of interest, a correlation of the degree of severity of the Parkinson's disease with the outcome was not found. This may be due to the small numbers in the series in conjunction with overall fairly poor results.

PARAPLEGIA

The patient with paraplegia presents an entirely different set of challenges in management. These patients must rely on their upper extremities for all activities of daily living, transfers, and mobility. Loss of shoulder function from either pain or degeneration presents a severe challenge to the patient's mobility. In turn, any degradation of mobility that interferes with the patient's ability to remain independent affects the patient's quality of life, affects the family because of increased caregiving demands, and affects society with lost productivity and health care costs.[49] Shoulder dysfunction can be a serious issue for the paraplegic patient.

Shoulder symptoms in the paraplegic commonly result from the heightened physical demands on the shoulder causing overuse type symptoms. Within 6 to 18 months after their spinal cord injury, as many as 35% of patients complain of shoulder pain.[50] The incidence of shoulder pain continues to increase with age, and ultimately most patients have pain.[26,49,51,52] Gellman et al[53] found the incidence of chronic shoulder pain ranged from 12% in those patients less than 5 years from injury to 100% of patients evaluated 25 years or more from their injury. Similarly, Pentland and Twomey[49] found that shoulder pain was associated with the duration of injury, exclusive of patient age, with an overall prevalence of shoulder pain of 39%. Shoulder or other upper extremity pain was experienced by most individuals with mobility tasks, self-care measures, and general activities.

The cause of the pain can be rotator cuff tendonitis or impingement syndrome, but more substantial shoulder damage is frequent. The shoulder is subject to the stress from full-body weight-bearing repeatedly through the day in transfer activities. With 36% of 28 patients reporting recent shoulder pain, Boninger et al[54] found a significant positive relationship between imaging abnormalities, most commonly distal clavicular osteolysis, and body mass index. Bayley et al[55] found that 33% of patients had shoulder pain, and 45% of these had arthrographic evidence of a rotator cuff tear. Only symptomatic patients had arthrography; the true incidence of rotator cuff tearing could therefore be higher. An additional five patients (5.3%) had aseptic necrosis of the humeral head, but no other degenerative changes were described in these shoulders. Intra-articular pressure measurements in the shoulders of five paraplegic individuals revealed readings up to 280 mm Hg during transfers. These increased stresses in combination with the abnormal distribution of stress transmission in the subacromial region were thought to be responsible for the high incidence of soft tissue damage in the shoulder.

Wylie and Chakera[56] reported the presence of degenerative changes on shoulder radiographs in 32% of 51 patients with paraplegia. All patients were more than 20 years since their injury. There was evidence of mild shoulder degeneration in 18% and moderate to severe changes in 13%. In a similar-size study, Lal[57] found radiographic evidence of degeneration in 72% of 53 patients with spinal cord injury. Escobedo et al[58] studied 23 consecutive outpatients in their clinic with unilateral or bilateral MRI of the shoulder. Rotator cuff tearing was evident in 57% of the 37 shoulders imaged. The prevalence of degenerative changes around the shoulder seems to be related to age of the patient, time since the spinal cord injury, and body mass index.

Spinal cord injuries are most common in the young adult, and their life expectancy is reduced compared to that of the general population.[59] However, as treatment for spinal cord injury improves, the life expectancy of the paraplegic patient has increased as well.[59–61] Yeo et al[61] found the life expectancy for these individuals ranges from 84% to 92% that of normal, depending on the completeness of their injury. McColl et al,[60] in a retrospective review of patients who sustained a spinal cord injury between the ages of 25 and 34 years, found a median sur-

vival of 38 years after injury.[60] Over 40% survived a minimum of 40 years. Frankle et al[59] demonstrated that patients injured between 1983 and 1990 showed a considerable improvement in survival compared to those in the previous decade. Those earlier patients were 1.5 times as likely to die. Although the life expectancy for the patient with spinal cord injury still does not match that of the general population, improvement is occurring each successive decade and many patients have a long life after their injury. As the life expectancy of the paraplegic patient increases, the long-term consequences of the stresses on the shoulder become apparent and are superimposed on the effects of aging.

The paraplegic patient places a high demand on the shoulder yet at the same time has a definite need for a functional shoulder. The high demand leads to an increased incidence of pain, rotator cuff degeneration, and arthritic changes. Paraplegic patients are often reluctant to consider surgery because of the profound postoperative impact on their independence, but it can be necessary.[49] If arthroplasty is considered, routine MRI examination of the shoulder preoperatively should be obtained for cuff evaluation. If there is substantial cuff tearing, humeral head replacement would be the preferable option to total shoulder arthroplasty to avoid premature glenoid failure. However, if the rotator cuff is intact, glenoid resurfacing can offer improved pain relief, functional scores, and ROM.[62] There is concern over glenoid component loosening in the younger, heavy-demand patient, but there is evidence that total shoulder arthroplasty has superior long-term survival over hemiarthroplasty in patients under 50 years of age.[63] Recognizing that the issue of humeral head replacement versus total shoulder arthroplasty becomes increasingly unsettled the younger and more active the patient is, it is my preference to perform total shoulder arthroplasty to maximize the clinical outcome and provide some protection from the glenoid erosion often seen after hemiarthroplasty. Total shoulder arthroplasty remains relatively contraindicated when rotator cuff damage exists.

Recently, reverse shoulder arthroplasty has been introduced in the United States for the treatment of the severely rotator cuff deficient shoulder. Early clinical outcomes can be very good.[64] Given the concerns over durability of reverse shoulder arthroplasty in the context of the high physical demands on the paraplegic shoulder, this type of replacement does not appear to be a viable option for the paraplegic patients with advanced cuff tearing.[65] Perhaps as technology improves, inverse replacement will become a consideration in the future.

Rehabilitation after arthroplasty can proceed along the same time line as for the nonparaplegic shoulder. The major consideration is helping the patient adjust to the temporary loss of an extremity necessary for transfers and mobility. Use of the involved extremity for transfers is best deferred for a minimum of 3 months and preferably 6 months to allow the soft tissue repair to mature. A physiatrist should be involved early in the process to assist the patient in preparing for the adjustments needed in postoperative convalescence and potential management in a postsurgical rehabilitation facility.

The literature on shoulder replacement in the paraplegic patient is sparse. Bayley et al[55] replaced the shoulders of three patients with osteonecrosis of the humeral head. All were reported to be "doing well," with improved ROM. Garreau De Loubresse et al[66] accumulated five cases in a multicenter study. Four prostheses were total shoulder replacements, and the last was a humeral head replacement. Two patients had reparable rotator cuff tears, and one had an irreparable tear. Improvement was modest but present. Mean Constant scores improved from 30 to 52 after surgery, and pain was typically relieved as well. These authors recommended humeral head replacement for the patient under 65 years of age and for those with rotator cuff tearing. For the remainder they suggested total shoulder arthroplasty.

REFERENCES

1. Boyle CA, Decouflé P, Yeargin-Allsopp M. Prevalence and health impact of developmental disabilities in US children. *Pediatrics* 1994;3:399–403.
2. Majnemer A, Mazer B. New directions in the outcome evaluation of children with cerebral palsy. *Semin Pediatr Neurol* 2004;11:11–17.
3. Gorter JW, Rosenbaum PL, Hanna SE, et al. Limb distribution, motor impairment, and functional classification of cerebral palsy. *Dev Med Child Neurol* 2004;46:461–467.
4. Goldstein M. The treatment of cerebral palsy: what we know, what we don't know. *J Pediatr* 2004;145(suppl):S42–S46.
5. O'Brien CF. Treatment of spasticity with botulinum toxin. *Clin J Pain* 2002;18(suppl): S182–S190.
6. Aoki KR, Guyer B. Botulinum toxin type A and other botulinum toxin serotypes: a comparative review of biomechanical and pharmacological actions. *Eur J Neurol* 8(suppl 5):21–29.
7. Dolly JO, Aoki KR. The structure and mode of action of different botulinum toxins. *Eur J Neurol* 2006;13(suppl 4):1–9.
8. Aoki KR. Pharmacology and immunology of botulinum toxins. *Int Ophthalmol Clin* 2005;45:25–37.
9. Ramachandran M, Eastwood DM. Botulinum toxin and its orthopedic applications. *J Bone Joint Surg Br* 2006;88:981–987.
10. Alderson K, Holds JB, Anderson RL. Botulinum-induced alteration of nerve-muscle interactions in the human orbicularis oculi following treatment for blepharospasm. *Neurology* 1991;41:1800–1805.
11. de Paiva A, Meunier FA, Molgo J, et al. Functional repair of motor endplates after botulinum neurotoxin type-A poisoning: biphasic switch of synaptic activity between nerve spouts and their parent terminals. *Proc Natl Acad Sci USA* 1999;96:3200–3205.
12. Priess RA, Condie DN, Rowley DI, et al. The effects of botulinum toxin (BTX-A) on spasticity of the lower limb and on gait in cerebral palsy. *J Bone Joint Surg Br* 2003;85:943–948.
13. Wasiak J, Hoare B, Wallen M. Botulinum toxin A as an adjunct to treatment in the management of the upper limb in children with spastic cerebral palsy. *Cochrane Database Syst Rev* 2004;4:CD003469.
14. Welch MJ, Purkiss JR, Foster KA. Sensitivity of embryonic rat dorsal root ganglia neurons to *Clostridium botulinum* neurotoxins. *Toxicon* 2000;38:245–258.
15. Durham P, Cady R, Cady R. Regulation of calcitonin gene-related peptide secretion from trigeminal nerve cells by botulinum toxin type A: implications for migraine therapy. *Headache* 2004;44:35–42.
16. Wissel J, Müller J, Dressnandt J, et al. Management of spasticity associated pain with botulinum toxin. *J Pain Symptom Manage* 2000;20:44–49.
17. Barwood S, Bailleiu C, Boyd RN, et al. Analgesic effects of botulinum toxin A: a randomized placebo-controlled clinical trial. *Dev Med Child Neurol* 2000;42:116–121.
18. Morton RE, Hankinson J, Nicholson J. Botulinum toxin for cerebral palsy; where are we now? *Arch Dis Child* 2004;89:1133–1137.
19. Shapiro BK. Cerebral palsy: a reconceptualization of the spectrum. *J Pediatr* 2004;145 (suppl):S3–S7.
20. Parish JL. Commercial preparations and handling of botulinum toxin type-A and type-B. *Clin Dermatol* 2003;21:481–484.
21. Foster KA, Bigalke H, Aoki KR. Botulinum neurotoxin: from laboratory to bedside. *Neurotox Res* 2006;9:133–140.
22. Gerber C, Yian EH, Pfirrmann CAW, et al. Subscapularis muscle function and structure after total shoulder replacement with lesser tuberosity osteotomy and repair. *J Bone Joint Surg Am* 2005;87:1739–1745.
23. Hattrup SJ, Cofield RH, Evidente VH, et al. Total shoulder arthroplasty for patients with cerebral palsy. *J Shoulder Elbow Surg* 2007;16:e5–9.
24. Albin RL. Parkinson's disease: background, diagnosis, and initial management. *Clin Geriatr Med* 2006;22:735–751.
25. de Lau LM, Giesbergen PC, de Rijk MC, et al. Incidence of parkinsonism and Parkinson's disease in a general population: the Rotterdam Study. *Neurology* 2004;63:1240–1244.
26. Elbaz A, Bower JH, Peterson BJ, et al. Survival study of Parkinson's disease in Olmsted County, Minnesota. *J Clin Epidemiol* 2002;55:25–31.
27. Gelb DJ, Oliver E, Gilman S. Diagnostic criteria for Parkinson's disease. *Arch Neurol* 1999;56:33–39.
28. Nutt JG, Wooten GF. Clinical practice: diagnosis and initial management of Parkinson's disease. *N Engl J Med* 2005;353:1021–1027.
29. Rao G, Fisch L, Srinivasan S, et al. Does this patient have Parkinson's disease? *JAMA* 2003;289:251.
30. Ahlskog JE, Muenter MD. Frequency of levodopa-related dyskinesias and motor fluctuations as estimated from the cumulative literature. *Mov Disord* 2001;16:448–458.
31. Van Gerpen JA, Kumar N, Bower JH, et al. Levodopa-associated dyskinesia risk among Parkinson's disease patients in Olmsted County, Minnesota, 1976–1990. *Arch Neurol* 2006;63:205–209.
32. McKeith JG, Dickson DW, Lowe J, et al. Diagnosis and management of dementia with Lewy bodies: third report of the DLB consortium. *Neurology* 2005;65:1863–1872.
33. Rongve A, Aarsland D. Management of Parkinson's disease dementia. *Drugs Aging* 2006;23:807–822.
34. Aarsland D, Larsen JP, Lim NG, et al. Range of neuropsychiatric disturbances in patients with Parkinson's disease. *J Neurol Neurosurg Psychiatry* 1999;67:492–496.
35. Aarsland D, Zaccai J, Brayne C. A systematic review of prevalence studies of dementia in Parkinson's disease. *Mov Disord* 2005;20:1255–1263.
36. Singh N, Pillay V, Choonara YE. Advances in the treatment of Parkinson's disease. *Prog Neurobiol* 2007;81:29–44.
37. Ahlskog JE. Parkinson's disease: is the initial treatment established? *Curr Neurol Neurosci Rep* 2003;3:289–295.
38. Hermanowicz N. Drug therapy for Parkinson's disease. *Semin Neurol* 2007;27:97–105.
39. Sheffield JK, Jankovic J. Botulinum toxin in the treatment of tremors, dystonias, sialorrhea, and other symptoms associated with Parkinson's disease. *Expert Rev Neurother* 2007;7: 637–647.
40. Giroux ML. Parkinson's disease: Managing a complex, progressive disease at all stages. *Cleve Clinic J Med* 2007;74:313–323.
41. Nutt JG. Levodopa-induced dyskinesia: review, observations, and speculations. *Neurology* 1990;40:340–345.
42. Uitti RJ, Ahlskog JE, Maraganore DM, et al. Levodopa therapy and survival in idiopathic Parkinson's disease: Olmsted County project. *Neurology* 1993;43:1918–1926.
43. D'Amelio, M. Ragonese, P. Morgante, et al. Long-term survival of Parkinson's disease: a population-based study. *J Neurol* 2006;253:33–37.
44. Coughlin L, Templeton J. Hip fractures in patients with Parkinson's disease. *Clin Orthop* 1980;148:192–195.
45. Rothermal JE, Garcia A. Treatment of hip fractures in hip patients with Parkinson's syndrome on levodopa therapy. *J Bone Joint Surg Am* 1972;54:1251–1254.
46. Staeheli JW, Frassica FJ, Sim FH. Prosthetic replacement of the femoral head for fracture of the femoral neck in patients who have Parkinson's disease. *J Bone Joint Surg Am* 1988;70:565–568.
47. Turcotte R, Godin C, Duchesne R, et al. Hip fractures and Parkinson's disease. *Clin Orthop* 1990;256:132–136.
48. Koch LD, Cofield RH, Ahlskog JE. Total shoulder arthroplasty in patients with Parkinson's disease. *J Shoulder Elbow Surg* 1997;6:24–28.
49. Pentland WE, Twomey LT. Upper limb function in persons with long-term paraplegia and implications for independence: Part I. *Paraplegia* 1994;32:211–218.
50. Silfverskjold J, Waters RL. Shoulder pain and functional disability in spinal cord injury patients. *Clin Orthop* 1991;272:141–145.
51. Nichols PJ, Nordan PA, Ennis JR. Wheelchair users shoulder. *Scand J Rehabil Med* 1979;11: 29–32.
52. Pentland WE, Twomey LT. The weight-bearing upper extremity in women with long-term paraplegia. *Paraplegia* 1991;29:521–530.
53. Gellman H, Sie I, Waters RL. Late complications of the weight-bearing upper extremity in the paraplegic patient. *Clin Orthop* 1988;233:132–135.
54. Boninger ML, Towers JD, Cooper RA, et al. Shoulder imaging abnormalities in individuals with paraplegia. *J Rehabil Res Dev* 2001;38:401–408.
55. Bayley JC, Cochran TP, Sledge CB. The weight-bearing shoulder: the impingement syndrome in paraplegics. *J Bone Joint Surg Am* 1987;69:676–678.
56. Wylie EJ, Chakera TM. Degenerative joint abnormalities in patients with paraplegia of duration greater than 20 years. *Paraplegia* 1988;26:101–106.
57. Lal S. Premature degenerative shoulder changes in spinal cord injury patients. *Spinal Cord* 1998;36:186–189.
58. Escobedo EM, Hunter JC, Hollister MC, et al. MR imaging of rotator cuff tears in individuals with paraplegia. *Am J Roentgenol* 1997;168:919–923.
59. Frankel HL, Coll JR, Charlifue SW, et al. Long-term survival in spinal cord injury: a 50-year investigation. *Spinal Cord* 1998;36:266–274.
60. McColl MA, Walker J, Stirling P, et al. Expectations of life and health among spinal cord injured adults. *Spinal Cord* 1997;35:818–828.
61. Yeo J D, Walsh J, Rutkowski S, et al. Mortality following spinal cord injury. *Spinal Cord* 1998;36:329–336.
62. Bryant D, Litchfield R, Sandow M, et al. A comparison of pain, strength, range of motion, and functional outcomes after hemiarthroplasty and total shoulder arthroplasty in patients with osteoarthritis of the shoulder: a systematic review and meta-analysis. *J Bone Joint Surg Am* 2005;87:1946–1957.
63. Sperling JW, Cofield RH, Rowland CM. Neer hemiarthroplasty and Neer total shoulder arthroplasty in patients 50 years old or less: long-term results. *J Bone Joint Surg Am* 1998; 80:464–473.
64. Wall B, Nové-Josserand L, O'Connor DP, et al. Reverse total shoulder arthroplasty: a review of results according to etiology. *J Bone Joint Surg Am* 2007;89:1476–1485.
65. Guery J, Favard L, Sirveaux F, et al. Reverse total shoulder arthroplasty: survivorship analysis of 80 replacements followed for 5 to 10 years. *J Bone Joint Surg Am* 2006;88: 1742–1747.
66. Garreau De Loubresse C, Norton MR, et al. Replacement arthroplasty in the weight-bearing shoulder of paraplegic patients. *J Shoulder Elbow Surg* 2004;13:369–372.

Robert H. Cofield
John W. Sperling

Epilogue

We, as editors, have been deeply impressed by the high quality of the contributions, the insights, of the contributing authors to this three-part text. The information is quite clear and typically very succinct.

In the first segment identifying the problems of failed shoulder arthroplasty, the subject has been approached in several ways to afford the readers a clear set of directions to define the issues. The first is the unique tack in defining the unsatisfactory shoulder arthroplasty, helping us understand poor results are a part of this picture, in addition to the expected complications creating the need for revision surgery. The second technique applied is Joint Registry analysis. This is really embryonic throughout the world and particularly neglected in North America. Using this method allows one to recognize the types of implants that do well and those that do not, in addition to understanding the factors that contribute to implant failure. The third approach taken to understanding the problems of shoulder arthroplasty is the traditional assessment of complications and failures, focusing on evaluation methodology for the individual patient. Low grade occult infections are increasingly recognized as an important contributor to failed arthroplasty. This has been emphasized in a separate chapter. As time goes by and the quality of surgical application in arthroplasty continues to improve we may find that this problem is the dominant reason for failure of shoulder arthroplasties. Finally in this introductory setting of the book what is known of the outcome of revision surgery in shoulder arthroplasty is enumerated—supplying the ground work, the base of knowledge for the next segment of the text.

The second section in the book deals specifically with techniques in revision arthroplasty—incorporating expanded materials on surgical exposure, details about implant characteristics that are continually shifting, and organized materials on the benefits and limitations of various types of component fixation to bone. From a structural standpoint, it has become clear that one of the two major problems is fixation of the glenoid component to bone and implant durability. The chapter on morphology of the glenoid leads us to understanding the limitations of this bony anatomy. The materials on revision of the glenoid component pinpoint the options now available. The second major problem is the contribution of the soft tissues to postoperative complications including not only the capsule and the rotator cuff tendons but also muscle contributions to shoulder stability and function.

Surgical options continually evolve. We all must have a contemporary and expanded understanding of the failures of reverse-type arthroplasties. Arthroscopy is ubiquitous in shoulder surgery; understanding applications of arthroscopy to failed arthroplasty is explained. Orthopedic surgeons understand tissue healing, postoperative limb support, and contributions of rehabilitation to success or failure. The depth of thinking by a knowledgeable physiatrist further develops rehabilitation concepts for us. Concluding this segment of the text is an analysis of the actual problems in reconstructive techniques used at the Mayo Clinic over approximately a quarter of a century. In reading this material one understands the problems and their treatment can be quite focused or unduly complex with many issues contributing to failure in one shoulder—requiring multiple technical maneuvers that are defined in this chapter.

The third component of the book addresses specific types of reconstruction that are not typically pinpointed when defining the problems that exist nor the basic reconstructive techniques. This includes the treatment of periprosthetic fractures that can vary greatly, and the specifics on surgical management of infected shoulder arthroplasty. Instability after arthroplasty is a major, if not the major, complication that currently exists. Shockingly, those in the field have recognized instability can be acute, chronic, or recurrent and in any direction just like instability without arthroplasty. Instability without arthroplasty is very complex and this subject is too. The main subject of this book is the failure of total shoulder arthroplasty. Hemiarthroplasty fails too. The reasons for and treatment of that are amplified in a separate chapter. In our practice the reverse type arthroplasty is used more commonly for treatment of failed anatomic shoulder arthroplasty than it is for treatment of primary diseases such as cuff tear arthropathy. Understanding when and how to apply the reverse arthroplasty in this setting is necessary information for the reconstructive surgeon in some instances, even planning a staged approach rather than a reconstruction in one operation. Prosthetic shoulder arthroplasty began for the care of acute trauma. It also has an important role in the management of old trauma: malunions, nonunions, instability, and locked dislocations, all conditions that require special definition and have been so developed in the text. Finally, we are pleased that authors with special knowledge and practice were able to contribute information on developmental dysplasia and acquired neuromuscular disorders, such as Parkinsonism.

We, as editors, are very pleased that all of the contributions in this text could be so completely developed, so there is in one place a greatly expanded body of contemporary knowledge on revision and complex shoulder arthroplasty that can be accessed. Not only in text but even in meetings often the fundamentals of shoulder arthroplasty are taught—and rightfully so. The nuances are more often beyond what meetings can deliver and what texts have covered in the past. The collection of information in this text should clearly expand the information and thinking on this subject and directly and positively influence patient care.

Index

Pages in italic denote figures; those followed by a *t* denote tables.